DECISION MAKING IN
MEDICINE

An Algorithmic Approach

CLINICAL DECISION MAKING™ SERIES

Berman:
Pediatric Decision Making

Bready, Smith:
Decision Making in Anesthesiology

Bucholz:
Orthopaedic Decision Making

Cohn, Doty, McElvein:
Decision Making in Cardiothoracic Surgery

Greene, Johnson, Lemcke:
Decision Making in Medicine

Korones, Bada-Ellzey:
Neonatal Decision Making

Levine:
Decision Making in Gastroenterology

Ramamurthy, Rogers:
Decision Making in Pain Management

van Heuven, Zwaan:
Decision Making in Ophthalmology

Weisberg, Strub, Garcia:
Decision Making in Adult Neurology

DECISION MAKING IN
MEDICINE
An Algorithmic Approach

HARRY L. GREENE II, M.D.

Executive Vice-President
Massachusetts Medical Society
Waltham, Massachusetts

WILLIAM P. JOHNSON, M.D.

Department of Medicine
The University of Arizona Health Sciences Center
Tucson, Arizona

DAWN LEMCKE, M.D.

Department of Medicine
The University of Arizona Health Sciences Center
Tucson, Arizona

SECOND EDITION

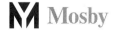 Mosby

A Harcourt Health Sciences Company

St. Louis   London   Philadelphia   Sydney   Toronto

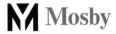

A Harcourt Health Sciences Company

Publisher: Susie Baxter
Senior Managing Editor: Lynne Gery
Editorial Assistant: Amanda Starr
Project Manager: Patricia Tannian
Project Specialist: Suzanne C. Fannin
Book Design Manager: Gail Morey Hudson
Manufacturing Manager: Karen Lewis
Cover Design: Liz Rudder

SECOND EDITION

Mosby, Inc.
11830 Westline Industrial Drive
St. Louis, Missouri 63146

Library of Congress Cataloging-in-Publication Data

Decision making in medicine / [edited by] Harry L. Greene II, William
    P. Johnson, Dawn Lemcke. — 2nd ed.
        p.   cm. — (Clinical decision making series)
    Includes bibliographical references and index.
    ISBN 0-323-00029-0
    1. Medical protocols.   I. Greene, Harry L. (Harry Lemoine),   .
    II. Johnson, William P.,   . III. Lemcke, Dawn P.
IV. Series.
    [DNLM: 1. Diagnosis. 2. Therapeutics. 3. Judgment.   WB   141D294
1998]
RC64.D43   1998
616—dc21
DNLM/DLC   98-28593

00 01 02 / 9 8 7 6 5 4 3 2

SECTION EDITORS

JACK E. ANSELL, M.D.

Professor, and Vice-Chairman for Clinical Affairs, Department of Medicine, Boston University Medical Center, Boston, Massachusetts

Hematology

THOMAS W. BOYDEN, M.D.

Associate Professor, Department of Medicine, University of Arizona College of Medicine; Chief, Endocrinology, VA Medical Center, Tucson, Arizona

Endocrinology

ANTHONY CAMILLI, M.D.

Clinical Associate Professor of Medicine, The University of Arizona Health Sciences Center, and University of Arizona Medical Center, Tucson, Arizona

Pulmonary Disease

†WILLIAM M. FEINBERG, M.D.

Professor, Department of Neurology, University of Arizona College of Medicine, Tucson, Arizona

Neurology

M. BRIAN FENNERTY, M.D.

Associate Professor of Medicine, and Section Chief, Gastroenterology, Oregon Health Sciences University, Portland, Oregon

Gastroenterology

JERRY M. GREENE, M.D.

Instructor of Medicine, Harvard Medical School, Boston; Chief, Rheumatology Section, Medical Service, Brockton/West Roxbury VA Medical Center, West Roxbury, Massachusetts

Rheumatology

MICHAEL D. KATZ, PHARM. D.

Associate Professor, Department of Pharmacy Practice and Service, University of Arizona College of Pharmacy; Clinical Pharmacist, Department of Internal Medicine, University Medical Center, Tucson, Arizona

Pharmacology

LISA KAUFMANN, M.D.

Associate Professor, Department of Medicine, State University of New York Health Science Center at Syracuse, Syracuse, New York

General Medicine

SAMUEL M. KEIM, M.D.

Associate Professor and Residency Director, Department of Emergency Medicine, University of Arizona College of Medicine; Attending Physician, Emergency Department, University Medical Center, Tucson, Arizona

Emergency Medicine

KARL B. KERN, M.D.

Professor of Medicine (Cardiology), University of Arizona College of Medicine; Associate Director, Cardiac Catheterization Lab, University Medical Center, Tucson, Arizona

Cardiology

DAWN LEMCKE, M.D., F.A.C.P.

Assistant Professor of Clinical Medicine, Section of General Internal Medicine, The University of Arizona Health Sciences Center, Tucson, Arizona

Women's Health

RICHARD M. MANDEL, M.D.

Assistant Professor of Clinical Medicine, Department of Internal Medicine, University of Arizona College of Medicine, and University Medical Center, Tucson, Arizona

Infectious Disease

REBECCA L. POTTER, M.D.

Professor of Clinical Psychiatry, University of Arizona College of Medicine, Tucson, Arizona

Behavioral Medicine

MARK J. SCHARF, M.D.

Associate Professor of Medicine, Division of Dermatology, University of Massachusetts Medical Center, and University of Massachusetts Memorial Health Care, Worcester, Massachusetts

Dermatology

DAVID B. VAN WYCK, M.D.

Associate Professor, Department of Medicine, University of Arizona College of Medicine; Clinical Director of Medicine and Subspecialties, VA Medical Center, Tucson, Arizona

Nephrology

HUNTER WESSELLS, M.D.

Assistant Professor of Clinical Surgery, Section of Urology, University of Arizona College of Medicine; Director of Urodynamics and Sexual Dysfunction Unit, Department of Urology, Arizona Health Sciences Center, Tucson, Arizona

Urology

---

†Deceased.

CONTRIBUTORS

JAMES L. ABBRUZZESE, M.D.

Professor and Chairman, Gastrointestinal Oncology and Digestive Diseases, University of Texas M.D. Anderson Cancer Center, Houston, Texas
Carcinoma of Unknown Primary Site

MARIE C. ABBRUZZESE, M.B.A.

Senior Data Coordinator, Research, Department of Clinical Investigation, University of Texas M.D. Anderson Cancer Center, Houston, Texas
Carcinoma of Unknown Primary Site

RODNEY D. ADAM, M.D.

Associate Professor of Medicine, Department of Microbiology and Immunology, Infectious Disease, The University of Arizona Health Sciences Center; Director, Travel Clinic, Infectious Disease Consultant, Department of Internal Medicine, Section of Infectious Disease, University Medical Center, Tucson, Arizona
Foreign Travel: Immunizations and Infections

GEOFFREY L. AHERN, M.D., PH.D.

Associate Professor of Neurology and Psychology, and Director, Behavioral Neuroscience and Alzheimer's Clinic, The University of Arizona Health Sciences Center, Tucson, Arizona
Memory Loss
Acute Behavior Change
Chronic Behavior Change
Coma

FREDERICK R. AHMANN, M.D.

Associate Professor of Medicine and Surgery, Division of Medical Oncology and Urology, University of Arizona College of Medicine, Tucson, Arizona
Superior Vena Caval Syndrome

ANWAR AL-HAIDARY, M.D., M.R.C.P., M.Sc.

Department of Nephrology, Wilson Memorial Medical Center, Wilson, North Carolina
Chronic Renal Failure
Acute Renal Failure
Proteinuria
Hematuria
Hyponatremia
Hypernatremia
Hypomagnesemia

ELAINE J. ALPERT, M.D., M.P.H.

Assistant Professor of Medicine and Public Health, Assistant Dean for Student Affairs, Boston University School of Medicine; Physician, Department of Medicine, Boston Medical Center, Boston, Massachusetts
Domestic Violence

HOMEIRA BAGHDADI, M.D.

Chief Resident, Department of Internal Medicine, The University of Arizona Health Sciences Center, Tucson, Arizona
Nipple Discharge

IRIS R. BELL, M.D., PH.D.

Associate Professor, Department of Psychiatry, University of Arizona College of Medicine; Director, Program in Geriatric Psychiatry, Tucson VA Medical Center, Tucson, Arizona
Depression

JAMES B. BENJAMIN, M.D.

Associate Professor of Surgery, Section of Orthopedics, The University of Arizona Health Sciences Center; Active Staff, Department of Surgery Section of Orthopedics, University Medical Center and VA Medical Center, Tucson, Arizona
Shoulder Pain
Hip Pain

RITA BLANCHARD, M.D.

Associate Professor, Department of Medicine, Boston University School of Medicine, and Boston Medical Center, Boston, Massachusetts
Adjuvant Therapy Choices in Breast Cancer

BARBARA BODE, M.D.

Clinical Instructor, Department of Internal Medicine, Rheumatology, University of Arizona College of Medicine; Physician, Department of Rheumatology, Tucson Medical Center, Tucson, Arizona
Low Back Pain
Scleroderma

THOMAS W. BOYDEN, M.D.

Associate Professor, Department of Medicine, University of Arizona College of Medicine; Chief, Endocrinology, VA Medical Center, Tucson, Arizona
Dyslipidemia
Hyperglycemia
Hypercalcemia
Test of Thyroid Function
Hypothyroidism
Hyperthyroidism
Goiter
Thyroid Nodule
Gynecomastia

RIEMKE BRAKEMA, M.D., F.A.C.E.P.

Clinical Lecturer, University of Arizona College of Medicine; Medical Director, Sexual Assault Resource Center; Staff Physician, Department of Emergency Medicine, El Dorado Hospital and Medical Center, Tucson, Arizona
Foreign Body Ingestion

SAMUEL M. BUTMAN, M.D.
Associate Professor, Department of Medicine, University of Arizona College of Medicine; Director, Cardiac Catheterization Laboratory, University Medical Center, Tucson, Arizona
Stable Angina
Unstable Angina

ANTONIO C. BUZAID, M.D.
Executive Director, Oncology Center, Hospital Sírio Labanês, São Paolo, Brazil
Abnormal Serum Protein Electrophoresis
Carcinoma of Unknown Primary Site
Neutropenia and Fever

JESSICA BYRON, M.D.
Coordinator, Women's Health Care, University of Arizona Campus Health Services; Staff Physician, Department of Obstetrics and Gynecology, Tucson Medical Center, Tucson, Arizona
Premenstrual Dysphoric Disorder

ANTHONY CAMILLI, M.D.
Clinical Associate Professor of Medicine, The University of Arizona Health Sciences Center, and University of Arizona Medical Center, Tucson, Arizona
Hemoptysis
Pulmonary Dyspnea
Mediastinal Adenopathy
Diffuse Interstitial Lung Disease
Positive Tuberculin Skin Test
Respiratory Symptoms and Occupational Exposure to Asbestos

J. KEVIN CARMICHAEL, M.D.
Unit Chief, El Rio Special Immunology Associates, El Rio Community Health Center, Tucson, Arizona
Approach to the Newly Diagnosed HIV-Positive Patient

SHARI CARNEY, M.D.
Clinical Assistant Instructor, State University of New York Health Science Center at Syracuse, Syracuse, New York
The Red Eye

M. KANTER CAROLIN, M.D.
Associate Professor, Department of Medicine (Neurology), University of Texas Health Science Center at San Antonio, and University Hospital, San Antonio, Texas
Transient Ischemic Attacks
Transient Monocular Visual Loss
Completed Stroke
Progressing Stroke

ANTHONY C. CARUSO, M.D.
Physician, Department of Cardiology, Chippenham Medical Center, Richmond, Virginia
Narrow QRS Complex Tachycardia
Wide QRS Complex Tachycardia
Syncope

LYNN CLEARY, M.D.
Professor of Medicine, and Associate Dean of Curriculum, State University of New York Health Science Center at Syracuse; Professor of Medicine, University Hospital, Syracuse, New York
Involuntary Weight Loss

JUNE CLEMENTS, M.D.
Staff Pathologist, Tucson Medical Center, Tucson, Arizona
Transfusion Therapy: Platelets
Transfusion Therapy: Red Blood Cells
Transfusion Therapy: Granulocytes
Transfusion Reactions and Complications

NEIL C. CLEMENTS, Jr., M.D., F.C.C.P.
Private Practice, Tucson Pulmonology, Tucson, Arizona
Stridor
Wheezing

DAVID M. CLIVE, M.D.
Associate Professor of Medicine, Department of Renal Medicine, University of Massachusetts Medical Center, Worcester, Massachusetts
Hypokalemia
Hyperkalemia

NANCY A. CUROSH, M.D.
Attending Physician, Endocrinology, Providence Portland Medical Center, Portland, Oregon
Hypoglycemia
Painful Thyroid
Adrenal Mass
Cushing's Syndrome
Hirsutism
Gynecomastia
Secondary Amenorrhea

PAMELA J. DAVIS, M.D.
Clinical Assistant Professor, Department of Internal Medicine, University of Arizona College of Medicine, Tucson; Regional Medical Director, South Central Region, Medical and Scientific Affairs, U.S. Human Health, Merck & Co., Scottsdale, Arizona
Hypertension

MARK J. DiNUBILE, M.D.
Associate Professor of Medicine, Division of Infectious Diseases, University of Medicine and Dentistry of New Jersey/Robert Wood Johnson Medical School of Camden; Physician, Cooper Health System, Camden, New Jersey
Chronic Meningitis
Pulmonary Infiltrates in HIV-Infected Patients
Staphylococcus Aureus Bacteremia
Hepatitis Exposure

HILLARY DON, M.D.

Professor, Department of Anesthesiology, University of California, San Francisco, School of Medicine; Staff Anesthetist, VA Medical Center, San Francisco, California

Metabolic Acidosis
Metabolic Alkalosis

DEBORAH DOUD, M.D.

Physician in Private Practice, Rheumatology, Internal Medicine Associates, Omaha, Nebraska

Monoarticular Arthritis
Polyarticular Arthritis

GEORGE W. DRACH, M.D.

Visiting Professor of Urology, University of Texas Southwestern Medical School; Physician, Department of Urology, Parkland Memorial Hospital, Dallas, Texas

Prostate Nodule or Enlargement
Prostatitis

GREGORY L. EASTWOOD, M.D.

President, and Dean, College of Medicine, State University of New York Health Science Center at Syracuse, Syracuse, New York

Belching
Gastrointestinal Bleeding
Flatulence

BRIAN L. ERSTAD, B.S., PHARM.D.

Associate Professor, Pharmacy Practice and Science, University of Arizona College of Pharmacy, and University Medical Center, Tucson, Arizona

Antimicrobial Prophylaxis in Surgical Patients
Use and Monitoring of Aminoglycoside Antibiotics
Use and Evaluation of Serum Drug Levels

LAURIE L. FAJARDO, M.D.

Vice Chair of Research, Department of Radiology, University of Virginia School of Medicine, Charlottesville, Virginia

Breast Mass

†WILLIAM M. FEINBERG, M.D.

Professor, Department of Neurology, University of Arizona College of Medicine, Tucson, Arizona

Brain Death

M. BRIAN FENNERTY, M.D.

Associate Professor of Medicine, and Section Chief, Gastroenterology, Oregon Health Sciences University, Portland, Oregon

Noncardiac Chest Pain
Acute Diarrhea
Guaiac-Positive Stools
Elevated Serum Iron

PAUL E. FENSTER, M.D.

Associate Professor, Department of Medicine, University of Arizona College of Medicine; Director of Adult Echocardiography, University Medical Center, Tucson, Arizona

Bradycardia
Palpitations
Acute Pulmonary Edema
Cardiac Dyspnea
Acute Myocardial Infarction

DAVID FRAMM, M.D., F.A.C.C.

Director of Vascular and Cardiac Ultrasound, Department of Cardiology, Mecklenberg Medical Group, Charlotte, North Carolina

Bradycardia
Cardiac Dyspnea

COLLIN FREEMAN, PHARM.D., B.C.P.S.

Assistant Professor, Department of Medicine, Clinical Pharmacology Section, University of Missouri-Kansas City School of Medicine; Clinical Pharmacologist, Department of Medicine, Truman Medical Center-West, Kansas City, Missouri

Nonsurgical Antimicrobial Prophylaxis
Use and Evaluation of Serum Drug Levels

ERIC P. GALL, M.D.

Professor and Chairman, Department of Medicine, Finch University of the Health Sciences/Chicago Medical School, North Chicago, Illinois

Hyperuricemia and Gout

JAMES M. GALLOWAY, M.D., F.A.C.C., F.A.C.P.

Assistant Professor of Clinical Medicine, Department of Cardiology, and Clinical Assistant Professor of Public Health; University of Arizona College of Medicine; Director, Native American Cardiology Program, Indian Health Service, University Medical Center, Tucson, Arizona

Acute Pulmonary Edema
Cardiac Arrest
Acute Myocardial Infarction

LAWRENCE A. GARCIA, M.D.

Fellow, Department of Medicine, Division of Cardiology, Harvard Medical School/Beth Israel Deaconess Medical Center, Boston, Massachusetts

Smoking Cessation

ALAN J. GELENBERG, M.D.

Professor and Head of Department of Psychiatry, The University of Arizona Health Sciences Center; Department of Psychiatry, University Medical Center, Tucson, Arizona

Psychosis

DAVID W. GIBSON, M.D.

Private Practice, Cardiology, Saint Thomas Hospital Group, Nashville, Tennessee

Edema

---

†Deceased.

STEPHEN J. GLUCKMAN, M.D.

Chief, Infectious Disease Clinical Service, Department of Medicine, University of Pennsylvania School of Medicine; Physician, Hospital of the University of Pennsylvania, Philadelphia, Pennsylvania

Hepatitis Exposure

MARK C. GOLDBERG, M.D., F.A.C.C.

Tucson Heart Group, Tucson, Arizona

Hypotension
Cor Pulmonale
Right Ventricular Failure

DEBORAH L. GOLDSMITH, M.D.

Assistant Professor of Clinical Medicine, and Director, Special Immunology Program, Section of Infectious Disease, University of Arizona College of Medicine, Tucson, Arizona

Aseptic Meningitis
The Acutely Ill HIV-Positive Patient
Central Nervous System Infection in the HIV-Infected Patient

GUILLERMO GONZALEZ-OSETE, M.D.

Clinical Associate Professor of Medicine, Southern Arizona Cancer Care Center, Tucson, Arizona

Deep Venous Thrombosis
Lymphadenopathy
Spinal Cord Compression

HARRY L. GREENE II, M.D.

Executive Vice-President, Massachusetts Medical Society, Waltham, Massachusetts

Edema
Smoking Cessation

KRISTYN M. GREIFER, M.D.

Assistant Professor, Department of General Medicine, State University of New York Health Science Center at Syracuse, Syracuse, New York

Sexual Dysfunction

IRWIN E. HARRIS, M.D.

Formerly Assistant Professor of Surgery, The University of Arizona Health Sciences Center; Formerly Physician and Orthopedic Surgeon, University Medical Center, Tucson, Arizona

Pathologic Fractures

STEVEN T. HARRIS, M.D.

Formerly Associate Clinical Professor of Medicine and Radiology; University of California, San Francisco, School of Medicine; Formerly Attending Physician, University of California Hospitals and Clinics, San Francisco, California

Hypophosphatemia

LEE J. HIXSON, M.D.

Department of Internal Medicine, Dixie Regional Medical Center, St. George, Utah

Dyspepsia
Chronic Abdominal Pain
Chronic Diarrhea

RICHARD F. HOFFMAN, M.D.

Clinical Assistant Professor, Department of Medicine, University of Arizona College of Medicine, and University Medical Center, Tucson, Arizona

Acute Dysuria or Pyuria in Men

PHILIP E. JAFFE, M.D.

Associate Professor of Medicine, GI Section, University of Arizona College of Medicine; Medical Director, GI Endoscopy, University Medical Center, Tucson, Arizona

Dysphagia
Biliary Colic
Constipation
Fecal Incontinence

WILLIAM P. JOHNSON, M.D.

Assistant Professor of Clinical Medicine, The University of Arizona Health Sciences Center, Tucson, Arizona

Preventive Health Services for Adults
Chronic Pain
Scrotal Mass
Snake Venom Poisoning

MICHAEL D. KATZ, PHARM.D.

Associate Professor, Department of Pharmacy Practice and Service, University of Arizona College of Pharmacy; Clinical Pharmacist, Department of Internal Medicine, University Medical Center, Tucson, Arizona

Urinary Tract Infection in Women
Acute Anticoagulation
Long-Term Anticoagulation
Anaphylaxis
Evaluation of Adverse Drug Reactions
Choosing Appropriate Antimicrobial Therapy

LISA KAUFMANN, M.D.

Associate Professor, Department of Medicine, State University of New York Health Science Center at Syracuse, Syracuse, New York

Fatigue
Persistent Excessive Sweating

SAMUEL M. KEIM, M.D.

Associate Professor and Residency Director, Department of Emergency Medicine, University of Arizona College of Medicine; Attending Physician, Emergency Department, University Medical Center, Tucson, Arizona

Drowning and Near-Drowning

KARL B. KERN, M.D.

Professor of Medicine (Cardiology), University of Arizona College of Medicine; Associate Director, Cardiac Catheterization Lab, University Medical Center, Tucson, Arizona

Bradycardia
Unstable Angina
Palpitations
Congestive Heart Failure
Cor Pulmonale
Right Ventricular Failure
Cardiac Arrest
Cardiac Dyspnea
Acute Myocardial Infarction
Counseling after Myocardial Infarction
Narrow QRS Complex Tachycardia

ROBERT F. KLEIN, M.D.

Formerly Associate Professor of Medicine, Division of Endocrinology, Diabetes and Clinical Nutrition, Oregon Health Sciences University School of Medicine; Formerly Staff Physician, VA Medical Center, Portland, Oregon

Hypophosphatemia

STEVEN R. KNOPER, M.D.

Research Assistant Professor, Department of Medicine, Section of Pulmonary and Critical Care, University of Arizona College of Medicine, Tucson, Arizona

Cough
Pleural Effusion

MARCIA KO, M.D.

Clinical Assistant Professor, Department of Medicine, Mayo Clinic Arizona, Scottsdale, Arizona

Keratoconjunctivitis Sicca (Sjögren's Syndrome)
Positive Antinuclear Antibody Test

WILLIAM H. KREISLE, M.D.

Clinical Instructor, Department of Medicine, University of Washington School of Medicine, Seattle, Washington; Physician, Department of Hematology/Oncology, St. Luke's Regional Medical Center, Mountain States Tumor Institute, Boise, Idaho

Leukopenia

JOHN W. LACE, M.D., F.C.C.P.

Medical Director, Departments of Respiratory Care and Critical Care, Providence General Medical Center, Everett, Washington

Solitary Pulmonary Nodule
Multiple Pulmonary Nodules

DAWN LEMCKE, M.D., F.A.C.P.

Assistant Professor of Clinical Medicine, Section of General Internal Medicine, The University of Arizona Health Sciences Center, Tucson, Arizona

Chest Pain in Women

NORMAN LEVINE, M.D.

Professor and Chief of Dermatology, Department of Medicine, University of Arizona College of Medicine, Tucson, Arizona

Pigmented Lesions
Urticaria
Generalized Pruritus
Palpable Purpura

RICHARD LIEBOWITZ, M.D.

Assistant Professor of Clinical Medicine, Department of Medicine, University of Arizona College of Medicine, Tucson, Arizona

Perioperative Evaluation

DOUGLAS LINDSEY, M.D., Dr.P.H.

Professor Emeritus, Departments of Surgery and Emergency Medicine, The University of Arizona Health Sciences Center, Tucson, Arizona

Human and Animal Bites

ROBERT J. LIPSY, M.D.

Pharmacy Services Department, Intergroup, Tucson, Arizona

Adverse Drug Reactions

MICHAEL LOEW, M.D.

Attending Physician, Department of Emergency Medicine, Penrose-St. Francis Hospital, Front Range Emergency Specialists, Colorado Springs, Colorado

Drowning and Near-Drowning

JOY L. LOGAN, M.D.

Associate Professor, Department of Medicine, University of Arizona College of Medicine; Staff Nephrologist, Medical Service, VA Medical Center, Tucson, Arizona

Chronic Renal Failure

ANA MARIA LÓPEZ, M.D., M.P.H.

Assistant Professor of Medicine and Pathology, Department of Hematology and Oncology, University of Arizona/ Arizona Cancer Center and University Medical Center, Tucson, Arizona

Contraceptive Choices

PHILIP A. LOWRY, M.D.

Physician Coordinator, Stem Cell Transplant, Saint Barnabas Cancer Center, Saint Barnabas Medical Center, Livingston, New Jersey

Clinical Considerations for Bone Marrow or Stem Cell Transplantation
Secondary Malignancies in Patients Previously Treated for Cancer

CYNTHIA MADDEN, M.D., M.P.H.

Clinical Associate Professor of Emergency Medicine, University of North Carolina at Chapel Hill School of Medicine, Chapel Hill; Attending Physician, Department of Emergency Medicine, Wake Medical Center, Raleigh, North Carolina

Caustic Ingestion and Exposure
Hypothermia

RICHARD M. MANDEL, M.D.

Assistant Professor of Clinical Medicine, Department of Internal Medicine, University of Arizona College of Medicine, and University Medical Center, Tucson, Arizona

Acute and Subacute Meningitis
Aseptic Meningitis
The Acutely Ill HIV-Positive Patient
Sepsis
Toxic Shock Syndrome
Fever of Unknown Origin

MICHAEL J. MARICIC, M.D.

Chief, Section of Rheumatology, Department of Medicine, The University of Arizona Health Sciences Center; Physician, University Medical Center, Tucson, Arizona

Seronegative Arthritis
Soft Tissue Pain
Neck Pain
Hand and Wrist Pain
Knee Pain
Osteopenia
Diffuse Muscle Pain and Stiffness: Polymyalgia Rheumatica and Giant Cell Arteritis
Temporomandibular Pain
Elevated Serum Alkaline Phosphate Level

LORNA A. MARSHALL, M.D.

Assistant Clinical Professor, Department of Obstetrics and Gynecology, University of Washington School of Medicine; Section Head, Reproductive Endocrinology, Virginia Mason Medical Center, Seattle, Washington

Female Infertility

PATRICIA MAYER, M.D., F.A.C.R.

Department of Rheumatology, North Colorado Medical Center, Greeley, Colorado

Raynaud's Phenomenon
Joint Hypermobility
Elevated Creatine Kinase Level

ANGELA MURPHY McGHEE, M.D.

Formerly Staff Dermatologist, Thomas-Davis Medical Center, Tucson, Arizona

Livedo Reticularis

†JAMES L. McGUIRE, M.D.

Formerly Associate Professor, Department of Medicine, Stanford University School of Medicine, Stanford; Formerly Director, Rheumatology Clinic, and Fellowship Chief, Rheumatology Section, Palo Alto VA Medical Center, Palo Alto, California

Kidney Stones

KENNETH E. McINTYRE, JR., M.D.

Professor of Surgery, Division of Vascular Surgery, University of Texas Southwestern Medical Center; Chief, Department of Vascular Surgery, St. Paul Medical Center, Dallas, Texas

Acute Pulseless Extremity

SUSAN McKENZIE, R.N., M.S.

Formerly Cardiac Rehabilitation Staff, The University of Arizona Health Sciences Center, Tucson, Arizona

Counseling after Myocardial Infarction

HUGH S. MILLER, M.D.

Clinical Associate Professor, Maternal-Fetal Division, Department of Obstetrics and Gynecology, University of Arizona College of Medicine

Cervicitis
Abnormal Vaginal Bleeding
Abnormal Pap Smear

JEFFREY I. MILLER, M.D.

Vice Chief of Surgery, Boca Raton Community Hospital, Boca Raton, Florida

Prostate Nodule or Enlargement
Prostatitis

JOHN MISIASZEK, M.D.

Associate Professor of Psychiatry, and Medical Director, Psychiatry Outpatient Clinic, The University of Arizona Health Sciences Center, Tucson, Arizona

Emotional Disorders with Somatic Expression

MANUEL MODIANO, M.D.

Chief of Staff, Carondelet St. Mary's Hospital, Tucson, Arizona

Leukopenia
Deep Venous Thrombosis
Coagulation Abnormalities
Lymphadenopathy
Spinal Cord Compression

ERWIN B. MONTGOMERY, Jr., M.D.

Formerly Associate Professor of Neurology, and formerly Attending Staff Neurologist, The University of Arizona Health Sciences Center, Tucson, Arizona

Tremor
Parkinson's Disease
Hyperkinesias

JANET MOORE, M.D.

Clinical Assistant Professor, Department of Obstetrics and Gynecology, University of Arizona College of Medicine, Tucson, Arizona

Vaginal Bleeding in Pregnancy

---

†Deceased

KARAM C. MOUNZER, M.D.

Assistant Clinical Professor of Medicine, Division of Infectious Diseases, University of Medicine and Dentistry of New Jersey/Robert Wood Johnson Medical School; Physician, Cooper Hospital, Camden, New Jersey
Pulmonary Infiltrates in HIV-Infected Patients

MYRA L. MURAMOTO, M.D.

Assistant Professor, Department of Family and Community Medicine, University of Arizona College of Medicine, Tucson, Arizona
Alcoholism

AMIR NASSERI, M.D.

Physician, Department of Obstetrics and Gynecology, The University of Arizona Health Sciences Center, Tucson, Arizona
Vaginal Discharge

SCOTT W. NOWLIN, M.D.

Resident, Department of Surgery, Section of Emergency Medicine, University of Arizona College of Medicine/University Medical Center, Tucson, Arizona
Obesity

EUGENIE A.M.T. OBBENS, M.D., Ph.D.

Chief, Pain Section, and Co-Director, Neuro-Oncology, Department of Neurology, Barrow Neurological Institute, Phoenix, Arizona
Disturbances of Smell and Taste

CYNTHIA A. O'NEIL, M.D.

Staff Physician, Department of Dermatology, Davis Monthan Air Force Base, Tucson, Arizona
Leg Ulcer

K. J. OOMMEN, M.D.

Associate Professor, Department of Neurology, University of Oklahoma Health Science Center, Oklahoma City, Oklahoma
Seizures
Status Epilepticus

PHILIP R. ORLANDER, M.D.

Professor and Clinical Director, Department of Internal Medicine, Division of Endocrinology, University of Texas Health Science Center at Houston; Professor, Department of Internal Medicine, Division of Endocrinology, Hermann Hospital and Lyndon B. Johnson General Hospital, Houston, Texas
Hyperglycemia
Hypocalcemia
Hypercalcemia
Pituitary Tumor

STEVEN PALLEY, M.D.

Clinical Assistant Professor, Department of Medicine, University of Arizona College of Medicine, Tucson; Active Staff, Department of Medicine, Flagstaff Medical Center, Flagstaff, Arizona
Acute Abdominal Pain
Nausea and Vomiting
Rectal Bleeding
Asymptomatic Increased Transaminases

CAROL S. PORTLOCK, M.D.

Associate Professor, Department of Clinical Medicine, Cornell University Medical Center; Attending Physician, Lymphoma Service, Department of Medicine, Memorial Sloan-Kettering Cancer Center, New York, New York
Hodgkin's Disease

REBECCA L. POTTER, M.D.

Professor of Clinical Psychiatry, University of Arizona College of Medicine, Tucson, Arizona
Suicidal Patient

ISSAM RAAD, M.D.

Associate Professor of Medicine, Chief, Section of Infection Control, Clinical Infection Control Officer, and Internist, Department of Medical Specialties, Sections of Infectious Diseases and Infection Control, University of Texas M.D. Anderson Cancer Center, Houston, Texas
Neutropenia and Fever

LYNN M. RANKIN, M.D.

Clinical Neurologist, Iowa Methodist Medical Center, and Iowa Lutheran Hospital, Des Moines, Iowa
Weakness
Peripheral Neuropathy

NAOMI RAPPAPORT, M.D.

Community Group Practice, Internal Medicine, Lahey Clinic, Fall River, Massachusetts
Rhinitis

ERIC M. REIMAN, M.D.

Professor of Psychiatry, University of Arizona College of Medicine, Tucson; Scientific Director, Samaritan PET Center, Good Samaritan Regional Medical Center, Phoenix, Arizona
Anxiety

JULIE I. RIFKIN, M.D.

Assistant Professor, Department of General Internal Medicine, University of Colorado School of Medicine; Medical Director, Outpatient Primary Care, HealthONE, Presbyterian/St. Luke's Hospital, Denver, Colorado
Test of Thyroid Function
Thyroid Nodule
Thyroid Function Tests in Nonthyroidal Illness

ROBERT M. RIFKIN, M.D., F.A.C.P.

Director, Blood and Marrow Transplant Program, Department of Internal Medicine, Columbia Presbyterian/St. Luke's Medical Center, Rocky Mountain Cancer Center, Denver, Colorado

Leukocytosis
Chronic Myelogenous Leukemia

TERRA A. ROBLES, B.S., PHARM.D.

Clinical Faculty, Department of Pharmacy Practice, University of Arizona College of Pharmacy, Tucson, Arizona

Use of Oral Contraceptives
Evaluation of a Drug for Clinical Use or Inclusion in a Formulary

DIANNA L. RYNKIEWICZ, M.D.

Senior Fellow, Section of Infectious Disease, University of Arizona Medical Center, Tucson, Arizona

Sexually Transmitted Diseases

RICHARD E. SAMPLINER, M.D.

Professor, Department of Medicine, University of Arizona College of Medicine; Chief, Gastroenterology, VA Medical Center, and University Medical Center, Tucson, Arizona

Heartburn
Jaundice
Ascites

ROBERT N. SAMUELSON, M.D.

Physician, Department of Obstetrics and Gynecology, Waterbury/St. Mary's Hospital, Waterbury, Connecticut

Acute Abdominal Pain in Women

SUSAN FISK SANDER, M.D.

Private Practice, Danville, California

Hearing Loss
Tinnitus

MARK J. SCHARF, M.D.

Associate Professor of Medicine, Division of Dermatology, University of Massachusetts Medical Center, and University of Massachusetts Memorial Health Care, Worcester, Massachusetts

Pigmented Lesions

GAIL L. SCHWARTZ, M.D.

Formerly Clinical Assistant Professor of Psychiatry, The University of Arizona Health Sciences Center, Tucson, Arizona

Grief

MICHAEL E. SCOTT, M.D.

Clinical Assistant Professor, Department of Psychiatry, University of Arizona College of Medicine; Medical Director, Clinical Psychiatry, Sierra Tucson Hospital, Tucson, Arizona

Alcoholism

JOSEPH I. SHAPIRO, M.D.

Formerly Assistant Professor of Medicine, University of Colorado School of Medicine; Formerly Director, Nuclear Magnetic Resonance Spectroscopy, University of Colorado Health Sciences Center, Denver, Colorado

Selection of Patients for Transplantation
Choosing a Chronic Dialysis Modality
Fever in a Transplant Patient

WILLIAM A. SIBLEY, M.D.

Professor, Department of Neurology, University of Arizona College of Medicine; Attending Physician, Department of Neurology, University Hospital, Tucson, Arizona

Dizziness
Gait Disturbances

JEFFREY L. SILBER, M.D.

Formerly Assistant Professor of Medicine, Division of Infectious Diseases, University of Medicine and Dentistry of New Jersey/Robert Wood Johnson Medical School at Camden; Formerly Hospital Epidemiologist, Department of Medicine, Cooper Hospital/University Medical Center, Camden, New Jersey

Chronic Meningitis
Staphylococcus Aureus Bacteremia

MARK S. SISKIND, M.D.

Formerly Clinical Assistant Professor of Medicine, The University of Arizona Health Sciences Center, Tucson, Arizona

Hypophosphatemia

MARTIN SNYDER, D.P.M.

Formerly Senior Clinical Lecturer, Department of Medicine, The University of Arizona Health Sciences Center, Tucson, Arizona

Foot Pain

JAMES R. STANDEN, M.D., F.R.C.P.C.

Professor of Clinical Radiology, University of Arizona College of Medicine; Head of Thoracic Radiology, University Medical Center, Tucson, Arizona

Large Cardiac Silhouette

LAWRENCE Z. STERN, M.D.

Professor, Department of Medicine, The University of Arizona Health Sciences Center, Tucson, Arizona

Muscle Cramps and Aches

RAYMOND TAETLE, M.D.

Professor of Medicine and Pathology, and Chief, Section of Hematology/Oncology, University of Arizona/Arizona Cancer Center, and University Medical Center, Tucson, Arizona

Anemia
Polycythemia
Disseminated Intravascular Coagulation

CATHERINE S. THOMPSON, M.D.

Formerly Associate Professor of Medicine, Division of Nephrology, University of Texas Medical School at Houston, Houston, Texas

Hypokalemia
Hyperkalemia

STEPHEN P. THOMSON, M.D.

Assistant Professor of Clinical Medicine, University of Arizona College of Medicine; Endocrinologist, Department of Medicine, VA Medical Center, Tucson, Arizona

Dyslipidemia
Hypothyroidism
Hyperthyroidism
Goiter

M. ANGELO TRUJILLO, M.D.

Clinical Assistant Professor of Medicine, Gastroenterology Section, University Medical Center, Tucson; Chairman, Department of Medicine, and Staff Physician, Flagstaff Medical Center, Flagstaff, Arizona

Anorexia
Anorectal Pain
Elevated Serum Amylase

DAVID B. VAN WYCK, M.D.

Associate Professor, Department of Medicine, University of Arizona College of Medicine; Clinical Director of Medicine and Subspecialties, VA Medical Center, Tucson, Arizona

Acute Renal Failure
Proteinuria
Hematuria
Kidney Stones
Renal Cysts and Masses
Hypomagnesemia

ALBERTA L. WARNER, M.D.

Formerly Clinical Assistant Professor, and Cardiologist, Section of Cardiology, The University of Arizona Health Sciences Center, Tucson, Arizona

Systolic Murmur
Diastolic Murmur

DONNA WEBER, M.D.

Assistant Professor, and Assistant Internist, Department of Lymphoma and Myeloma, University of Texas M.D. Anderson Cancer Center, Houston, Texas

Abnormal Serum Protein Electrophoresis

ROBERT W. WEISENTHAL, M.D.

Clinical Associate Professor, Department of Ophthalmology, State University of New York Health Science Center at Syracuse; Chief of Ophthalmology, VA Hospital, Syracuse, New York

The Red Eye

SETH D. WEISSMAN, M.D.

Clinical Assistant Professor of Medicine, Stanford University School of Medicine; Staff Physician, Stanford Medical Group, Stanford University Hospital, Stanford, California

Fever of Unknown Origin

JEANETTE K. WENDT, M.D.

Neurological Associates of Tucson, Tucson, Arizona

Acute Headache
Chronic Headache

HUNTER WESSELLS, M.D.

Assistant Professor of Clinical Surgery, Section of Urology, University of Arizona College of Medicine; Director of Urodynamics and Sexual Dysfunction Unit, Department of Urology, Arizona Health Sciences Center, Tucson, Arizona

Urinary Incontinence
Male Infertility

CAROL A. WOLFE, M.D.

Clinical Assistant Professor, Department of Internal Medicine, University of Arizona College of Medicine and University Medical Center, Tucson, Arizona

Eating Disorders

IAN WOOLLEY, M.B., B.S., F.R.A.C.P.

Fellow, Division of Infectious Diseases, Case Western Reserve University School of Medicine, and University Hospitals of Cleveland, Cleveland, Ohio

Pulmonary Infiltrates in HIV-Infected Patients

PREFACE

Decision Making in Medicine is a book for the practitioner, resident physician, medical student, nurse practitioner, or physician assistant seeking guidelines for diagnosis and therapy. It endeavors to bridge the gap between the didactics of a larger textbook and the practice of seasoned clinicians.

The topics are organized by sign, symptom, problem, or laboratory abnormality. One then follows a decision-tree approach to arrive at the proper diagnosis or family of diagnoses to consider. In other cases the algorithm leads to the appropriate therapy or course of action.

A book of this type assumes that there can be an orderliness to medicine and to the workup of common complaints. Such an approach offers uniformity, a means to control costs and order tests in an appropriate manner, and the possibility of a consistent quality approach to the same presenting complaints.

Medicine cannot be taught by cookbooks. Much of the flavor of medicine comes from the interplay of individual physician style and patient preference; we cannot put that in a book. The approaches presented here reflect the expertise and preferences of the individual authors, but there is much latitude for the reader's art of medicine.

I want to thank the contributing authors and editors who have successfully put their daily practice and best practices into a systematic approach and provided solid patterns to follow. My co-editors for this edition, William P. Johnson, M.D., and Dawn Lemcke, M.D., have done a superb job with review and revision of the manuscripts. I also want to thank Lynne Gery, Senior Managing Editor at Mosby, for outstanding support for this book. Suzanne Copple, Production Editor at Graphic World, has done a solid job with manuscript revision, page management, and preparation for final printing. Lesley M. Traver at Massachusetts Medical Society has been a valuable asset on the details of technical and administrative support. Linda M. Healy has been a constant support throughout the process.

This edition is dedicated to my father, Harry L. Greene, M.D., and mother, Helen B. Greene, R.N., and their physician, William P. Johnson, M.D., who through their lives have shown that serving others is the greatest gift of all.

Harry L. Greene II

CONTENTS

GENERAL MEDICINE

Preventive Health Services for Adults, 2
William P. Johnson, M.D.

Fatigue, 4
Lisa Kaufmann, M.D.

Eating Disorders, 8
Carol A. Wolfe, M.D.

Involuntary Weight Loss, 10
Lynn Cleary, M.D.

Obesity, 12
Scott W. Nowlin, M.D.

Sexual Dysfunction, 14
Kristyn M. Greifer, M.D.

Edema, 18
David W. Gibson, M.D., and Harry L. Greene II, M.D.

Chronic Pain, 22
William P. Johnson, M.D.

Persistent Excessive Sweating, 24
Lisa Kaufmann, M.D.

The Red Eye, 26
Shari Carney, M.D., and Robert W. Weisenthal, M.D.

Rhinitis, 32
Naomi Rappaport, M.D.

Tinnitus, 36
Susan Fisk Sander, M.D.

Hearing Loss, 40
Susan Fisk Sander, M.D.

Perioperative Evaluation, 44
Richard Liebowitz, M.D.

INTERNAL MEDICINE
CARDIOLOGY

Bradycardia, 60
David Framm, M.D., Paul E. Fenster, M.D., and Karl B. Kern, M.D.

Narrow QRS Complex Tachycardia, 62
Anthony C. Caruso, M.D., and Karl B. Kern, M.D.

Wide QRS Complex Tachycardia, 64
Anthony C. Caruso, M.D.

Stable Angina, 66
Samuel M. Butman, M.D.

Unstable Angina, 68
Samuel M. Butman, M.D., and Karl B. Kern, M.D.

Systolic Murmur, 70
Alberta L. Warner, M.D.

Diastolic Murmur, 72
Alberta L. Warner, M.D.

Hypertension, 74
Pamela J. Davis, M.D.

Hypotension, 78
Mark C. Goldberg, M.D., F.A.C.C.

Palpitations, 80
Karl B. Kern, M.D., and Paul E. Fenster, M.D.

Syncope, 82
Anthony C. Caruso, M.D.

Large Cardiac Silhouette, 84
James R. Standen, M.D.

Congestive Heart Failure, 86
Karl B. Kern, M.D.

Acute Pulmonary Edema, 88
James M. Galloway, M.D., and Paul E. Fenster, M.D.

Cor Pulmonale, 90
Mark C. Goldberg, M.D., and Karl B. Kern, M.D.

Right Ventricular Failure, 92
Mark C. Goldberg, M.D., and Karl B. Kern, M.D.

Cardiac Arrest, 94
James M. Galloway, M.D., and Karl B. Kern, M.D.

Cardiac Dyspnea, 96
David Framm, M.D., Paul E. Fenster, M.D., and Karl B. Kern, M.D.

Acute Myocardial Infarction, 98
Paul E. Fenster, M.D., James M. Galloway, M.D., and Karl B. Kern, M.D.

Counseling after Myocardial Infarction, 102
Susan McKenzie, R.N., M.S., and Karl B. Kern, M.D.

DERMATOLOGY
Pigmented Lesions, 104
Mark J. Scharf, M.D., and Norman Levine, M.D.

Leg Ulcer, 106
Cynthia A. O'Neil, M.D.

Urticaria, 108
Norman Levine, M.D.

Generalized Pruritus, 110
Norman Levine, M.D.

Palpable Purpura, 112
Norman Levine, M.D.

Livedo Reticularis, 114
Angela Murphy McGhee, M.D.

ENDOCRINOLOGY
Dyslipidemia, 116
Stephen P. Thomson, M.D., and Thomas W. Boyden, M.D.

Hypoglycemia, 120
Nancy A. Curosh, M.D.

Hyperglycemia, 122
Philip R. Orlander, M.D., and Thomas W. Boyden, M.D.

Hypocalcemia, 126
Philip R. Orlander, M.D.

Hypercalcemia, 128
Philip R. Orlander, M.D., and Thomas W. Boyden, M.D.

Test of Thyroid Function, 130
Julie I. Rifkin, M.D., and Thomas W. Boyden, M.D.

Hypothyroidism, 131
Stephen P. Thomson, M.D., and Thomas W. Boyden, M.D.

Hyperthyroidism, 134
Stephen P. Thomson, M.D., and Thomas W. Boyden, M.D.

Goiter, 136
Stephen P. Thomson, M.D., and Thomas W. Boyden, M.D.

Thyroid Nodule, 138
Julie I. Rifkin, M.D., and Thomas W. Boyden, M.D.

Painful Thyroid, 140
Nancy A. Curosh, M.D.

Thyroid Function Tests in Nonthyroidal Illness, 142
Julie I. Rifkin, M.D.

Adrenal Mass, 144
Nancy A. Curosh, M.D.

Cushing's Syndrome, 146
Nancy A. Curosh, M.D.

Pituitary Tumor, 148
Philip R. Orlander, M.D.

Hirsutism, 150
Nancy A. Curosh, M.D.

Gynecomastia, 152
Nancy A. Curosh, M.D., and Thomas W. Boyden, M.D.

GASTROENTEROLOGY
Acute Abdominal Pain, 154
Steven Palley, M.D.

Chronic Abdominal Pain, 156
Lee J. Hixson, M.D.

Nausea and Vomiting, 158
Steven Palley, M.D.

Anorexia, 160
M. Angelo Trujillo, M.D.

Dysphagia, 162
Philip E. Jaffe, M.D.

Heartburn, 164
Richard E. Sampliner, M.D.

Noncardiac Chest Pain, 166
M. Brian Fennerty, M.D.

Belching, 168
Gregory L. Eastwood, M.D.

Dyspepsia, 170
Lee J. Hixson, M.D.

Jaundice, 172
Richard E. Sampliner, M.D.

Ascites, 174
Richard E. Sampliner, M.D.

Biliary Colic, 176
Philip E. Jaffe, M.D.

Gastrointestinal Bleeding, 178
Gregory L. Eastwood, M.D.

Rectal Bleeding, 182
Steven Palley, M.D.

Acute Diarrhea, 184
M. Brian Fennerty, M.D.

Chronic Diarrhea, 186
Lee J. Hixson, M.D.

Constipation, 188
Philip E. Jaffe, M.D.

Irritable Bowel Syndrome, 190
William P. Johnson, M.D.

Anorectal Pain, 192
M. Angelo Trujillo, M.D.

Guaiac-Positive Stools, 194
M. Brian Fennerty, M.D.

Flatulence, 196
Gregory L. Eastwood, M.D.

Fecal Incontinence, 198
Philip E. Jaffe, M.D.

Asymptomatic Increased Transaminases, 200
Steven Palley, M.D.

Elevated Serum Iron, 202
M. Brian Fennerty, M.D.

Elevated Serum Amylase, 204
M. Angelo Trujillo, M.D.

HEMATOLOGY/ONCOLOGY
Anemia, 206
Raymond Taetle, M.D.

Polycythemia, 210
Raymond Taetle, M.D.

Leukocytosis, 212
Robert M. Rifkin, M.D., F.A.C.P.

Leukopenia, 214
William H. Kreisle, M.D., and Manuel Modiano, M.D.

Disseminated Intravascular Coagulation, 216
Raymond Taetle, M.D.

Deep Venous Thrombosis, 218
Guillermo Gonzalez-Osete, M.D., and Manuel Modiano, M.D.

Coagulation Abnormalities, 220
Manuel Modiano, M.D.

Transfusion Therapy: Platelets, 224
June Clements, M.D.

Transfusion Therapy: Red Blood Cells, 226
June Clements, M.D.

Transfusion Therapy: Granulocytes, 228
June Clements, M.D.

Transfusion Reactions and Complications, 230
June Clements, M.D.

Hodgkin's Disease, 232
Carol S. Portlock, M.D.

Chronic Myelogenous Leukemia, 234
Robert M. Rifkin, M.D.

Abnormal Serum Protein Electrophoresis, 236
Antonio C. Buzaid, M.D., and Donna Weber, M.D.

Lymphadenopathy, 240
Guillermo Gonzalez-Osete, M.D., and Manuel Modiano, M.D.

Carcinoma of Unknown Primary Site, 242
Antonio C. Buzaid, M.D., Marie C. Abbruzzese, M.B.A., and
James L. Abbruzzese, M.D.

Neutropenia and Fever, 246
Antonio C. Buzaid, M.D., and Issam Raad, M.D.

Pathologic Fractures, 248
Irwin E. Harris, M.D.

**Clinical Considerations for Bone Marrow or Stem
Cell Transplantation,** 252
Philip A. Lowry, M.D.

**Secondary Malignancies in Patients Previously Treated
for Cancer,** 254
Philip A. Lowry, M.D.

Superior Vena Caval Syndrome, 256
Frederick R. Ahmann, M.D.

Spinal Cord Compression, 258
Guillermo Gonzalez-Osete, M.D., and Manuel Modiano, M.D.

INFECTIOUS DISEASE
Foreign Travel: Immunizations and Infections, 260
Rodney D. Adam, M.D.

Acute and Subacute Meningitis, 262
Richard M. Mandel, M.D.

Chronic Meningitis, 266
Jeffrey L. Silber, M.D., and Mark J. DiNubile, M.D.

Aseptic Meningitis, 268
Deborah L. Goldsmith, M.D., and Richard M. Mandel, M.D.

Sexually Transmitted Diseases, 270
Dianna L. Rynkiewicz, M.D.

**Approach to the Newly Diagnosed HIV-Positive
Patient,** 276
J. Kevin Carmichael, M.D.

The Acutely Ill HIV-Positive Patient, 280
Deborah L. Goldsmith, M.D., and Richard M. Mandel, M.D.

Pulmonary Infiltrates in HIV-Infected Patients, 282
Karam C. Mounzer, M.D., Ian Woolley, M.D., B.S., F.R.A.C.P., and
Mark J. DiNubile, M.D.

**Central Nervous System Infection in the HIV-Infected
Patient,** 286
Deborah L. Goldsmith, M.D.

Sepsis, 288
Richard M. Mandel, M.D.

Toxic Shock Syndrome, 290
Richard M. Mandel, M.D.

***Staphylococcus Aureus* Bacteremia,** 292
Jeffrey L. Silber, M.D., and Mark J. DiNubile, M.D.

Hepatitis Exposure, 294
Stephen J. Gluckman, M.D., and Mark J. DiNubile, M.D.

Fever of Unknown Origin, 296
Seth D. Weissman, M.D., and Richard M. Mandel, M.D.

NEPHROLOGY

Chronic Renal Failure, 298
Anwar Al-Haidary, M.D., M.R.C.P., M.Sc., and Joy L. Logan, M.D.

Acute Renal Failure, 300
*Anwar Al-Haidary, M.D., M.R.C.P., M.Sc., and
David B. Van Wyck, M.D.*

Proteinuria, 302
*Anwar Al-Haidary, M.D., M.R.C.P., M.Sc., and
David B. Van Wyck, M.D.*

Hematuria, 304
*Anwar Al-Haidary, M.D., M.R.C.P., M.Sc., and
David B. Van Wyck, M.D.*

Kidney Stones, 306
James L. McGuire, M.D., and David B. Van Wyck, M.D.

Renal Cysts and Masses, 308
David B. Van Wyck, M.D.

Metabolic Acidosis, 310
Hillary Don, M.D.

Metabolic Alkalosis, 312
Hillary Don, M.D.

Hyponatremia, 314
Anwar Al-Haidary, M.D., M.R.C.P., M.Sc.

Hypernatremia, 316
Anwar Al-Haidary, M.D., M.R.C.P., M.Sc.

Hypokalemia, 318
Catherine S. Thompson, M.D., and David M. Clive, M.D.

Hyperkalemia, 320
Catherine S. Thompson, M.D., and David M. Clive, M.D.

Hypomagnesemia, 322
*Anwar Al-Haidary, M.D., M.R.C.P., M.Sc., and
David B. Van Wyck, M.D.*

Hypophosphatemia, 324
*Mark S. Siskind, M.D., Robert F. Klein, M.D., and
Steven T. Harris, M.D.*

Choosing a Chronic Dialysis Modality, 326
Joseph I. Shapiro, M.D.

Selection of Patients for Transplantation, 328
Joseph I. Shapiro, M.D.

Fever in a Transplant Patient, 330
Joseph I. Shapiro, M.D.

NEUROLOGY

Acute Headache, 332
Jeanette K. Wendt, M.D.

Chronic Headache, 334
Jeanette K. Wendt, M.D.

Transient Ischemic Attacks, 336
M. Kanter Carolin, M.D.

Transient Monocular Visual Loss, 338
M. Kanter Carolin, M.D.

Completed Stroke, 340
M. Kanter Carolin, M.D.

Progressing Stroke, 342
M. Kanter Carolin, M.D.

Memory Loss, 344
Geoffrey L. Ahern, M.D., Ph.D.

Dizziness, 348
William A. Sibley, M.D.

Seizures, 350
K. J. Oommen, M.D.

Status Epilepticus, 352
K. J. Oommen, M.D.

Weakness, 356
Lynn M. Rankin, M.D.

Gait Disturbances, 360
William A. Sibley, M.D.

Tremor, 362
Erwin B. Montgomery, Jr., M.D.

Parkinson's Disease, 364
Erwin B. Montgomery, Jr., M.D.

Peripheral Neuropathy, 366
Lynn M. Rankin, M.D.

Hyperkinesias, 370
Erwin B. Montgomery, Jr., M.D.

Muscle Cramps and Aches, 374
Lawrence Z. Stern, M.D.

Acute Behavior Change, 376
Geoffrey L. Ahern, M.D.

Chronic Behavior Change, 378
Geoffrey L. Ahern, M.D.

Disturbances of Smell and Taste, 382
Eugenie A.M.T. Obbens, M.D., Ph.D.

Coma, 384
Geoffrey L. Ahern, M.D.

Brain Death, 386
William M. Feinberg, M.D.

PULMONARY DISEASE
Hemoptysis, 388
Anthony Camilli, M.D.

Stridor, 390
Neil C. Clements, Jr., M.D., F.C.C.P.

Wheezing, 392
Neil C. Clements, Jr., M.D., F.C.C.P.

Cough, 394
Steven R. Knoper, M.D.

Pulmonary Dyspnea, 396
Anthony Camilli, M.D.

Pleural Effusion, 398
Steven R. Knoper, M.D.

Mediastinal Adenopathy, 400
Anthony Camilli, M.D.

Solitary Pulmonary Nodule, 402
John W. Lace, M.D., F.C.C.P.

Multiple Pulmonary Nodules, 404
John W. Lace, M.D., F.C.C.P.

Diffuse Interstitial Lung Disease, 406
Anthony Camilli, M.D.

Positive Tuberculin Skin Test, 408
Anthony Camilli, M.D.

**Respiratory Symptoms and Occupational Exposure
to Asbestos,** 410
Anthony Camilli, M.D.

RHEUMATOLOGY
Monoarticular Arthritis, 412
Deborah Doud, M.D.

Polyarticular Arthritis, 414
Deborah Doud, M.D.

Seronegative Arthritis, 416
Michael J. Maricic, M.D.

Soft Tissue Pain, 418
Michael J. Maricic, M.D.

Neck Pain, 420
Michael J. Maricic, M.D.

Shoulder Pain, 422
James B. Benjamin, M.D.

Low Back Pain, 424
Barbara Bode, M.D.

Hip Pain, 426
James B. Benjamin, M.D.

Hand and Wrist Pain, 428
Michael J. Maricic, M.D.

Knee Pain, 430
Michael J. Maricic, M.D.

Foot Pain, 432
Martin Snyder, D.P.M.

Scleroderma, 434
Barbara Bode, M.D.

**Keratoconjunctivitis Sicca (Sjögren's
Syndrome),** 436
Marcia Ko, M.D.

Raynaud's Phenomenon, 438
Patricia Mayer, M.D., F.A.C.R.

Osteopenia, 440
Michael J. Maricic, M.D.

Hyperuricemia and Gout, 442
Eric P. Gall, M.D.

**Diffuse Muscle Pain and Stiffness: Polymyalgia
Rheumatica and Giant Cell Arteritis,** 444
Michael J. Maricic, M.D.

Joint Hypermobility, 446
Patricia Mayer, M.D., F.A.C.R.

Temporomandibular Pain, 450
Michael J. Maricic, M.D.

Positive Antinuclear Antibody Test, 452
Marcia Ko, M.D.

Elevated Serum Alkaline Phosphate Level, 454
Michael J. Maricic, M.D.

Elevated Creatine Kinase Level, 456
Patricia Mayer, M.D., F.A.C.R.

WOMEN'S HEALTH
Vaginal Discharge, 458
Amir Nasseri, M.D.

Cervicitis, 460
Hugh S. Miller, M.D.

Secondary Amenorrhea, 462
Nancy A. Curosh, M.D.

Abnormal Vaginal Bleeding, 464
Hugh S. Miller, M.D.

Vaginal Bleeding in Pregnancy, 466
Janet Moore, M.D.

Acute Abdominal Pain in Women, 470
Robert N. Samuelson, M.D.

Chest Pain in Women, 472
Dawn Lemcke, M.D., F.A.C.P.

Urinary Tract Infection in Women, 476
Michael D. Katz, Pharm.D.

Breast Mass, 478
Laurie L. Fajardo, M.D.

Adjuvant Therapy Choices in Breast Cancer, 480
Rita Blanchard, M.D.

Nipple Discharge, 484
Homeira Baghdadi, M.D.

Abnormal Pap Smear, 486
Hugh S. Miller, M.D.

Premenstrual Dysphoric Disorder, 488
Jessica Byron, M.D.

Contraceptive Choices, 490
Ana Maria López, M.D., M.P.H.

Use of Oral Contraceptives, 494
Terra A. Robles, B.S., Pharm.D.

Female Infertility, 498
Lorna A. Marshall, M.D.

Domestic Violence, 502
Elaine J. Alpert, M.D., M.P.H.

UROLOGY
Acute Dysuria or Pyuria in Men, 506
Richard F. Hoffman, M.D.

Scrotal Mass, 508
William P. Johnson, M.D.

Prostate Nodule or Enlargement, 510
Jeffrey I. Miller, M.D., and George W. Drach, M.D.

Prostatitis, 512
Jeffrey I. Miller, M.D., and George W. Drach, M.D.

Urinary Incontinence, 514
Hunter Wessells, M.D.

Male Infertility, 518
Hunter Wessells, M.D.

EMERGENCY MEDICINE
Acute Pulseless Extremity, 522
Kenneth E. McIntyre, Jr., M.D.

Foreign Body Ingestion, 524
Riemke Brakema, M.D., F.A.C.E.P.

Caustic Ingestion and Exposure, 528
Cynthia Madden, M.D., M.P.H.

Human and Animal Bites, 530
Douglas Lindsey, M.D., Dr.P.H.

Snake Venom Poisoning, 532
William P. Johnson, M.D.

Hypothermia, 534
Cynthia Madden, M.D.

Drowning and Near-Drowning, 536
Samuel M. Keim, M.D., and Michael Loew, M.D.

BEHAVIORAL MEDICINE
Alcoholism, 542
Michael E. Scott, M.D., and Myra L. Muramoto, M.D.

Anxiety, 544
Eric M. Reiman, M.D.

Depression, 548
Iris R. Bell, M.D., Ph.D.

Emotional Disorders with Somatic Expression, 552
John Misiaszek, M.D.

Grief, 554
Gail L. Schwartz, M.D.

Psychosis, 556
Alan J. Gelenberg, M.D.

Smoking Cessation, 558
Harry L. Greene II, M.D., and Lawrence A. Garcia, M.D.

Suicidal Patient, 562
Rebecca L. Potter, M.D.

PHARMACOLOGY
Acute Anticoagulation, 566
Michael D. Katz, Pharm.D.

Long-Term Anticoagulation, 570
Michael D. Katz, Pharm.D.

Anaphylaxis, 574
Michael D. Katz, Pharm.D.

Evaluation of Adverse Drug Reactions, 578
Robert J. Lipsy, M.D., and Michael D. Katz, Pharm.D.

Nonsurgical Antimicrobial Prophylaxis, 580
Collin Freeman, Pharm.D., B.C.P.S.

Antimicrobial Prophylaxis in Surgical Patients, 584

Brian L. Erstad, B.S., Pharm.D.

Choosing Appropriate Antimicrobial Therapy, 586

Michael D. Katz, Pharm.D.

Use and Monitoring of Aminoglycoside Antibiotics, 588

Brian L. Erstad, B.S., Pharm.D.

Use and Evaluation of Serum Drug Levels, 590

Collin Freeman, Pharm.D., B.C.P.S., and Brian L. Erstad, B.S., Pharm.D.

Evaluation of a Drug for Clinical Use or Inclusion in a Formulary, 592

Terra A. Robles, B.S., Pharm.D.

GENERAL MEDICINE

PREVENTIVE HEALTH SERVICES FOR ADULTS

William P. Johnson

Preventive services require a high standard of evidence before being widely applied. Because everyone is a potential candidate for preventive services, the aggregate cost is high. Because people are theoretically healthy when they seek advice, the obligation to make recommendations based on high-quality evidence is even more stringent. The guiding principle should be *Primum certior fe, tunc mone* (first understand, then advise). When evidence from large, well-designed random controlled trials (RCTs) is lacking, expert panels come together to give advice based on the best available evidence. Three expert panels have evaluated the full range of preventive services: the Canadian Task Force on the Periodic Health Examination, the U.S. Preventive Services Task Force, and the American College of Physicians. All three insist on comprehensive literature searches, background articles that evaluate the evidence critically, clear rationales for their recommendations, and review by external experts.

A. Questions about adult preventive services usually fall into one of four categories: the periodic health examination, screening, immunizations/prophylaxis, and counseling.

B. Risk generally refers to the probability of some untoward event. In terms of prevention, we generally use the term *risk* in a more restricted sense to indicate the likelihood that people who are exposed to certain factors (i.e., risk factors) will subsequently develop a particular disease. Risk factors, by definition, predict for some future event. This discussion considers only two forms of risk: average and increased.

C. The major expert panels agree on the following policies for "average risk" adults:
    - Blood pressure (BP) measurement—every medical visit and at least once every 2 years
    - Breast examination by a physician—annual examination for women > 40 years old
    - Serum cholesterol—every 5 years beginning at age 35 in men and age 40 in women
    - Mammography—yearly beginning at age 50
    - Cervical cytologic screening—every 1–3 years starting at the age of first intercourse, if there has been regular screening with normal results, screening is unnecessary after age 65

    - Vaccinations—annual influenza and pneumococcal vaccinations after age 65
    - Counseling—tobacco cessation, use of seat belts, alcohol consumption

D. Patients at "increased risk" for a disease should have an appropriately thorough examination, and/or testing, and/or prophylaxis, and/or counseling. Because the prevalence of disease is theoretically higher in this group, one can justify a more aggressive approach.

E. Many controversies (marked with an asterisk on decision tree) surround preventive health recommendations for "average risk" patients including the following:
    - Breast cancer—Should women at average risk be screened in their 40s? At what age should screening stop?
    - Colorectal cancer—Fecal occult blood testing (FOBT) and flexible sigmoidoscopy are effective but in what combination, and why not a single full colonoscopy every 10 years?
    - Hormone replacement therapy—Given risks/benefits should this be a routine recommendation, especially in women with average risk for CAD?
    - Hypercholesterolemia—What is the best age to begin? Is there any evidence that primary prevention is effective?
    - Prostate cancer—The results of the ongoing RCT must justify recommending screening for this disease.

Because these recommendations are subject to change, the best way to find the latest recommendation is via the internet. The best current internet site for prevention is *http://odphp.osophs.dhhs.gov/pubs/guidecps/tcpstoc.htm.*

References

Guide to Clinical Preventive Services. Report of the US Preventive Services Task Force. 2nd ed. Baltimore: Williams & Wilkins, 1996.

Molberg P. Prevention in adults. Prim Care 1995; 22:653.

Sox HC. Preventive health services in adults. N Engl J Med 1994; 330:1589.

Patient for PREVENTIVE HEALTH SERVICES

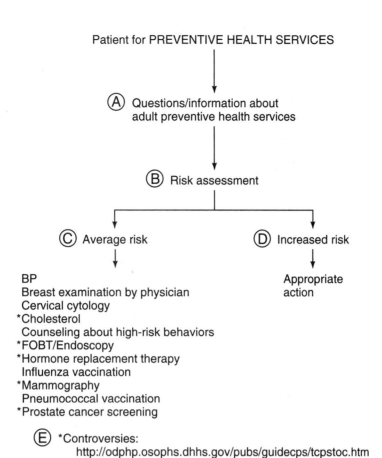

Ⓐ Questions/information about
  adult preventive health services

Ⓑ Risk assessment

Ⓒ Average risk

Ⓓ Increased risk

BP
Breast examination by physician
Cervical cytology
*Cholesterol
Counseling about high-risk behaviors
*FOBT/Endoscopy
*Hormone replacement therapy
Influenza vaccination
*Mammography
Pneumococcal vaccination
*Prostate cancer screening

Appropriate
action

Ⓔ *Controversies:
    http://odphp.osophs.dhhs.gov/pubs/guidecps/tcpstoc.htm

FATIGUE

Lisa Kaufmann

Acute (<6 months' duration) and chronic (>6 months' duration) fatigue are associated with many diseases, but most patients have signs and symptoms of the primary disease process. In a large urban internal medicine practice, 25% of patients admitted to at least 6 months of fatigue that interfered with their daily activities. Fatigue is the chief complaint in 1–7% of office visits by adults. Acute fatigue is more likely than chronic fatigue to be associated with a clear-cut cause or to resolve spontaneously.

A. Although 75% of patients with a chief complaint of chronic fatigue have a psychiatric diagnosis and 20% have no definable diagnosis, about 7% have significant physical disease (4% have both medical and psychiatric disease, and 3% have only a medical diagnosis). Because fatigue is so nonspecific, a careful history and physical are essential and should include a description of the fatigue (e.g., is it exhaustion, breathlessness, lack of interest), precipitating and palliative factors (is it related to work, less on vacations or weekends, affected by bed rest, onset, relationship to activities), and any associated physical or psychological symptoms.

B. Physiologic fatigue results from a situation that would cause most people to become fatigued. It is common in sleep-deprived new parents, working mothers of toddlers, and workers doing rotating shifts or overtime, but it also can result from overtraining in athletes, malnutrition, and exposure to high noise levels. Rest, improved scheduling, and/or ear protection usually resolve the fatigue. Boring, low paying jobs are more likely to be experienced as fatiguing than are more stimulating jobs, especially if they involve low levels of physical activity (perhaps they fall below the level needed to maintain arousal).

C. Consider drugs or toxins (alcohol, illicit drugs, sedating medications, such as antihistamines, β blockers, or non-steroidals, including over-the-counter and herbal medications, and occupational toxin exposures). Neurologic (e.g., multiple sclerosis, Parkinson's, postpolio, seizures), as well as medical disease can cause fatigue. Adrenal insufficiency may present as fatigue but usually is associated with orthostatic hypotension. Hypothyroidism, hypopituitarism, asthma, sarcoidosis, anemia, lupus, hepatitis, chronic infections, and malignancy have all been identified in case series. Many illnesses produce severe fatigue, but usually other symptoms are more prominent (e.g., heart failure, tuberculosis).

D. Unless another cause of the fatigue is obvious on initial evaluation, carefully question all fatigued patients for risk factors for HIV, syphilis, and hepatitis B and C, all of which can present as isolated fatigue.

E. Lyme disease occurs in temperate wooded climates. Coccidioidomycosis is caused by a fungus endemic in the desert southwest and can be acquired with brief exposure such as driving through the area. Both illnesses may present as isolated fatigue.

F. Fibromyalgia affects about 3% of adult women in the general population and is characterized by aching muscles both above and below the waist, multiple tender points, and the absence of other disease to explain the symptoms. Although the American Rheumatologic Association criteria require 11 tender points of 18 tested, population studies show a spectrum of symptoms with aching muscles and increasing numbers of tender points being correlated with sleep disturbance, fatigue, and depression. Up to 70% of patients who meet criteria for chronic fatigue syndrome (Fig. 1) also meet criteria for fibromyalgia. Because other rheumatologic conditions may cause similar symptoms, add a careful joint and skin examination as well as screening rheumatologic laboratory testing (creatine phosphokinase [CPK], C-reactive protein [CRP], ANA, and rheumatoid factor [RF]) to the usual laboratory evaluation of fatigue when fibromyalgia is suspected.

G. Because most patients with a presenting symptom of fatigue have a psychiatric diagnosis, perform a careful psychosocial assessment (Table 1). Because few of these patients think that their symptoms are psychiatric in origin, it is helpful to the maintenance of a strong therapeutic relationship for the primary physician to do the assessment if possible.

(Continued on page 7)

TABLE 1 Areas of Psychosocial Assessment for Symptoms of Fatigue

Historical data	Current functioning
Work history	Current work experience
Past or current substance abuse	Quality of relationships or support networks
Addictive behavior patterns	Sexual activity and function
Depression, anxiety, or other psychiatric diagnosis	Appetite and diet
Abuse (physical, sexual, emotional)	Life goals
	Self-esteem
Family history of chronic health problems	Exercise or recreational activities
Significant life changes or losses	Coping skills
	Relaxation techniques

From Ruffin MT, Cohen M. Evaluation and management of fatigue. Am Fam Physician 1994; 50:625, as adapted from Holmes GP. Defining the chronic fatigue syndrome. Rev Infect Dis 1991; 13(suppl 1):S53.

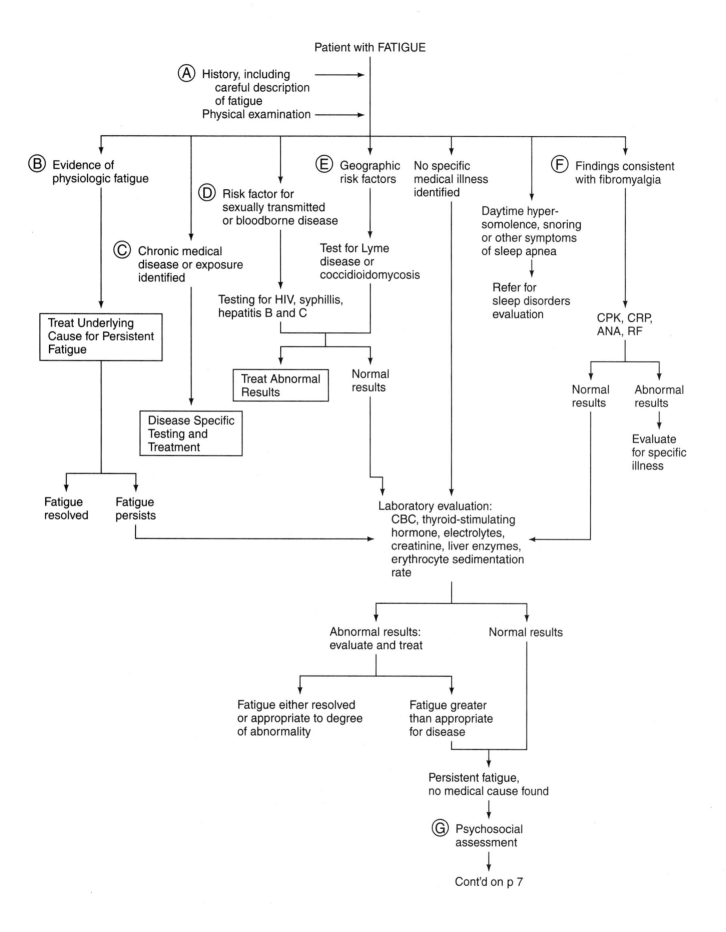

Patient with FATIGUE

A History, including careful description of fatigue
Physical examination

B Evidence of physiologic fatigue

D Risk factor for sexually transmitted or bloodborne disease

E Geographic risk factors

No specific medical illness identified

F Findings consistent with fibromyalgia

C Chronic medical disease or exposure identified

Test for Lyme disease or coccidioidomycosis

Daytime hyper-somolence, snoring or other symptoms of sleep apnea

Testing for HIV, syphillis, hepatitis B and C

Refer for sleep disorders evaluation

Treat Underlying Cause for Persistent Fatigue

CPK, CRP, ANA, RF

Treat Abnormal Results

Normal results

Disease Specific Testing and Treatment

Normal results

Abnormal results

Fatigue resolved

Fatigue persists

Evaluate for specific illness

Laboratory evaluation: CBC, thyroid-stimulating hormone, electrolytes, creatinine, liver enzymes, erythrocyte sedimentation rate

Abnormal results: evaluate and treat

Normal results

Fatigue either resolved or appropriate to degree of abnormality

Fatigue greater than appropriate for disease

Persistent fatigue, no medical cause found

G Psychosocial assessment

Cont'd on p 7

Major criteria
(Patient must have both major criteria)

Persistent or relapsing fatigue or easy fatigability
for at least 6 months that:
- Does not resolve with bed rest.
- Is severe enough to reduce average daily activity
by at least 50%.
Other chronic conditions are excluded.

Minor criteria
(Patient must have at least six of the minor criteria)

Mild fever or chills
Sore throat
Lymph node pain in anterior or posterior cervical
or axillary chains
Unexplained generalized muscle weakness
Myalgia
Prolonged (>24 hr) generalized fatigue following
previously tolerable levels of exercise
New, generalized headaches
Migratory, noninflammatory arthralgia
Neuropsychologic symptoms
Photophobia
Transient visual scotomata
Forgetfulness
Excessive irritability
Confusion
Difficulty thinking
Inability to concentrate
Depression
Sleep disturbance (hypersomnia or insomnia)
Patient describes initial onset as acute or subacute

Physical criteria
(Must be documented by a physician
on at least two occasions at least 1
month apart)

Low-grade fever
Nonexudative pharyngitis
Palpable or tender anterior
or posterior cervical
or axillary lymph nodes
(<2 cm in diameter)

Plus two additional
minor criteria

Figure 1   Criteria for chronic fatigue syndrome. To meet the diagnosis of chronic fatigue syndrome, the patient must have two major criteria plus eight minor criteria (for a total of 10) or two major criteria plus six minor criteria plus two physical criteria (for a total of 10). (From Ruffin MT, Cohen M. Evaluation and management of fatigue. Am Fam Physician 1994; 50:625, as adapted from Holmes GP. Defining the chronic fatigue syndrome. Rev Infect Dis 1991; 13[suppl 1]:S53.)

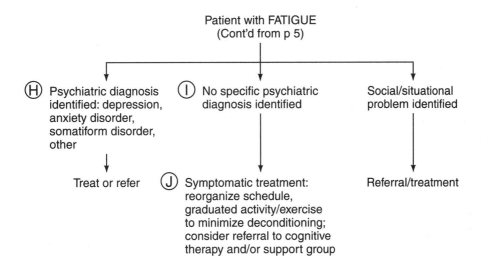

Patient with FATIGUE
(Cont'd from p 5)

(H) Psychiatric diagnosis identified: depression, anxiety disorder, somatiform disorder, other

(I) No specific psychiatric diagnosis identified

Social/situational problem identified

Treat or refer

(J) Symptomatic treatment: reorganize schedule, graduated activity/exercise to minimize deconditioning; consider referral to cognitive therapy and/or support group

Referral/treatment

H. The most common cause of chronic fatigue is major depression, followed by anxiety disorders and somatiform disorders. Treatment of these conditions is described elsewhere in this book. Many patients in this group with fatigue rather than complaints of depressed or anxious mood prefer to conceptualize their illness as physical and may be more willing to take appropriate medications if possible improvements of the physical symptoms such as insomnia and fatigue are emphasized. Sometimes presenting a psychiatric referral as helping with coping with an overall difficult life situation may make it more acceptable.

I. Patients who are chronically fatigued for >6 months with no specific cause identified may meet criteria for the chronic fatigue syndrome (see Fig. 1). These criteria are useful for research purposes, but because there is no specific cause or treatment associated with the criteria, these patients should be treated like any other patients with chronic fatigue of unknown cause.

J. About 20% of chronically fatigued patients have no identifiable medical or psychiatric cause, a situation frustrating to both the patient and physician. Encourage patients to remain as active as possible because exces-

sive rest results in deconditioning, which exacerbates the fatigue. This can be accomplished by scheduling important activities when fatigue is least severe (a symptom diary is helpful) and encouraging regular mild exercise (calibrated by the patient to avoid severe exhaustion). For patients with fibromyalgia, stretching and swimming are useful. Chronic fatigue and the inability to perform activities previously taken for granted cause major social stress and grief. Brief cognitive therapy geared toward refocusing goals and expectations has proven useful, and patient support groups can help. These modalities also can help patients with chronic fatigue of a known cause.

References

Bates DW, Schmitt W, Buchwald D, et al. Prevalence of fatigue and chronic fatigue syndrome in a primary care practice. Arch Intern Med 1993; 153:2759.

Manu P, Lane TJ, Matthews DA. Chronic fatigue and chronic fatigue syndrome: clinical epidemiology and aetiological classification. CIBA Foundation Symposium 1993; 173:23.

Ruffin MT, Cohen M. Evaluation and management of fatigue. Am Fam Physician 1994; 50:625.

EATING DISORDERS

Carol A. Wolfe

A. The primary care physician (PCP) has an important role in detecting eating disorders during routine medical examinations. The patient with an eating disorder typically is an adolescent or young adult white female of middle to upper-middle socioeconomic class. Males also have eating disorders but much less commonly. These patients are often secretive or in denial about their disorder; therefore careful history from family members concerning food rituals, weight swings, and/or excessive exercise is helpful if an eating disorder is suspected. Several tools have been used to assess the presence of an eating disorder; the most common is the Eating Attitudes Test (EAT). An overwhelming preoccupation with body image suggests an eating disorder.

B. Bulimia tends to start at a later age than anorexia, and patients present much later in the course of the disease. They are embarrassed by their abnormal eating habits and try to hide them. They usually are of normal or slightly above normal weight. The two most common complaints on review of systems are swelling of the hands and feet and abdominal bloating. These are vague and indirect complaints, so clues on physical examination are often important to attain an early diagnosis. Ulceration or calluses on the dorsum of the hand or on the proximal interphalangeal joints can be caused by the teeth during manual triggering of the gag reflex to induce vomiting. This is more often seen early in the disease because most patients are soon able to vomit spontaneously. A dull gray discoloration or dental erosions of teeth caused by recurrent exposure to gastric acid are often present. Salivary gland hypertrophy is common. Subconjunctival hemorrhages can be seen. Unexplained muscle weakness should trigger suspicion of ipecac use, which if absorbed in large enough doses can cause a primary myositis. Hypokalemia may be due to vomiting or laxative and/or diuretic use. Male bulimics are often wrestlers or jockeys who purge to lose weight quickly before sporting events.

C. Evaluate bulimic patients for life-threatening medical problems. The most common are fluid and electrolyte abnormalities, dehydration, hypotension, hypokalemia, and alkalosis. Other rare medical emergencies are esophageal rupture, pneumomediastinum, cardiac myositis from emetine overdose, and pancreatitis. If amenorrhea is present, order a bone density study to assess the need for estrogen replacement.

D. Anorexia nervosa is easiest to detect during physical examination. Weight continually 15% below that expected for height is required for diagnosis. These patients rarely ask for help and are unaware of their malnutrition because denial is a large part of the disease. Usually there is a history of an attempt at weight loss starting in the teenage years, and abnormal eating habits develop from that time with severe restriction of food.

Food rituals (e.g., storing food in a certain place in the refrigerator) can occur. There is an intense fear of gaining weight and an abnormal self-image. Although very thin, these patients perceive themselves as fat. They often have a history of amenorrhea. Anorexics engage in excess physical activity, often predating the onset of overt anorexia nervosa. They often participate in purging activities, including self-induced vomiting, excessive diuretic use, and cathartic use. History from the family will confirm whether the patient is involved in many of these activities. There is an association with childhood trauma.

E. Anorexics often are hospitalized because of severe malnutrition or for fluid and electrolyte disorders (seen more commonly with the bulimic variant). These patients often need tube feeding to regain a minimal weight and to be stabilized. Refeeding, whether by nasogastric tube or by behavior therapy, is associated with congestive heart failure (CHF) and severe hypophosphatemia. There may be multiple physical problems, mostly relating to malnutrition, and sudden death from cardiac arrest associated with prolongation of the QT interval may occur. Other physical problems are amenorrhea, osteoporosis, euthyroid sick syndrome, hypercarotenemia, abnormal temperature regulation, decreased gastric emptying, constipation, elevated liver enzymes, anemia, and hypoalbuminemia. Most are treated by providing adequate nutrition. This must be done gradually to decrease the risk of CHF. A bone density study and estrogen replacement are essential for patients with osteoporosis and amenorrhea.

F. After hospitalization or if hospitalization is unnecessary, psychiatric evaluation and treatment with help from an experienced nutritionist are begun. Often there is an associated depression that requires antidepressant medication. The only medications that have undergone placebo-controlled prospective study are fluoxitene and desipramine. Both have been found to be effective. Many patients have problems with alcohol or other substance abuse and sexual promiscuity. A team approach, including a psychotherapist, a PCP, and an experienced nutritionist, is necessary for success. Goals should be agreed on by the treatment group. Cognitive therapy has been the most successful and should include family therapy. If relapse occurs, goals and types of therapy should be re-evaluated. If there are recurrent medical emergencies, contracts with patients to limit high-risk behavior and mandatory hospitalization for failure to comply can be helpful. Frequent monitoring by the PCP is essential. A nonjudgmental approach is helpful in permitting the patient to contact the PCP before an emergency occurs.

G. There are many atypical presentations of eating disorders. Many women are distressed with their body shape

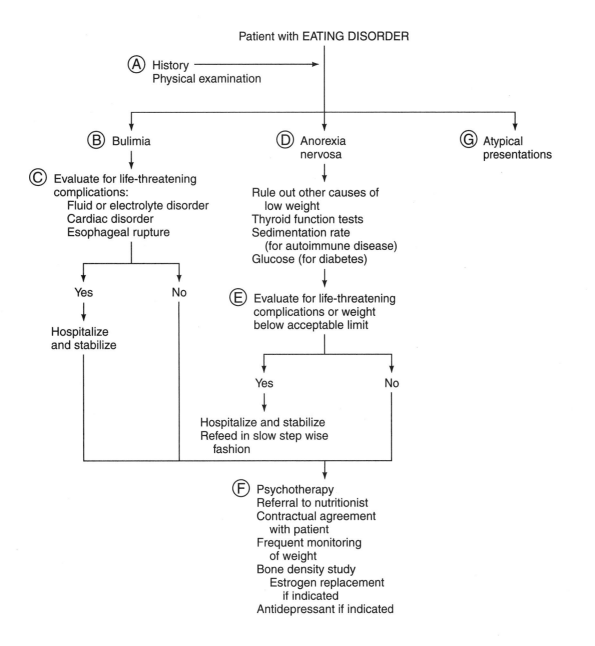

Patient with EATING DISORDER

(A) History
Physical examination

(B) Bulimia

(C) Evaluate for life-threatening
complications:
Fluid or electrolyte disorder
Cardiac disorder
Esophageal rupture

Yes

No

Hospitalize
and stabilize

(D) Anorexia
nervosa

Rule out other causes of
low weight
Thyroid function tests
Sedimentation rate
(for autoimmune disease)
Glucose (for diabetes)

(E) Evaluate for life-threatening
complications or weight
below acceptable limit

Yes

No

Hospitalize and stabilize
Refeed in slow step wise
fashion

(F) Psychotherapy
Referral to nutritionist
Contractual agreement
with patient
Frequent monitoring
of weight
Bone density study
Estrogen replacement
if indicated
Antidepressant if indicated

(G) Atypical
presentations

without having an eating disorder, but if they are abnormally thin, consider a psychiatric evaluation. Many women set abnormally low weight goals to compete in ballet, sports, or modeling. Unlike typical anorexia nervosa patients, these women know they are thin. If they are unwilling to achieve a healthy minimal weight, refer them for psychiatric evaluation. There is a subclinical group of patients with eating disorders who intermittently, when under stress, have binge-purge episodes. Many women are binge eaters during times of stress, but purging suggests self-destructive behavior that should be evaluated by a psychiatrist.

References

Blinder BJ, et al. The eating disorders: medical and psychological basis of diagnosis and treatment. New York: PMA Publishing, 1988.

Mitchell JE, Seim HC, Colon E, Pomeroy C. Medical complications and medical management of bulimia. Ann Intern Med 1987; 107:71.

Yager J, ed. Symposium on eating disorders. Psychiatr Clin North Am 1996; 19(4).

INVOLUNTARY WEIGHT LOSS

Lynn Cleary

Involuntary weight loss (IWL) is defined as >5% loss of usual body weight within 6 months. It is significantly associated with older age, poorer health status, smoking, lower body mass index, and in men, widowhood and less education. It is also associated with higher mortality rates in patients with and without established disease and merits diagnostic and therapeutic intervention.

Medical literature documenting IWL is scant. Clinical studies looking at underlying causes have studied small numbers of patients with wide variability in their demographic characteristics (e.g., age, inpatients vs. outpatients, long-term care residents, veterans). Generalization in the diagnostic approach to IWL is therefore limited in its applicability to different populations.

Diagnostic causes are found in 65–90% of cases. Inpatients on medical service have a high proportion of physical causes, whereas ambulatory patients are found to have psychiatric disease almost as often as physical causes. Geriatrics studies have shown a high prevalence of both. In 10–35% of cases, no cause can be found.

A. It is important to document the complaint of weight loss or to look for indirect evidence of weight loss if documentation is unavailable. Many patients complaining of weight loss do not in fact have any documented loss.

B. Common underlying causes include neoplasm, primary gastroenterologic disease, chronic underlying illness (cardiovascular, metabolic, pulmonary), poor nutrition, hyperthyroidism, dementia, depression, and anxiety. The prevalence of each diagnosis greatly depends on the group being studied.

C. Review risks, symptoms, and examination results for evidence of cancer, diabetes, heart/lung disease, oral/dental disease, GI pathology, hyperthyroidism, dementia, and psychiatric illness.

D. Physical causes often are apparent early in the investigation. This may not be as applicable to the elderly, in whom disease often presents in nonspecific ways and IWL is more prevalent. Although there are no data to support more aggressive testing in the elderly, it may be reasonable to focus more attention on the oral/dental/gastroenterologic as well as psychosocial contributions to IWL if the initial evaluation is unrevealing.

E. Whether or not a diagnostic cause is confirmed, the patient with IWL should be followed closely because there is an association with higher mortality and lower health status regardless of specific cause.

References

Meltzer AA, Everhart JE. Unintentional weight loss in the United States. Am J Epidemiol 1995; 142:10.

Wise GR, Craig D. Evaluation of involuntary weight loss. Where do you start? Postgrad Med 1994; 95:4.

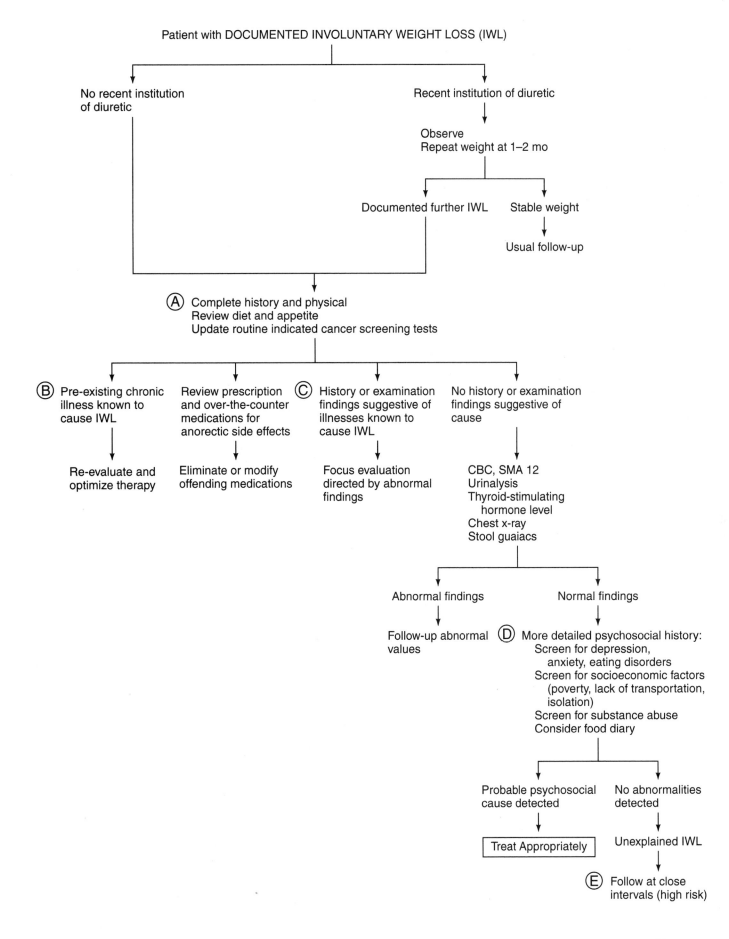

Patient with DOCUMENTED INVOLUNTARY WEIGHT LOSS (IWL)

No recent institution of diuretic

Recent institution of diuretic

Observe
Repeat weight at 1–2 mo

Documented further IWL

Stable weight

Usual follow-up

(A) Complete history and physical
Review diet and appetite
Update routine indicated cancer screening tests

(B) Pre-existing chronic illness known to cause IWL

Review prescription and over-the-counter medications for anorectic side effects

(C) History or examination findings suggestive of illnesses known to cause IWL

No history or examination findings suggestive of cause

Re-evaluate and optimize therapy

Eliminate or modify offending medications

Focus evaluation directed by abnormal findings

CBC, SMA 12
Urinalysis
Thyroid-stimulating hormone level
Chest x-ray
Stool guaiacs

Abnormal findings

Normal findings

Follow-up abnormal values

(D) More detailed psychosocial history:
Screen for depression, anxiety, eating disorders
Screen for socioeconomic factors (poverty, lack of transportation, isolation)
Screen for substance abuse
Consider food diary

Probable psychosocial cause detected

No abnormalities detected

Treat Appropriately

Unexplained IWL

(E) Follow at close intervals (high risk)

11

OBESITY

Scott W. Nowlin

In the United States obesity affects about 34 million adults between the ages of 20 and 74 years. Morbidity and mortality rates are high. Effective treatment is difficult.

A. *Overweight* can be defined as an increase in body weight above some arbitrary standard defined in relation to height. Up to 20% above the upper limits of "ideal" is considered overweight. Obesity means an abnormally high proportion of body fat (Table 1). Anthropometric measurements such as height, weight, and skin fold thickness are useful for determining the degree of overweight or obesity in a patient. A person >20% above the upper limits of ideal body weight can be considered obese. The Metropolitan Life Insurance Company's Tables of Heights and Weights commonly are used to determine ideal body weight, the ideal weight for height being that weight at which longevity is the greatest.

B. On initial evaluation of the obese patient, one must consider a variety of possible causes. Unfortunately, <1% of obese patients have an identifiable endocrine dysfunction. In most cases, obesity results from an imbalance of energy intake versus energy expenditure. Multiple twin and adoption studies have indicated that human fatness is under strong genetic control. Rare genetic diseases such as the Laurence-Moon-Biedl syndrome are associated with obesity through unknown mechanisms.

C. Medications such as the phenothiazines and the tricyclic antidepressants can lead to obesity by increasing appetite. Corticosteroids also increase appetite and are associated with central or truncal obesity.

D. Obesity predisposes individuals to many diseases. Diabetes mellitus, hypertension, and cardiovascular disease are more common in obese individuals. About 85% of patients in the United States with type 2 diabetes mellitus are obese. Obesity is an independent risk factor for the development of coronary artery disease. Other associated disorders include cholesterol, gallstones, hyperlipidemia, venous circulatory disease, osteoarthritis, gout, and cancer. Women have an increased incidence of cancer of the breast, endometrium, ovary, and biliary system. Men have an increased incidence of cancer of the colon, rectum, and prostate.

E. Before beginning a treatment program for obesity, assess the patient's motivation and commitment. Educate the patient about the benefits of weight loss and the health benefits attained. Long-term success depends on a combination approach using diet, exercise, and behavior modification. Social and psychological support also are important.

F. Exercise should (1) promote increased energy expenditure, (2) promote fat loss and the maintenance of lean body mass, (3) be safe for the participant, and (4) promote increases in activity levels within the individual's lifestyle.

G. Low calorie diets should be nutritionally balanced and provide macronutrients in the following distribution: carbohydrates (≥50% of total energy intake), fat (<30%), and protein (15–20%). The usual energy intake for such diets is 1000–1200 kcal/day. When energy intake is <1000 kcal/day, vitamin and mineral supplements usually are necessary.

H. Very low calorie diets (VLCDs) provide 400–800 kcal/day. They supply protein of high biologic value and are prescribed for severely or morbidly obese patients (body mass index [BMI] >35). Medical supervision and supplementation with vitamins and minerals are necessary. The VLCD allows rapid weight loss while preserving lean body mass by providing dietary protein; it usually lasts 12–16 weeks. Behavior modifications and close follow-up also are necessary.

I. Behavior changes in eating patterns to affect weight loss are the crux of behavior modification. Behavioral assessment of obese persons involves attention to three points: (1) the antecedents of eating that promote excessive intake, (2) slowing the act of eating, and (3) selectively emphasizing the consequences of certain behaviors (e.g., rewarding appropriate eating behaviors).

J. Drug therapy can be considered in the compliant, motivated individual in conjunction with dietary measures. Relatively weak CNS stimulants such as phentermine have been successful at reducing weight in the short term.

K. Gastric surgery should be considered only in morbidly obese patients who have been unsuccessful with conventional means of weight loss. The other approaches to weight loss, including dietary management and exercise, are still important in those who undergo surgery.

TABLE 1 Parameters of Obesity

	Men	Women
Triceps plus subscapular skinfold (mm)	>43	>58
Body fat (% body weight)	>25	>30
BMI $\frac{\text{weight in kg}}{(\text{height in m})^2}$	>30	>30

Adapted from Bray GA. Obesity: an endocrine perspective. In: DeGroot LJ, ed. Endocrinology. 2nd ed. Philadelphia: WB Saunders, 1989:2303.

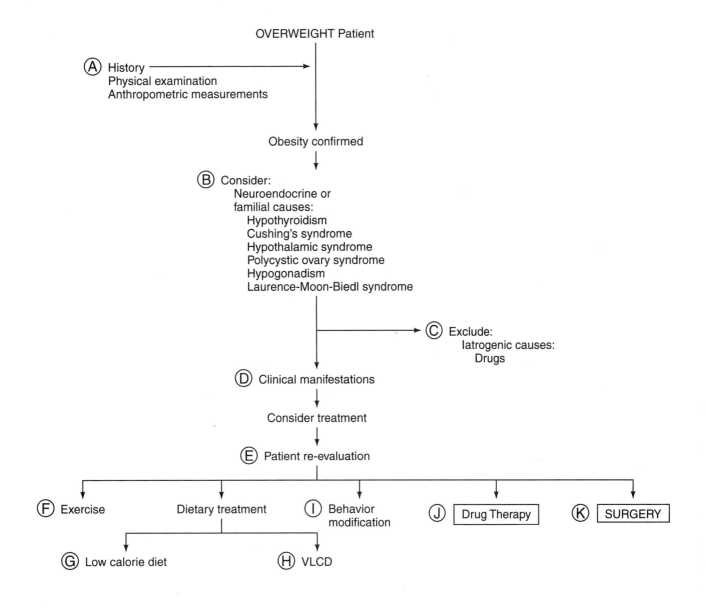

OVERWEIGHT Patient

Ⓐ History
Physical examination
Anthropometric measurements

Obesity confirmed

Ⓑ Consider:
Neuroendocrine or
familial causes:
Hypothyroidism
Cushing's syndrome
Hypothalamic syndrome
Polycystic ovary syndrome
Hypogonadism
Laurence-Moon-Biedl syndrome

Ⓒ Exclude:
Iatrogenic causes:
Drugs

Ⓓ Clinical manifestations

Consider treatment

Ⓔ Patient re-evaluation

Ⓕ Exercise

Dietary treatment

Ⓘ Behavior
modification

Ⓙ Drug Therapy

Ⓚ SURGERY

Ⓖ Low calorie diet

Ⓗ VLCD

References

Bray GA. The syndromes of obesity: an endocrine approach. In: DeGroot LJ, ed. Endocrinology. 3rd ed. Philadelphia: WB Saunders, 1995:2651.

Council on Scientific Affairs. Treatment of obesity in adults. JAMA 1988; 260:2547.

The Surgeon General's report on nutrition and health. Washington, DC: US Department of Health and Human Services, Public Health Service, 1988:275.

Wadden TA, Van Itallie TB, Blackburn GL. Responsible and irresponsible use of very-low calorie diets in the treatment of obesity. JAMA 1990; 263.

SEXUAL DYSFUNCTION

Kristyn M. Greifer

A. Although a few patients will volunteer sexual difficulties, most will not. A detailed medical history should include a sexual history to elicit complaints. Ask general, nonjudgmental questions, including effects on current relationships, to open the discussion. Make no assumptions about a patient's sexual preferences or experiences.

B. Decreased libido can be associated with depression or other psychiatric disorders or their medical treatment. Stress in relationships or work also can contribute. Psychiatric evaluation and counseling can help. Medical causes of decreased sexual desire include medications (e.g., antihypertensives), substance abuse, and acute or chronic illness. Sex and/or marital therapy should be considered for patients with significant relationship problems (as either a cause or a result).

C. Erectile dysfunction or impotence can be classified as organic or psychogenic, although many men have a mixture of both. The presence of morning erections is highly specific for psychogenic impotence, although not very sensitive. There are a number of organic causes for erectile dysfunction, including endocrine, vascular, and neurologic causes. Some surgical procedures such as radical prostatectomy may result in erectile dysfunction. Routine serologic screening for endocrine disorders is not warranted in the absence of other indicators in the history or physical examination. Medications (e.g., antihypertensives) also have been implicated. Acute and chronic illness can contribute both organically and psychologically. A nocturnal penile tumescence test using stamps or an inexpensive strain gauge will more reliably differentiate psychogenic from organic dysfunction. In either case, one might consider injection or topical treatment with prostaglandin agents. Newer oral agents may also prove effective (e.g., sildenafil [Viagra]). Devices to enhance erections (e.g., penile rings or vacuum pumps) can be used. Sex therapy also can be useful for patients with a psychological component. Referral to a urologist for evaluation and treatment is appropriate in refractory cases.

D. Premature ejaculation is a common complaint among young, sexually inexperienced men. It also is seen in patients having relationship or situational stresses and is well known to occur with fatigue. Therapy is limited to the pause (or hold) and squeeze technique in addition to increasing sexual stimulation, which is thought to increase the latency period. Sex therapy can be helpful. Drugs may be available in the near future. Absent ejaculation may be organic and a result of hypogonadism. Retrograde ejaculation requires referral to a urologist. Rarely, anorgasmia occurs in the absence of hypogonadism and is best addressed by sex therapy-

(Continued on page 16)

Patient with SEXUAL DYSFUNCTION

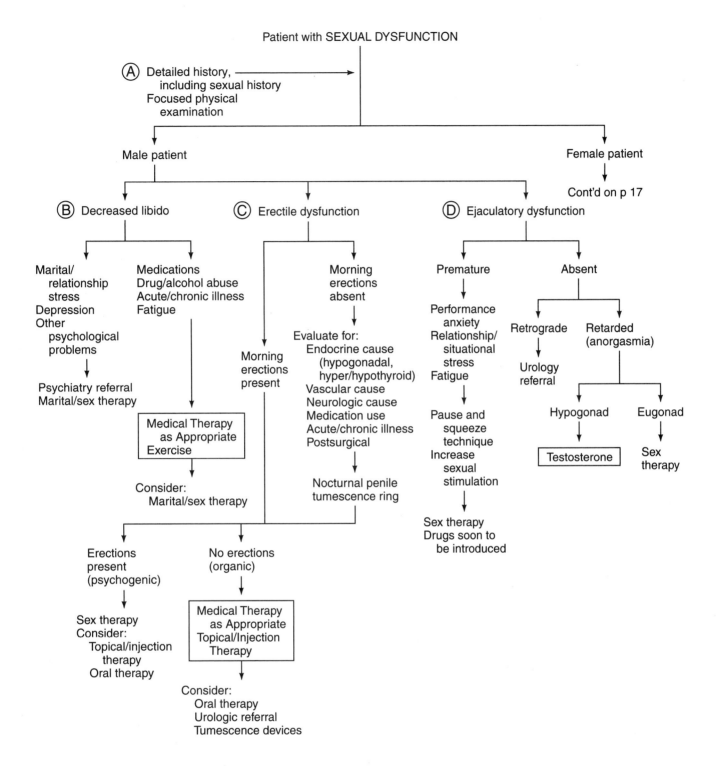

A Detailed history, including sexual history Focused physical examination

Male patient

Female patient

Cont'd on p 17

B Decreased libido

C Erectile dysfunction

D Ejaculatory dysfunction

Marital/ relationship stress
Depression
Other psychological problems

↓

Psychiatry referral
Marital/sex therapy

Medications
Drug/alcohol abuse
Acute/chronic illness
Fatigue

Medical Therapy as Appropriate Exercise

Consider:
Marital/sex therapy

Morning erections present

Morning erections absent

↓

Evaluate for:
Endocrine cause (hypogonadal, hyper/hypothyroid)
Vascular cause
Neurologic cause
Medication use
Acute/chronic illness
Postsurgical

↓

Nocturnal penile tumescence ring

Premature

↓

Performance anxiety
Relationship/ situational stress
Fatigue

↓

Pause and squeeze technique
Increase sexual stimulation

↓

Sex therapy
Drugs soon to be introduced

Absent

Retrograde

Retarded (anorgasmia)

Urology referral

Hypogonad

Eugonad

Testosterone

Sex therapy

Erections present (psychogenic)

Sex therapy
Consider:
Topical/injection therapy
Oral therapy

No erections (organic)

Medical Therapy as Appropriate Topical/Injection Therapy

Consider:
Oral therapy
Urologic referral
Tumescence devices

E. Hypoactive sexual desire in women, as in men, can be associated with medications, substance abuse, and illness. It can also accompany menopause, natural or surgical. Appropriate hormone replacement therapy (HRT) can improve sexual desire, especially if lack of desire is related to dyspareunia (painful intercourse) from inadequate lubrication. Women who have been oophorectomized may also benefit from androgen replacement at low dosages. Depression, difficulties with body image, and the maternal role also can decrease female desire. Fatigue can be reduced with the addition of regular exercise (often accompanied by an increase in sexual desire). A history of sexual abuse or domestic violence may present as hypoactive sexual desire and avoidance of sexual contact. Depression can be treated medically, although many antidepressants have decreased sexual desire as a side effect. Psychiatric referral is appropriate for all women with a history of sexual abuse.

F. Anorgasmia is much more common in women than in men. Often it is a combination of inhibition relating to sex itself and a lack of knowledge about female sexual arousal. Education about anatomy and encouragement to use self-stimulation coupled with erotic materials often enhance a woman's sexual experience. Sex therapy can also be used in these cases.

G. Dyspareunia is a common sexual complaint of women. It is important to distinguish between insertional (just before or during penile penetration) and deep thrust dyspareunia. Insertional pain has a number of easily reversed causes such as vulvovaginitis, urethritis, and inadequate lubrication. Treatment with antibiotics when indicated and HRT (topical, transdermal, or oral) in perimenopausal or postmenopausal women can eliminate the problem. Vulvar dystrophies, vulvar vestibulitis, and urethral syndrome require gynecologic referral. Most causes of deep thrust dyspareunia require gynecologic evaluation. Pelvic inflammatory disease can be treated with antibiotics. Atrophic vaginitis and inadequate lubrication often respond to HRT.

H. Vaginismus is a severe type of insertional dyspareunia. The patient complains of inability to achieve penetration—she may be unable to insert a tampon or tolerate a speculum examination—secondary to involuntary muscle contraction. If there is no history of sexual abuse, it may be related to fear and inhibition surrounding sex. Education about anatomy and sexual response, coupled with insertion of progressively larger vaginal dilators, may allow receptive penetration. Sex therapy and/or psychiatric evaluation also may be required. A history of sexual abuse demands psychiatric referral.

References

Bachmann GA, Ayers CA. Psychosexual gynecology. Med Clin North Am 1995; 79:1299.

O'Keefe M, Hunt DK. Assessment and treatment of impotence. Med Clin North Am 1995; 79:415.

Skolnick A. Guidelines for treating erectile dysfunction issued. JAMA 1997; 277(1):7.

Steege JF, Ling FW. Dyspareunia. Obstet Gynecol Clin North Am 1993; 20:779.

Female patient with SEXUAL DYSFUNCTION
(Cont'd from p 15)

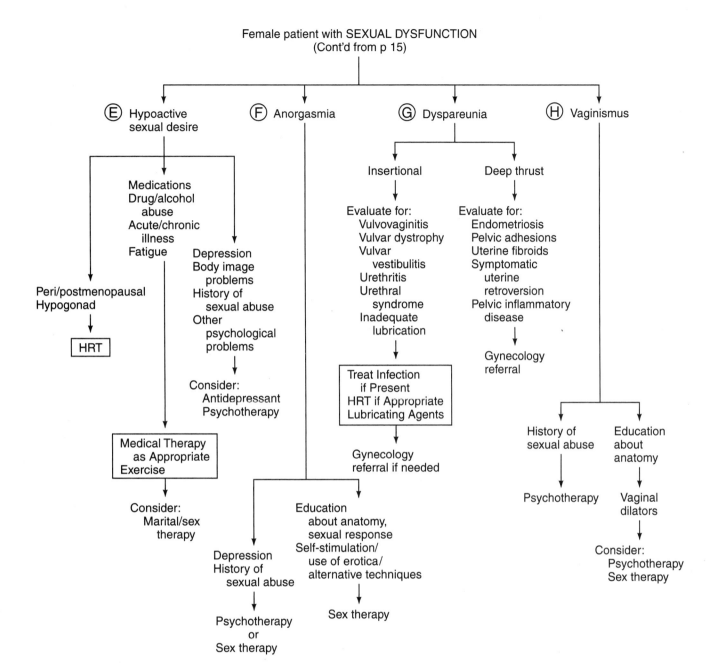

Ⓔ Hypoactive sexual desire

Ⓕ Anorgasmia

Ⓖ Dyspareunia

Ⓗ Vaginismus

Medications
Drug/alcohol
abuse
Acute/chronic
illness
Fatigue

Depression
Body image
problems
History of
sexual abuse
Other
psychological
problems

Peri/postmenopausal
Hypogonad

HRT

Consider:
Antidepressant
Psychotherapy

Medical Therapy
as Appropriate
Exercise

Consider:
Marital/sex
therapy

Depression
History of
sexual abuse

Psychotherapy
or
Sex therapy

Education
about anatomy,
sexual response
Self-stimulation/
use of erotica/
alternative techniques

Sex therapy

Insertional

Deep thrust

Evaluate for:
Vulvovaginitis
Vulvar dystrophy
Vulvar
vestibulitis
Urethritis
Urethral
syndrome
Inadequate
lubrication

Evaluate for:
Endometriosis
Pelvic adhesions
Uterine fibroids
Symptomatic
uterine
retroversion
Pelvic inflammatory
disease

Gynecology
referral

Treat Infection
if Present
HRT if Appropriate
Lubricating Agents

Gynecology
referral if needed

History of
sexual abuse

Education
about
anatomy

Psychotherapy

Vaginal
dilators

Consider:
Psychotherapy
Sex therapy

17

EDEMA

David W. Gibson
Harry L. Greene II

Edema is an abnormal collection of fluid in the interstitial space that may be localized or generalized. Fluid movement between the intra- and extravascular space is related to the interacting forces of hydrostatic pressure, colloid oncotic pressure, and capillary permeability, as well as to the effects of lymphatic drainage. Normally, there exists an equilibrium among these forces, and no net fluid accumulation takes place. Edema occurs when there is a decrease in plasma oncotic pressure, an increase in hydrostatic pressure, an increase in capillary permeability, or a combination of these factors. Edema also can be present when lymphatic flow is obstructed.

A. The history and physical examination focus on the causes of edema and seek to ascertain whether it is generalized or localized.

B. Generalized edema can be documented by weight gain and often is associated with increased capillary hydrostatic pressure as seen in congestive heart failure (CHF), in renal failure with increased sodium and water load, after expansion of the intravascular volume from IV fluids, or in conditions of sodium retention. Edema may occur after corticosteroid therapy or with estrogens or other medications. Edema involving the whole body (e.g., anasarca) may extend to involve the peritoneal cavity (e.g., ascites) or the pleural space (e.g., hydrothorax). In patients with generalized edema the first step is to estimate central venous pressure by determining jugular venous pressure (JVP). The distance from the manubrium sterni to the fluid meniscus in the jugular vein should be ≤2 cm at 45° or 5 cm from the left atrium.

C. Determine serum albumin and urinary protein in patients with generalized edema and normal JVP.

D. If serum albumin is normal, perform urinalysis, looking for abnormal urinary sediment, and check BUN and creatinine to evaluate the possibility of renal pathology. If urinalysis findings are normal, order thyroid function tests (TFTs) to look for myxedema. Remaining patients should be considered as possibly having idiopathic edema or drug-induced edema.

E. If serum albumin is decreased, perform urinalysis to check for proteinuria. More than 3.5 g protein suggests nephrotic syndrome; <3.5 g in a normal urinalysis suggests another cause, such as hepatitis or hepatic infiltration disease. Order liver function tests (LFTs); if results are abnormal, evaluate for liver pathology. If LFT results are normal, check prealbumin and cholesterol to evaluate for malnutrition. If the prealbumin is <20 mg/dl and the cholesterol level is low, malnutrition is suggested. If the prealbumin is >20 mg/dl, a capillary leak, abnormal protein synthesis, and protein-losing enteropathy are all possibilities.

F. In patients with an elevated JVP and generalized edema, order chest radiographs to look for cardiomegaly.

G. If cardiomegaly is found, order an echocardiogram to look for pericardial effusion; pericardial thickening, as in acute or chronic pericarditis; abnormal contractility of the heart, as might be seen in CHF; or signs of infiltrative cardiac problems, such as hypertrophic obstructive cardiomyopathy, amyloid, or neoplasm.

H. If cardiac size is normal on the chest film, evaluate the lung fields for pulmonary hypertension. Such a finding should lead to evaluation for cor pulmonale. Clear lung fields should prompt echocardiography to seek pericardial constriction.

I. Regional edema or localized edema often is caused by increased capillary pressure. Some causes include chronic venous insufficiency; incompetent venous valves; vascular obstructions, either extrinsic because of neoplasm, lymph nodes, surgery, fibrosis, or radiation, or intrinsic because of deep venous thrombosis, surgery, infection, immobility, trauma, or a hypercoagulable state (e.g., protein C deficiency, protein S deficiency, antithrombin 3 deficiency, the presence of neoplasms, or secondary to the venodilating effects of drugs such as calcium channel blockers).

(Continued on page 20)

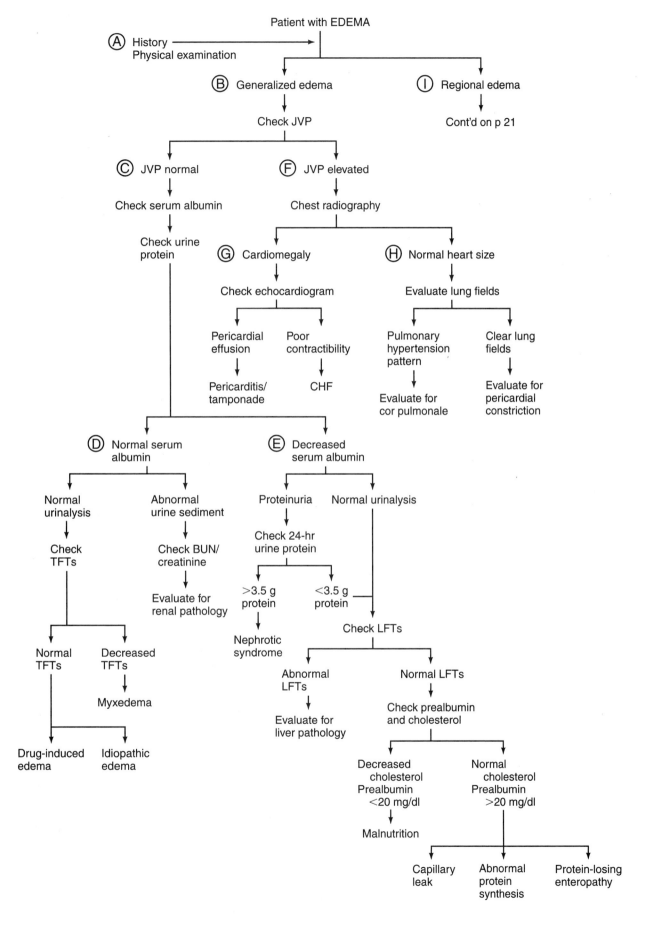

Patient with EDEMA

(A) History
Physical examination

(B) Generalized edema

Check JVP

(C) JVP normal

Check serum albumin

Check urine protein

(F) JVP elevated

Chest radiography

(G) Cardiomegaly

Check echocardiogram

Pericardial effusion → Pericarditis/tamponade

Poor contractibility → CHF

(H) Normal heart size

Evaluate lung fields

Pulmonary hypertension pattern → Evaluate for cor pulmonale

Clear lung fields → Evaluate for pericardial constriction

(I) Regional edema

Cont'd on p 21

(D) Normal serum albumin

Normal urinalysis → Check TFTs

Normal TFTs

Decreased TFTs → Myxedema

Drug-induced edema

Idiopathic edema

Abnormal urine sediment → Check BUN/creatinine → Evaluate for renal pathology

(E) Decreased serum albumin

Proteinuria → Check 24-hr urine protein

>3.5 g protein → Nephrotic syndrome

<3.5 g protein

Normal urinalysis

Check LFTs

Abnormal LFTs → Evaluate for liver pathology

Normal LFTs → Check prealbumin and cholesterol

Decreased cholesterol Prealbumin <20 mg/dl → Malnutrition

Normal cholesterol Prealbumin >20 mg/dl

Capillary leak

Abnormal protein synthesis

Protein-losing enteropathy

J. When regional edema is present, note its location. If it is in one or both upper extremities, determine JVP.

K. Patients with upper extremity edema and normal JVP should undergo a Doppler study, impedance plethysmography (IPG), or venography to look for venous obstruction from either intrinsic or extrinsic causes with a negative study for lymphatic obstruction.

L. Evaluate patients with upper extremity edema and elevated JVP for superior vena cava syndrome with a chest radiograph, CT scan, or MRI of the chest.

M. If the regional edema is confined to the lower extremities, note whether it is unilateral or bilateral. Seek historical features specifically directed toward trauma, a hypercoagulable state, history of neoplasm, or conditions that might cause lymphatic or venous obstruction.

N. If the history is negative, order a Doppler study or IPG. If this study is positive, venography may be indicated to evaluate venous thrombosis versus extrinsic compression. If the Doppler study is negative, rhabdomyolysis, musculoskeletal edema, or localized vascular defects may be present.

O. Patients with a positive history of lower extremity edema should undergo IPG, Doppler study, or venography of the lower extremity. Again, a positive study may suggest venous thrombosis, with treatment for this. A negative study may suggest lymphatic obstruction. This can be evaluated with lymphangiography.

References

Berczeller PH. Idiopathic edema. Hosp Pract (Off Ed) 1994; 29:115.

Braunwald E. Edema. In: Fauci AS, Braunwald E, Isselbacher KJ, et al, eds. Harrison's principles of internal medicine. 14th ed. New York: McGraw-Hill, 1997:210.

Ciocon JO, Fernandez BB, Ciocon DG. Leg edema: clinical clues to the differential diagnosis. Geriatrics 1993; 48:34.

Goroll AH, May LA, Mulley AG. Primary care medicine. 3rd ed. Philadelphia: Lippincott-Raven, 1995:105.

Greene HL, Kreis SR, Kahn KL. Edema. In: Greene HL, ed. Clinical medicine. 2nd ed. St. Louis: Mosby, 1996:138.

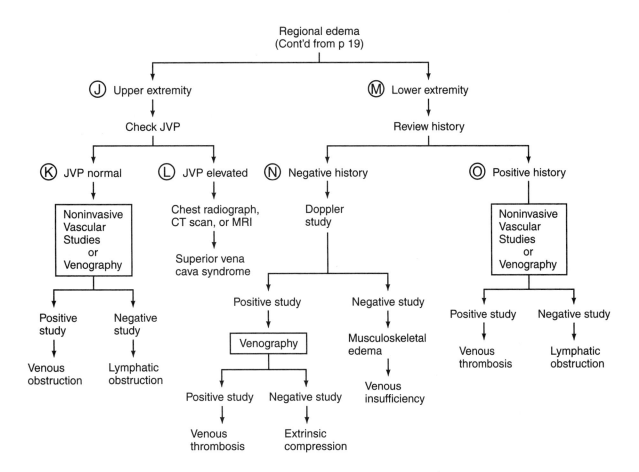

Regional edema
(Cont'd from p 19)

Ⓙ Upper extremity

Check JVP

Ⓚ JVP normal

Noninvasive
Vascular
Studies
or
Venography

Positive
study

Negative
study

Venous
obstruction

Lymphatic
obstruction

Ⓛ JVP elevated

Chest radiograph,
CT scan, or MRI

Superior vena
cava syndrome

Ⓜ Lower extremity

Review history

Ⓝ Negative history

Doppler
study

Positive study

Venography

Positive study

Venous
thrombosis

Negative study

Extrinsic
compression

Negative study

Musculoskeletal
edema

Venous
insufficiency

Ⓞ Positive history

Noninvasive
Vascular
Studies
or
Venography

Positive study

Venous
thrombosis

Negative study

Lymphatic
obstruction

CHRONIC PAIN

William P. Johnson

A. The information needed to evaluate the patient includes a detailed history of the pain complaint(s), an understanding of pain characteristics, response to past treatments, a thorough understanding of the patient's history (i.e., a review of the often voluminous medical records and psychosocial history), and the temporal relationship of all these factors to the onset and exacerbation of pain.

B. Acute pain often is associated with an increase in circulation, ventilation, and metabolism and a decrease in urinary and GI function. Patients are in obvious pain, and often there are associated findings of pallor, diaphoresis, and nausea.

C. Chronic pain is defined as any pain continuing beyond the usual course of an acute injury process. It can be dangerous to place an arbitrary time limit, such as 6 months, on this definition. For example, the pain of a broken wrist should last, at most, 2 weeks. Any continuing pain may indicate a reflex sympathetic dystrophy. This is a cause of chronic pain in which early recognition and treatment lead to complete recovery. Waiting 6 months to consider this pain chronic could leave the patient with a permanent disability. Patients with constant pain develop vegetative signs: disturbances in sleep and appetite, constipation, increased irritability, decreased libido, psychomotor retardation, and lowered pain tolerance. Patients with intermittent chronic pain (e.g., those with recurrent bouts of neuralgia, headaches, or angina) may have responses similar to those with acute pain.

D. Chronic benign pain is a diagnostic and management challenge. If possible, it sometimes is useful to localize the pain to the target organ most affected.

E. Some patients do not fit nicely into any of the usual chronic benign pain subcategories. The approach to this group of patients needs to be individualized.

F. All chronic pain patients go through proven psychological changes while coping with their pain. Psychological and environmental factors play a great role in chronic pain, with 30% of patients becoming clinically depressed. However, psychogenic pain occurs when the pain is a result of psychological mechanisms. The fact that a physician cannot find a specific organic cause for the pain is insufficient, by itself, to warrant a psychiatric diagnosis. Positive evidence for a psychiatric diagnosis must be found. (DSM-IV criteria should be applied.)

G. A multidisciplinary pain center (MPC) should have on its staff a variety of health care providers capable of assessing and treating physical, psychosocial, medical, vocational, and social aspects of chronic pain. A multidisciplinary pain team may include an internist, psychiatrist, physiatrist, pharmacist, anesthesiologist, neurosurgeon, nurse, dentist, psychologist, physical therapist, and occupational therapist. At least three medical specialties should be represented on the staff of an MPC. If one of the physicians is not a psychiatrist, physicians from two specialties and a clinical psychologist are the minimum required. The MPC may exist in either an inpatient or outpatient setting. An MPC should establish protocols for patient management and assess their efficiency periodically. With benign pain the emphasis should be on pain management and rehabilitation, with little or no use of controlled medications.

H. Effective pain management requires consistent strategies: (1) establishing treatment goals in terms of outcomes with a definite timeline, (2) regularly scheduling follow-up appointments, (3) establishing medication refill guidelines, and (4) establishing patient behavior guidelines.

I. This group of patients may cause licensing and legal headaches unless certain guidelines are followed:
- Do an initial comprehensive clinical examination, which results in an explicit working diagnosis.
- Call the last treating physician and discuss the case.
- Review all outside records.
- Establish a written treatment plan with recorded measurable objectives.
- If habituating medications are used, informed consent must be given, making explicit the material risks of treatment, including alternative treatments, treatment side effects and potential interactions, risk of tolerance, how to withdraw treatment, risk of addiction, and risk of impaired judgement.
- Review current treatment and modify as indicated.
- Consult as indicated.
- Be comprehensive and compulsive in record keeping.

References

Bonica JJ, ed. The management of pain. 2nd ed. Philadelphia: Lea & Febiger, 1990.

Godfrey RG. A guide to the understanding and use of tricyclic antidepressants in the overall management of fibromyalgia and other chronic pain syndromes. Arch Intern Med 1996; 156:1047.

Levy MH. Pharmacologic treatment of cancer pain. N Engl J Med 1996; 335:1124.

Vasudevan SV, Lynch NT. Pain centers: organization and outcome. In: Rehabilitation medicine—adding life to years (special issue). West J Med 1991; 154:532.

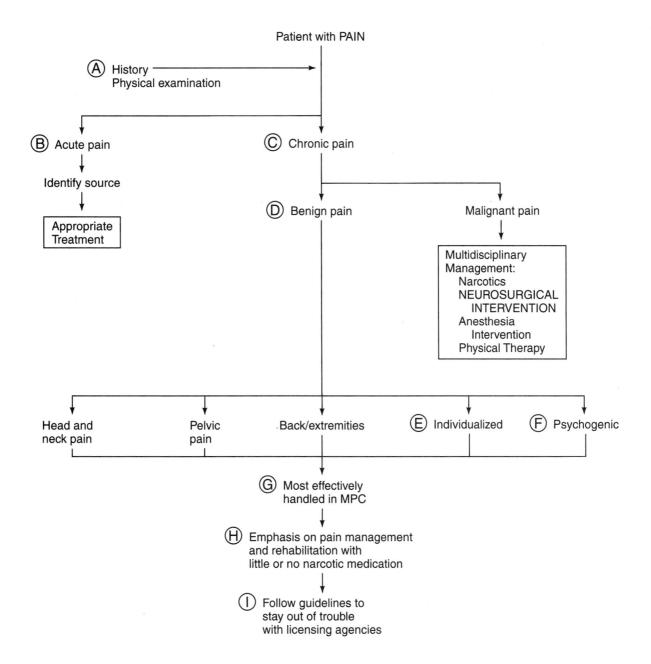

Patient with PAIN

Ⓐ History
Physical examination

Ⓑ Acute pain

Identify source

Appropriate
Treatment

Ⓒ Chronic pain

Ⓓ Benign pain

Malignant pain

Multidisciplinary
Management:
　Narcotics
　NEUROSURGICAL
　　INTERVENTION
　Anesthesia
　　Intervention
　Physical Therapy

Head and
neck pain

Pelvic
pain

Back/extremities

Ⓔ Individualized

Ⓕ Psychogenic

Ⓖ Most effectively
handled in MPC

Ⓗ Emphasis on pain management
and rehabilitation with
little or no narcotic medication

Ⓘ Follow guidelines to
stay out of trouble
with licensing agencies

PERSISTENT EXCESSIVE SWEATING

Lisa Kaufmann

A. Several dermatologic conditions are associated with localized hyperhidrosis: increased sweating in areas of vitiligo, granulosis, rubra nasi, dyshidrotic eczema, pachydermoperiostosis, epidermolysis, bullosa, pachyonychia congenita, nail-patella syndrome, palmoplantar keratodermas, and others. These conditions should be detectable on physical examination.

B. Although anxiety or stimulants may increase sweating, some people have severe hyperhidrosis without an obvious psychiatric disorder. Such patients often have a family history of hyperhidrosis. Severe hyperhidrosis may cause difficulty with hand work, infection caused by the moist environment (especially in the feet), and considerable social distress. Topical treatments have varying success. Removal of the axillary sweat glands or sympathectomy have been reported to give good results in severe cases (see references).

C. A structural lesion in the sympathetic nervous system may cause abnormalities in sweating. Cerebrocortical tumors, stroke, or infection may cause contralateral hyperhidrosis through release of inhibition. When injured sympathetic nerves regrow, connections may develop between the parasympathetic and sympathetic nerves. This can result in sweating of the innervated skin, as seen with gustatory sweating. Spinal cord disease (including syringomyelia, spinal cord injury, tabes dorsalis) may cause segmental areas of hyperhidrosis. Thoracic sympathetic nerve trunk injury may also cause localized hyperhidrosis. A large area of anhidrosis, as in severe diabetic autonomic neuropathy or after a sympathectomy involving more than one limb, may result in compensatory hyperhidrosis of other areas.

D. Many chemicals may cause sweating, either during withdrawal states (as from alcohol or opiates) or with use (e.g., alcohol, some tricyclic antidepressants, cholinergic and adrenergic agents, and acetylcholinesterase inhibitors). Chronic ingestion of mercury or arsenic can cause excessive sweating.

E. Malaria, tuberculosis, brucellosis, abdominal abscesses, rheumatic fever, and endocarditis are commonly seen with fevers and sweats as the predominant symptoms, but any infection producing a fever may cause sweating through the hypothalamic temperature regulatory centers as the fever falls. Even after a severe febrile illness resolves, patients may continue to have sweats for days to months.

F. Certain malignant conditions, including lymphoma, monocytic leukemia, and renal carcinoma, classically cause fevers, but fever with associated sweats also may be found in other malignancies. Carcinoid syndrome may cause excessive sweating. Rheumatologic diseases associated with excessive sweating include rheumatoid arthritis and Raynaud's phenomenon.

G. Other endocrine causes of hyperhidrosis include menopause, pregnancy, diabetes mellitus, gout, obesity, porphyria, rickets, and hyperpituitarism. In some cases of hypoglycemia, CNS dysfunction and sweats may occur in the absence of other adrenergic symptoms.

References

Champion RH. Disorders of the sweat glands. In: Champion RH, Burton JL, Ebling FJG, eds. Rook/Wilkinson/Ebling textbook of dermatology. London: Blackwell Scientific, 1992:1745.

Drott C, Göthberg G, Clae G. Endoscopic transthoracic sympathectomy: an efficient and safe method for the treatment of hyperhidrosis. J Am Acad Dermatol 1995; 33:78.

Herbst F, Plas EG, Függer R, Fritsch A. Endoscopic thoracic sympathectomy for primary hyperhidrosis of the upper limbs: a critical analysis and long-term results of 480 operations. Ann Surg 1994; 220:86.

Hurley HJ. The eccrine sweat glands. In: Moschella SC, Hurley HJ, eds. Dermatology. Philadelphia: WB Saunders, 1985:1341.

Patient with PERSISTENT EXCESSIVE SWEATING

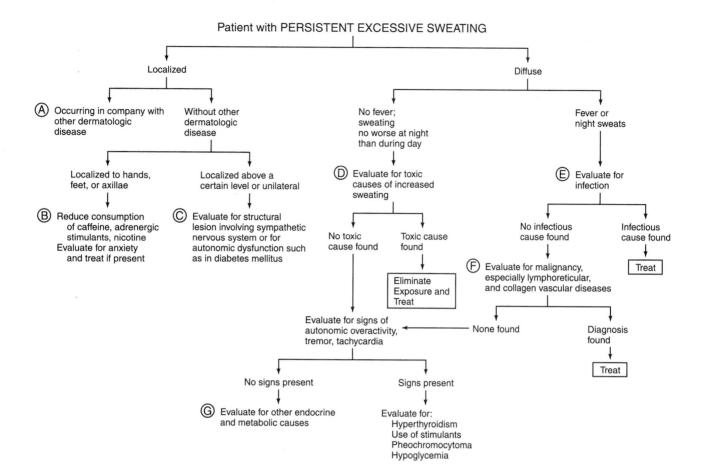

Localized

Ⓐ Occurring in company with other dermatologic disease

Without other dermatologic disease

Localized to hands, feet, or axillae

Ⓑ Reduce consumption of caffeine, adrenergic stimulants, nicotine
Evaluate for anxiety and treat if present

Localized above a certain level or unilateral

Ⓒ Evaluate for structural lesion involving sympathetic nervous system or for autonomic dysfunction such as in diabetes mellitus

Diffuse

No fever; sweating no worse at night than during day

Ⓓ Evaluate for toxic causes of increased sweating

No toxic cause found

Toxic cause found

Eliminate Exposure and Treat

Evaluate for signs of autonomic overactivity, tremor, tachycardia

No signs present

Ⓖ Evaluate for other endocrine and metabolic causes

Signs present

Evaluate for:
Hyperthyroidism
Use of stimulants
Pheochromocytoma
Hypoglycemia

Fever or night sweats

Ⓔ Evaluate for infection

No infectious cause found

Infectious cause found

Treat

Ⓕ Evaluate for malignancy, especially lymphoreticular, and collagen vascular diseases

None found

Diagnosis found

Treat

THE RED EYE

Shari Carney
Robert W. Weisenthal

Many patients present with a red eye to an emergency room or their primary care physician instead of an ophthalmologist. It is important to determine which cases need referral and which cases can be managed by the primary care physician. A thorough ocular and systemic history is extremely helpful in making this decision. Key questions include loss of vision, presence of deep versus superficial pain, trauma, history of angle closure glaucoma, uveitis or systemic illness, and recent ocular history such as surgery. Physical examination also is important. It is essential in all patients with ocular complaints to check visual acuity. Many patients with tearing or discharge note blurred vision, but they can improve it by blinking. If patients have forgotten their glasses, using a pinhole to check vision will compensate for uncorrected refractive error. Patients with deep pain, truly decreased vision, severe perilimbal injection, corneal opacification, and recent ocular surgery all need ophthalmology evaluation. See decision tree for details on timing.

A. Orbital cellulitis presents with lid erythema, proptosis, and restricted eye movements. The lid may look ptotic (pseudoptosis) secondary to the swelling. The patient also may give a history of sinusitis. In children orbital cellulitis may easily spread from preseptal cellulitis. These patients need to be admitted for IV antibiotics. Some patients may have a real ptosis and a red eye. The examiner needs to look further for cranial nerve palsies. Orbital congestion secondary to a cavernous sinus thrombosis will present with a red, congested eye and an isolated or combined III, IV, V, or VI nerve palsy. A VII nerve palsy may cause a red eye secondary to exposure.

B. A history of thyroid abnormalities, lid retraction, proptosis, and injection over the rectus muscles may indicate Graves' orbitopathy. These patients require a thyroid work-up and an ophthalmic evaluation to determine optic nerve involvement on a semi-urgent basis.

C. Scleritis presents as a severe, deep pain similar to a toothache. If left undiagnosed and untreated, it can have significant visual morbidity. The globe is tender to touch. The sclera appears violaceous in sunlight because of involvement of the sclera as compared with the superficial vessels overlying it. The redness may be either focal or diffuse. It often is associated with systemic immunologic disease. Semi-urgent referral is required.

(Continued on page 28)

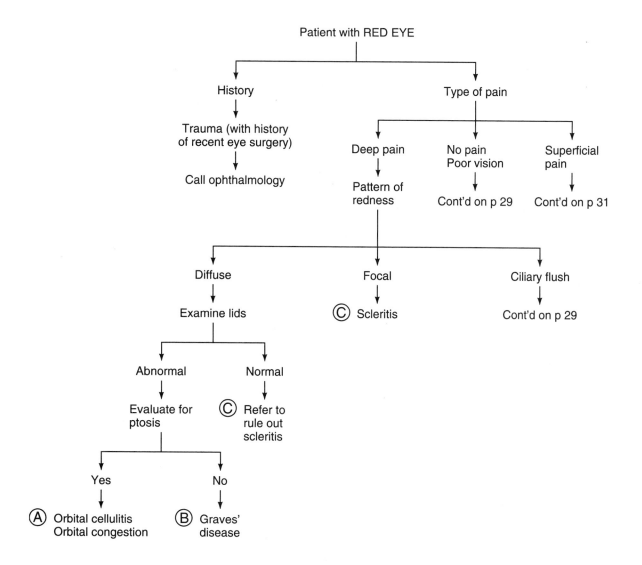

Patient with RED EYE

History
↓
Trauma (with history
of recent eye surgery)
↓
Call ophthalmology

Type of pain

Deep pain
↓
Pattern of
redness

No pain
Poor vision
↓
Cont'd on p 29

Superficial
pain
↓
Cont'd on p 31

Diffuse
↓
Examine lids

Focal
↓
Ⓒ Scleritis

Ciliary flush
↓
Cont'd on p 29

Abnormal
↓
Evaluate for
ptosis

Normal
↓
Ⓒ Refer to
rule out
scleritis

Yes
↓
Ⓐ Orbital cellulitis
Orbital congestion

No
↓
Ⓑ Graves'
disease

D. Acute angle closure glaucoma presents with a red eye, decreased vision, eye pain, headache, a mid-dilated pupil, and corneal edema. The patient may be able to give a history of prior episodes. Immediate (within 1–2 hours) referral to an ophthalmologist is indicated.

E. If the patient has injection primarily around the cornea (ciliary flush), decreased vision, and a small pupil compared with the contralateral eye, the patient may have a anterior uveitis (iritis). Inquire about other systemic symptoms such as arthritis, back pain, and coexisting medical conditions such as ulcerative colitis. These patients need referral for proper diagnosis and treatment on a semi-urgent basis (within 24 hours).

F. If the cornea has a white opacity, the patient may have a corneal ulcer, which should be referred to an ophthalmologist urgently for cultures and intensive treatment. Herpes simplex keratits also may present with a dendritic figure that will highlight with fluorescein, with an underlying clear cornea.

G. A hypopyon is layered WBCs in the anterior chamber and may indicate an infection throughout the eye (endopththalmitis) or may be secondary to a corneal ulcer. The patient may give a history of recent ophthalmic surgery or trauma. This requires immediate referral for cultures and proper treatment.

H. It is essential to examine the anterior chamber in a patient with a red eye. Layered blood in the anterior chamber (hyphema) may also be associated with a flat or shallow anterior chamber, a possible sign of a ruptured globe, requiring immediate referral. A hyphema with a well-formed chamber and no other signs of a ruptured globe should be referred that day.

I. A patient with a red eye, decreased vision, and no other obvious signs may have a retinitis, vitritis, or posterior scleritis. These are rare causes of a red eye. Refer these patients to an ophthalmologist on a semi-urgent basis.

(Continued on page 30)

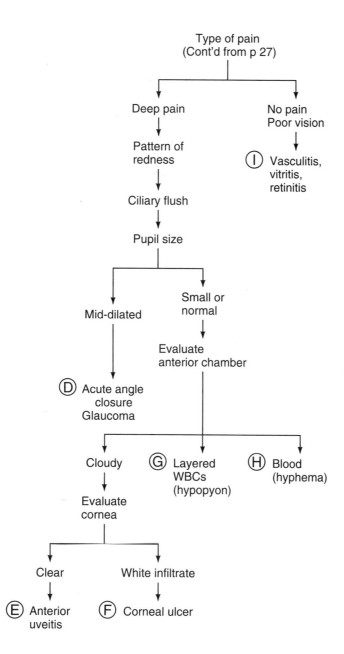

Type of pain
(Cont'd from p 27)

Deep pain

No pain
Poor vision

Pattern of
redness

Ⓘ Vasculitis,
vitritis,
retinitis

Ciliary flush

Pupil size

Mid-dilated

Small or
normal

Evaluate
anterior chamber

Ⓓ Acute angle
closure
Glaucoma

Cloudy

Ⓖ Layered
WBCs
(hypopyon)

Ⓗ Blood
(hyphema)

Evaluate
cornea

Clear

White infiltrate

Ⓔ Anterior
uveitis

Ⓕ Corneal ulcer

J. If the patient was working with metal or wood, inspect the eye for a foreign body. Irrigating the eye with normal saline may help remove a foreign body. Removal of a conjunctival foreign body may be attempted by rolling a cotton swab over it. An embedded corneal foreign body, which does not irrigate out, should be referred to an ophthalmologist within 24 hours for removal. Start the patient on topical antibiotics to prevent infection. If there is a residual rust ring, the patient should follow up with an ophthalmologist in 24–48 hours for removal. If the vision is significantly decreased or there is a question of a globe laceration from the foreign body, urgent referral is necessary.

K. Exposure to chemicals warrants immediate copious saline irrigation (500 ml). If the chemical injury is mild and characterized by mild injection without fluorescein uptake, start topical antibiotics and follow up in 1–2 days. If the chemical injury is severe with corneal clouding and loss of conjunctival blood vessels (porcelain sclera), the patient should be seen by an ophthalmologist immediately.

L. Corneal abrasions present with a severe foreign body sensation, and on Wood's lamp examination show fluorescein uptake in an otherwise clear cornea. Treatment consists of topical antibiotic ointment and patching. Recheck these patients in 24 hours, and if not dramatically improved, refer them to an ophthalmologist.

M. Blepharitis is an inflammation of the eyelids characterized by redness of the eyelids, crusting, and foreign body sensation. The treatment is warm compresses and lid hygiene. Acne rosacea can cause a secondary blepharitis, which should be treated with oral tetracycline or doxycycline. A hordeolum (stye) or chalazion should also be treated with warm compresses and topical antibiotic ointment. Chalazia need to be incised and drained only if they do not respond to a 2-week course of medical therapy.

N. The most common cause of conjunctivitis is a viral infection. The eyes are diffusely red with a watery discharge. Many patients have a preauricular lymph node on the affected side. Treatment is palliative; cool compresses and astringent drops are used because the condition is self-limited. The patient should follow up on a routine basis if the condition does not resolve in 1 week to 10 days.

O. Allergic conjunctivitis is typically seasonal and always presents with itching and occasionally with mild foreign body sensation. Topical antihistamine drops relieve the symptoms. Follow-up is indicated only if symptomatic treatment is ineffective.

P. Bacterial conjunctivitis comprises <5% of all conjunctivitis. Sight-threatening disease can occur with a virulent bacterial species such as gonococcus. Usually the onset is hyperacute (<24 hours) with a fulminant mucopurulent discharge and requires urgent work-up with cultures/gram stain. *Streptococcus pneumoniae, Haemophilus influenzae,* and *Chlamydia* are other common pathogens and present as a less purulent conjunctivitis. The appropriate topical and, in severe cases, systemic antibiotic is based on results of the Gram stain/culture. Initially, use a broad-spectrum antibiotic, altering therapy according to culture results if the conjunctivitis does not respond to initial therapy. Patients who develop corneal or scleral thinning require urgent referral to an ophthalmologist.

Q. Nonspecific conjunctivitis results from mild inflammation of the ocular surface and can be treated with a topical antihistamine or mild topical antibiotic.

R. A pterygium is a fibrovascular growth that extends onto the nasal portion of the cornea. It can sometimes become inflamed or may grow slowly over the pupil (taking months to years). If it extends into the central cornea, reducing the patient's vision, excision is necessary. Pingueculae are degenerative lesions of the bulbar conjunctiva that do not extend onto the cornea. They occur secondary to actinic exposure. They usually are nasal in location and are yellow-white in appearance. They are benign. If they become inflamed, artificial tears are helpful. Routine follow-up is indicated only if symptoms persist.

S. A subconjunctival hemorrhage consists of blood trapped under the conjunctiva. It can occur with any injury to the globe or with Valsalva's maneuvers. It usually is benign; however, a history of trauma with a flat anterior chamber requires an ophthalmic evaluation on an urgent basis. If a patient has recurring subconjunctival hemorrhage with no known cause, a work-up for a hematologic disorder is indicated. Episcleritis is localized inflammation of the episcleral blood vessels that responds to topical steroids. Be certain that the patient does not have herpetic keratitis before starting treatment.

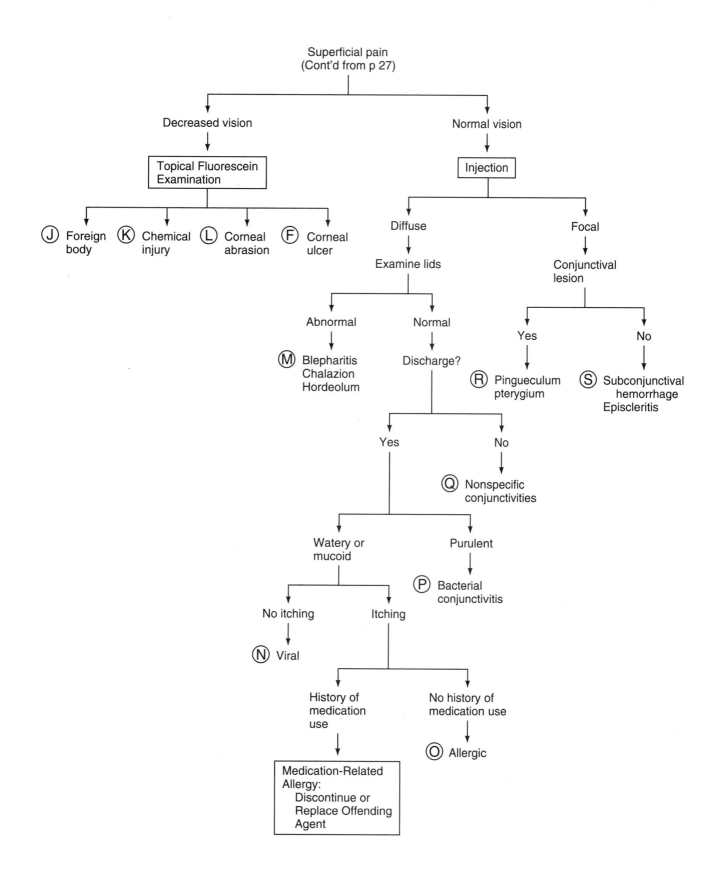

Superficial pain
(Cont'd from p 27)

Decreased vision

Topical Fluorescein Examination

Ⓙ Foreign body Ⓚ Chemical injury Ⓛ Corneal abrasion Ⓕ Corneal ulcer

Normal vision

Injection

Diffuse

Examine lids

Abnormal

Ⓜ Blepharitis Chalazion Hordeolum

Normal

Discharge?

Yes

Watery or mucoid

No itching

Ⓝ Viral

Itching

History of medication use

Medication-Related Allergy: Discontinue or Replace Offending Agent

No history of medication use

Ⓞ Allergic

Purulent

Ⓟ Bacterial conjunctivitis

No

Ⓠ Nonspecific conjunctivities

Focal

Conjunctival lesion

Yes

Ⓡ Pingueculum pterygium

No

Ⓢ Subconjunctival hemorrhage Episcleritis

RHINITIS

Naomi Rappaport

Rhinitis is inflammation of the mucous membrane of the nose characterized by one or more of the following symptoms: nasal congestion, rhinorrhea, sneezing, or itching of eyes and/or nose.

A. The cause usually can be determined through a detailed history and physical examination. Assess for environmental and occupational exposures and personal and family history of allergies. Note onset of symptoms, especially age, frequency, duration, and severity of symptoms. Carefully examine conjunctiva, nares, tympanic membranes, and pharynx. Transillumination of sinuses in a completely dark room with a good light and percussion for tenderness may result in a false-positive result and is of questionable use.

B. Clues to diagnosis include acute onset; others ill at home, school, or work; and confirming physical findings. Symptomatic treatment includes hydration and a cold care kit geared toward alleviating symptoms. Cough syrup (include expectorant, suppressant, mucolytic, etc. depending on symptoms), analgesics, and/or nasal decongestant (topical or systemic) can be included. Cost-effectiveness of intranasal ipratropium has yet to be determined.

C. There are no pathognomonic features for sinusitis. It can be confused with allergic rhinitis, upper respiratory infections, dental disorders, and any other causes of facial or head pain. In one study the overall clinical impression was superior to any single historical or physical finding. Reserve imaging studies for patients who fail to respond to empiric treatment or who have an unusual presentation.

D. Of bacterial isolates, 70% are *Streptococcus pneumoniae* and *Haemophilus influenzae*. β-Lactamase producing *H. influenzae* or *Moraxella catarrhalis* are unusual in untreated adults. Of symptomatic patients, 30% have negative bacterial cultures, suggesting either viral or allergic disease. Treatment with macrolides or trimethoprim-sulfamethoxazole for 7–10 days results in symptomatic and bacteriologic improvement in 80–90% of patients. Community-acquired drug-resistant *S. pneumoniae* are emerging, and the use of amoxicillin is questionable. Treatment for 2–3 weeks may result in fewer incompletely treated patients. Topical or systemic decongestants and saline nasal spray that target the underlying ostial obstruction should be included in treatment. Consider adding mucolytic therapy. Avoid use of antihistamines; they may thicken nasal mucus and cause further obstruction.

E. Treat incomplete resolution or early relapse with an additional 7-day course of the same antibiotic, other first-line antibiotic, or second-line antibiotic like second- or third-generation cephalosporin. Then consider reassessment, imaging studies, or referral to allergist or ENT. Limited CT of the sinuses is more sensitive than conventional x-rays. However, specificity may be low because many symptomatic patients undergoing CT for other reasons have some sinus abnormalities. Recurrent sinusitis may indicate an underlying process such as allergic rhinitis causing ostial obstruction, anatomic abnormality, cystic fibrosis, or immune deficiency.

F. Fungal or other opportunistic infections can be lethal in the immunocompromised host. Use a low threshold for referral to a specialist for diagnosis and treatment.

G. Prolonged use of intranasal decongestants can result in rebound congestion. Topical or systemic steroids and saline lavage can be used while slowly withdrawing the topical decongestant. Explore reasons why patient started taking decongestants.

H. Numerous medications can cause rhinitis, including antihypertensives, methyldopa, reserpine, hydralazine, angiotensin-converting enzyme (ACE) inhibitors, α-adrenoceptor antagonists, oral contraceptives, aspirin, and other NSAIDs. Use of intranasal cocaine can also cause these symptoms.

(Continued on page 34)

Patient with RHINITIS

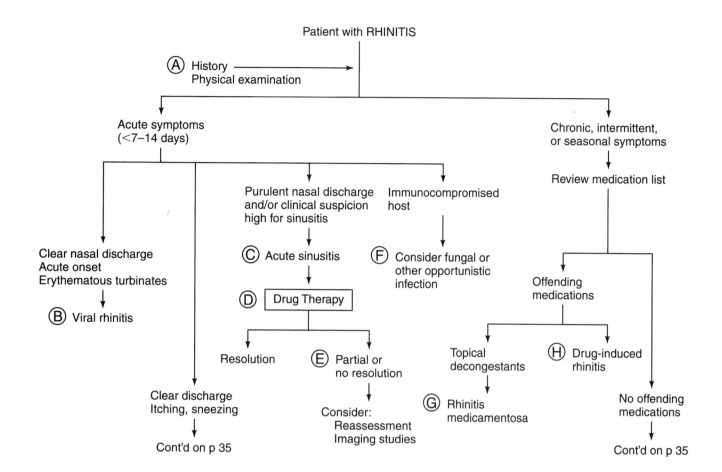

Cont'd on p 35

Cont'd on p 35

I. History of eczema and family history of allergies may help in the diagnosis. Allergen may be one or many, pollen or nonpollen, or seasonal or perennial. Physical examination may reveal violacious mucosa, boggy turbinates, allergic shiners, injected conjunctivae, and clear nasal discharge. Treatment depends on symptoms. Allergen avoidance is most important but may be impossible. Pharmacotherapy consists of antihistamines, intranasal or oral steroids, and topical or oral decongestants. In select patients with a clearly identifiable seasonal allergy, nasal cromolyn started several weeks before the appearance of the allergen may help. If medical measures fail, refer for skin testing and immunotherapy.

J. Diagnosis of occupational rhinitis is challenging because symptoms may occur 6–8 hours after exposure. With chronic exposure, symptoms may not improve on weekends and longer periods of avoidance may be needed for symptom improvement. Institute a trial of avoidance, increased ventilation and/or conventional pharmacotherapy for allergy. Use a low threshold to refer to an allergist or occupational physician.

K. Chronic sinusitis usually is secondary to an underlying cause such as allergic rhinitis, mucociliary disturbance, immune deficiency, or polyps. However, consider infection with specific organisms such as anaerobes, *Mycobacterium tuberculosis, Klebsiella rhinoscleroma, M. leprae, Treponema pallidum,* and fungal agents. Referral to a specialist may be necessary.

L. Perennial allergic rhinitis is most often caused by indoor allergens (house dust mites, animal dander, molds). Nasal blockage predominates and may present with symptoms of sinusitis or a permanent cold. Treatment consists of allergen avoidance and topical nasal steroids.

M. Idiopathic rhinitis is commonly called *vasomotor rhinitis,* which implies a cause is known. Patients complain of watery rhinorrhea or nasal obstruction after exposure to a nonspecific trigger. Triggers can include irritants such as strong odors or fumes, change in temperature, or air conditioning. Diagnosis is by exclusion. Skin testing is negative. Treatment includes patient education and symptomatic treatment.

N. Less common or rare causes of rhinitis are CSF leak in patients with unilateral rhinorrhea and a history of head trauma or surgery; nonallergic rhinitis with eosinophilia syndrome (these patients have perennial symptoms or sneezing, itching, and rhinorrhea; however, they lack evidence of allergic disease by skin testing and IgE levels); structural abnormalities (tumor, deviated septum, foreign objects); systemic disorders (defect of mucus production [cystic fibrosis or Young syndrome], ciliary dysfunction [Kartagener's syndrome or primary ciliary dyskinesia], immunodeficiency, sarcoidosis, or Wegener's granulomatosis); pregnancy; or hypothyroidism.

References

Guarderas JC. Rhinitis and sinusitis: office management. Mayo Clin Proc 1996; 71:882.

International Rhinitis Management Working Group. International consensus report on the diagnosis and management of rhinitis. Allergy 1994; 49(suppl 19):1.

Willett LR, Carson JL, Williams JW. Current diagnosis and management of sinusitis. J Gen Intern Med 1994; 9:38.

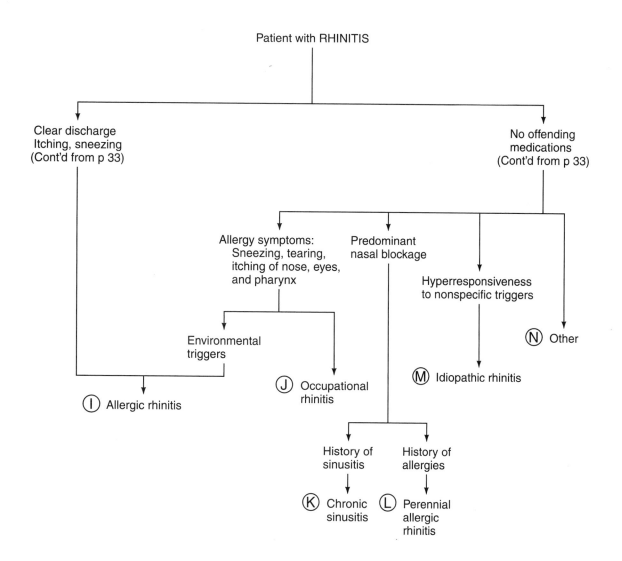

TINNITUS

Susan Fisk Sander

Tinnitus is a perceived sound that is not related to an external source. It usually is described by patients as a ringing, clicking, humming, or blowing sound. Most patients with tinnitus have an underlying otologic problem, most commonly hearing loss. It is postulated that tinnitus is the result of an imbalance between excitation and inhibition of auditory pathways. The imbalance may occur at any level, including cochlear hair cells, midbrain, and cortical central auditory pathways.

A. Diagnosing the cause of tinnitus requires a detailed history. Onset, duration, frequency, and localization are helpful in the evaluation for the underlying cause. Tinnitus may be caused by systemic disease, infection, metabolic abnormalities, medication exposure, or inflammatory conditions. Review exposure to aminoglycosides, loop-diuretics, salicylates, quinine, antimalarials, nonsteroidal anti-inflammatory drugs, and any history of toxic exposure to heavy metals with the patient.

B. The physical examination should include a check of the blood pressure, a head and neck examination, and an auscultation for vascular bruits and heart murmurs.

C. Tinnitus cerebre is a perceived sound that is diffuse and not localized to either ear. Consider encephalitis of the temporal lobe and psychiatric illnesses. Auditory hallucinations are noted primarily in patients with psychosis.

D. Tinnitus aurium is a perceived nonexternal sound that is localized to one or both ears. It occurs in vibratory (perceived by the examiner and patient) and nonvibratory (subjective) forms.

E. Subjective tinnitus is more common than objective tinnitus, but diagnosis of the underlying cause is more difficult. The differential diagnoses of subjective tinnitus are metabolic abnormalities, pathologic condition in the peripheral (cochlear) or central (retrococlear) pathways, anxiety, depression, and dental disorders. Metabolic abnormalities include hypothyroidism, hyperthyroidism, hyperlipidemia, anemia, and zinc deficiency. The initial work-up of a patient should include a CBC, fasting glucose, triglycerides, cholesterol, and thyroid-stimulating hormone. Pathologic conditions of the ear associated with subjective tinnitus include otosclerosis, chronic suppurative otitis media, Meniere's disease, presbycusis, and noise-induced hearing loss.

F. Objective tinnitus is rare. Causes include acquired and congenital vascular malformations, neuromuscular disorders (palatal myoclonus, stapedius muscle spasm, and temporomandibular disorders), intracranial tumors, and structural defects of the ear. Objective tinnitus is of two types: vascular and mechanical.

G. Pusatile tinnitus refers to nonexternal sounds that are amplified and synchronous with the patient's pulse. Benign intracranial hypertension, jugular bulb abnormalities, and aberrant carotid artery are included in the differential diagnoses. High-resolution CT of the temporal bones is needed when a retrotympanic mass is noted on examination. MRI and angiography are indicated for patients with normal otoscopic examination to evaluate for dural venous thromboses and to look for the empty sella and small ventricles associated with benign intracranial hypertension. Angiography is used when atherosclerotic carotid artery disease, fibromuscular dysplasia, and small dural arteriovenous (AV) malformations are suspected and the patient is a surgical candidate.

H. Stapedial muscle spasm–induced tinnitus is amplified with external noise and is intermittent. Stapedial muscle spasm is associated with facial nerve palsies, although it can occur without them. Division of the stapedius muscle and tensor tympani tendons is reserved for severe cases. Long-term use of benzodiazepines for stapedial muscle spasm is not recommended.

I. Palatal myoclonus is apparent on examination of the oral cavity. The tinnitus is thought to be generated from the opening and closing of the eustachian tube and the rubbing of mucosal surfaces. Electromyography (EMG) of the palatal muscles confirming the diagnosis. Treatment with benzodiazepines results in a decrease in anxiety. Surgery to modify palatal function is considered in severe cases. There have been case reports of botulinum injection into the palatal muscles with good results.

J. Tinnitus associated with patulous eustachian tube is synchronous with breathing. The patient may experience autophony (hearing of their own voice or breathing). Rapid weight loss and high estrogen states (e.g., use of birth control pills, postpartum) are associated with patulous eustachian tubes. Tympanography is diagnostic. On examination, if the patient has a reduction in his symptoms when the head is placed in a dependent position, suspect a patulous eustachian tube. Long-term therapy for patients with significant disability include applying caustics to the nasopharynx, applying irritants to the mucosa, or injecting Teflon into the eustachian tube wall.

(Continued on page 38)

Patient with TINNITUS

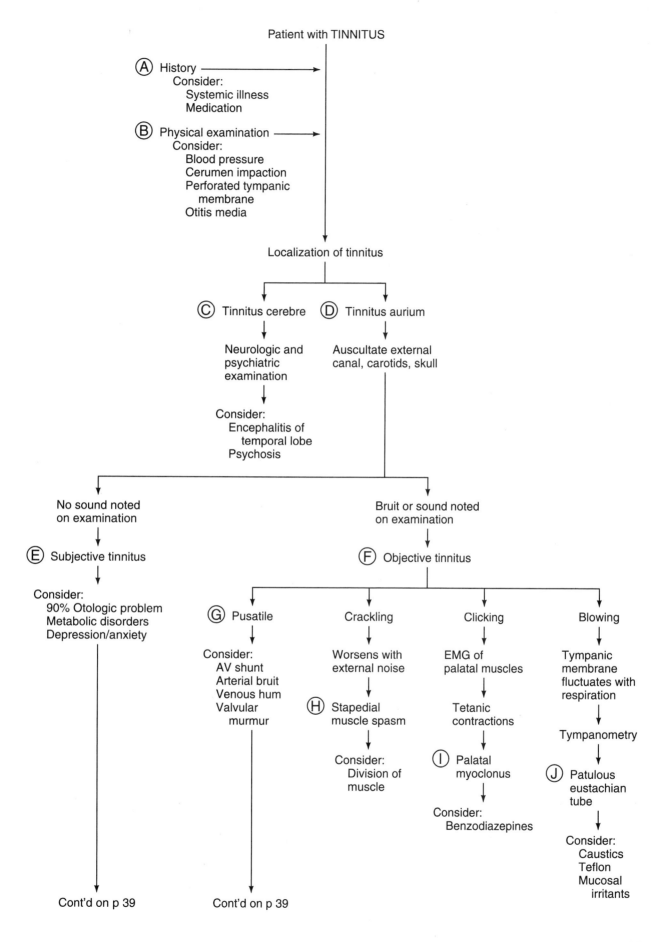

(A) History
Consider:
Systemic illness
Medication

(B) Physical examination
Consider:
Blood pressure
Cerumen impaction
Perforated tympanic
membrane
Otitis media

Localization of tinnitus

(C) Tinnitus cerebre

(D) Tinnitus aurium

Neurologic and
psychiatric
examination

Auscultate external
canal, carotids, skull

Consider:
Encephalitis of
temporal lobe
Psychosis

No sound noted
on examination

Bruit or sound noted
on examination

(E) Subjective tinnitus

(F) Objective tinnitus

Consider:
90% Otologic problem
Metabolic disorders
Depression/anxiety

(G) Pusatile

Crackling

Clicking

Blowing

Consider:
AV shunt
Arterial bruit
Venous hum
Valvular
murmur

Worsens with
external noise

EMG of
palatal muscles

Tympanic
membrane
fluctuates with
respiration

(H) Stapedial
muscle spasm

Tetanic
contractions

Tympanometry

Consider:
Division of
muscle

(I) Palatal
myoclonus

(J) Patulous
eustachian
tube

Consider:
Benzodiazepines

Consider:
Caustics
Teflon
Mucosal
irritants

Cont'd on p 39

Cont'd on p 39

K. Hearing evaluations include assessment of sensorineural hearing impedance testing, and speech discrimination. These tests assist in localizing the otologic deficit. Nonvibratory tinnitus lesions can be attributed to defects in the cochlea (75%), CNS (18%) and middle ear (4%). Peripheral tinnitus is associated with symmetric hearing loss, usually gradual in onset. Presbycusis is common with this condition. As hearing loss increases, tinnitus increases. Treating the hearing loss may result in a decrease in tinnitus because ambient background noise is amplified.

L. In patients with hearing loss that is not treatable by a surgical procedure, a hearing aid may improve the tinnitus. Hearing aids and masking devices may be used together in patients who do not respond to hearing aids alone. Medications should be given to patients with severe disability. Lidocaine injection in uncontrolled studies has a 65–80% success rate. Clinically, lidocaine is impractical because it is not oral and has a short half-life. Oral tocainide and mexilitine have not been shown to be of benefit in controlled studies. The antidepressant nortriptyline has been found to improve disability related to tinnitus and tinnitus loudness. In a controlled study, the patients who benefitted most were those with insomnia, who noted improved sleep with nortriptyline. Controlled studies of carbamazepine have shown no improvement of tinnitus compared with controls. Benzodiazepine use has long been thought to treat anxiety in patients with tinnitus. A double-blind study of alprazolam revealed improvement in tinnitus loudness (76%) compared with placebo (5%). Long-term benzodiazepine therapy for tinnitus is not recommended.

M. Central tinnitus requires an evaluation for posterior fossa problems, including cerebellopontine angle tumors. The most common cerebellopontine tumor is the acoustic neuroma. Symptoms of an acoustic neuroma include unilateral hearing loss, tinnitus, and disequilibrium. MRI with gadolinium contrast to assess for posterior masses is indicated for abnormal auditory brainstem response (ABR) tests. The sensitivity for acoustic neuromas <15 mm is greater with MRI with gadolinium contrast than with high-resolution CT. In patients with unilateral hearing loss and normal ABR tests, surveillance is required at 6 months and 1 year to assess for progression of symptoms. ENT referrals are indicated for all patients with asymmetric hearing loss. Treatment for tumors depends on the size, location, and the patient's preoperative state.

N. Distinguishing Meniere's disease from acoustic neuromas is difficult clinically. Meniere's tinnitus is intermittent, whereas the tinnitus of acoustic neuroma is constant. Meniere's disease is associated with vertigo as distinguished from the disequilibrium of an acoustic neuroma.

O. Conductive hearing loss requires evaluation for a pathologic condition of the external and middle ear, malignancy, glomus tumor, and cholesteatoma. Early referral to ENT is recommended.

References

Dobie RA, Sakai CS, Sullivan MD, et al. Antidepressant treatment of tinnitus patients: report of a randomized clinical trial and clinical prediction of benefit. Am Otol 1993; 14:18.

Johnson RM, Brummett R, Scheuning A. Use of alprazolam for relief of tinnitus. Arch Otolaryngol Head Neck Surg 1993; 119:842.

Marai K, Tyler RS, Harker LA, Stouffer JL. Review of pharmacologic treatment of tinnitus. Am J Otol 1992; 13:454.

Schleuning AJ II. Management of the patient with tinnitus. Med Clin North Am 1991; 75:1225.

Sismanis A, Smoker WRK. Pulsatile tinnitus: recent advances in diagnosis. Laryngoscope 1994; 104:681.

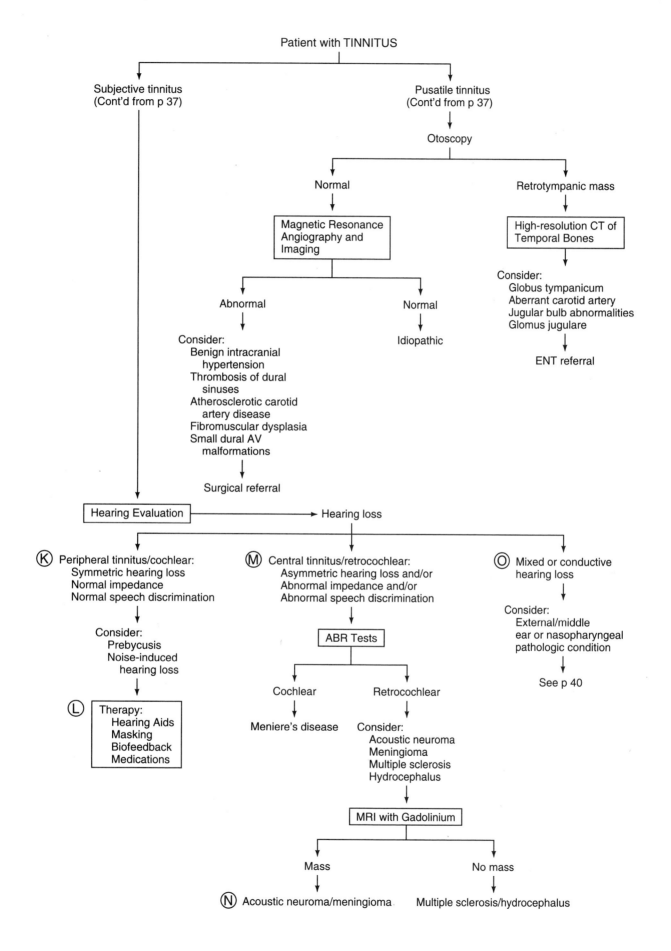

Patient with TINNITUS

Subjective tinnitus
(Cont'd from p 37)

Pusatile tinnitus
(Cont'd from p 37)

Otoscopy

Normal

Retrotympanic mass

Magnetic Resonance
Angiography and
Imaging

High-resolution CT of
Temporal Bones

Consider:
  Globus tympanicum
  Aberrant carotid artery
  Jugular bulb abnormalities
  Glomus jugulare

ENT referral

Abnormal

Normal

Idiopathic

Consider:
  Benign intracranial
    hypertension
  Thrombosis of dural
    sinuses
  Atherosclerotic carotid
    artery disease
  Fibromuscular dysplasia
  Small dural AV
    malformations

Surgical referral

Hearing Evaluation → Hearing loss

Ⓚ Peripheral tinnitus/cochlear:
  Symmetric hearing loss
  Normal impedance
  Normal speech discrimination

Ⓜ Central tinnitus/retrocochlear:
  Asymmetric hearing loss and/or
  Abnormal impedance and/or
  Abnormal speech discrimination

Ⓞ Mixed or conductive
  hearing loss

Consider:
  Prebycusis
  Noise-induced
    hearing loss

ABR Tests

Consider:
  External/middle
  ear or nasopharyngeal
  pathologic condition

See p 40

Cochlear

Retrocochlear

Ⓛ Therapy:
  Hearing Aids
  Masking
  Biofeedback
  Medications

Meniere's disease

Consider:
  Acoustic neuroma
  Meningioma
  Multiple sclerosis
  Hydrocephalus

MRI with Gadolinium

Mass

No mass

Ⓝ Acoustic neuroma/meningioma

Multiple sclerosis/hydrocephalus

HEARING LOSS

Susan Fisk Sander

A. Approximately 50% of the 16 million hearing-impaired Americans are >65 years old. A history of acoustic or physical trauma; barotrauma; deafness; exposure to ototoxins, including medications, recent upper respiratory infection, or associated symptoms such as otalgia, tinnitus, or vertigo helps direct the evaluation.

B. Physical examination of the ear must include otoscopy and evaluation of the external auditory canal, tympanic membrane, and ossicles to exclude underlying external and middle ear pathology. Otitis externa, foreign body in the external canal, cerumen impaction, canal cholesteatoma, exostosis, tympanic membrane perforation, and effusions (hemorrhagic, purulent, or serous) can be observed directly. Weber's and Rinne's tests can further define the hearing loss as sensorineural, conductive, or mixed. Perform Weber's test by placing a tuning fork on the central forehead. Lateralization of the sound to one ear is consistent with either a conductive defect to the affected ear or a sensorineural defect to the opposite ear. No lateralization indicates either a normal result or bilaterally symmetric sensorineural or conductive defects. This test, in conjunction with Rinne's test, supports either a sensorineural or a conductive disorder. The underlying causes and the evaluation process for sensorineural and conductive hearing loss are different. Subsequent testing is determined by the type of hearing loss.

C. Hearing evaluation includes audiography (pure tone testing of air and bone thresholds), speech reception and discrimination, and acoustic impedance. In sensorineural loss (SNHL) both air and bone thresholds are depressed compared with normal. In conductive hearing loss the bone conduction threshold is greater than air conduction thresholds. In mixed deficits air conduction is less than bone conduction, both being depressed.

D. SNHL is a lesion in the organ of Corti or in the central pathways, including the eighth nerve and auditory cortex. SNHL may be the result of an inherited disorder, congenital abnormality, and/or acquired deficit. Acquired causes include metabolic disorders, vascular insufficiency, autoimmune disease, infection, degenerative disorder, or neoplasm. The metabolic work-up of patients with bilateral progressive sensorineural deficits includes evaluation for diabetes mellitus, hyper- and hypothyroidism, anemia, hyperlipidemia, and renal disease. Exclude sources of infection. Neurosyphilis may present with a waxing and waning bilateral SNHL; therefore, initial laboratory evaluation should include a FTA-Abs. Exposure to medications also is in the differential diagnosis. Aminoglycoside antibiotics, loop-diuretics, and salicylates are the most common drugs causing hearing loss; others are quinine, chloroquine, and antineoplastics such as *cis*-platinum. Autoimmune disorders that cause SNHL include Cogan's syndrome,

giant-cell arteritis, systemic lupus erythematosus, polyarteritis nodosum, and Wegener's granulomatosis. Autoimmune SNHL without evidence of systemic symptoms has been observed. An assay for antibodies to inner ear proteins is available. Neoplasms cause SNHL, including acoustic neuroma and metastatic carcinoma of the breast, prostate, and kidney. Degenerative disorders of the auditory pathways include presbycusis, noise-induced hearing loss, and Meniere's disease. Vascular disorders include occlusive disease (vertebrobasilar insufficiency), basilar migraine, embolism, and occlusion secondary to hypercoagulable states. Therapy is aimed at the underlying cause: removal of the offending drug; treatment of the autoimmune disease; a trial of steroids for idiopathic sudden SNHL; either surgery, radiation therapy, or chemotherapy for a neoplasm; surgical repair of membrane rupture; and antibiotics and steroids for syphilis. For acoustic trauma surgical evaluation is warranted. Hearing aids are the treatment of choice for presbycusis and disorders not improved by medical and surgical intervention.

E. Congenital hearing deficits may be due to maternal viral infections during pregnancy (e.g., cytomegalovirus [CMV], rubella, and mumps). Other possibilities include Rh incompatibility, maternal hypothyroidism, anoxia at birth, and exposure to fetal ototoxins.

F. Hereditory disorders of hearing loss are numerous. The three most common inherited forms of SNHL are Waardenburg's syndrome (laterally displaced medial canthi, broad nasal root, white forelock and heterochromia iridis, and sensorineural deafness), Alport's syndrome (nephritis and SNHL), and Usher's syndrome (retinitis pigmentosa and congenital sensorineural deafness).

G. Sudden-onset SNHL is hearing loss of variable severity that develops in ≤3 days. Profound hearing loss is associated with poor prognosis for recovery of hearing. Several etiologies are proposed. A history of trauma and sudden onset of hearing loss suggests temporal fracture. Temporal bone fractures occur longitudinally or transversely. Longitudinal fracture results in middle ear damage (tympanic membrane, cochlea, and auditory nerve damage) and is associated with a conductive hearing loss. Transverse fracture may damage the facial nerve and the labyrinth and result in a sensorineural deficit. Both require referral to an otolaryngologist. Concussion alone may result in a temporary SNHL as a result of acoustic trauma.

H. Heavy lifting may result in a leak of inner ear fluid from a membranous rupture at the oval or round windows, leading to hearing loss and vestibular symptoms. Referral to an otolaryngologist for surgical repair with a graft is indicated.

(Continued on page 42)

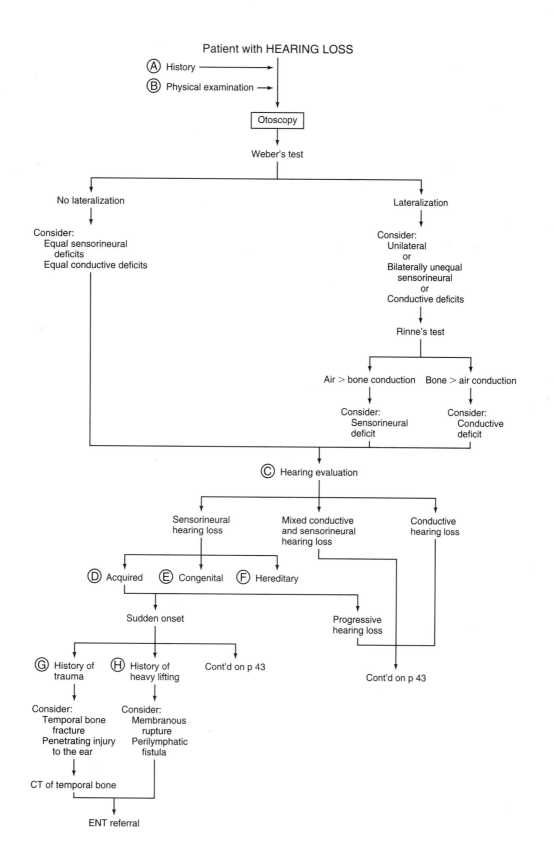

Patient with HEARING LOSS

Ⓐ History ⟶
Ⓑ Physical examination ⟶

Otoscopy

Weber's test

No lateralization

Consider:
    Equal sensorineural
      deficits
    Equal conductive deficits

Lateralization

Consider:
    Unilateral
      or
    Bilaterally unequal
      sensorineural
      or
    Conductive deficits

Rinne's test

Air > bone conduction   Bone > air conduction

Consider:
    Sensorineural
    deficit

Consider:
    Conductive
    deficit

Ⓒ Hearing evaluation

Sensorineural
hearing loss

Mixed conductive
and sensorineural
hearing loss

Conductive
hearing loss

Ⓓ Acquired   Ⓔ Congenital   Ⓕ Hereditary

Sudden onset

Progressive
hearing loss

Ⓖ History of
trauma

Ⓗ History of
heavy lifting

Cont'd on p 43

Consider:
    Temporal bone
      fracture
    Penetrating injury
      to the ear

Consider:
    Membranous
      rupture
    Perilymphatic
      fistula

Cont'd on p 43

CT of temporal bone

ENT referral

I. Infectious causes of sudden-onset SNHL include suppurative labyrinthitis from otitis media, mastoiditis, and viral infections (mumps, CMV, Epstein-Barr virus, rubella, rubeola, herpes zoster, and herpes simplex). Vascular causes include vertebrobasilar insufficiency, embolism, hypercoagulable states, and basilar migraines. Some medications (see D) cause sudden-onset hearing loss. Hearing loss from aminoglycoside antibiotics and loop-diuretics usually is irreversible. Salicylate withdrawal results in improved hearing in most patients.

J. Treatment of sudden-onset SNHL is directed at the underlying disorder. In the past when the cause was not found, bed rest, head elevation, avoidance of loud sound, and steroids were prescribed. Controlled studies of steroid therapy for idiopathic sudden-onset hearing loss show a statistically significant improvement in hearing with steroids (89% vs. 44%). Consider referral to an otolaryngologist.

K. Progressive SNHL that is unilateral or asymmetric requires auditory brainstem response (ABR) testing to localize abnormalities in the retrocochlear areas. MRI with gadolinium contrast is required for all patients suspected of having a retrocochlear lesion. MRI has a higher sensitivity for acoustic neuromas <15 mm than does high-resolution CT. Posterior fossa meningioma and primary cholesteatoma are other masses that cause progressive SNHL in the retrocochlear area. Treatment of acoustic neuromas depends on the size of the tumor, cranial nerve involvement, and the patient's preoperative state. Radiation therapy is used for patients who are not surgical candidates. If ABR testing does not reveal an abnormality, continue surveillance of patients with asymmetric SNHL.

L. Mixed conductive and sensorineural hearing loss is the result of advanced disease. Patients with chronic otitis media, tuberculosis, otosclerosis, skull fractures, penetrating injury of the ear, Wegener's granulomatosis, and squamous cell carcinoma all have been observed to have a conductive and sensorineural deficit in advanced stages of the diseases.

M. Conductive hearing loss, defined as a lesion involving the outer and middle ear to the level of the oval window, results from mechanical disruption of the transmitted sound through the external auditory canal, tympanic membrane, and ossicles. Direct observation of the external canal during physical examination allows evaluation of conditions causing mechanical disruption: atresias of the external canal, cerumen impaction, exostosis, foreign bodies, canal cholesteatoma, external otitis, tympanic membrane perforation or sclerosis, effusions, and ossicular damage. Multiple perforations of the tympanic membrane suggests tuberculous infection of the middle ear. Acoustic stapedius reflex testing for fixation of the stapedius is part of the evaluation of conductive hearing loss. Otosclerosis, the most common congenital form of conductive hearing loss, is diagnosed with this test and treated with stapedectomy. Cholesteatoma, glomus tumor, and nasopharyngeal malignancies (squamous cell carcinoma, adenocarcinoma, and basal cell carcinoma) can produce conductive hearing loss. Barotrauma resulting from unequal air pressure in the external auditory canal and the middle ear can result in an effusion and a temporary conductive hearing loss. High-resolution CT of the temporal bones is the study of choice to evaluate for masses in the middle ear. Therapy of the underlying problem may improve the conductive hearing loss: removal of the foreign body or cerumen, antituberculous drugs, tympanoplasty, ossiculoplasty, stapedectomy, and removal of excessive cartilage (exostosis). Treatment of masses within the middle ear depend on the site, pathologic condition, and preoperative evaluation of the patient. Referral to an otolaryngologist is indicated.

References

Arts HA. Differential diagnosis of sensorineural hearing loss. In: Cummings CW, et al, eds. Otolaryngology head and neck surgery. 4th ed. St. Louis: Mosby, 1998.

Backous D, Niparko J. Differential diagnosis of conductive hearing loss. In: Cummings CW, et al, eds. Otolaryngology head and neck surgery. 4th ed. St. Louis: Mosby, 1998.

Grandis JR, Hirsch BE, Wagener MM. Treatment of idiopathic sudden sensorineural hearing loss. Am J Otol 1993; 14:183.

Nadol JB. Hearing loss. N Engl J Med 1993; 329:1092.

Shikowitz MJ. Sudden sensorineural hearing loss. Med Clin North Am 1991; 75:1239.

Patient with HEARING LOSS

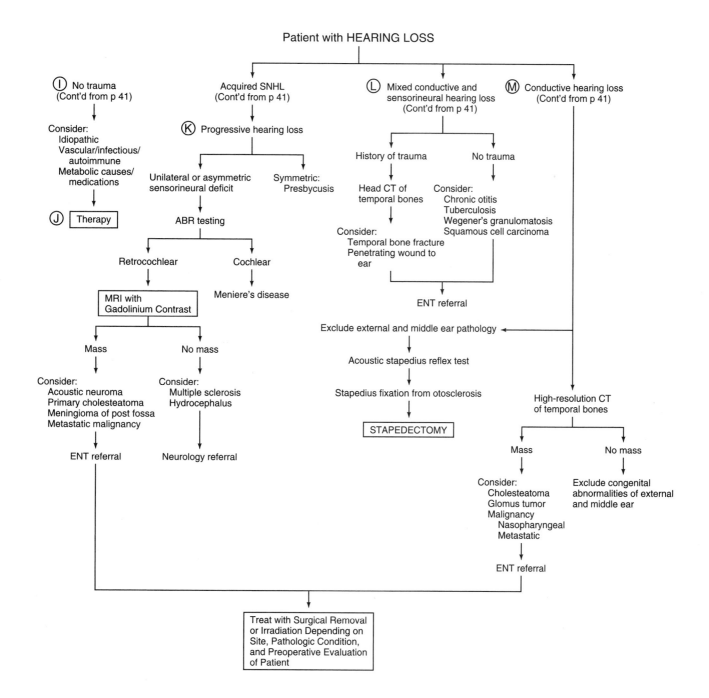

I No trauma
(Cont'd from p 41)

Consider:
Idiopathic
Vascular/infectious/
autoimmune
Metabolic causes/
medications

J Therapy

Acquired SNHL
(Cont'd from p 41)

K Progressive hearing loss

Unilateral or asymmetric
sensorineural deficit

Symmetric:
Presbycusis

ABR testing

Retrocochlear

Cochlear

MRI with
Gadolinium Contrast

Meniere's disease

Mass

No mass

Consider:
Acoustic neuroma
Primary cholesteatoma
Meningioma of post fossa
Metastatic malignancy

Consider:
Multiple sclerosis
Hydrocephalus

ENT referral

Neurology referral

L Mixed conductive and
sensorineural hearing loss
(Cont'd from p 41)

History of trauma

No trauma

Head CT of
temporal bones

Consider:
Chronic otitis
Tuberculosis
Wegener's granulomatosis
Squamous cell carcinoma

Consider:
Temporal bone fracture
Penetrating wound to
ear

ENT referral

Exclude external and middle ear pathology

Acoustic stapedius reflex test

Stapedius fixation from otosclerosis

STAPEDECTOMY

M Conductive hearing loss
(Cont'd from p 41)

High-resolution CT
of temporal bones

Mass

No mass

Consider:
Cholesteatoma
Glomus tumor
Malignancy
Nasopharyngeal
Metastatic

Exclude congenital
abnormalities of external
and middle ear

ENT referral

Treat with Surgical Removal
or Irradiation Depending on
Site, Pathologic Condition,
and Preoperative Evaluation
of Patient

PERIOPERATIVE EVALUATION

Richard Liebowitz

The evaluation of patients before surgery entails a process of risk assessment based on three independent factors. The first two relate to the skill of the surgeon and the specific risk of the procedure and thus are outside the purview of the consulting physician. The third risk factor, however, is patient related. This chapter deals with the perioperative evaluation and interventions required to minimize morbidity and mortality resulting from patient-related risks. Consultants must remember that their role is not to "clear" patients for surgery but rather to identify modifiable conditions and potential problems suggested by risk factors. Postoperative assistance with medical problems is commonly required of the consultant. The consultant must establish whether his or her role is limited to making recommendations in the medical record or includes writing orders and thereby directly assuming management. Communication between consulting and attending physicians is paramount and is the responsibility of the consultant.

A. The overall risk of death and permanent sequelae from operative procedures continues to decline with advances in anesthetic and surgical techniques. Low-risk procedures associated with general anesthesia have a mortality rate of about 0.01–0.27%, whereas mortality from high-risk operations ranges from 9–20%. Emergent surgery doubles the standard mortality. Complications most often occur >24 hours after surgery, leading some to speculate about a loss of a "protective" anesthetic effect. The American Society of Anesthesiologists' physical status classification (ASA) helps one to rapidly determine anticipated patient outcomes (Table 1). The role of the consulting physician is not only to recognize the patient's ASA class and determine the risk of morbidity, but also to ascertain whether any preoperative interventions are indicated. The risks and benefits of postponing surgery in patients with active medical problems must be considered. Complications may be generalized, such as deep venous thrombosis (DVT), or specific to the particular procedure. Medication use unrelated to the surgery is a crucial problem in this period; some agents may increase the risk of morbidity and mortality and must be discontinued, whereas others may need dosage adjustments.

B. Noncardiac surgery in the cardiac patient is the most common indication for medical consultation. Goldman and subsequent authors have attempted to predict the likelihood of postoperative complications in this patient group. A system of points given for recognized risk variables attempts to stratify patients from low to high risk (Table 2). The American College of Cardiology has published a task force report addressing this issue. Evidence from their study is convincing that operative intervention for coronary disease need not be considered solely because of the patient's need for noncardiac surgery. Similarly, a noninvasive work-up is not indicated for patients with class I or II angina unless activity is limited by noncardiac causes. Pharmacologic stress testing may be helpful in patients with physical limitations. Careful postoperative monitoring of all cardiac patients, including serial ECGs, is essential, but no advantage to the use of pulmonary artery catheters has yet been demonstrated. Consider administering atenolol to patients with known cardiac disease or those with at least two cardiac risk factors; this intervention has been documented to decrease short- and long-term operative mortality.

(Continued on page 46)

TABLE 1   ASA Classification

Class I	No organic, physiologic, biochemical, or psychiatric abnormality
Class II	Mild to moderate systemic disturbance such as hypertension or mild controlled diabetes
Class III	Severe systemic disturbance or disease such as symptomatic coronary artery disease or pneumonia
Class IV	Severe systemic disorders that are life threatening on their own and not always correctable by surgery such as diabetic ketoacidosis or status asthmaticus
Class V	Moribund patient with little chance of survival such as ruptured aortic aneurysm
E	Emergency surgery is denoted by an E following the class and is associated with increased risk

TABLE 2   Multifactorial Cardiac Risk Index

Variable	Points
S_3 gallop or increased jugular venous distension (JVD)	11
Myocardial infarction in past 6 mo	10
Rhythm other than sinus	7
Age >70 yr	5
Emergency surgery	4
Intraperitoneal, intrathoracic, or aortic operation	3
Suspected critical aortic stenosis	3
Poor general medical condition (K^+ <3.0, Po_2 <60 mm Hg or Pco_2 >50 mm Hg, BUN ≥50, creatinine 3 mg/dl, chronic liver disease or patient bedridden)	3

Operative risks may be classed as:	I (low)	0–5 points
	II	6–12 points
	III	13–25 points
	IV (high)	>25 points

From Goldman L. Cardiac risks and complications of noncardiac surgery. Ann Intern Med 1983; 98:504.

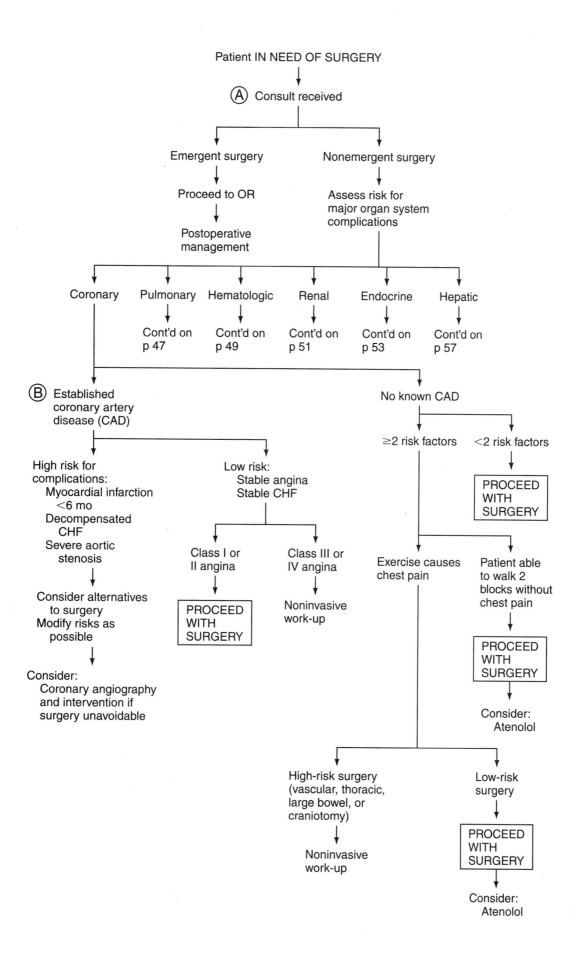

Patient IN NEED OF SURGERY

Ⓐ Consult received

Emergent surgery

Proceed to OR

Postoperative management

Nonemergent surgery

Assess risk for major organ system complications

Coronary

Pulmonary — Cont'd on p 47

Hematologic — Cont'd on p 49

Renal — Cont'd on p 51

Endocrine — Cont'd on p 53

Hepatic — Cont'd on p 57

Ⓑ Established coronary artery disease (CAD)

No known CAD

High risk for complications:
Myocardial infarction <6 mo
Decompensated CHF
Severe aortic stenosis

Consider alternatives to surgery
Modify risks as possible

Consider:
Coronary angiography and intervention if surgery unavoidable

Low risk:
Stable angina
Stable CHF

Class I or II angina

PROCEED WITH SURGERY

Class III or IV angina

Noninvasive work-up

≥2 risk factors

<2 risk factors

PROCEED WITH SURGERY

Exercise causes chest pain

Patient able to walk 2 blocks without chest pain

PROCEED WITH SURGERY

Consider: Atenolol

High-risk surgery (vascular, thoracic, large bowel, or craniotomy)

Noninvasive work-up

Low-risk surgery

PROCEED WITH SURGERY

Consider: Atenolol

C. Chronic obstructive pulmonary disease (COPD) is the most common risk factor for postoperative pulmonary complications. Smoking raises the risk for pneumonia and hypoxemia. After 6 months of cessation, smoking is no longer a risk factor. Obesity, age >60 years, duration of anesthesia >4 hours, presence of an upper respiratory infection, and asthma all increase the risk of postoperative pulmonary complications. Primary pulmonary-based elevations of Pa_{CO_2} >45 mm Hg portend significantly increased risk of death and other pulmonary complications. The site of surgery plays a major role: Thoracic and upper abdominal surgery have significantly higher rates of complications. Pulmonary function tests (PFTs) are recommended for patients at risk for complications, but their sensitivity is <40%. Pulmonary resection surgery in patients with abnormally low volumes may require sophisticated testing such as split lung studies to determine the ultimate effect of the proposed surgery. Although there is no absolute cutoff value for FEV_1 in nonthoracic surgery, a volume <0.5 L is associated with a high risk of pulmonary complications. General and regional anesthesia have similar rates of postoperative pulmonary complications, and other factors should be considered in the choice of anesthesia.

(Continued on page 48)

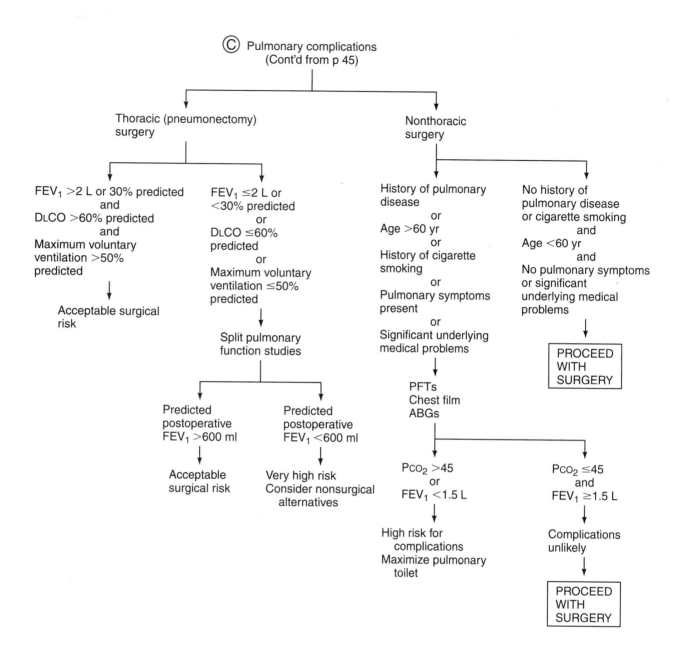

D. Postoperative hematologic concerns include excessive bleeding, risk of DVT, and the results of surgery in the anemic patient. The absence of a history of serious postoperative bleeding does not eliminate future risk. Although commonly ordered, there is little evidence that a bleeding time successfully predicts patients at risk for bleeding. Pulmonary embolism (PE) and DVT are the most preventable causes of hospital-associated morbidity and mortality; consider prophylaxis for all hospitalized patients, withholding it only for those at low risk (Table 3). The role of low-molecular-weight heparin in the transition of chronically anticoagulated patients to surgery has yet to be determined. Individual decisions must be made concerning the need for pre- and postoperative IV heparin in these patients, weighing the risk of bleeding against the risk of thrombosis and embolization.

(Continued on page 50)

TABLE 3 Thromboembolism Prophylaxis in Surgical Patients

Type of Surgery	Agent	Regimen
General, urologic, gynecologic, extracranial neurosurgery	Unfractionated heparin	5000–7500 U SC bid
Intracranial surgery	Pneumatic compression	
Hip replacement	LMW heparin	Enoxaparin 30 mg bid
	or	
	Low-intensity warfarin	INR 2.0–3.0
	or	
	Adjusted-dose heparin	PTT 31–36 sec
Hip fracture	LMW heparin	Enoxaparin 30 mg bid
	or	
	Low-intensity warfarin	INR 2.0–3.0
Total knee replacement	LMW heparin	Enoxaparin 30 mg bid
	or	
	Pneumatic compression	

LMW, Low molecular weight; *INR,* International Normalized Ratio; *PTT,* partial thromboplastic time.

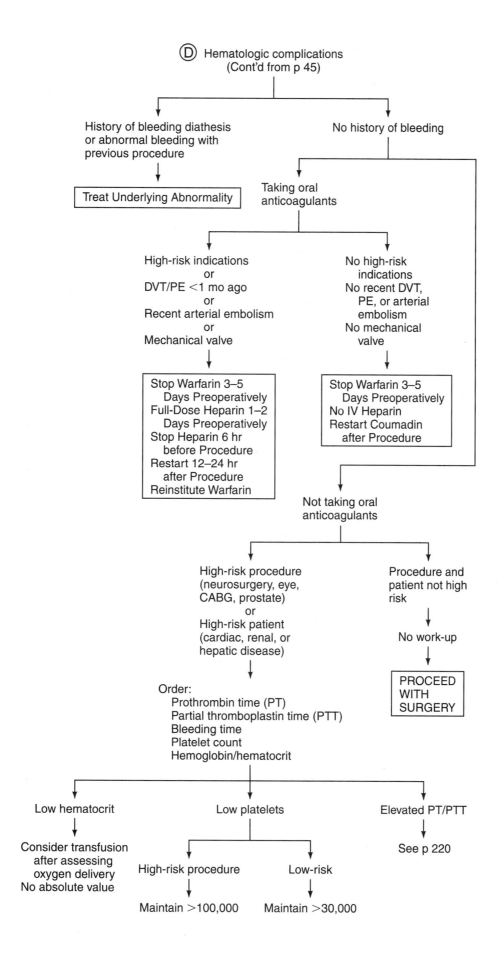

D Hematologic complications
(Cont'd from p 45)

History of bleeding diathesis
or abnormal bleeding with
previous procedure

No history of bleeding

Treat Underlying Abnormality

Taking oral
anticoagulants

High-risk indications
or
DVT/PE <1 mo ago
or
Recent arterial embolism
or
Mechanical valve

No high-risk
indications
No recent DVT,
PE, or arterial
embolism
No mechanical
valve

Stop Warfarin 3–5
    Days Preoperatively
Full-Dose Heparin 1–2
    Days Preoperatively
Stop Heparin 6 hr
    before Procedure
Restart 12–24 hr
    after Procedure
Reinstitute Warfarin

Stop Warfarin 3–5
    Days Preoperatively
No IV Heparin
Restart Coumadin
    after Procedure

Not taking oral
anticoagulants

High-risk procedure
(neurosurgery, eye,
CABG, prostate)
or
High-risk patient
(cardiac, renal, or
hepatic disease)

Procedure and
patient not high
risk

No work-up

PROCEED
WITH
SURGERY

Order:
    Prothrombin time (PT)
    Partial thromboplastin time (PTT)
    Bleeding time
    Platelet count
    Hemoglobin/hematocrit

Low hematocrit

Low platelets

Elevated PT/PTT

Consider transfusion
after assessing
oxygen delivery
No absolute value

High-risk procedure

Low-risk

See p 220

Maintain >100,000

Maintain >30,000

E. Acute renal failure (ARF) greatly increases postoperative mortality. Renal insufficiency, especially with glomerular filtration rates <25 ml/min, is the most significant risk factor for the development of ARF in the postoperative period. Other recognized risk factors include advanced age, congestive heart failure (CHF), vascular surgery, hypotension, and known nephrotoxic agents. Chronic dialysis does not greatly increase the mortality associated with planned surgery. Dialysis required immediately before surgery should be terminated at least 4 hours before the procedure to minimize bleeding risk. The most common postoperative complication in patients with chronic renal insufficiency is hyperkalemia. Vascular access must be maintained in these patients for means of appropriate antibiotic prophylaxis and avoidance of vascular devices in the ipsilateral extremity. Despite appropriate precautions, the thrombosis rate of the vascular access approaches 3%.

(Continued on page 52)

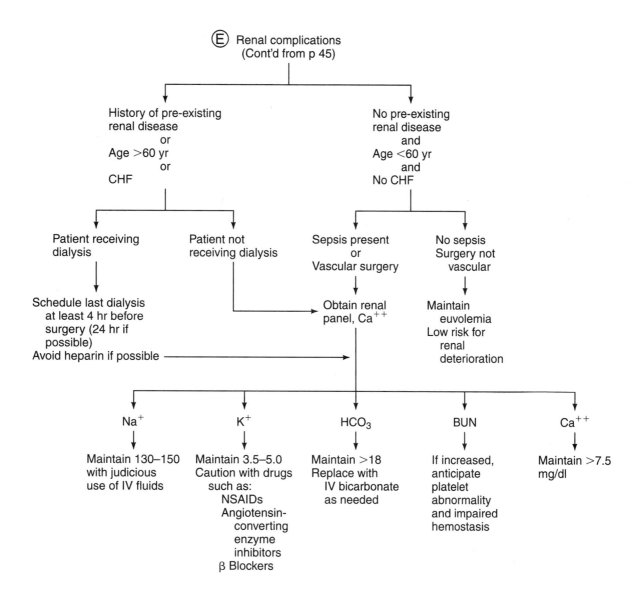

E Renal complications
(Cont'd from p 45)

History of pre-existing
renal disease
or
Age >60 yr
or
CHF

No pre-existing
renal disease
and
Age <60 yr
and
No CHF

Patient receiving
dialysis

Patient not
receiving dialysis

Sepsis present
or
Vascular surgery

No sepsis
Surgery not
vascular

Schedule last dialysis
at least 4 hr before
surgery (24 hr if
possible)
Avoid heparin if possible

Obtain renal
panel, Ca^{++}

Maintain
euvolemia
Low risk for
renal
deterioration

Na^+

K^+

HCO_3

BUN

Ca^{++}

Maintain 130–150
with judicious
use of IV fluids

Maintain 3.5–5.0
Caution with drugs
such as:
NSAIDs
Angiotensin-
converting
enzyme
inhibitors
β Blockers

Maintain >18
Replace with
IV bicarbonate
as needed

If increased,
anticipate
platelet
abnormality
and impaired
hemostasis

Maintain >7.5
mg/dl

F. Diabetes is the most common endocrinopathy in surgical patients. Diabetic patients may be at risk for up to 50% greater surgical mortality than the general population. Ensure adequate glucose control before surgery and evaluate end-organ dysfunction. Oral agents generally are discontinued 24–36 hours before surgery. Multiple approaches exist for insulin dosing on the day of surgery; most common is a dose of half the usual intermediate-acting insulin in the morning, accompanied by a glucose drip. Ideal surgical glucose levels are debated; the general principle is to avoid episodes of hypoglycemia and maintain levels <250 mg/dl. Readings above this level are associated with impaired host factors leading to increased risk of postoperative infection. Sliding-scale insulin offers no benefits alone or in conjunction with standing longer-acting insulin. Strongly consider the use of insulin drips in patients undergoing major surgery (e.g., laparotomy, open heart, vascular, thoracic).

G. Adrenal suppression occurs most often in patients receiving pharmacologic steroid therapy. Consider stress dosing in any patient who has received ≥7.5 mg/day of prednisone equivalent for >1 week. Further management of these patients is discussed elsewhere.

(Continued on page 54)

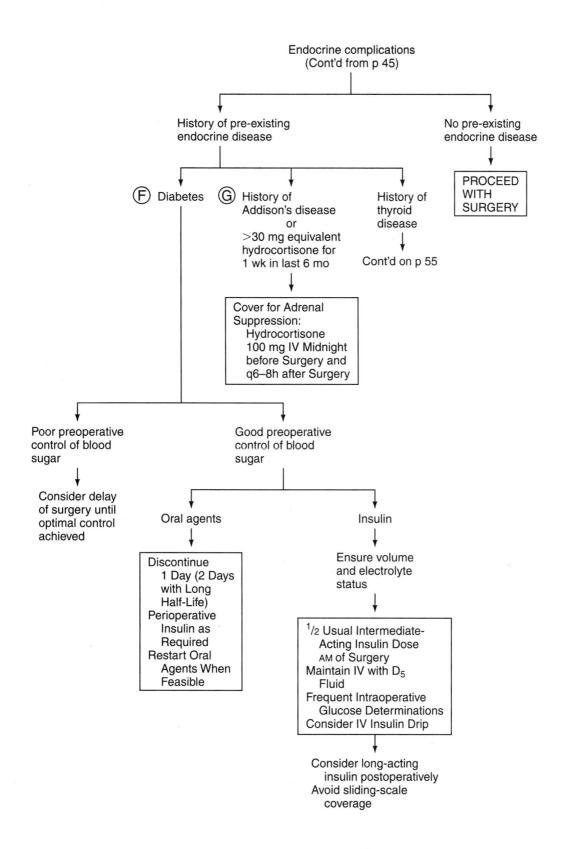

Endocrine complications
(Cont'd from p 45)

History of pre-existing
endocrine disease

No pre-existing
endocrine disease

PROCEED
WITH
SURGERY

(F) Diabetes

(G) History of
Addison's disease
or
>30 mg equivalent
hydrocortisone for
1 wk in last 6 mo

History of
thyroid
disease

Cont'd on p 55

Cover for Adrenal
Suppression:
Hydrocortisone
100 mg IV Midnight
before Surgery and
q6–8h after Surgery

Poor preoperative
control of blood
sugar

Good preoperative
control of blood
sugar

Consider delay
of surgery until
optimal control
achieved

Oral agents

Insulin

Discontinue
1 Day (2 Days
with Long
Half-Life)
Perioperative
Insulin as
Required
Restart Oral
Agents When
Feasible

Ensure volume
and electrolyte
status

$1/2$ Usual Intermediate-
Acting Insulin Dose
AM of Surgery
Maintain IV with D_5
Fluid
Frequent Intraoperative
Glucose Determinations
Consider IV Insulin Drip

Consider long-acting
insulin postoperatively
Avoid sliding-scale
coverage

H. Mild to moderate thyroid disease poses less risk in the perioperative period than previously thought. The main risk in hyperthyroidism is precipitation of thyroid storm. β Blockers are safe and indicated in this period. If surgery cannot be delayed, use of these agents, along with propylthiouracil (PTU) and potassium iodide (SSKI), decreases the risk of storm. Treat hypothyroidism before surgery; if this is not possible, give L-thyroxine. Complications such as CHF, hypoxemia, hypotension, and ileus are noted. Starting thyroid replacement in mildly hypothyroid individuals before coronary artery bypass surgery (CABG) may increase the risk of cardiovascular events; consider postponing this until the postoperative period.

(Continued on page 56)

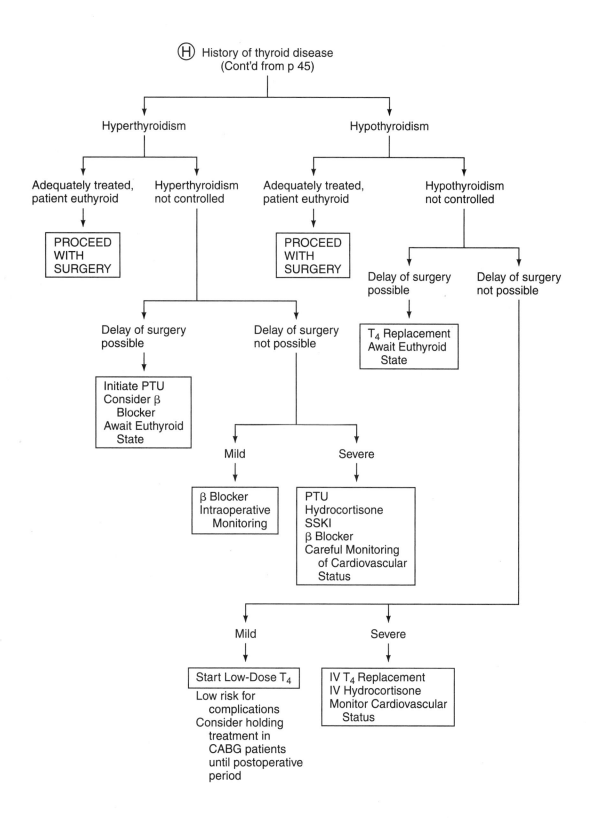

TABLE 4   Modified Childs' Index for Grading Severity of Liver Disease

Clinical or Laboratory Feature	Points Scored for Increasing Abnormality*		
	1	2	3
Encephalopathy	None	Mild–moderate	Severe
Ascites	None	Slight	Moderate
Bilirubin	<2 mg/dl	2–3 mg/dl	>3 mg/dl
Albumin	>3.5 g/L	2.8–3.4 g/L	<2.8 g/L
Prothrombin time	<4 sec	4–6 sec	>6 sec

*A, 5–6 points, good risk; B, 7–9 points, moderate risk; C, 10–15 points, poor risk. Adapted from Pugh RNH, Murray-Lyon IM, Dawson JL, et al. Transection of the oesophagus for bleeding oesophageal varices. Br J Surg 1973; 60:646, by permission of the publishers Butterworth-Heinemann Ltd.

I. Patients with known liver disease are at risk for worsening of their underlying abnormality because all anesthetics currently used decrease hepatic blood flow. None of these agents, however, is directly hepatotoxic. If possible, postpone surgery for patients with acute hepatitis. Patients with severe chronic hepatitis probably are at increased risk for postoperative morbidity and mortality, although mild disease may not predispose them to significant problems. Common complications include ARF, upper GI bleeding, pneumonia, and wound infections. Take special care in monitoring fluid status, electrolytes, coagulation, encephalopathy, and nutritional status in these patients. The most accepted classification for risk stratification is the Pugh modification of the classic Childs' criteria (Table 4). Patients in the lowest risk group need no specific intervention preoperatively, whereas all other groups need careful evaluation before elective surgery. Specific symptoms of liver disease are discussed in other chapters.

References

Clagett GP, Anderson FA Jr, Heit J, et al. Prevention of venous thromboembolism. Chest 1995; 108(suppl 4):312S.

Eagle KA, Brundage BH, Chaitman BR, et al. Guidelines for perioperative cardiovascular evaluation for noncardiac surgery. Report of the American College of Cardiology/American Heart Association Task Force on Practice Guidelines Committee on Perioperative Cardiovascular Evaluation for Noncardiac Surgery. Circulation 1996; 93:1280.

Goldman L. Cardiac risks and complications of noncardiac surgery. Ann Intern Med 1983; 98:504.

Mangano DT, Layug EL, Wallace A, Tateo I. Effect of atenolol on mortality and cardiovascular morbidity after noncardiac surgery. N Engl J Med 1996; 335:1713.

Novis BK, Roizen MF, Aronson S, Thisted RA. Association of preoperative risk factors with postoperative acute renal failure. Anesth Analg 1994; 78:143.

Pugh RN, Murray-Lyon IM, Dawson JL, et al. Transection of the oesophagus for bleeding oesophageal varices. Br J Surg 1973; 60:646.

Queale WS, Seidler AJ, Brancati FL. Glycemic control and sliding scale insulin use in medical inpatients with diabetes mellitus. Arch Intern Med 1997; 157:545.

Schiff RL, Emanuele MA. The surgical patient with diabetes mellitus: guidelines for management. J Gen Intern Med 1995; 10:154.

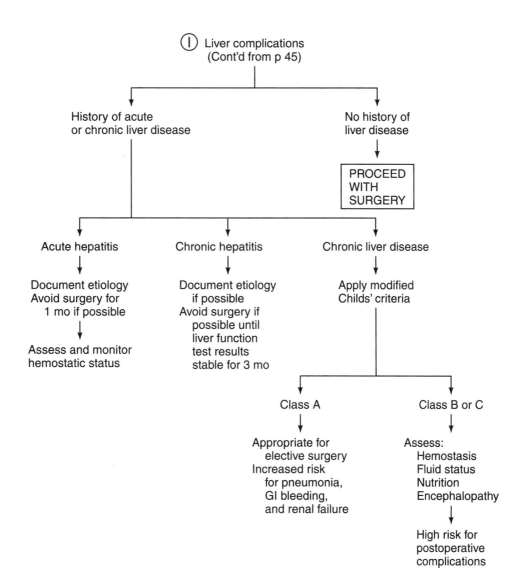

INTERNAL MEDICINE

CARDIOLOGY

BRADYCARDIA

David Framm
Paul E. Fenster
Karl B. Kern

Bradycardia is a common clinical problem, particularly in the elderly. It is most important in the selection of therapy to be certain that the described symptoms are the result of a slow heart rate (HR). No definitive rate requirement can be established because some athletes may do well with rates at 30–40 beats/min, whereas some patients with underlying cardiac or CNS disease may be truly symptomatic when the rate falls below 60 beats/min.

A. History is crucial in establishing a relationship between the observed rate and symptoms. Subtle symptoms, often mental or personality changes, can often best be observed and documented by family members. Medication use is critical in the consideration of reversible causes for bradycardia. A history of underlying heart disease, ischemic or valvular, also is helpful.

B. If reversible causes for the bradycardia are found, they should be eliminated and the resolution of the slow arrhythmia documented. If the bradycardia persists, further work-up is indicated.

C. If no precipitating or reversible cause for the bradycardia can be identified, a rhythm strip or ECG should be examined to distinguish patients with sinus node disease or Mobitz I atrioventricular (AV) block from those with higher-degree AV block (Mobitz II and complete heart block).

D. Patients with sinus node disease or Mobitz I AV block should be carefully evaluated for symptoms. If they are asymptomatic, an exercise test (treadmill) can be helpful to document appropriate increases in HR with exercise. If no increase is seen, careful periodic monitoring to ascertain any worsening of rhythm disturbance is warranted.

E. Symptomatic patients with sinus node disease or low-grade AV block (Mobitz I) should undergo Holter monitoring. If evidence for tachy-brady syndrome is found, a pacemaker probably will be needed to allow adequate therapy for both the rapid rhythm (using drugs) and the slow rhythm (using a permanent pacemaker). If only bradycardia is evident, a pacemaker may be indicated, depending on the symptoms and their correlation with the bradycardia.

F. High-grade AV block (Mobitz II or greater) has a poor long-term prognosis, often proceeding to complete heart block. A permanent pacer is indicated for such patients.

G. Immediately treat any hemodynamic instability secondary to a slow HR. Initial therapy could include a trial of atropine at 0.5–1.0 mg. Transcutaneous pacing is often rapid and can be effective. Transvenous pacing is the most stable solution if the bradycardia persists.

References

Dreifus LS, Fisch C, Griffin JC, et al. Guidelines for implantation of cardiac pacemakers and antiarrhythmia devices. J Am Coll Cardiol 1991; 18:1.

Emergency Cardiac Care Committee and Subcommittees, American Heart Association. Guidelines for cardiopulmonary resuscitation and emergency cardiac care. III. Adult advanced cardiac life support. JAMA 1992; 268:2171.

Hayes DL, Osborn MJ. Pacing: antibradycardia devices. In: Giuliani ER, Gersh BJ, McGoon MD, et al, eds. Mayo Clinic practice of cardiology. 3rd ed. St. Louis: Mosby, 1996:909.

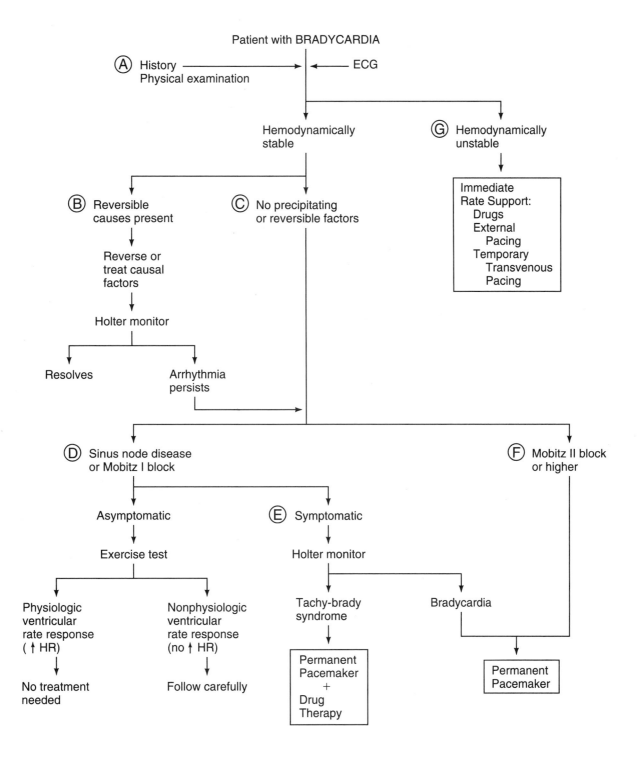

Patient with BRADYCARDIA

Ⓐ History
Physical examination ——→ ←—— ECG

Hemodynamically stable   Ⓖ Hemodynamically unstable

Immediate
Rate Support:
   Drugs
   External
      Pacing
   Temporary
      Transvenous
      Pacing

Ⓑ Reversible causes present   Ⓒ No precipitating or reversible factors

Reverse or treat causal factors

Holter monitor

Resolves   Arrhythmia persists

Ⓓ Sinus node disease or Mobitz I block   Ⓕ Mobitz II block or higher

Asymptomatic   Ⓔ Symptomatic

Exercise test   Holter monitor

Physiologic ventricular rate response (↑ HR)   Nonphysiologic ventricular rate response (no ↑ HR)   Tachy-brady syndrome   Bradycardia

No treatment needed   Follow carefully

Permanent Pacemaker + Drug Therapy

Permanent Pacemaker

NARROW QRS COMPLEX TACHYCARDIA

Anthony C. Caruso
Karl B. Kern

Evaluation of patients with narrow complex tachycardia poses a challenge to the physician, for clearly, many different tachyarrhythmias appear to be identical on superficial examination. *Supraventricular tachycardia* is a broad term for a variety of rhythm disturbances that originate at or above the atrioventricular (AV) node. This includes atrial fibrillation and atrial flutter, which usually are rather distinct in presentation, as well as sinus tachycardia, sinus node re-entry tachycardia (SNRT), ectopic atrial tachycardia, accelerated junctional rhythm, multifocal atrial tachycardia, AV node re-entrant tachycardia (AVNRT), and sometimes new accessory pathway-mediated tachycardias such as the orthodromic atrioventricular re-entrant tachycardia (AVRT) found in Wolff-Parkinson-White (WPW) syndrome.

A. The foremost consideration in evaluating narrow complex tachycardia is hemodynamic stability. If the patient is unstable, immediate cardioversion is warranted, regardless of the QRS morphology or exact diagnosis.

B. Stable patients can be more carefully evaluated with a 12-lead ECG. The major initial decision is whether P waves are visible.

C. If P waves are present and identical to the sinus P seen previous to the tachycardia, sinus tachycardia is likely. The hallmark of SNRT is an abrupt onset and offset of narrow complex tachycardia in which the P wave has the same axis configuration as the P wave during sinus rhythm.

D. The appearance of P waves distinctly different from the sinus P wave is helpful. Ectopic atrial tachycardia is characterized by a single P wave morphology distinct from that of the sinus P wave. This tachycardia often is initiated by a premature atrial beat late in diastole. An inverted P wave (retrograde P) (often best seen in leads II, III, or AVF) indicates paroxysmal supraventricular tachycardia (PSVT). PSVT in the elderly population is most commonly AVNRT in which the P wave usually is seen buried within the ST segment. This tachycardia, along with orthodromic AVRT of WPW,

responds well to vagal maneuvers, with 50% of patients returning to sinus rhythm. A delta wave on a resting ECG alerts the clinician to an accessory pathway, but in patients with a concealed accessory pathway, there is no antegrade conduction and consequently no delta wave. Atrial flutter is recognized by the typical sawtooth pattern of atrial waves at a rate of 280–300 beats/min. Atrial flutter P waves are best seen in leads II, III, AVF, or V.

E. If multiple distinct forms of P waves are evident, the likely diagnosis is multifocal atrial tachycardia (MAT).

F. If distinct P waves are absent, carefully consider the baseline between QRS complexes and the regularity of the RR interval. If a chaotic baseline and irregularly irregular RR intervals are found, the diagnosis is most likely atrial fibrillation.

G. If the baseline is smooth and the RR interval remains regular, the diagnosis is almost certainly an accelerated junctional tachycardia.

References

Bär FW, Brugada P, Dossen WRM, Wellens HJJ. Differential diagnosis of tachycardia with narrow QRS complex. Am J Cardiol 1984; 54:555.

Brugada P, Smeets JLRM, Wellens HJJ. Spectrum of supraventricular tachycardias. Am J Cardiol 1989; 62:4L.

Emergency Cardiac Care Committee and Subcommittee, American Heart Association. Advanced cardiac life support 1997; 1.

Levine JH, Michael JR, Guarnieri T. Treatment of multifocal atrial tachycardia with verapamil. N Engl J Med 1985; 312:21.

Mehta D, Ward DE, Wafa S, Camm AJ. Relative efficacy of various physical maneuvers in the termination of junctional tachycardia. Lancet 1988; 1:1187.

Rankin AC, McGovern BA. Adenosine or verapamil for the acute treatment of supraventricular tachycardia? Ann Intern Med 1991; 114:513.

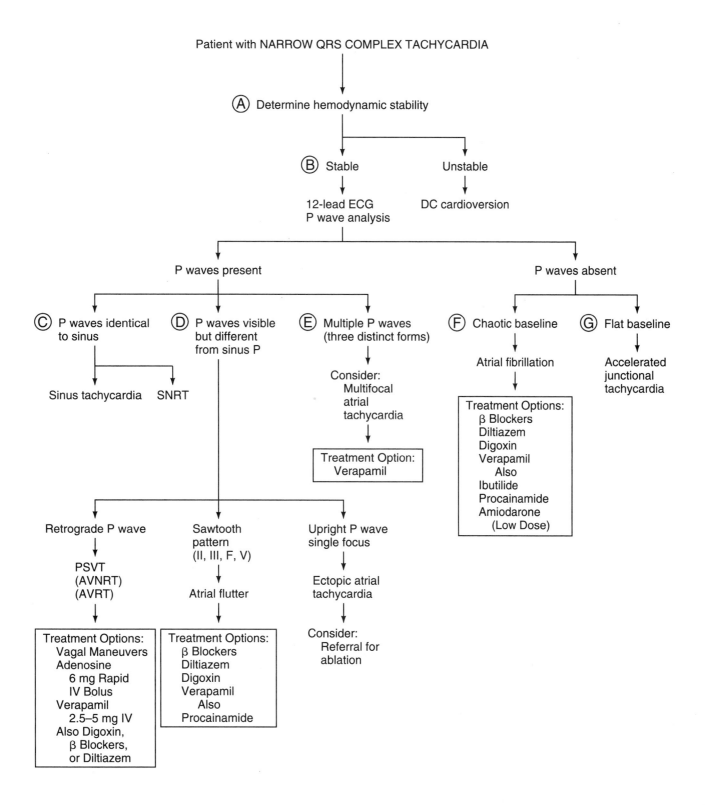

Patient with NARROW QRS COMPLEX TACHYCARDIA

(A) Determine hemodynamic stability

(B) Stable   Unstable

12-lead ECG   DC cardioversion
P wave analysis

P waves present   P waves absent

(C) P waves identical (D) P waves visible (E) Multiple P waves   (F) Chaotic baseline   (G) Flat baseline
to sinus   but different   (three distinct forms)
              from sinus P

Sinus tachycardia   SNRT   Consider: Atrial fibrillation   Accelerated
                                 Multifocal   junctional
                                 atrial   tachycardia
                                 tachycardia

Consider:
Multifocal
atrial
tachycardia

Treatment Option:
Verapamil

Treatment Options:
β Blockers
Diltiazem
Digoxin
Verapamil
Also
Ibutilide
Procainamide
Amiodarone
(Low Dose)

Retrograde P wave   Sawtooth   Upright P wave
                      pattern   single focus
                      (II, III, F, V)

PSVT   Atrial flutter   Ectopic atrial
(AVNRT)   tachycardia
(AVRT)

Consider:
Referral for
ablation

Treatment Options:
Vagal Maneuvers
Adenosine
6 mg Rapid
IV Bolus
Verapamil
2.5–5 mg IV
Also Digoxin,
β Blockers,
or Diltiazem

Treatment Options:
β Blockers
Diltiazem
Digoxin
Verapamil
Also
Procainamide

WIDE QRS COMPLEX TACHYCARDIA

Anthony C. Caruso

Wide QRS tachycardia poses a complex set of problems because the treatment of supraventricular tachycardias with aberrant conduction is clearly different from that of acute ventricular tachycardia. Inability to distinguish one from the other may have catastrophic consequences.

A. The first step in the management of all tachycardias is an assessment of hemodynamic stability. In patients with a wide QRS complex tachycardia who are hemodynamically unstable, immediate cardioversion with 200 joules is appropriate; pharmacologic interventions at this point would only delay a safe and effective therapy. In hemodynamically stable patients, a 12-lead ECG provides valuable information in distinguishing a supraventricular from a ventricular cause of wide QRS complex tachycardia.

B. Patients with an irregular RR interval must be distinguished from those with a regular RR interval.

C. In those with an irregular RR interval who have a history of either congenital or an acquired long QT and are found to have atrioventricular (AV) dissociation, the diagnosis is one of probable polymorphic ventricular tachycardia (VT), and the appropriate therapy is administration of 2 g magnesium sulfate IV. Should this fail to convert the patient to sinus rhythm, isoproterenol infusion to shorten QT intervals is effective. In patients with recent myocardial infarction or unstable angina, this therapy may be hazardous. An equally effective approach is the use of transient cardiac pacing to maintain adequate QT reduction. Correction of electrolyte abnormalities is essential.

D. In patients with an irregular RR rate with classic bundle branch block (BBB) morphology in which no AV dissociation is obvious, the most likely cause is atrial fibrillation with aberrancy, and esmolol, digitalis, or verapamil may be initiated to control ventricular response. This should be performed only if there is no evidence of a delta wave. In patients with rapid ventricular response across an accessory pathway, cardiac collapse has been known to occur with the administration of verapamil.

E. In patients with a regular RR interval, an attempt should be made to identify P waves on a 12-lead ECG; in patients with clear AV dissociation, the diagnosis is one of probable VT. Treatment at this point would be lidocaine with an initial bolus of 1.5 mg/kg followed by 0.8 mg/kg at 8-, 16-, and 24-min intervals. A maintenance infusion of 30 μg/kg/min is then initiated with appropriate titration via plasma levels of lidocaine. If this is unsuccessful, it is recommended to proceed with procainamide: a 15-mg/kg loading dose administered at 35 mg/min followed by a maintenance dose of 4 mg/min. This regimen achieves adequate steady state levels quickly with dose adjustment via drug level determination. If lidocaine or procainamide fails to control VT, bretylium may be administered at a 5-mg/kg loading dose administered over 30 minutes followed by 1–2 mg/min constant infusion.

F. In patients who have wide complex tachycardia with a regular RR interval and AV synchrony, supraventricular tachycardia (SVT) may be suspected. However, in all cases of wide complex tachycardia, one should always be wary of VT. Consequently, in patients with suspected SVT with aberrant conduction, it is recommended that adenosine rather than verapamil be used for management. Although AV dissociation virtually establishes a diagnosis of VT, the presence of AV association does not exclude VT. In patients in whom an assessment of AV synchrony cannot be made, procainamide should be administered. This successfully treats most cases of paroxysmal supraventricular tachycardia (PSVT) and provides reasonable management of VT.

References

Li HJ, Morillo CA, Zardini M, et al. Effect of adenosine or adenosine triphosphate on antidromic tachycardia. J Am Coll Cardiol 1994; 24:728.

McGovern B, Garan H, Ruskin JN. Precipitation of cardiac arrest by verapamil in patients with Wolff-Parkinson-White syndrome. Ann Intern Med 1986; 104:791.

Rankin AC, Goldroyd K, Chong E, et al. Value and limitations of adenosine in the diagnosis and treatment of narrow and broad complex tachycardias. Br Heart J 1989; 62:195.

Tzivoni D, Banai S, Schuger C, et al. Treatment of torsades de pointes with magnesium sulfate. Circulation 1988; 77:392.

Woosley RL, Shand DG. Pharmacokinetics of antiarrhythmic drugs. Am J Cardiol 1978; 41:986.

Patient with WIDE QRS COMPLEX TACHYCARDIA

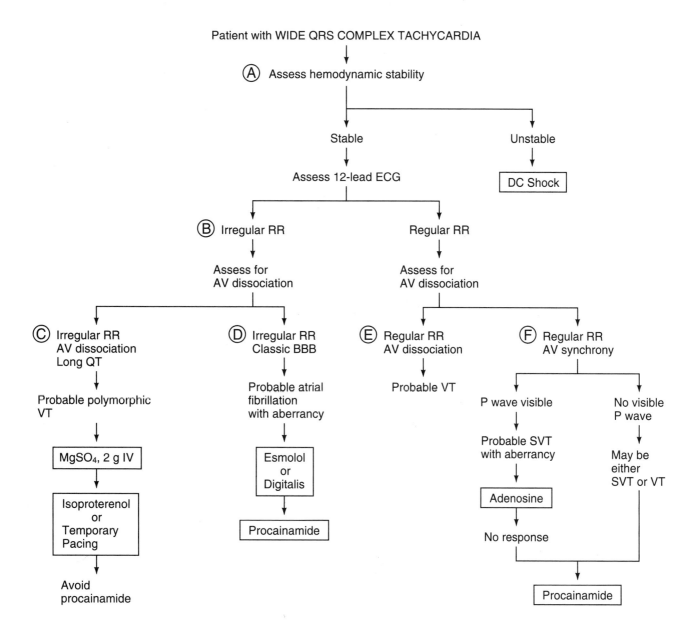

STABLE ANGINA

Samuel M. Butman

A. The evaluation of chronic stable angina should provide the clinician with documentation of coronary disease as the cause of chest pain, determine the efficacy of therapy, and select patients at high risk for infarction or death so that revascularization can be performed early and safely. When the diagnosis of chronic stable angina is made, evaluation and modification of risk factors should begin with cholesterol reduction, control of hypertension, weight loss, and smoking cessation.

B. The choice of stress testing is determined by the patient's resting ECG and ability to exercise and the clinician's familiarity with the study.

C. The most common stress test is the exercise treadmill test (ETT) in which the grade and rate of the treadmill are increased incrementally to achieve an increase in heart rate (HR) that correlates with an increase in oxygen consumption. The sensitivity of this test is about 65% (35% false-negative) and the specificity 90% (10% false-positive) when at least 85% of the predicted maximal HR is achieved. False-positive results are particularly common in patients taking digitalis and diuretics or who have hypertensive disease, hypertrophy, hypokalemia, Wolff-Parkinson-White syndrome, interventricular conduction defects, and left bundle branch block.

D. When a false-positive result is likely, the study can be performed with thallium imaging (Th-ETT), radionuclide angiography, or stress echocardiography.

E. Patients with a good chance of completing an exercise test proceed with Th-ETT, but if exercise tolerance or ability is questionable, an alternative is dipyridamole-thallium testing.

F. A nondiagnostic study is one in which an adequate HR is not achieved because of poor conditioning, other medical factors, or cardiac medications (β blockers and calcium channel blockers). A nondiagnostic study should be followed by a dipyridamole-thallium study. Patients with claudication, lung disease, arthritis, or other debilitating diseases should be spared a probable nondiagnostic study, and a dipyridamole-thallium study should be performed.

G. A positive stress test provides information to enable the clinician to stratify patients into high- and low-risk groups.

H. The criteria for high-risk patients with ETT include early onset of ST depression, >2 mm ST depression, ST changes at a low HR and level of exercise, or a drop in systolic blood pressure. Studies show that the degree of ST depression correlates with a higher incidence of left main and multivessel disease. Patients in the high-risk group are more likely to have a cardiac event and poorer survival than those in the low-risk group. Likewise, with thallium studies the increasing number of segments with reperfusion defects correlates with increasing severity of coronary disease (i.e., more myocardium at risk), and the same has been shown with wall motion abnormalities with stress echocardiography. Using radionuclide angiography, an exercise ejection fraction (EF) ≥50% is associated with a very good prognosis (regardless of resting EF), but one ≤35% is substantially worse (50% risk of cardiac event in 3 years). Irrespective of the method of stress testing chosen, all patients who fall into the high-risk group should undergo cardiac catheterization and appropriate revascularization with percutaneous coronary angioplasty (PTCA) or coronary artery bypass grafting (CABG), if needed.

I. The decision of which patients should have surgical therapy or medical therapy for coronary artery disease has been evaluated by three large, ongoing studies. Clearly, patients with refractory angina on maximally tolerated medical therapy should receive PTCA or CABG for symptom relief. Patients with left main disease have prolonged survival with surgical therapy, as do those with three-vessel disease and two-vessel disease with proximal left-anterior descending (LAD) stenosis and who have decreased EF and evidence of ischemia. Studies comparing CABG with PTCA for multivessel disease show fairly equivalent results, except in diabetic patients, in whom CABG is a better choice.

References

Bonow RO. Prognostic implications of exercise radionuclide angiography in patients with coronary artery disease. Mayo Clin Proc 1988; 63:630.

Brown KA. Prognostic value of thallium 201 myocardial perfusion imaging: a diagnostic tool comes of age. Circulation 1991; 83:363.

Helfant RH. Stable angina pectoris: risk stratification and therapeutic options. Circulation 1990; 82(Suppl II):66.

King SB 3rd, Lembo NJ, Weintraub WS, et al. A randomized trial comparing coronary angioplasty with coronary bypass surgery. Emory Angioplasty versus Surgery Trial. N Engl J Med 1994, 331:1044.

Kirklin JW, Akins CW, Blackstone EH, et al. Guidelines and indications for coronary artery bypass graft surgery. J Am Coll Cardiol 1991; 17:543.

Schlant RC, Blomquist CG, Brandenberg RO, et al. Guidelines for exercise testing. J Am Coll Cardiol 1986; 8:725.

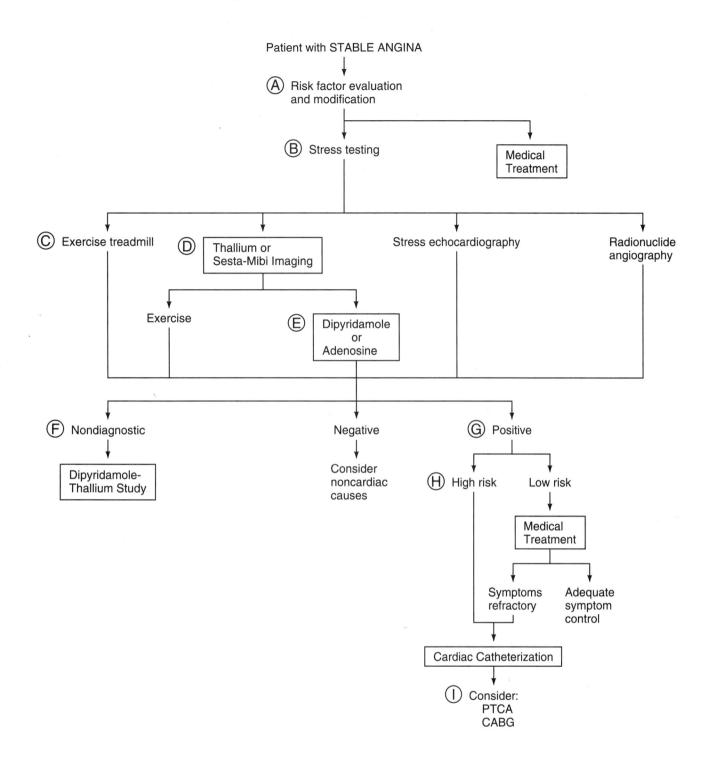

Patient with STABLE ANGINA

Ⓐ Risk factor evaluation and modification

Ⓑ Stress testing

Medical Treatment

Ⓒ Exercise treadmill

Ⓓ Thallium or Sesta-Mibi Imaging

Stress echocardiography

Radionuclide angiography

Exercise

Ⓔ Dipyridamole or Adenosine

Ⓕ Nondiagnostic

Dipyridamole-Thallium Study

Negative

Consider noncardiac causes

Ⓖ Positive

Ⓗ High risk

Low risk

Medical Treatment

Symptoms refractory

Adequate symptom control

Cardiac Catheterization

Ⓘ Consider: PTCA CABG

UNSTABLE ANGINA

Samuel M. Butman
Karl B. Kern

Unstable angina is a clinical syndrome defined by one of the following entities: (1) new-onset angina or ischemia, (2) intensification (quality, duration, or inciting factors) of pre-existing angina, or (3) angina that occurs at rest. The natural history of unstable angina has been studied. Approximately 10–15% of patients with unstable angina have an acute myocardial infarction (MI) during that hospitalization, and 10–40% experience an MI within the next year. The incidence of death is 1–5% in the hospital, and 5–25% over the next year. Approximately one third of patients with unstable angina undergo coronary artery bypass grafting (CABG) within 1 year. In addition, 40–60% of patients with acute infarctions experience antecedent unstable angina. The goal of therapy for unstable angina should be to decrease the risk of infarction and death.

A. Diagnosis of unstable angina depends on a careful clinical history, physical examination, and examination of a resting 12-lead ECG. Therefore the initial evaluation of patients with symptoms consistent with ischemic pain usually should not be done by telephone. The most common ECG changes with unstable angina are T wave changes (present 62% of the time), including T-wave inversion, flattening, or pseudonormalization (upright T waves with angina that are inverted at baseline). ST segment depression is present in 20–30% of patients with unstable angina chest pain. The absence of ECG changes does not rule out significant coronary disease.

B. "Unstable" angina can be subclassified by history, physical examination, and the resting ECG. Persons with new-onset angina and those who experience a change in symptoms have a better prognosis than those who develop angina at rest. New-onset angina probably represents progressive luminal narrowing that has advanced to a critical obstruction of coronary blood flow. Persons with new-onset angina have less severe coronary disease, higher left ventricular ejection fractions, and lower mortality rates.

C. Those with significant (>20 minutes) ongoing rest pain associated with signs of heart failure, new valvular regurgitation, hypotension, or ST depression on ECG are at especially high risk for MI or death.

D. High- and intermediate-risk patients should be hospitalized and treated aggressively with IV medication.

E. If the patient continues to have significant chest pain despite IV medication, urgent cardiac catheterization should be done with the idea of offering some form of acute revascularization, catheter based or surgical.

F. If the patient can be stabilized, it is optimal to wait 24–48 hours before performing revascularization secondary to decreased complications at angioplasty.

G. Patients without high- or intermediate-risk features can be safely treated and evaluated as outpatients. This includes patients with an increase in angina or those with "new-onset" angina beginning >2 weeks before their seeking medical assistance. Adequate follow-up is critical to the outpatient approach. Re-evaluate within 72 hours.

H. If the patient is stabilized, outpatient work-up, either exercise stress testing or catheterization, is acceptable. If still symptomatic, the patient should be hospitalized and treated more aggressively.

References

Ambrose JA, Winters SL, Arora RR, et al. Angiographic evolution of coronary artery morphology in unstable angina. J Am Coll Cardiol 1986; 7:472.

Braunwald E. Unstable angina: a classification. Circulation 1989; 80:410.

Braunwald E, Brown J, Brown L, et al. Clinical practice guideline, unstable angina: diagnosis and management. (Agency for Health Care Policy and Research Publication No. 94-0602).

Butman SM, Olson HG, Butman LK. Early exercise testing after stabilization of unstable angina: correlation with coronary angiographic findings and subsequent cardiac events. Am Heart J 1986; 111:11.

Calvin JE, Klein LW, Vandenberg BJ, et al. Risk stratification in unstable angina, prospective validation of the Braunwald Classification. JAMA 1995; 273:136.

Myler RK, Shaw RE, Stertzer SH, et al. Unstable angina and coronary angioplasty. Circulation 1990; 82(Suppl II):11.

Théroux P, Duimet H, McCans J, et al. Aspirin, heparin, or both to treat acute unstable angina. N Engl J Med 1988; 319:1105.

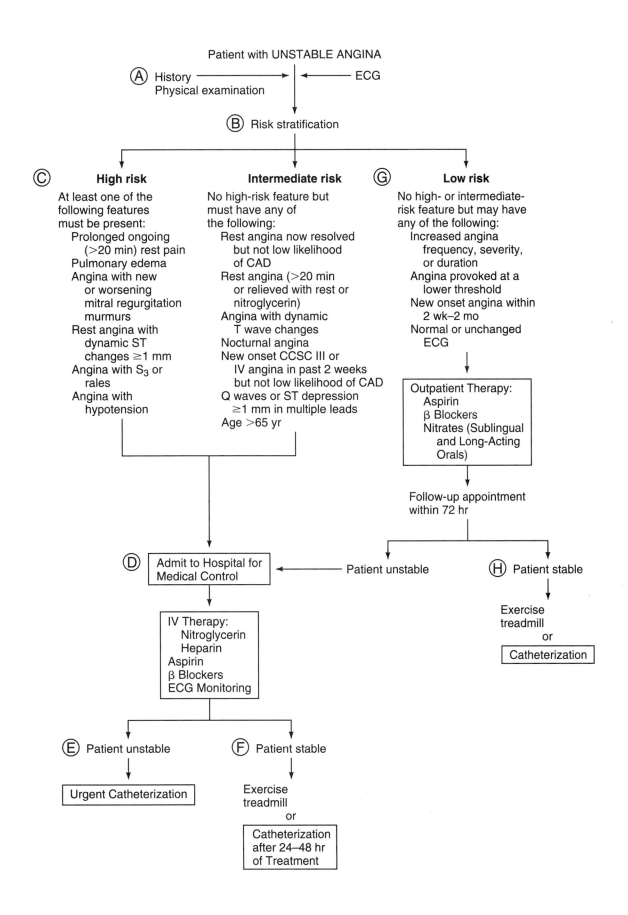

Patient with UNSTABLE ANGINA

Ⓐ History ——————→ ←—————— ECG
Physical examination

Ⓑ Risk stratification

High risk Ⓒ

At least one of the
following features
must be present:
  Prolonged ongoing
    (>20 min) rest pain
  Pulmonary edema
  Angina with new
    or worsening
    mitral regurgitation
    murmurs
  Rest angina with
    dynamic ST
    changes ≥1 mm
  Angina with S_3 or
    rales
  Angina with
    hypotension

Intermediate risk

No high-risk feature but
must have any of
the following:
  Rest angina now resolved
    but not low likelihood
    of CAD
  Rest angina (>20 min
    or relieved with rest or
    nitroglycerin)
  Angina with dynamic
    T wave changes
  Nocturnal angina
  New onset CCSC III or
    IV angina in past 2 weeks
    but not low likelihood of CAD
  Q waves or ST depression
    ≥1 mm in multiple leads
  Age >65 yr

Low risk Ⓖ

No high- or intermediate-
risk feature but may have
any of the following:
  Increased angina
    frequency, severity,
    or duration
  Angina provoked at a
    lower threshold
  New onset angina within
    2 wk–2 mo
  Normal or unchanged
    ECG

Outpatient Therapy:
  Aspirin
  β Blockers
  Nitrates (Sublingual
    and Long-Acting
    Orals)

Follow-up appointment
within 72 hr

Ⓓ Admit to Hospital for
Medical Control ←—————— Patient unstable

Ⓗ Patient stable

IV Therapy:
  Nitroglycerin
  Heparin
  Aspirin
  β Blockers
  ECG Monitoring

Exercise
treadmill
or
Catheterization

Ⓔ Patient unstable

Urgent Catheterization

Ⓕ Patient stable

Exercise
treadmill
or
Catheterization
after 24–48 hr
of Treatment

SYSTOLIC MURMUR

Alberta L. Warner

A. After it has been determined whether a murmur occurs during systole or diastole, the next step is to listen carefully during respiration. Systolic murmurs of right-side origin usually increase during inspiration, whereas left-sided systolic murmurs increase during expiration.

B. It may be difficult to identify a murmur as regurgitant or ejection. If the patient has occasional ectopy or an irregular rhythm, listen for a change in intensity after a pause. An ejection or outflow murmur increases in intensity after a pause, whereas a regurgitant murmur remains unchanged. One must also identify the relationship of the murmur to the first and second heart sounds. An ejection murmur cannot begin until the aortic or pulmonic valve opens, after the isovolumetric contraction period, and thus well after S_1. In contrast, a regurgitant murmur usually begins as soon as the pressure in the ventricle rises above that in the atrium, and thus with S_1. Furthermore, regurgitant murmurs usually do not end until after the aortic component of S_2 into the isovolumetric relaxation period. Although the classic regurgitant murmur is holosystolic, regurgitant murmurs may be early systolic (as in acute mitral regurgitation [MR]) or late systolic (as in mitral valve prolapse [MVP]). Hence, a systolic murmur that begins with S_1 or continues into S_2 usually is regurgitant.

C. The presence of other heart sounds gives clues to the origin of a systolic murmur. An ejection sound, which is high pitched and occurs shortly after S_1, may be present with pulmonic stenosis (PS) or aortic stenosis (AS). Abnormal splitting of S_2, such as the wide fixed split S_2 of an atrial septal defect, or the paradoxically split S_2 of severe AS, aids in diagnosis. The clicks of MVP are distinguished by their movement away from S_1 with squatting and toward S_1 with standing.

D. An "innocent" murmur is one caused by normal turbulence across the pulmonic or aortic valve in a patient with a normal cardiovascular system. Murmurs that occur in high-output states such as anemia or sepsis are caused by turbulent flow, but they are not necessarily innocent by definition. Innocent murmurs are ejection murmurs that decrease or even disappear with maneuvers that decrease venous return (Valsalva, standing) and increase with maneuvers that increase venous return (squatting). The presence of an ejection sound or abnormal splitting of S_2 identifies AS or PS. Innocent flow murmurs can be identified by their soft quality, short duration, occurrence only in early systole, and localiza-tion along the left sternal border. The key is the absence of apparent cardiac pathology on history taking or thorough examination. ECG and chest films are normal, whereas left ventricular hypertrophy is evident with AS. Echo-Doppler evaluation is a reliable diagnostic tool for clarification or confirmation of a diagnosis and a means to quantitate more accurately the severity of a valvular lesion.

E. To further characterize a systolic murmur, dynamic auscultation should be used during Valsalva, squatting, and standing maneuvers. The murmur of hypertrophic cardiomyopathy (HCM) can be especially distinguished with these maneuvers. Maneuvers that decrease venous return (e.g., Valsalva or standing from a squatting position) increase the intensity of the murmur of HCM. The murmur of AS may decrease in intensity, whereas that of MR or ventricular septal defect (VSD) may remain unchanged. Conversely, maneuvers that increase venous return (e.g., squatting) decrease the murmur of HCM, whereas other systolic murmurs increase or remain unchanged. An exception to this is the murmur of MVP, which may begin earlier in systole with the Valsalva maneuver and later in systole with the squatting maneuver. This is distinguished from the murmur of HCM, which varies in intensity rather than in timing with these maneuvers.

F. The murmurs of MR and VSD demonstrate similar changes in response to maneuvers. MR is distinguished by its localization at the apex, whereas the murmur of VSD is localized at the lower left sternal border. Furthermore, the presence of right ventricular hypertrophy on ECG or chest film supports the diagnosis of VSD, as opposed to that of MR in which left ventricular and left atrial enlargement predominate.

References

Ewy GA. Bedside evaluation of the cardiac patient. Hosp Med 1980; 16:11.

Grewe K, Crawford MH, O'Rourke RA. Differentiation of cardiac murmurs by dynamic auscultation. Curr Probl Cardiol 1988; 10:671.

Lembo NJ, Dell'Italia LJ, Crawford JH, et al. Bedside diagnosis of systolic murmurs. N Engl J Med 1988; 318:1572.

Warner AL, Ewy GA. Using the cardiovascular physical exam to full advantage. Contemp Intern Med 1992; Feb:51.

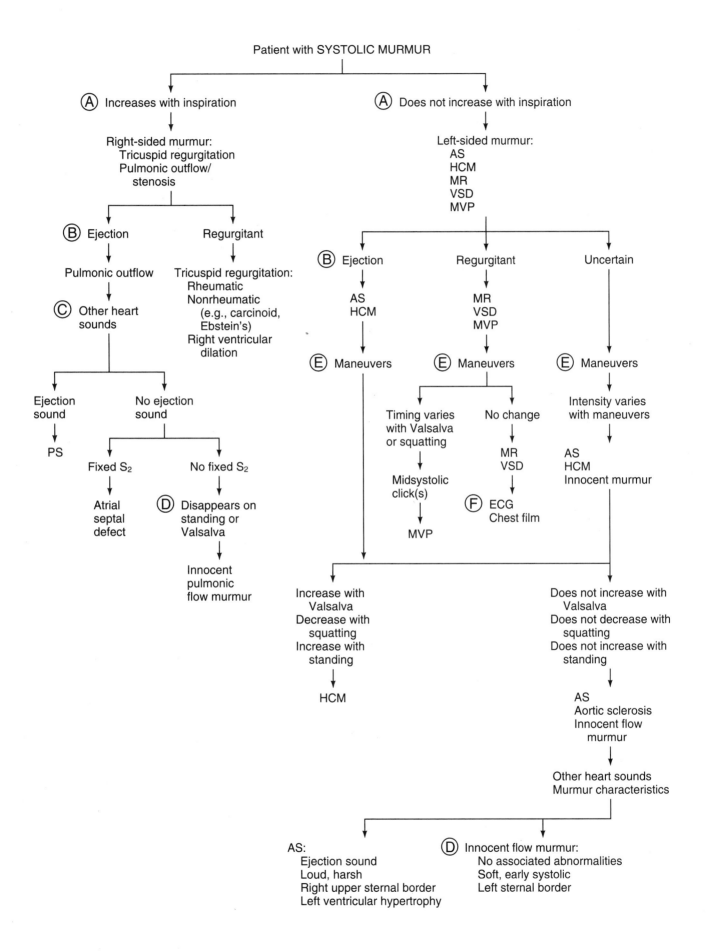

Patient with SYSTOLIC MURMUR

Ⓐ Increases with inspiration

Right-sided murmur:
 Tricuspid regurgitation
 Pulmonic outflow/
  stenosis

Ⓑ Ejection

Pulmonic outflow

Ⓒ Other heart
 sounds

Ejection
sound

PS

No ejection
sound

Fixed S₂

Atrial
septal
defect

No fixed S₂

Ⓓ Disappears on
 standing or
 Valsalva

Innocent
pulmonic
flow murmur

Regurgitant

Tricuspid regurgitation:
 Rheumatic
 Nonrheumatic
  (e.g., carcinoid,
  Ebstein's)
 Right ventricular
  dilation

Ⓐ Does not increase with inspiration

Left-sided murmur:
 AS
 HCM
 MR
 VSD
 MVP

Ⓑ Ejection

AS
HCM

Ⓔ Maneuvers

Regurgitant

MR
VSD
MVP

Ⓔ Maneuvers

Timing varies
with Valsalva
or squatting

Midsystolic
click(s)

MVP

No change

MR
VSD

Ⓕ ECG
 Chest film

Uncertain

Ⓔ Maneuvers

Intensity varies
with maneuvers

AS
HCM
Innocent murmur

Increase with
Valsalva
Decrease with
squatting
Increase with
standing

HCM

Does not increase with
Valsalva
Does not decrease with
squatting
Does not increase with
standing

AS
Aortic sclerosis
Innocent flow
murmur

Other heart sounds
Murmur characteristics

AS:
 Ejection sound
 Loud, harsh
 Right upper sternal border
 Left ventricular hypertrophy

Ⓓ Innocent flow murmur:
 No associated abnormalities
 Soft, early systolic
 Left sternal border

DIASTOLIC MURMUR

Alberta L. Warner

A. The presence of a diastolic murmur usually indicates cardiovascular pathology. As with systolic murmurs, careful auscultation during respiration should be performed. Augmentation of a diastolic murmur during inspiration suggests a right-sided murmur, either tricuspid stenosis or pulmonic regurgitation. Left-sided diastolic murmurs, as mitral stenosis or aortic regurgitation (AR), soften with inspiration and increase during expiration.

B. Tricuspid stenosis and pulmonic regurgitation may be distinguished by their differences in location and pitch. Tricuspid stenosis is heard as a low-pitched diastolic rumble along the lower left sternal border, whereas pulmonic regurgitation presents with a higher-pitched murmur at the upper left sternal border. Tricuspid stenosis, which is relatively rare, almost always is rheumatic in origin and usually is associated with rheumatic mitral valve disease. The presence of prominent A waves in the jugular venous pulse and of ascites supports a diagnosis of significant tricuspid stenosis, which may be masked by concomitant mitral stenosis on auscultation.

C. Pulmonic regurgitation often occurs secondary to pulmonary hypertension and is called a *Graham Steell murmur*. A right ventricular lift along the left sternal border, an increased pulmonic component of the second heart sound, and associated tricuspid regurgitation suggest pulmonic regurgitation from pulmonary hypertension.

D. As with right-sided murmurs, the murmurs of mitral stenosis and aortic regurgitation usually can be distinguished by their quality and localization. AR is heard best along the left sternal border, with the patient upright or leaning forward, and has a high-pitched blowing quality. AR from aortic root dilation rather than leaflet incompetence often is heard best at the right upper sternal border. In contrast, mitral stenosis is low-pitched, requiring the bell of the stethoscope to hear the characteristic "rumble," and is heard best at the apex with the patient in a left lateral decubitus position.

E. An Austin Flint murmur is a low-pitched diastolic murmur that occurs in severe AR because of impaired opening of the anterior leaflet of the mitral valve against the regurgitant aortic jet. The absence of an opening snap or the presence of left ventricular (LV) enlargement support the diagnosis of an Austin Flint murmur from AR, rather than that of mitral stenosis. Amyl nitrate, which lowers systemic vascular resistance, increases the murmur of mitral stenosis but decreases diastolic murmurs from AR.

F. Acute AR caused by aortic dissection, infective endocarditis, or trauma presents clinically differently from chronic AR and must be identified. Because the increase in LV load, congestive heart failure may occur early and suddenly. The pulse pressure usually is not increased in acute AR; hence peripheral findings of chronic AR such as Duroziez' sign or Quincke's sign are not present. On auscultation, S_1 may be soft because of early closure of the mitral valve, and an S_3 sound often is present. The murmur of acute AR is shorter and lower-pitched than that of chronic AR because of the rapid rise in LV pressure. Indeed, a shortening or diminishing AR murmur may herald acute worsening of AR.

References

Braunwald E. Valvular heart disease. In: Braunwald E, ed. Heart disease: a textbook of cardiovascular medicine. 5th ed. Philadelphia: WB Saunders, 1997:1007.

Grewe K, Crawford MH, O'Rourke RA. Differentiation of cardiac murmurs by dynamic auscultation. Curr Probl Cardiol 1988; 10:671.

Warner AL, Ewy GA. Using the cardiovascular physical exam to full advantage. Contemp Intern Med 1992; Feb:51.

Patient with DIASTOLIC MURMUR

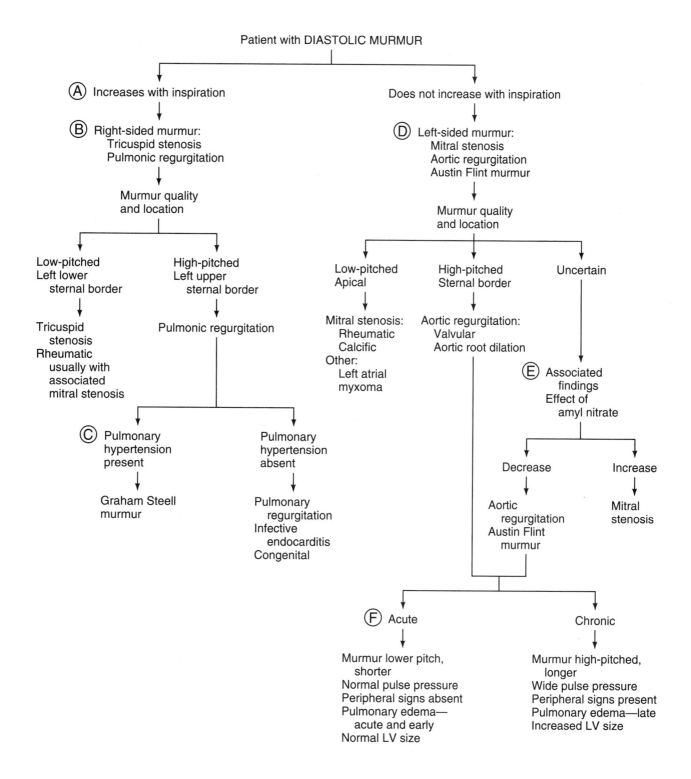

A Increases with inspiration

B Right-sided murmur:
   Tricuspid stenosis
   Pulmonic regurgitation

Murmur quality
and location

Low-pitched
Left lower
sternal border

High-pitched
Left upper
sternal border

Tricuspid
stenosis
Rheumatic
usually with
associated
mitral stenosis

Pulmonic regurgitation

C Pulmonary
hypertension
present

Pulmonary
hypertension
absent

Graham Steell
murmur

Pulmonary
regurgitation
Infective
endocarditis
Congenital

Does not increase with inspiration

D Left-sided murmur:
   Mitral stenosis
   Aortic regurgitation
   Austin Flint murmur

Murmur quality
and location

Low-pitched
Apical

High-pitched
Sternal border

Uncertain

Mitral stenosis:
   Rheumatic
   Calcific
Other:
   Left atrial
   myxoma

Aortic regurgitation:
   Valvular
   Aortic root dilation

E Associated
findings
Effect of
amyl nitrate

Decrease

Increase

Aortic
regurgitation
Austin Flint
murmur

Mitral
stenosis

F Acute

Chronic

Murmur lower pitch,
   shorter
Normal pulse pressure
Peripheral signs absent
Pulmonary edema—
   acute and early
Normal LV size

Murmur high-pitched,
   longer
Wide pulse pressure
Peripheral signs present
Pulmonary edema—late
Increased LV size

HYPERTENSION

Pamela J. Davis

Hypertension (HTN) is the most common reason for a patient to see a physician in the United States today and is the most common indication for the use of prescription medication. The primary care physician plays a key role in the detection, assessment, and treatment of HTN. About 58 million Americans have HTN, defined as elevated blood pressure (BP): systolic pressure (SBP) ≥140 mm Hg and/or diastolic pressure (DBP) ≥90 mm Hg. The prevalence of HTN and HTN-related complications (stroke, heart failure, end-stage renal disease) increases with age and degree of elevation of BP and is greater in African-Americans than in whites. HTN with no definable cause is termed *primary, idiopathic,* or *essential HTN.* HTN caused by a specific organ or metabolic defect is termed *secondary HTN.*

A. HTN should not be diagnosed on the basis of a single BP reading or a single visit, unless severe HTN (SBP ≥180 mm Hg) or target organ damage (TOD) is present. Individuals commonly experience a transient, moderate elevation in BP when under stress (e.g., in an emergency department or doctor's office or while in pain). Elevated BP readings in this setting may be spurious and should be repeated. The following measurement techniques are recommended: (1) The patient should be seated, back supported, with arm bared and positioned at heart level, and should rest quietly for 5 minutes before measurement; (2) there should be no caffeine or tobacco intake within 30 minutes before measurement; (3) measurements should be taken with a mercury sphygmomanometer; (4) an appropriate cuff size should be used to ensure an accurate measurement (the bladder within the cuff should encircle at least 80% of the arm); (5) SBP and DBP should be recorded at least twice, separated by 2 minutes and averaged using the disappearance of sound (phase V) for DBP reading. Patients should be informed and taught the meaning of their BP readings and advised of the need for periodic measurement. Screening for HTN is cost-effective for all adults. BP should be measured at all initial contacts, no matter how brief.

B. The objectives in evaluating a patient with HTN are (1) to identify the specific cause of HTN, looking for secondary causes; (2) to assess the presence or absence of TOD and cardiovascular disease (CVD), the extent of disease, and the response to therapy; and (3) to estimate the patient's risk profile for the development of CVD and concomitant disorders that may affect prognosis and treatment. The history should emphasize the onset of HTN and prior BP levels; family history of CVD; personal history of diabetes mellitus, renal disease, hyperlipidemia, medications (herbal remedies, nonprescription drugs, prior HTN medications); weight loss or gain; lifestyle factors such as alcohol, tobacco, and illicit drug use; sodium intake; and pertinent psychosocial and environmental factors such as stress and food preferences. In the review of systems, secondary HTN symptoms may be elicited. Headache, sweating, weight loss, palpitations (pheochromocytoma), muscle cramps, weakness, polyuria (hyperaldosteronism), leg claudication (coarctation), menstrual irregularities, easy bruising, or personality changes (Cushing's syndrome) are a few symptoms that may be revealed.

C. Observe the patient's appearance, noting any stigmata of disease. Focus on height and weight measurements, body mass index (BMI), funduscopic examination, palpation of the thyroid, careful cardiopulmonary review, evaluation of peripheral vasculature, and neurologic assessment. Most patients with established HTN of several years' duration may exhibit varying degrees of TOD. Narrowing of the arteriolar wall and obscuring of veins as they cross behind arteries (grade I, II) are seen in early stages of HTN. More serious disease is indicated by hemorrhages and exudate (grade III), which may progress to papilledema (grade IV). Examine the neck for carotid bruits and increased jugular venous pressure; the lungs for bibasilar rales; the heart for increased rate and size, clicks, murmurs, and S_3 and S_4 heart sounds; and the abdomen for bruits and masses. Measure BP in both arms and perform simultaneous radiofemoral pulse palpation. Finally, a simple neurologic examination may uncover evidence of a previous stroke or neurologic deficit. On the basis of the history and physical examination, most secondary causes of HTN can be excluded and overall cardiovascular status determined.

D. The diagnostic tests ordered may depend on the patient's presentation, but these tests are essential in the routine evaluation of HTN: CBC; urinalysis; determinations of serum potassium, creatinine, BUN, calcium, fasting glucose, cholesterol, and high-density lipoprotein levels; and ECG. These tests usually provide sufficient information about the presence of TOD and the likelihood that complications will develop from BP elevation. When the history, physical examination, or laboratory evaluation suggests a secondary cause of HTN, obtain additional specific studies as indicated.

(Continued on page 76)

Patient with ELEVATED BLOOD PRESSURE (≥140/90)

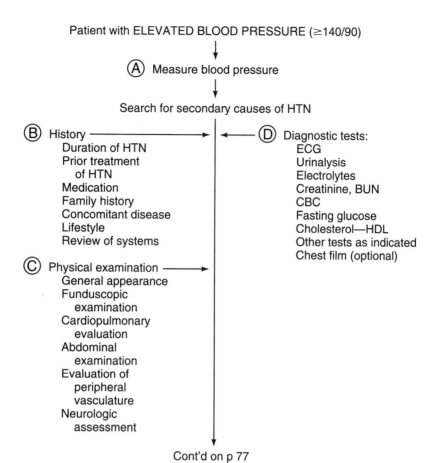

Ⓐ Measure blood pressure

Search for secondary causes of HTN

Ⓑ History
    Duration of HTN
    Prior treatment
      of HTN
    Medication
    Family history
    Concomitant disease
    Lifestyle
    Review of systems

Ⓒ Physical examination
    General appearance
    Funduscopic
      examination
    Cardiopulmonary
      evaluation
    Abdominal
      examination
    Evaluation of
      peripheral
      vasculature
    Neurologic
      assessment

Ⓓ Diagnostic tests:
    ECG
    Urinalysis
    Electrolytes
    Creatinine, BUN
    CBC
    Fasting glucose
    Cholesterol—HDL
    Other tests as indicated
    Chest film (optional)

Cont'd on p 77

E. Renovascular disease, a common cause of secondary HTN (1–5% of HTN patients), results in renal hypoperfusion and renovascular HTN (RVH). Suspect RVH when there is an abrupt onset of severe, difficult-to-control HTN in a woman <30 or >50 years of age, abdominal or flank bruits, HTN refractory to three-drug regimen, azotemia induced by angiotensin-converting enzyme inhibitors or angiotensin II receptor blockers, and evidence of TOD. The two main causes of RVH are fibromuscular dysplasia and atheromatous stenosis. Fibromuscular dysplasia usually is confined to the renal arteries, where it is characterized by one or more fibrous bands that partly occlude the lumen. Atheromatous stenosis commonly is bilateral and associated with stenosis in other arteries. In patients <50 years old fibromuscular dysplasia predominates, and in older patients RVH results from atheroma. The diagnosis is suggested by the captopril stimulation test. The patient should consume a normal amount of salt and discontinue all antihypertension medications, including diuretics, for at least 1 week before the test. The patient is seated for 30 minutes before and throughout the test. Plasma renin activity (PRA) is determined at baseline and 60 minutes after oral administration of 50 mg captopril. An increase in PRA at 60 minutes is the hallmark of RVH. Other diagnostic tools used to confirm RVH are duplex Doppler flow studies, magnetic resonance angiography, and renal arteriography.

F. Primary aldosteronism (Conn's syndrome) results from excessive aldosterone production from a unilateral adrenocortical adenoma, occurring with equal frequency on either side. Aldosterone-producing adenomas occur more commonly in women than in men, ages 30–50 years. Many patients have clinical and biochemical features characteristic of primary aldosteronism, but a solitary adenoma is not found at surgery. Instead, these patients have bilateral adrenocortical hyperplasia. Clinical features include refractory HTN, spontaneous hypokalemia, sensitivity to potassium-wasting diuretics, excessive urinary potassium, weakness, headache, muscle cramping, and polydipsia. The ECG shows signs of left ventricular enlargement and prominent U waves, denoting potassium depletion. Edema usually is absent. Patients with significant hypokalemia, suppressed PRA, or increased aldosterone excretion rate are unequivocal evidence of primary aldosteronism. Patients with equivocal findings require salt loading.

G. Pheochromocytoma occurs in ≤1% of HTN patients, generally in the fourth to sixth decades of life. It is a catecholamine-producing tumor arising from the adrenal medulla (only a small percentage originate in extra-adrenal sites). The distinctive clinical features of pheochromocytoma are related to excessive production of catecholamines. Clinical features are extremely variable, with paroxysmal HTN occurring in 50% of cases. Typical paroxysms consist of marked BP elevation, headache, sweating, palpitations, pallor, nausea, and abdominal discomfort. Attacks may be spontaneous or precipitated by emotion, smoking, exercise, or postural change. Pheochromocytomas are associated with neurofibromatosis, von Hippel-Lindau syndrome, and med-

ullary carcinoma of the thyroid. The diagnosis is based on elevated levels of catecholamines and their metabolites in the urine. Assays of urinary catecholamines and metanephrines usually are sufficient to diagnose pheochromocytoma in most patients, but when results are equivocal and pheochromocytoma is suggested clinically, plasma catecholamines should be measured. After diagnosis the tumor is located by abdominal CT scan. About 90% of pheochromocytomas are in an adrenal gland, with a 2:1 preference for the right over the left side.

H. Cushing's syndrome is caused by cortisol excess. The syndrome has an excessive mortality rate because of its association with CVD. HTN, present in >80% of patients with Cushing's syndrome, is the major risk factor for the development of premature CVD. Bruising, myopathy, HTN, edema, hirsutism, striae, and various neuropsychiatric disturbances ranging from a mild decrease in energy to severe depression are found in the syndrome. The extent of the work-up of patients with suspected Cushing's syndrome varies with the clinical situation. Although it is cumbersome to perform, 24-hour urinary free cortisol determination is the best available test for documenting endogenous hypercortisolism. If pituitary and ectopic sources cannot be differentiated on the basis of plasma cortisol levels alone, adrenocorticotropic hormone (ACTH) secretion should be manipulated pharmacologically. The overnight dexamethasone suppression test requires a blood collection only for serum cortisol at 8 AM after the patient has taken a 1-mg dose of dexamethasone at 11 PM the previous evening.

I. Coarctation of the aorta is a constriction of the lumen of the aorta, just below the origin of the left subclavian artery. The lesion occurs in 7% of patients with congenital heart disease and is twice as common in males than in females. The most striking finding is a systolic murmur best heard over the back, between the left scapula and the spine. Symptoms may include headache, cold extremities, fatigue, and claudication of lower extremities. HTN in the upper extremities and marked delay or diminution of femoral pulses are detected on physical examination. The ECG may reveal left ventricular hypertrophy of varying degree. Chest radiographs may show cardiomegaly, rib notching, and the "3" sign from dilation of the aorta above and below the constriction. Two-dimensional echocardiography is used to identify the site of the coarctation.

References

Braunwald E, Hollenberg NK. Hypertension: mechanisms and therapy. Atlas of heart diseases. Vol 1. Philadelphia: Current Medicine, 1995.

Joint National Committee on Detection, Evaluation and Treatment of High Blood Pressure. JNC V. Arch Intern Med 1993; 53:154.

Kaplan NM. Clinical hypertension. 6th ed. Baltimore: Williams & Wilkins, 1994.

Mann SJ, Pickering TG. Detection of renovascular hypertension: state of the art. Ann Intern Med 1992; 117:845.

Patient with ELEVATED BLOOD PRESSURE (≥140/90)
(Cont'd from p 75)

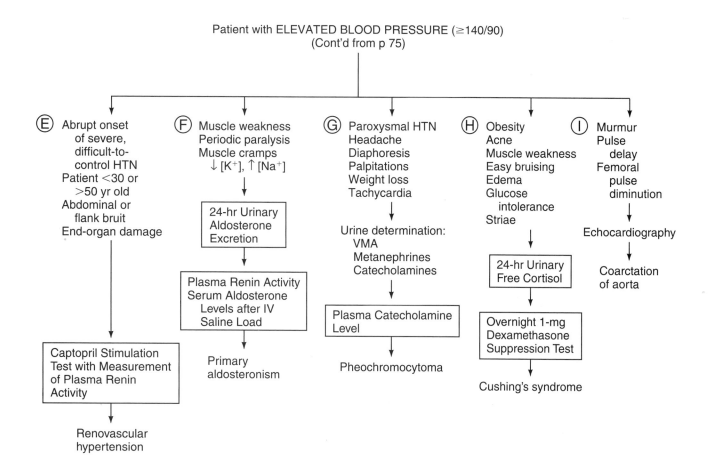

Ⓔ Abrupt onset
of severe,
difficult-to-
control HTN
Patient <30 or
>50 yr old
Abdominal or
flank bruit
End-organ damage

Captopril Stimulation
Test with Measurement
of Plasma Renin
Activity

Renovascular
hypertension

Ⓕ Muscle weakness
Periodic paralysis
Muscle cramps
↓ [K$^+$], ↑ [Na$^+$]

24-hr Urinary
Aldosterone
Excretion

Plasma Renin Activity
Serum Aldosterone
Levels after IV
Saline Load

Primary
aldosteronism

Ⓖ Paroxysmal HTN
Headache
Diaphoresis
Palpitations
Weight loss
Tachycardia

Urine determination:
VMA
Metanephrines
Catecholamines

Plasma Catecholamine
Level

Pheochromocytoma

Ⓗ Obesity
Acne
Muscle weakness
Easy bruising
Edema
Glucose
intolerance
Striae

24-hr Urinary
Free Cortisol

Overnight 1-mg
Dexamethasone
Suppression Test

Cushing's syndrome

Ⓘ Murmur
Pulse
delay
Femoral
pulse
diminution

Echocardiography

Coarctation
of aorta

HYPOTENSION

Mark C. Goldberg

The systolic pressure at which a patient can be considered hypotensive is variable. When systolic blood pressure drops below 80 mm Hg, symptoms and signs of a generalized inadequacy in tissue perfusion often are noted. Chronically hypertensive patients may manifest these symptoms and signs long before their systolic pressure reaches 80 mm Hg.

A. If the cause of hypotension does not declare itself immediately on presentation, the symptoms and signs of inadequate tissue perfusion will alert the examiner to the rapid need for investigation. An altered sensorium; diaphoresis; tachycardia; a drop in urine output; tachypnea; and cool, clammy skin typically are present. A history and physical examination in conjunction with basic laboratory studies (including chest films and ECG) usually provide a diagnosis.

B. ECG monitoring begins on presentation of the hypotensive patient. The prevalence of coronary artery disease makes acute myocardial infarction (MI) a likely cause of hypotension in the middle-aged and elderly population. In the setting of acute MI, malignant arrhythmias may be effectively treated with DC cardioversion if they need to be treated immediately. In situations unrelated to an ischemic event, supraventricular and ventricular arrhythmias may cause hypotension by reducing the ventricular filling period. Pharmacologic therapy occasionally is indicated, but cardioversion is most often preferred in hypotensive patients.

C. In patients with acute MI and hypotension, Swan-Ganz catheterization is used to direct therapy. A moderately elevated left-sided filling pressure suggests substantial loss of left ventricular (LV) muscle, which may result in progression to cardiogenic shock. Conversely, a normal-to-low pulmonary capillary wedge pressure (PCWP) with an elevated right ventricular (RV) pressure is found in RV infarction. This usually arises when an inferior infarction involves the right ventricle. If the PCWP tracing shows large V waves, acute papillary muscle rupture must be suspected. Oxygen saturations may be performed on blood withdrawn from ports located at various positions on the catheter. If RV saturation exceeds right atrial (RA) saturation, a ventricular septal defect may be diagnosed.

D. The chest film in cardiac tamponade often shows an enlarged cardiac silhouette. Patients in congestive heart failure have Kerley B lines, interstitial edema, and pulmonary effusions in addition to an enlarged cardiac silhouette.

E. A crude gauge of volume status may be obtained from the BUN/creatinine ratio. The hemoglobin may be followed in a bleeding patient, although it is not useful in acute situations.

F. Cardiac tamponade may be considered a state of relative volume depletion in that ventricular filling is compromised although the patient is euvolemic. Both echocardiography and Swan-Ganz catheterization may be used to confirm the diagnosis. On echocardiography, evidence of RA or RV collapse in addition to specific Doppler flow patterns are diagnostic. The Swan-Ganz catheter shows an equalization of pressures throughout the heart brought about by external compression of the heart.

G. Pneumothorax may be diagnosed on chest film by a shift in mediastinal location and loss of pulmonary markings in the periphery of the affected hemithorax.

References

Forrester JS, Diamond MD, Chatterjee K, Swan HJ. Medical therapy of acute myocardial infarction by application of hemodynamic subsets. N Engl J Med 1976; 295:1356.

Fox AC, Glassman E. Surgical remediable complications of myocardial infarction. Prog Cardiovasc Dis 1979; 21:461.

Yakaitis RW, Ewy GA, Otto CW, et al. Influence of time and therapy on ventricular defibrillation in dogs. Crit Care Med 1986; 8:157.

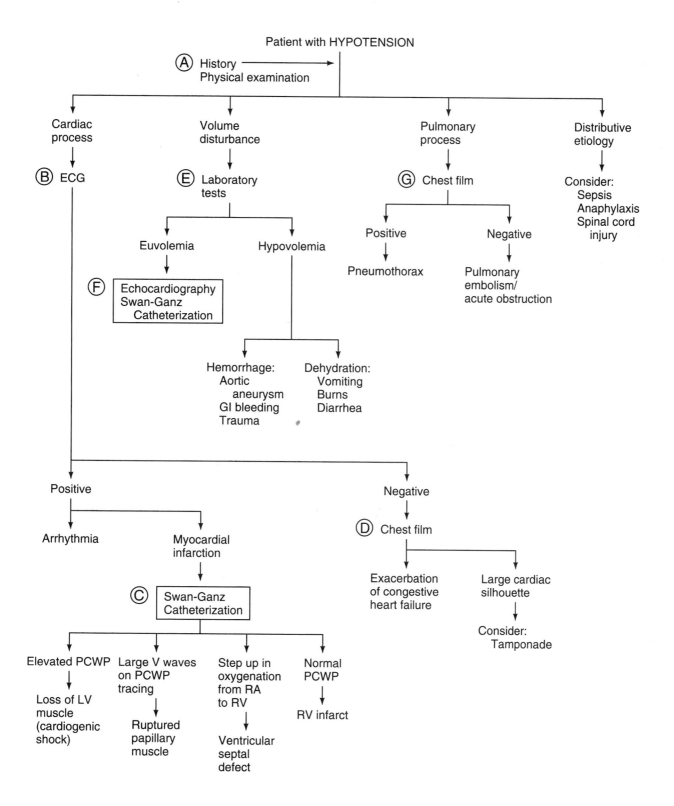

Patient with HYPOTENSION

(A) History
Physical examination

Cardiac process

Volume disturbance

Pulmonary process

Distributive etiology

(B) ECG

(E) Laboratory tests

(G) Chest film

Consider:
Sepsis
Anaphylaxis
Spinal cord injury

Euvolemia

Hypovolemia

Positive

Negative

(F) Echocardiography
Swan-Ganz
Catheterization

Pneumothorax

Pulmonary embolism/ acute obstruction

Hemorrhage:
Aortic aneurysm
GI bleeding
Trauma

Dehydration:
Vomiting
Burns
Diarrhea

Positive

Negative

Arrhythmia

Myocardial infarction

(D) Chest film

Exacerbation of congestive heart failure

Large cardiac silhouette

(C) Swan-Ganz Catheterization

Consider:
Tamponade

Elevated PCWP

Large V waves on PCWP tracing

Step up in oxygenation from RA to RV

Normal PCWP

Loss of LV muscle (cardiogenic shock)

Ruptured papillary muscle

Ventricular septal defect

RV infarct

PALPITATIONS

Karl B. Kern
Paul E. Fenster

Palpitations are a common problem. Recent evidence suggests a more cautious approach to antiarrhythmic therapy in dealing with such problems.

A. The history and physical examination should be targeted toward revealing any reversible cause for the palpitations. Most important is the patient's current use of medications. Stimulants, including caffeine and smoking, should also be reviewed carefully. Metabolic, pulmonary, and neurologic/psychiatric causes should then be considered.

B. Important in the work-up of palpitations is the relative frequency at which they occur. If they are infrequent but bothersome, an event monitor may help. Such a device can be worn for up to 1 week and has the ability to continuously monitor the patient's rhythm, but it records the rhythm only when specific buttons are activated. Some devices can even "go back in time" and record up to 15–30 seconds before the moment when the recording button is activated. If the palpitations are associated with exercise, an ETT can help.

C. Results from the monitoring period may vary. Some patients may experience their symptoms and yet show no correlation on the monitor to a rhythm disturbance. No cardiac treatment is then necessary.

D. Supraventricular arrhythmias may cause palpitations. If atrial fibrillation is discovered, an assessment of underlying organic heart disease is helpful because thromboembolism is common in patients with heart disease and atrial fibrillation.

E. Discovery of atrial premature contractions (APCs) or even supraventricular tachycardia (SVT) may first be dealt with as benign and with reassurance. If symptoms are troublesome, therapy may be indicated. (See pp 62 and 63.)

F. If ventricular ectopy is the cause of palpitations, the underlying status of myocardial disease is an important factor in considering treatment. If there is no evidence of coronary artery disease (CAD) or left ventricular dysfunction, reassurance, even for nonsustained ventricular tachycardia, appears to be the best therapeutic choice.

G. If there is left ventricular dysfunction, treatment of the underlying condition is most helpful.

H. The presence of CAD should lead to Holter- or electrophysiologic study (EPS)-guided treatment for any serious form of ventricular ectopy. Alternatives are empiric amiodarone therapy or an implantable device (automatic implantable cardioverter-defibrillator [AICD]) if documented, serious ventricular ectopy is found.

I. Bradycardia can also cause palpitations. Most commonly, medications are involved. If bradycardia is not caused by a reversible cause (e.g., drugs) and the degree of block is advanced (Mobitz II or worse), pacemaker therapy is worth considering.

References

Burkart F, Pfisterer M, Kiowski W, et al. Effect of antiarrhythmic therapy on mortality in survivors of myocardial infarction with symptomatic complex ventricular arrhythmias: Basel Antiarrhythmic Study of Infarct Survival (BASIS). J Am Coll Cardiol 1990; 16:1711.
Cardiac Arrhythmia Suppression Trial. Preliminary report: effect of encainide and flecainide on mortality in a randomized trial of arrhythmia suppression after myocardial infarction. N Engl J Med 1989; 321:406.
SPAF Investigators. Preliminary report of the Stroke Prevention in Atrial Fibrillation Study. N Engl J Med 1990; 322:863.
SPAF Investigators. Warfarin versus aspirin for prevention of thromboembolism in atrial fibrillation: Stroke Prevention in Atrial Fibrillation II Study. Lancet 1994; 343:687.
Stanton MS, Prystowsky EN, Fineberg NS, et al. Arrhythmogenic effects of antiarrhythmic drugs: a study of 506 patients treated for ventricular tachycardia or fibrillation. J Am Coll Cardiol 1989; 14:209.

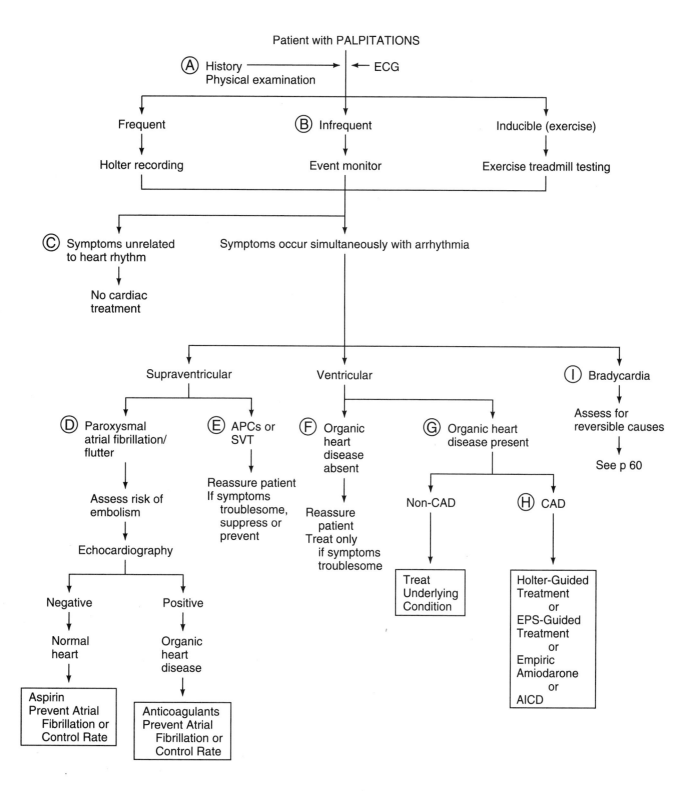

Patient with PALPITATIONS

(A) History → ECG
Physical examination

Frequent → Holter recording

(B) Infrequent → Event monitor

Inducible (exercise) → Exercise treadmill testing

(C) Symptoms unrelated to heart rhythm → No cardiac treatment

Symptoms occur simultaneously with arrhythmia

Supraventricular

(D) Paroxysmal atrial fibrillation/ flutter → Assess risk of embolism → Echocardiography

Negative → Normal heart → Aspirin Prevent Atrial Fibrillation or Control Rate

Positive → Organic heart disease → Anticoagulants Prevent Atrial Fibrillation or Control Rate

(E) APCs or SVT → Reassure patient If symptoms troublesome, suppress or prevent

Ventricular

(F) Organic heart disease absent → Reassure patient Treat only if symptoms troublesome

(G) Organic heart disease present

Non-CAD → Treat Underlying Condition

(H) CAD → Holter-Guided Treatment or EPS-Guided Treatment or Empiric Amiodarone or AICD

(I) Bradycardia → Assess for reversible causes → See p 60

SYNCOPE

Anthony C. Caruso

Syncope is a temporary loss of consciousness and postural tone with spontaneous resolution. Although syncope is common, accounting for up to 6% of medical admissions and 3% of all ER visits, the causes are myriad, the work-up seemingly unending, and the results often inconclusive. A reassuring point is that the patient who has a diagnosis of syncope of undetermined origin following an extensive work-up as described in this chapter is at low risk for having a fatal event, although the morbidity of frequent episodes of syncope should not be minimized.

A. A detailed history is important. The events leading up to syncope (e.g., micturition, postural changes, exercise), prodromal symptoms or auras, and the presence of witnesses and their impressions are extremely valuable. A history of other medical problems such as hypoglycemia and neurologic disease and a complete knowledge of current medications is essential. Physical examination should include orthostatic blood pressure determinations, cardiovascular examination, and thorough neurologic assessment. Although carotid hypersensitivity is an uncommon cause of syncope, carotid sinus massage may be performed at this time if there are no contraindications. Blood chemistry studies, including glucose and electrolytes, and a 12-lead ECG conclude the initial evaluation.

B. In patients with a history of seizure disorder, focal neurologic findings, a recent history of head trauma or other factors suggesting a neurologic etiology, CT of the head and EEG are beneficial.

C. In patients with a strong cardiac history or who show evidence of obstructive coronary disease, valvular heart disease, or arrhythmia, a careful cardiac work-up should be pursued before a neurologic work-up. A simple 12-lead ECG may reveal evidence of heart block or sinus node dysfunction but rarely leads to a diagnosis of tachyarrhythmias as the cause of syncope. Because 26% of all episodes of syncope are a result of cardiac causes and there is an increased risk of sudden death (up to 30% mortality) if syncope has a cardiac cause, it is prudent to screen carefully for a cardiac etiology if the history and physical examination do not suggest a neurologic basis.

D. Echocardiography is helpful for evaluation of structural cardiac defects associated with syncope, including aortic stenosis, hypertrophic cardiomyopathy (HCM), atrial myxomas, and mitral stenosis. If a cardiac cause seems possible and no history of cardiac disease is known, echocardiography can help determine the presence of normal or abnormal left ventricular (LV) function. In patients with preserved LV function, the head-up tilt test may be helpful but lacks specificity.

This method of assessing neurocardiac syncope has undergone a resurgence of interest recently, although the mechanism for neurocardiac syncope remains unclear. We recommend that the head-up tilt should be to at least 60° after a baseline supine assessment of at least 20 minutes (the initial tilt should be for up to 45 minutes if catecholamines are not to be used) or until the patient becomes symptomatic. After baseline assessment the patient is returned to the supine position for 5 minutes then returned to a 60° tilt with the administration of a 2-µg isoproterenol IV bolus. This should be repeated with incremental doses of isoproterenol at 4, 6, and 8 µg after rest periods of 5 minutes in the supine position or until symptomatic. The patient should remain in the upright tilt position for up to 10 minutes after each administration of isoproterenol or until symptoms develop.

E. The ambulatory Holter monitor is helpful when the patient has frequent episodes of syncope or presyncope, but in patients whose episodes are infrequent, a cardiac event monitor often is necessary. In patients with depressed LV function (LVEF <40%) and a history of myocardial infarction who are found to have nonsustained ventricular tachycardia, a signal-averaged ECG is often useful.

F. A negative signal-averaged ECG has excellent negative predictive accuracy and gives reassurance that the patient is at low risk for cardiac sudden death. Up to 50% of patients with a positive signal-averaged ECG will be found to have inducible ventricular tachycardia on electrophysiologic studies (EPS).

G. The use of invasive EPS in the work-up of syncope remains controversial. Clearly there are problems with the sensitivity and specificity of invasive testing of sinoatrial and atrioventricular nodal function. We recommend that EPS be reserved for patients with a high pretest probability of a tachyarrhythmia as the cause of syncope because the sensitivity and specificity of inducible ventricular tachycardia in patients with no structural heart disease are only 40 and 60%, respectively. It is strongly urged that patients with a positive signal-averaged ECG or a history of myocardial infarction, depressed LV function, and nonsustained ventricular tachycardia undergo EPS because the incidence of ventricular tachycardia in this population is increased and the consequence of missing this diagnosis may be catastrophic.

H. Exercise treadmill testing (ETT) often is helpful in a patient with a history of exercise-induced syncope, but it is otherwise of little value because myocardial ischemia is a rare cause of syncope.

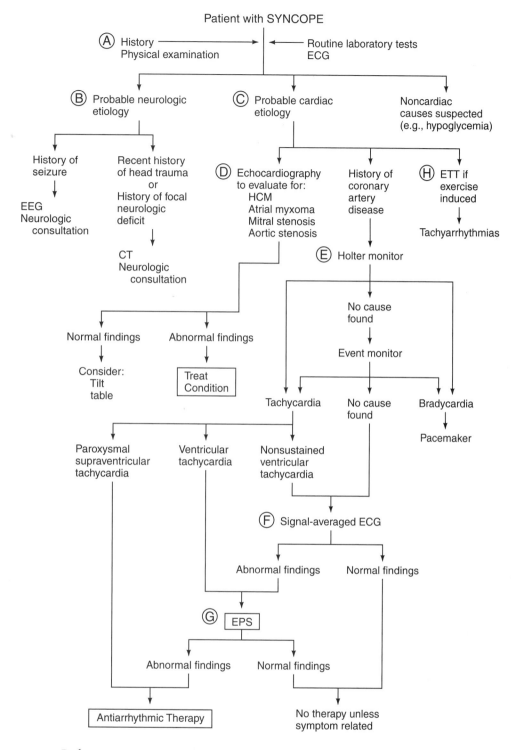

Patient with SYNCOPE

(A) History → ← Routine laboratory tests
Physical examination ECG

(B) Probable neurologic etiology

(C) Probable cardiac etiology

Noncardiac causes suspected (e.g., hypoglycemia)

History of seizure

↓

EEG
Neurologic consultation

Recent history of head trauma
or
History of focal neurologic deficit

↓

CT
Neurologic consultation

(D) Echocardiography to evaluate for:
HCM
Atrial myxoma
Mitral stenosis
Aortic stenosis

History of coronary artery disease

(H) ETT if exercise induced

↓

Tachyarrhythmias

(E) Holter monitor

No cause found

↓

Event monitor

Normal findings

↓

Consider:
Tilt table

Abnormal findings

↓

Treat Condition

Tachycardia

No cause found

Bradycardia

↓

Pacemaker

Paroxysmal supraventricular tachycardia

Ventricular tachycardia

Nonsustained ventricular tachycardia

(F) Signal-averaged ECG

Abnormal findings   Normal findings

(G) EPS

Abnormal findings   Normal findings

Antiarrhythmic Therapy

No therapy unless symptom related

References

Dimarco JP. Electrophysiologic studies in patients with unexplained syncope. Circulation 1987; 75:140.

Kapoor WN. Workup and management of patients with syncope. Med Clin North Am 1995; 79:1153.

Kapoor WN, Cha R, Petersen JR, et al. Prolonged electrocardiographic monitoring in patients with syncope. Am J Med 1987; 83:20.

Kapoor WN, Karpf M, Wieand S, et al. A prospective evaluation and follow-up of patients with syncope. N Engl J Med 1983; 309:197.

Strasberg B, Rechavie E, Sagie A, et al. The head-up tilt table test in patients with syncope of unknown origin. Am Heart J 1989; 118:923.

LARGE CARDIAC SILHOUETTE

James R. Standen

Cardiomegaly on chest films is a common finding in many heart diseases. In some conditions there is generalized enlargement of the cardiac silhouette; in others there is a dilation of some cardiac chambers and sparing of the rest. Chamber dilation may be caused by volume overload (e.g., aortic regurgitation) or decompensation from pressure overload (e.g., aortic stenosis). Identification of the pattern of enlargement and specifically of which individual chambers and great vessels are involved often provides a specific diagnosis.

A. The pulmonary vascular pattern gives useful insights into cardiac function. Decreased pulmonary vascularity is seen in severe forms of constrictive pericarditis, cardiac tamponade, and obstructive lesions of the right side of the heart (e.g., pulmonary stenosis and tetralogy of Fallot). Increased pulmonary vascularity, with normal upper and lower lobe distribution, is usually seen in left-to-right shunt lesions when the shunt ratio is >2:1 (e.g., atrial septal defect). Pulmonary venous hypertension with redistribution of flow to the upper lungs (with or without pulmonary edema) results from impaired diastolic function of the left ventricle and/or emptying of the left atrium. Vascular redistribution begins when the pulmonary venous pressure (wedge pressure) exceeds 15–20 mm Hg. In the acute situation, pulmonary edema results when the pressure exceeds the oncotic pressure of plasma at 25–30 mm Hg. In chronic states (e.g., mitral stenosis), compensatory mechanisms such as increased lymphatic drainage may prevent pulmonary edema even though the pulmonary venous pressure considerably exceeds that of the plasma proteins. Pulmonary arterial hypertension may be caused by postcapillary pulmonary venous hypertension (e.g., mitral stenosis), obliteration of the capillary bed (e.g., cor pulmonale in emphysema), or precapillary obstruction (e.g., primary pulmonary hypertension). When persistent, it causes dilation of the central pulmonary arteries, with oligemia or "pruning" of the smaller peripheral branches. Recognition of specific heart chamber, pulmonary vascular, and great vessel abnormalities on chest films can help direct which further investigations are appropriate (e.g., echocardiography, nuclear studies, cardiac catheterization) and what particular information is required from them. Localized enlargements of specific cardiac chambers may lead to distinct diagnoses.

B. Left ventricular (LV) enlargement alone results from decompensated aortic stenosis or systemic hypertension. In some cases of aortic stenosis, a prominent ascending aorta is seen from poststenotic dilation.

C. LV and aortic enlargement commonly results from aortic regurgitation.

D. LV and left atrial (LA) enlargement indicates mitral regurgitation.

E. LA and pulmonary artery (PA) enlargement with vascular redistribution to the upper lobes results from mitral stenosis. A "double density" sign for LA enlargement is often seen.

F. Increased pulmonary vascularity (i.e., shunt vascularity) may result from several lesions, with consequent increased left-to-right pulmonary flow. Right ventricular (RV) and sometimes right atrial (RA) enlargement with shunt vascularity is seen with atrial septal defect. LV and LA enlargement with shunt vascularity indicates ventricular septal defect. LV, LA, and aortic enlargement with shunt vascularity indicates patent ductus arteriosus.

G. RV and central PA enlargement with "pruning" of the pulmonary vascular pattern peripherally is seen with primary pulmonary hypertension, cor pulmonale, or multiple pulmonary emboli.

References

Fraser RG, Pare JAP. Diagnosis of diseases of the chest. 3rd ed. Philadelphia: WB Saunders, 1990.

Miller SW. Cardiac radiology: the requisites. St. Louis: Mosby, 1996.

Taveras JM, Ferrucci JT. Radiology: diagnosis—imaging—intervention. Philadelphia: JB Lippincott, 1990.

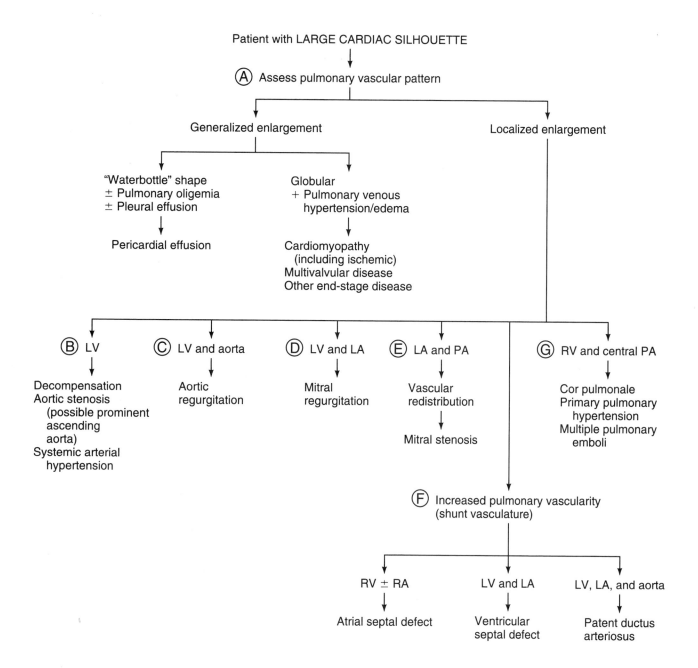

Patient with LARGE CARDIAC SILHOUETTE

(A) Assess pulmonary vascular pattern

Generalized enlargement

Localized enlargement

"Waterbottle" shape
± Pulmonary oligemia
± Pleural effusion

Pericardial effusion

Globular
+ Pulmonary venous
hypertension/edema

Cardiomyopathy
(including ischemic)
Multivalvular disease
Other end-stage disease

(B) LV

Decompensation
Aortic stenosis
(possible prominent
ascending
aorta)
Systemic arterial
hypertension

(C) LV and aorta

Aortic
regurgitation

(D) LV and LA

Mitral
regurgitation

(E) LA and PA

Vascular
redistribution

Mitral stenosis

(G) RV and central PA

Cor pulmonale
Primary pulmonary
hypertension
Multiple pulmonary
emboli

(F) Increased pulmonary vascularity
(shunt vasculature)

RV ± RA

Atrial septal defect

LV and LA

Ventricular
septal defect

LV, LA, and aorta

Patent ductus
arteriosus

CONGESTIVE HEART FAILURE

Karl B. Kern

Heart failure affects approximately 2 million Americans. The prevalence of this disease in persons 50–59 years of age is 1%. This number doubles every decade, so 10% of the U.S. population >80 years old is affected. Heart failure has a grave prognosis, with a 5-year mortality rate of 62% in men and 42% in women. Heart failure is not a single disease entity with one cause; rather, there are many causes. An improved clinical outcome can be achieved with many forms of heart failure, so it is important to determine the cause of heart failure and treat it appropriately.

A. Valvular heart disease accounts for 5–10% of cases of heart failure and includes lesions caused by rheumatic heart disease, myxomatous valves, and degenerative (usually calcified) valves. Both stenotic and regurgitant lesions can lead to heart failure by creating either pressure (stenotic) or volume (regurgitant) overload on the heart.

B. Approximately 40–60% of patients with heart failure have coronary artery disease (CAD). In patients with known or suspected CAD, an echocardiographic (ECHO) or radionuclide ventriculography (RVG) study is indicated to assess the ejection fraction (EF). Many patients with CAD have systolic failure with a low EF resulting from replacement of functioning myocardium with scar tissue created by myocardial infarction(s). Patients with systolic heart failure benefit from afterload reduction, diuretics, and digitalis therapy.

C. Many patients with documented heart failure have a normal EF. The cause of heart failure in these patients is diastolic dysfunction resulting from impaired relaxation and filling of the left ventricle. Diastolic dysfunction can be caused by acute ischemia, which may be silent and thus not detected on a resting ECHO study.

D. If there is no evidence of systolic or diastolic dysfunction, a cardiac stress test (treadmill, thallium, stress ECHO, or RVG) should be performed to rule out CAD. Right and left heart catheterization also may be indicated if the diagnosis of CAD and cause of heart failure are still in question.

E. Hypertensive heart disease is very prevalent, especially in the elderly, and may be found in up to 75% of heart failure patients. The initial problem is decreased ventricular compliance causing impaired relaxation and ventricular filling. This may be severe and is usually associated with ventricular hypertrophy. With appropriate antihypertensive therapy (angiotensin-converting enzyme inhibitors, calcium channel blockers, and to a lesser extent, β-adrenergic blockers), the hypertrophy regresses and an improvement in diastolic function may also occur. As the disease progresses, systolic failure may result, but this is much less common.

F. Even though a patient has hypertensive disease, CAD may also be contributing to the heart failure if wall motion abnormalities are demonstrated on ECHO. A combination of hypertension and CAD often are the cause of heart failure, and each should be appropriately treated.

G. When the history and physical examination do not help determine the cause of the heart failure, an ECHO can provide useful information. Evidence of restrictive, constrictive, and hypertrophic heart disease may be seen, and if so should be followed up with cardiac catheterization. One should consider obtaining a cardiac biopsy at the time of catheterization if an infiltrative disease process (e.g., amyloid) is suspected but not confirmed by ECHO.

H. Many diseases can cause a dilated cardiomyopathy, but the most common ones are postviral and idiopathic, accounting for 10–30% of patients with heart failure. The role of biopsy in this group of patients has been examined; when acute viral myocarditis is suspected, there is a moderate yield from the biopsy (20–65%). However, when the biopsy is performed to obtain a diagnosis of unexplained heart failure, the yield is low and does not warrant the risk of the procedure. Other causes of heart failure in this group are rare and include alcohol, metal intoxication, cardiotoxic medications, and other systemic diseases. When these rare causes are suspected, a prudent and exhaustive evaluation is warranted.

I. When the ECHO is normal in a patient with symptoms of heart failure, a right and left heart catheterization may provide useful information and uncover unsuspected coronary or pulmonary vascular disease. When this is not the case, chronic lung disease, anemia, obesity, physical deconditioning, depression, or an endocrine abnormality should be considered as the cause of the symptoms.

References

Applegate RJ, Little WC. Systolic and diastolic dysfunction in CHF. Cardiology 1991; 57.

Chow LC, Dittrich HC, Shabetai R. Endomyocardial biopsy in patients with unexplained heart failure. Ann Intern Med 1988; 109:535.

Kannel WB, Belanger AJ. Epidemiology of heart failure. Am Heart J 1991; 121:951.

Levy D, Larson MG, Vasan RS, et al. The progression from hypertension to congestive heart failure. JAMA 1996; 275:1557.

Redfield MM. Evaluation of congestive heart failure. In: Giuliani ER, Gersh BJ, McGoon MD, et al, eds. Mayo Clinic practice of cardiology. 3rd ed. St. Louis: Mosby, 1996:569.

Patient with CONGESTIVE HEART FAILURE

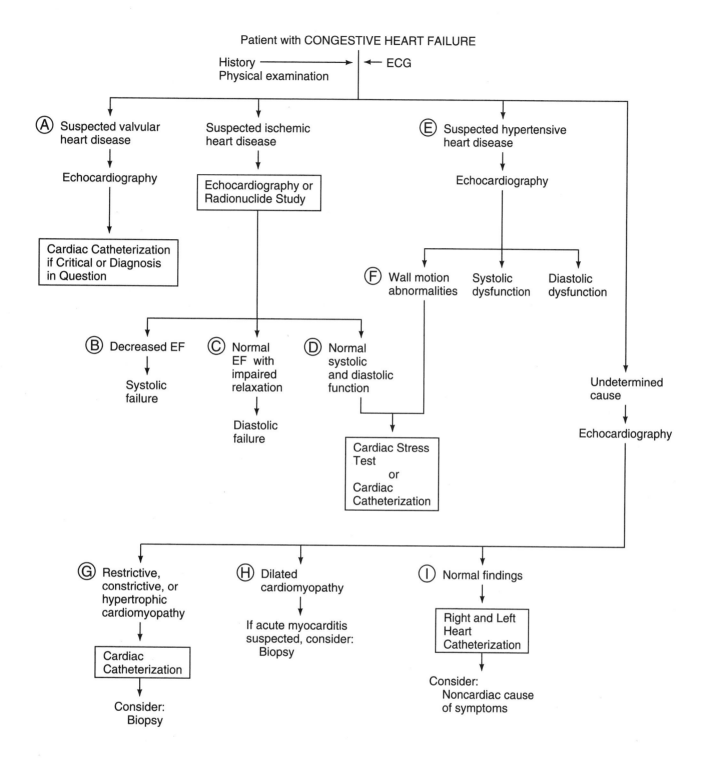

ACUTE PULMONARY EDEMA

James M. Galloway
Paul E. Fenster

A. Significant historical data include any history of heart disease (including ischemic, valvular, or congestive heart failure), pulmonary disease, recent acute illness, fevers, chills, sweats, sputum production, chronic renal failure, or other chronic illness. Also, determine current medication and drug usage.

B. Direct particular attention in the physical examination to BP, pulse rate, the presence or absence of a pulsus paradoxus, jugular venous pressure, pulmonary status, heart murmurs, the presence or absence of an S_3, and peripheral edema.

C. Initial laboratory evaluation should include arterial blood gases, CBC with differential, electrolytes, BUN, creatinine, ECG, and chest film. A pulse oximeter to determine peripheral oxygenation status may be helpful and provide a rapid assessment of the severity of the hypoxia.

D. A number of priorities can be addressed simultaneously. In urgent cases therapeutic interventions should be initiated immediately upon patient arrival, even while the history and physical examination are being performed. In most patients the assumption of a sitting position, IV administration of a potent diuretic, and high-flow O_2 and IV morphine and/or sublingual nitroglycerin results in significant clinical improvement. Diuretics commonly used include furosemide, 20–40 mg, or bumetanide, 0.5–1.0 mg. IV furosemide acutely exerts a direct venodilating effect that produces venous pooling and reduces central venous pressure (CVP) before the onset of diuresis. IV morphine is effective in reducing CVP and afterload as well as reducing anxiety. Sublingual nitroglycerin, 0.4–0.8 mg, also reduces CVP. Morphine or nitroglycerin may worsen hypotension. High concentrations of O_2 (50–100%) should be initiated at once. O_2 therapy should not be withheld in hypoxic patients with acute dyspnea despite a history of chronic obstructive pulmonary disease and concern about CO_2 retention, although initial low-concentration or low-flow rates may be prudent. If higher levels of O_2 are required, assess the need for intubation frequently.

E. Clinically, an adequate response to therapy is indicated by improvement in pulse rate, respiratory rate and depth, skin color, pulmonary status, and overall appearance. A reasonable goal for adequate oxygenation is to maintain Pao_2 of 90–100 mm Hg.

F. In patients believed to be in initially unresponsive cardiogenic pulmonary edema with adequate BP, the use of afterload reduction to improve cardiac output and reduce pulmonary congestion may be of significant benefit. A continuous infusion of IV nitroprusside or nitroglycerin can be given. IV nitroglycerin has the added advantage of antianginal properties. The IV use of positive inotropes also can be considered in this group of patients (as well as those with low BP) to increase cardiac output. Continuous infusions of dobutamine or dopamine may be given and titrated to optimal response. The placement of a pulmonary artery (PA) catheter is generally recommended to guide therapy while these agents are used.

G. Although the differential diagnosis of acute pulmonary edema is extensive, most patients who have this condition have a history of heart disease and have had progression of underlying disease (e.g., worsening valvular disease, recurrent ischemia), dietary indiscretion, a recent change in medications (through noncompliance, the addition of a cardiodepressant medication, or a recent decrease in needed cardiac medications), an increase in metabolic demands (including infection, anemia, pregnancy, atrioventricular [AV] shunt, hyperthyroidism), or (particularly in hospitalized patients) volume overload.

H. Myocardial causes include systolic and diastolic dysfunction resulting from primary or secondary myocardial disease. These conditions include dilated cardiomyopathies with many possible causes (hypertensive, ischemic, infectious, toxic, idiopathic), restrictive cardiomyopathies (amyloidosis, sarcoidosis, hemochromatosis), and hypertrophic cardiomyopathy.

I. Acute pulmonary edema with no easily discernible cause may have cardiac or noncardiac causes. Cardiogenic causes include transient ischemic or arrhythmic events, occult valvular disease (e.g., infectious endocarditis), pericardial disease (e.g., tamponade and constriction), metabolic causes (e.g., hyperthyroidism and hypothyroidism), initial late presentations of congenital heart disease, and heart disease related to connective tissue disorders. Noncardiac causes include diffuse pulmonary infections, aspiration, toxic pulmonary insults (e.g., smoke, chlorine gas), narcotic overdose, gram-negative septicemia, hemorrhagic pancreatitis, lymphatic blockage resulting from carcinomatosis, fibrosis or inflammatory disease, neurogenic disorders, and high-altitude pulmonary edema. Echocardiography can differentiate cardiogenic from noncardiogenic causes and thus determine further therapeutic interventions. If echocardiography is nondiagnostic, further evaluate noncardiogenic or transient cardiogenic causes.

J. Initial evaluation for transient arrhythmias (besides the initial ECG) generally should consist of a Holter monitor and/or a signal-averaged ECG. If these suggest significant ventricular arrhythmias, electrophysiologic evaluation may be in order to best define the arrhythmia and

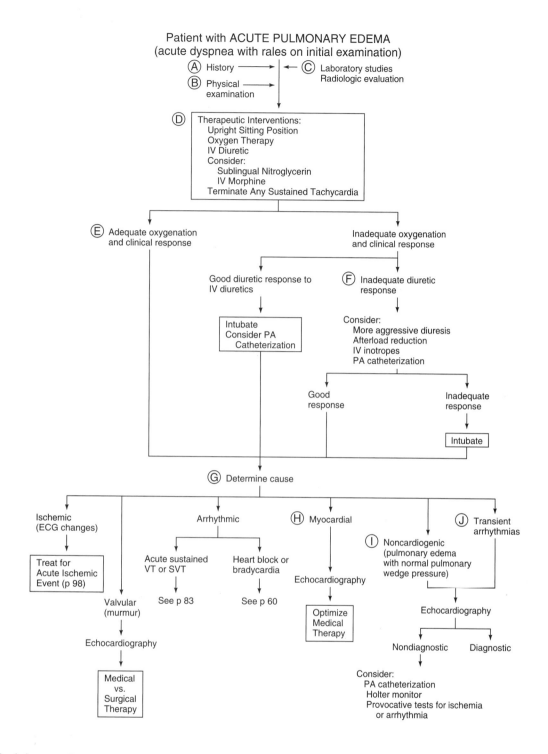

Patient with ACUTE PULMONARY EDEMA
(acute dyspnea with rales on initial examination)

Ⓐ History ⟶ ⟵ Ⓒ Laboratory studies
Ⓑ Physical ⟶ Radiologic evaluation
examination

Ⓓ Therapeutic Interventions:
Upright Sitting Position
Oxygen Therapy
IV Diuretic
Consider:
Sublingual Nitroglycerin
IV Morphine
Terminate Any Sustained Tachycardia

Ⓔ Adequate oxygenation
and clinical response

Inadequate oxygenation
and clinical response

Good diuretic response to
IV diuretics

Ⓕ Inadequate diuretic
response

Intubate
Consider PA
Catheterization

Consider:
More aggressive diuresis
Afterload reduction
IV inotropes
PA catheterization

Good
response

Inadequate
response

Intubate

Ⓖ Determine cause

Ischemic
(ECG changes)

Arrhythmic

Ⓗ Myocardial

Ⓙ Transient
arrhythmias

Ⓘ Noncardiogenic
(pulmonary edema
with normal pulmonary
wedge pressure)

Treat for
Acute Ischemic
Event (p 98)

Acute sustained
VT or SVT

Heart block or
bradycardia

Echocardiography

Valvular
(murmur)

See p 83

See p 60

Optimize
Medical
Therapy

Echocardiography

Echocardiography

Nondiagnostic

Diagnostic

Medical
vs.
Surgical
Therapy

Consider:
PA catheterization
Holter monitor
Provocative tests for ischemia
or arrhythmia

its ideal therapy. Provocative testing for transient ischemia generally consists of a treadmill exercise test, with or without the use of thallium or echocardiographic imaging.

References

Chesebro JG, Burnett JL. Cardiac failure: characteristics and clinical manifestations. In: Giuliani ER, Fuster V, Gersh BJ, et al, eds. Cardiology: fundamentals and practice. 2nd ed. St. Louis: Mosby, 1991.

Ingram RH Jr, Braunwald E. Dyspnea and pulmonary edema. In: Fauci AS, Braunwald E, Isselbacher KJ, et al, eds. Harrison's principles of internal medicine. 14th ed. New York: McGraw-Hill, 97:190.

Ruggie N. Congestive heart failure. Med Clin North Am 1986; 70:829.

COR PULMONALE

Mark C. Goldberg
Karl B. Kern

Cor pulmonale is cardiac dysfunction that occurs as a result of some process affecting respiratory structure or function, or both. The process responsible for right ventricular (RV) hypertrophy and ultimately dilation must be intrinsic to the lung. The most commonly implicated causes of cor pulmonale are (1) diseases of the pulmonary parenchyma such as emphysema, chronic bronchitis, asthma, or interstitial lung disease; (2) diseases of the pulmonary vasculature such as primary pulmonary hypertension (HTN) or recurrent thromboembolic events; (3) disorders in the mechanism or mechanics of respiration (e.g., sleep apnea or kyphoscoliosis); and (4) chronic exposure to low P_{O_2}. Disorders that cause RV failure but are not intrinsic to the lung (e.g., mitral stenosis or congenital cardiac defects) must be excluded before the diagnosis of cor pulmonale can be made.

A. The history and physical findings in chronic cor pulmonale vary widely, often overshadowed by those of the underlying disease. A 59-year-old man with emphysema may give a history of tobacco abuse and complain of dyspnea, cough, and sputum production; a 23-year-old woman with primary pulmonary HTN may give a history of dyspnea and exertional syncope. Likewise, the physical findings in cor pulmonale vary according to the cause. An accentuated pulmonary closure sound and the ability to feel the pulmonary valve close in the second intercostal space on the left are two of the earliest findings in pulmonary HTN. RV heave, an indication of RV hypertrophy, and the murmurs of tricuspid and pulmonic insufficiency tend to occur later in the course and indicate more severe disease. Other physical findings in cor pulmonale include tachypnea; cyanosis; increased jugular venous pressure with prominent A wave reflecting noncompliance of hypertrophied RV; RV heave; RV S_3, S_4; murmurs of tricuspid and pulmonic insufficiency; hepatomegaly; ascites; and peripheral edema.

B. The chest film is an integral part of the work-up. Cor pulmonale secondary to thoracic deformities such as kyphoscoliosis may be dramatically illustrated. The chest film may specifically suggest the diagnosis of chronic diffuse interstitial fibrosis, bronchiectasis, tuberculosis, or sarcoidosis. Often the chest film is normal, especially in cases of primary pulmonary HTN or chronic pulmonary embolism. Findings on chest films most often reflect the underlying disease process. However, if the pulmonary HTN is of long standing, the main pulmonary artery may have dilated. In the lateral chest film the hypertrophied RV may be seen occupying what was previously the retrosternal air space. Occasionally the "pruned tree" appearance of branching pulmonary arteries is observed. Pulmonary function testing may be useful in distinguishing between obstructive and restrictive disorders. Obstruction caused by emphysema and chronic bronchitis may be noted, as well as that caused by scarring or tumor in the tracheobronchial tree. Restrictive lung disease from thoracic cage, respiratory muscle, parenchymal, or pleural abnormalities can be diagnosed.

C. This diagnosis should most often be suspected in persons living at a high altitude. In many patients with mild or moderate disease the resting P_{O_2} is normal if the ABG testing is performed at a lower altitude. With exercise, desaturation will occur. This reflects the hyperactivity of the pulmonary vasculature in a group of patients who seem predisposed to pulmonary HTN when exposed to a low P_{O_2}.

D. The ECG in cor pulmonale should indicate RV hypertrophy. Criteria most commonly used include right axis deviation; delayed intrinsicoid deflection in V_1; R/S ratio in V_1 >1, or <1 in V_5, V_6; QR pattern in V_1; and R wave V_1 + S wave V_5 and V_6 >10.5. These findings are further supported when ST depression and T wave inversion are noted in the precordium and when P pulmonale is seen in the right atrium.

E. Echocardiography reveals the anatomic changes in RV function that have occurred as a result of pulmonary HTN. The RV may be hypertrophied or dilated. Color echocardiography may show tricuspid or pulmonic insufficiency. Pulmonary artery pressures may be quantitated on Doppler study.

F. If doubt remains that a congenital shunt may be the underlying cause of pulmonary HTN or RV failure, cardiac catheterization or a nuclear medicine shunt study is necessary.

References

Alpert JS, Kwin RS, Dalen JE. Pulmonary hypertension. Curr Prob Cardiol 1981; 5:1.

Brent BN, Berger HJ, Matthay RA, et al. Physiologic correlates of right ventricular ejection fraction in chronic obstructive pulmonary disease: a combined radionuclide and hemodynamic study. Am J Cardiol 1982; 50:255.

Dexter L. Pulmonary vascular disease in acquired and congenital heart disease. Arch Intern Med 1979; 139:922.

Fernandez-Bonetti P, Lupi-Herrera E, Martinez-Guerra ML, et al. Peripheral airways obstruction in idiopathic pulmonary artery hypertension (primary). Chest 1983; 83:732.

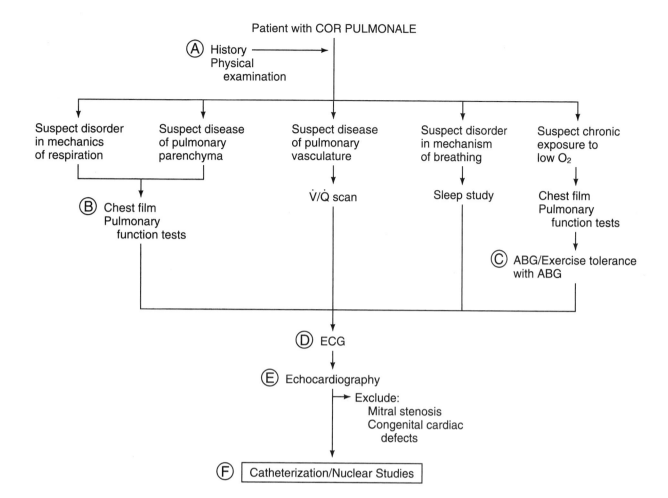

Patient with COR PULMONALE

Ⓐ History
Physical
examination

Suspect disorder
in mechanics
of respiration

Suspect disease
of pulmonary
parenchyma

Suspect disease
of pulmonary
vasculature

Suspect disorder
in mechanism
of breathing

Suspect chronic
exposure to
low O$_2$

Ⓑ Chest film
Pulmonary
function tests

$\dot{V}/\dot{Q}$ scan

Sleep study

Chest film
Pulmonary
function tests

Ⓒ ABG/Exercise tolerance
with ABG

Ⓓ ECG

Ⓔ Echocardiography

Exclude:
Mitral stenosis
Congenital cardiac
defects

Ⓕ Catheterization/Nuclear Studies

RIGHT VENTRICULAR FAILURE

Mark C. Goldberg
Karl B. Kern

Right ventricular (RV) failure describes failure of the right ventricle as a pump. In this state, pressure builds up in the venous system behind the right ventricle, hydrostatic forces exceed osmotic forces, and the net result is a transudation of fluid. The symptoms of RV failure reflect the underlying increase in venous pressures. The causes, however, are myriad. Almost any type of cardiac disease may lead to RV failure. Pulmonary processes also may lead to RV failure; when this occurs, the term *cor pulmonale* is applied. Regardless of the cause, approach to the diagnosis of RV failure begins with a complete history and physical examination, ECG, and chest film. Analysis of preliminary data leads to hypotheses concerning the cause of RV dysfunction, which can be more specifically targeted for investigation.

A. The distinction between right and left ventricular failure may become difficult late in the course of the disease when both ventricles have become dysfunctional. Early symptoms include fatigue and peripheral edema. Physical examination may reveal elevated jugular venous pressure, an enlarged and perhaps pulsatile liver, tricuspid regurgitation, and an RV S_3. An occasional patient may have ascites and jaundice.

B. The chest film in RV failure may be helpful. When the disease process involves a state in which pulmonary pressures are chronically elevated, the pulmonary artery may be dilated. Often the lateral chest film shows the right ventricle occupying what was previously the retrosternal air space. In cor pulmonale the chest film may specifically suggest an underlying cause (e.g., chronic diffuse interstitial fibrosis or bronchiectasis).

C. When RV failure is secondary to cor pulmonale, valvular heart disease, or a shunt, the ECG should show RV hypertrophy. If RV failure is secondary to ischemic heart disease, a concurrent inferior myocardial infarction is most often seen on ECG. If infarction is acute, a V4 R lead may show ST elevation consistent with RV infarction.

D. If history and physical are compatible with sleep apnea, a sleep study is in order.

E. If cor pulmonale is a likely cause of RV failure, pulmonary function testing may be useful in distinguishing between obstructive and restrictive disorders. Obstruction from emphysema and bronchitis, as well as tumor in the tracheobronchial tree, may be diagnosed. Restrictive lung disease from thoracic cage, respiratory muscle, parenchymal, or pleural abnormalities can also be diagnosed.

F. Pulmonary embolism initially is investigated with a ventilation-perfusion ($\dot{V}/\dot{Q}$) scan. Pulmonary angiography may be required in follow-up.

G. Echocardiography may show a hypertrophied or dilated right ventricle. Color echocardiography may show tricuspid and pulmonic insufficiency as well as mitral and pulmonic stenosis. Pulmonary artery pressures may be quantitated using Doppler. If doubt remains that a congenital shunt may be the underlying cause of pulmonary hypertension or RV failure, cardiac catheterization is necessary. Catheterization is always performed before shunt or valve repair.

References

Cintron GB, Hernandez E, Linares E, Aranda JM. Bedside recognition, incidence and clinical course of right ventricular infarction. Am J Cardiol 1981; 47:224.

Fishman AP. Chronic cor pulmonale. Am Rev Respir Dis 1976; 114:775.

Guilleminault C, Tilkian A, Dement WC. The sleep apnea syndromes. Annu Rev Med 1976; 27:465.

McDonald IG, Hirsh J, Hale GS, O'Sullivan EF. Major pulmonary embolism, a correlation of clinical findings, haemodynamics, pulmonary angiography, and pathological physiology. Br Heart J 1972; 34:356.

Shah PK, Maddahi J, Berman DS, et al. Scintigraphically detected predominant right ventricular dysfunction in acute myocardial infarction: clinical and hemodynamic correlates and implications for therapy and prognosis. J Am Coll Cardiol 1985; 6:1264.

Patient with RIGHT VENTRICULAR FAILURE

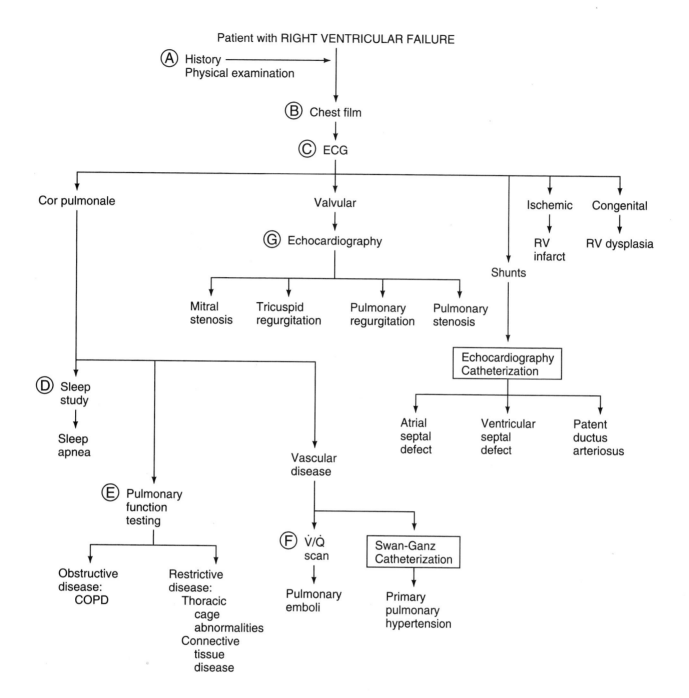

CARDIAC ARREST

James M. Galloway
Karl B. Kern

The following guidelines, as suggested by the American Heart Association's Advanced Cardiac Life Support Task Force, were written to provide useful help for most patients. However, they were not written to preclude other measures that may be indicated in a particular patient.

A. If the cardiac arrest is witnessed but a monitor-defibrillator is not immediately available and the patient is pulseless, a solitary precordial thump may be attempted in an effort to convert the patient. Although this rarely is successful, it may be of benefit and costs little time.

B. Cardiac arrest is a common final pathway of several arrhythmias amenable to defibrillation. In one report of cardiac arrest occurring in ambulatory patients during ECG monitoring, 62% had ventricular tachycardia as the initial rhythm that rapidly evolved into ventricular fibrillation, 8% had primary ventricular fibrillation, and 13% had torsades de pointes. Automatic external defibrillators capable of assessing the rhythm, charging, and then delivering a defibrillation shock are now available. These devices extend the opportunity to provide rapid defibrillation outside the usual medical or paramedical circle of care.

C. Because the probability of survival after a cardiac arrest declines rapidly as the time to defibrillation increases, early defibrillation is essential for a successful outcome. Therefore, as soon as a monitor-defibrillator is available, the patient's rhythm must be identified. If the rhythm is ventricular tachycardia or ventricular fibrillation and the pulse is absent, the patient should be defibrillated immediately. This step should take precedence if a defibrillator is available.

D. The importance of properly performed CPR cannot be overemphasized. Effective CPR is essential in the patient in whom early defibrillation either is not immediately available or is initially unsuccessful. External CPR is the most widely used technique to support the circulation and ventilation of a cardiac arrest patient. However, in a hospital setting, with individuals trained and experienced in the performance of thoracotomy, open chest or internal cardiac compression may be used. Standard closed-chest CPR is now recommended to be 80–100 compressions/min with 2-inch compression depth and an accompanying ventilator breath after every fifth compression. If resuscitative efforts are not immediately successful, a central line should be placed to ensure optimal delivery of medications in the central circulation.

E. The current recommended dosage of epinephrine is given in the decision tree. However, the ideal dosage of epinephrine is unknown. Animal studies have shown that higher dosages improved cerebral and myocardial blood flow. Human reports have been published suggesting no significant benefit with higher dosages.

F. Adequate ventilation can be accomplished in the early stages of cardiac arrest treatment with alternative measures (e.g., mouth to mouth, bag to mouth). However, if initial attempts to restore circulation fail, intubation should be performed. An additional benefit of intubation is the ability to then measure end-tidal carbon dioxide levels; these have proved the best available measure of CPR effectiveness in individual patients. Such information can be used to tailor CPR effects to the needs of each cardiac arrest victim.

G. Electromechanical dissociation (EMD) is determined to be present when there is evidence of an organized cardiac rhythm without the generation of a pulse. This rhythm carries a grave prognosis, and a careful search must be made for reversible causes. The most common causes include hypovolemia, hypoxia, tension pneumothorax, pericardial tamponade, massive myocardial infarction, and massive pulmonary embolus.

H. Fine ventricular fibrillation can mimic asystole and is more amenable to therapy. Therefore, it is important to check at least two different ECG leads to define this rhythm. If fine ventricular fibrillation is suspected, an attempt at defibrillation is reasonable.

I. In a pulseless patient, regardless of whether the arrest was witnessed, blind defibrillation (without documentation of the rhythm first) can be performed. In the unusual situation when a defibrillator is available but a monitor is not, blind defibrillation should be initiated at 200 J and subsequently, if no pulse returns, with 200–300 J, followed if necessary by 360 J.

References

Brown CG, Martin DR, Pepe PE, et al. A comparison of standard-dose and high-dose epinephrine in cardiac arrest outside the hospital: The Multicenter High-Dose Epinephrine Study Group. N Engl J Med 1992; 327:1051.

De Luna AB, Coumel P, Leclercq JF. Ambulatory sudden cardiac death: mechanism of production of fatal arrhythmia on the basis of data from 157 cases. Am Heart J 1989; 117:151.

Emergency Cardiac Care Committee and Subcommittees. American Heart Association: guidelines for cardiopulmonary resuscitation and emergency cardiac care, III: adult advanced cardiac life support. JAMA 1992; 268:2171.

Sanders AB, Kern KB, Otto CW, et al. End-tidal carbon dioxide monitoring during cardiopulmonary resuscitation: a prognostic indicator for survival. JAMA 1989; 262:1347.

Textbook of advanced cardiac life support. American Heart Association, 1997; 1:2.

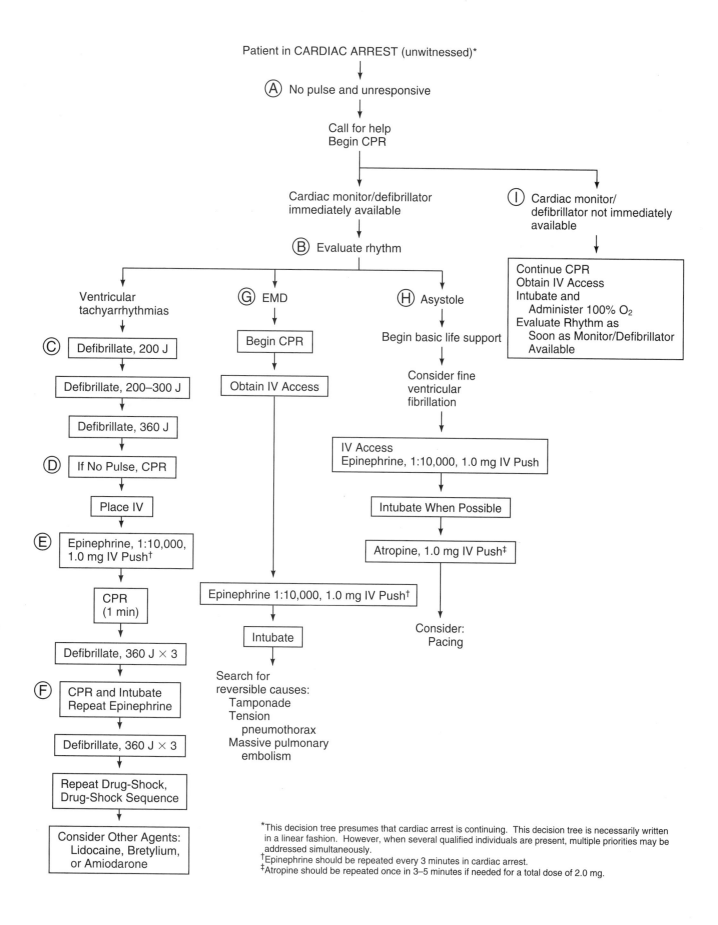

Patient in CARDIAC ARREST (unwitnessed)*

(A) No pulse and unresponsive

Call for help
Begin CPR

Cardiac monitor/defibrillator
immediately available

(I) Cardiac monitor/
defibrillator not immediately
available

(B) Evaluate rhythm

Continue CPR
Obtain IV Access
Intubate and
    Administer 100% O₂
Evaluate Rhythm as
    Soon as Monitor/Defibrillator
    Available

Ventricular
tachyarrhythmias

(G) EMD

(H) Asystole

(C) Defibrillate, 200 J

Begin CPR

Begin basic life support

Defibrillate, 200–300 J

Obtain IV Access

Consider fine
ventricular
fibrillation

Defibrillate, 360 J

(D) If No Pulse, CPR

IV Access
Epinephrine, 1:10,000, 1.0 mg IV Push

Place IV

Intubate When Possible

(E) Epinephrine, 1:10,000,
1.0 mg IV Push†

Atropine, 1.0 mg IV Push‡

CPR
(1 min)

Epinephrine 1:10,000, 1.0 mg IV Push†

Defibrillate, 360 J × 3

Intubate

Consider:
Pacing

(F) CPR and Intubate
Repeat Epinephrine

Defibrillate, 360 J × 3

Search for
reversible causes:
    Tamponade
    Tension
        pneumothorax
    Massive pulmonary
        embolism

Repeat Drug-Shock,
Drug-Shock Sequence

Consider Other Agents:
Lidocaine, Bretylium,
or Amiodarone

*This decision tree presumes that cardiac arrest is continuing. This decision tree is necessarily written
in a linear fashion. However, when several qualified individuals are present, multiple priorities may be
addressed simultaneously.
†Epinephrine should be repeated every 3 minutes in cardiac arrest.
‡Atropine should be repeated once in 3–5 minutes if needed for a total dose of 2.0 mg.

CARDIAC DYSPNEA

David Framm
Paul E. Fenster
Karl B. Kern

A. The history and physical examination of a patient with dyspnea can be helpful. Carefully explore any known cardiac or pulmonary disease. Also consider metabolic, hematologic, renal, or neuromuscular diseases. Physical examination may reveal such overt causes as congestive heart failure or pneumonia, thus directing the diagnostic work-up and therapeutic plan.

B. If the diagnosis remains uncertain, it is important to determine the severity of the symptoms. If these are mild or episodic, an exercise treadmill can provide a useful objective assessment of functional capacity.

C. If symptoms are severe and functional capacity is limited, a chest film is an important first step. Three distinct patterns may be identified, depending on the presence of pulmonary disease and the size of the cardiac silhouette.

D. A chest film showing evidence of pulmonary disease and a normal-sized heart can be followed up by specific tests as needed. Pulmonary function tests (PFTs) can help differentiate obstructive and restrictive disease as well as the location of the obstructive process.

E. If no evidence of overt pulmonary disease is seen on the chest film and the cardiac silhouette is likewise normal, PFTs, including ABGs are needed. When these are abnormal, a ventilation-perfusion ($\dot{V}/\dot{Q}$) scan or pulmonary angiography can define possible pulmonary emboli as the source of dyspnea.

F. When the chest film reveals an enlarged heart or vascular redistribution, an echocardiographic Doppler study can differentiate between several potential causes of dyspnea. Pericardial disease, represented by either pericardial fluid (and potential tamponade) or pericardial constriction (from scarring), can be identified by echocardiography. Valvular disease and its severity can be assessed by echocardiographic and Doppler studies. If left ventricular (LV) dysfunction is seen on echocardiography, Doppler studies can determine whether systolic dysfunction or both systolic and diastolic dysfunction are present. When systolic contraction is preserved, a Doppler study can demonstrate diastolic dysfunction, a potential cause of dyspnea that is often overlooked. Segmental wall motion abnormalities detected on echocardiography may be the result of ischemic disease and should be further evaluated with an exercise test or catheterization.

References

Dexter L, Richards CL. Dyspnea. In: Greene HL, ed. Clinical medicine. 2nd ed. St. Louis: Mosby, 1996:166.

Gillespie DJ, Staats BA. Unexplained dyspnea. Mayo Clin Proc 1994; 69:657.

Swan HJC, Ganz W, Forrester JS. Catheterization of the heart in man with the use of a flow-directed balloon-tipped catheter. N Engl J Med 1970; 283:447.

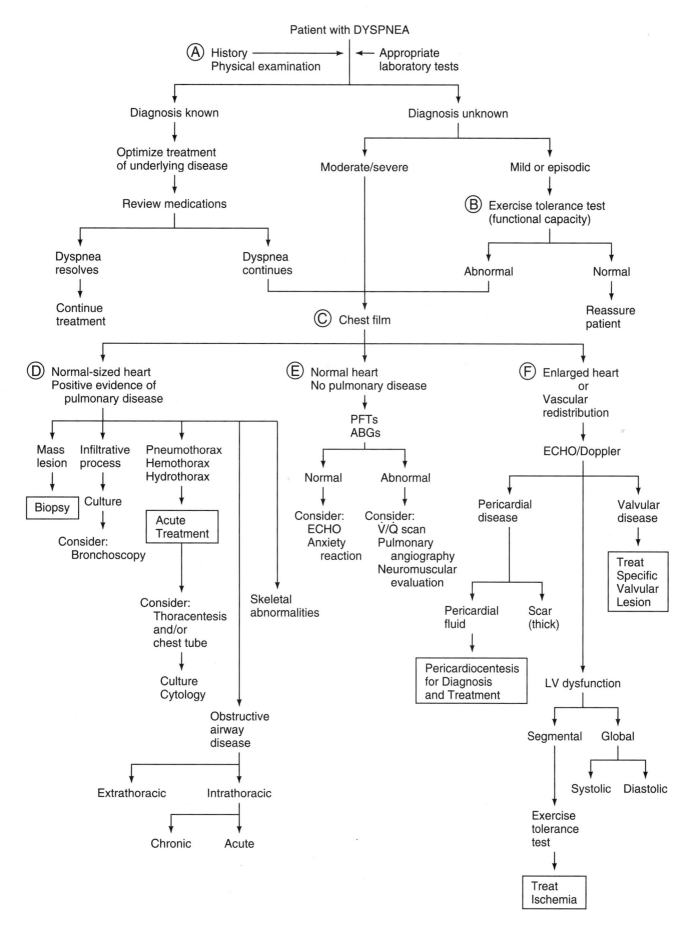

Patient with DYSPNEA

(A) History ——→ ←— Appropriate
Physical examination   laboratory tests

Diagnosis known   Diagnosis unknown

Optimize treatment
of underlying disease   Moderate/severe   Mild or episodic

Review medications   (B) Exercise tolerance test
                                                    (functional capacity)

Dypsnea   Dyspnea   Abnormal   Normal
resolves   continues

Continue   Reassure
treatment   (C) Chest film   patient

(D) Normal-sized heart   (E) Normal heart   (F) Enlarged heart
Positive evidence of   No pulmonary disease   or
pulmonary disease   Vascular
                                    PFTs   redistribution
                                    ABGs
                                                              ECHO/Doppler
Mass   Infiltrative   Pneumothorax   Normal   Abnormal
lesion   process   Hemothorax   Pericardial   Valvular
                          Hydrothorax   Consider: Consider: disease   disease
Biopsy   Culture   ECHO   V/Q scan
                                 Acute   Anxiety   Pulmonary   Treat
                    Acute   reaction   angiography   Specific
Consider: Treatment   Neuromuscular   Valvular
Bronchoscopy   evaluation   Pericardial   Scar   Lesion
                                                             fluid   (thick)
Consider: Skeletal
Thoracentesis   abnormalities   Pericardiocentesis
and/or   for Diagnosis
chest tube   and Treatment   LV dysfunction

Culture
Cytology   Segmental   Global

Obstructive   Systolic   Diastolic
airway
disease   Exercise
                                                               tolerance
Extrathoracic   Intrathoracic   test

                 Chronic   Acute   Treat
                                                               Ischemia

ACUTE MYOCARDIAL INFARCTION

Paul E. Fenster
James M. Galloway
Karl B. Kern

A. Important initial measures in the treatment of patients with suspected acute myocardial infarction (AMI) are 12-lead ECG, cardiac monitoring, pain and anxiety relief with IV morphine, bed rest, and adequate sedation. Aspirin should be given (160–325 mg) and chewed. Supplemental O_2 should be provided at least for the initial hours for all patients who have blood oxygen saturation <90% or pulmonary congestion. Low flow rates may be prudent in patients with chronic obstructive pulmonary disease. Pain after the initial hours may indicate continuing ischemia of jeopardized myocardium. Thus, efforts to limit myocardial O_2 demand (including adequate sedation, pain control, and anti-ischemic medication) are important.

B. Sublingual nitroglycerin is effective in the treatment of coronary artery spasm, another cause of ST segment elevation. If this causes resolution of the chest discomfort and ECG changes, admit the patient and evaluate for evidence of AMI. If infarction is ruled out, perform a stress test. If this is negative for ischemia, treat the patient for coronary artery spasm with calcium channel blockers and/or nitrates.

C. Thrombolytic therapy significantly reduces mortality in patients with AMI and ST segment elevation who are treated within 1 hour of the onset of symptoms. As time passes, however, its efficacy is dramatically reduced. Clinically significant benefit occurs up to 12 hours after onset of symptoms. The most widely studied thrombolytic drugs are streptokinase (STK) and tissue plasminogen activator (tPA). Although tPA has a higher early recanalization rate, the late patency of the infarct vessel is comparable for the two drugs. Clinical trials comparing the drugs document slightly greater reduction in mortality with tPA.

D. Maintenance of a patent infarct artery after thrombolytic therapy is important. In the Heparin-Aspirin Reperfusion Trial, early IV heparin significantly improved the early infarct artery patency rate in tPA-treated patients. However, heparin does not significantly improve the overall result with STK.

E. Primary angioplasty (PTCA), when feasible within a 60-minute "door-to-dilation" interval, is considered by many to be the reperfusion strategy of choice. Stroke risk is reduced compared with thrombolytic therapies. High-risk patients, especially the elderly, benefit most by PTCA, compared with thrombolysis.

F. Acute IV β blocker therapy followed by oral therapy reduces acute mortality and the rate of reinfarction and cardiac arrest in patients who are not receiving concomitant thrombolytic therapy. Combining a β blocker with thrombolytic therapy has resulted in a reduction in infarction and mortality rates. Chronic oral β blocker therapy begun in the first few days after AMI also improves survival rates and decreases the incidence of reinfarction.

G. Angiotensin-converting enzyme (ACE) inhibitors reduce mortality when administered early in AMI. The absolute benefit, overall, is small but is substantial in high-risk patients, especially those with heart failure or large infarctions. The ACE inhibitor can be stopped after 6 weeks but should be continued indefinitely in those with an ejection fraction (EF) of <40%.

(Continued on page 100)

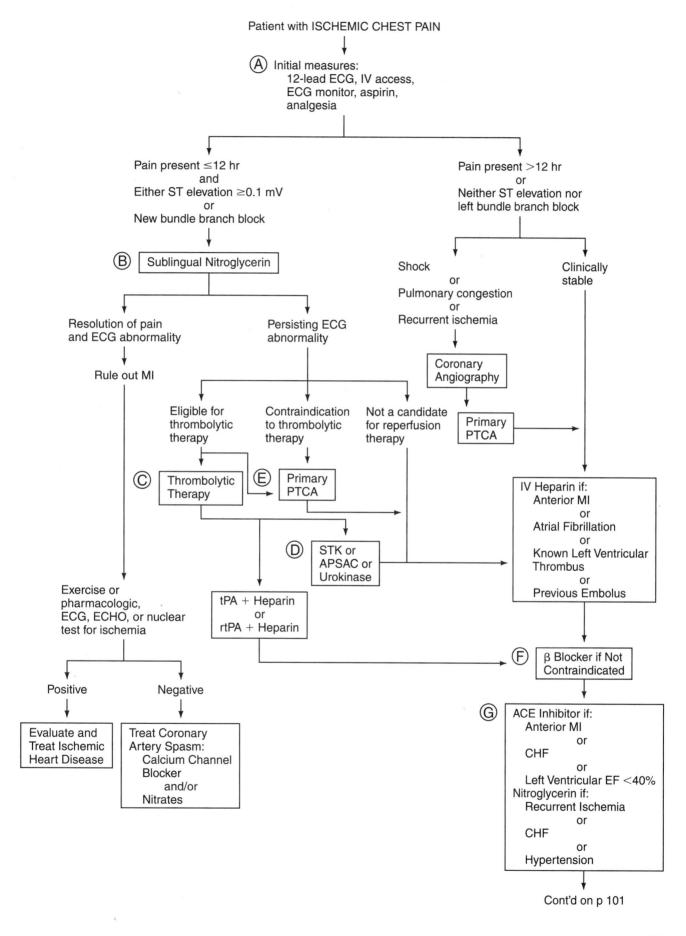

Patient with ISCHEMIC CHEST PAIN

(A) Initial measures:
12-lead ECG, IV access,
ECG monitor, aspirin,
analgesia

Pain present ≤12 hr
and
Either ST elevation ≥0.1 mV
or
New bundle branch block

Pain present >12 hr
or
Neither ST elevation nor
left bundle branch block

(B) Sublingual Nitroglycerin

Shock
or
Pulmonary congestion
or
Recurrent ischemia

Clinically
stable

Resolution of pain
and ECG abnormality

Persisting ECG
abnormality

Rule out MI

Coronary
Angiography

Eligible for
thrombolytic
therapy

Contraindication
to thrombolytic
therapy

Not a candidate
for reperfusion
therapy

Primary
PTCA

(C) Thrombolytic
Therapy

(E) Primary
PTCA

IV Heparin if:
Anterior MI
or
Atrial Fibrillation
or
Known Left Ventricular
Thrombus
or
Previous Embolus

(D) STK or
APSAC or
Urokinase

Exercise or
pharmacologic,
ECG, ECHO, or nuclear
test for ischemia

tPA + Heparin
or
rtPA + Heparin

(F) β Blocker if Not
Contraindicated

Positive

Negative

Evaluate and
Treat Ischemic
Heart Disease

Treat Coronary
Artery Spasm:
Calcium Channel
Blocker
and/or
Nitrates

(G) ACE Inhibitor if:
Anterior MI
or
CHF
or
Left Ventricular EF <40%
Nitroglycerin if:
Recurrent Ischemia
or
CHF
or
Hypertension

Cont'd on p 101

H. The prophylactic use of antiarrhythmic drugs is discouraged. In some studies, routine lidocaine administration was associated with a mortality rate higher than that in placebo-treated controls. Its use is currently recommended in patients with acute or suspected AMI with sustained ventricular tachyarrhythmias. Lidocaine may not be needed if a β blocker is administered.

I. Ventricular arrhythmias are a major cause of death in the first year after AMI. Electrophysiologic study (EPS) helps determine the risk of arrhythmic death but is invasive, so patients must be selected carefully. Noninvasive tests can indicate low-risk patients and can be combined to better define the high-risk patient, who may then undergo EPS. A reasonable approach is to sequentially perform a signal-averaged ECG, Holter monitoring to look for ventricular tachycardia (VT), and then an echocardiographic or nuclear study to determine if EF is <40%. If all three tests are abnormal, EPS is indicated. If any one test is normal, the arrhythmic risk is low, and further arrhythmia evaluation is unnecessary. Patients with VT and low EF may benefit from an automatic implantable cardiac defibrillator (AICD).

J. Although there are no uniform recommendations for an ideal time for stress testing after AMI, its importance in risk stratification cannot be overemphasized. Evidence for residual ischemia may be evaluated by exercise testing (treadmill or stationary bicycle), with assessment using ECG, echocardiography, radionuclide imaging (thallium or sestamibi), or positron emission tomography. Patients who have received thrombolytic therapy should undergo a submaximal stress test early, possibly before hospital discharge. Such patients may require a second (symptom-limited) stress test 4–8 weeks after AMI to determine safe activity levels or exercise prescription. However, for most patients a single symptom-limited stress test at 3 weeks is safe and cost-effective, with few deaths or reinfarctions occurring between hospital discharge and stress testing. Another alternative is submaximal testing 7–10 days after AMI (which can be performed on an outpatient basis), with a follow-up symptom-limited test at 4–6 weeks.

References

ACC/AHA Guidelines for the management of patients with acute myocardial infarction. A report of the American College of Cardiology/American Heart Association Task Force on Practice Guidelines (Committee on Management of Acute Myocardial Infarction). J Am Coll Cardiol 1996; 28:1328.

American Heart Association. Textbook of advanced cardiac life support. Dallas: American Heart Association, 1997; 9:1.

Grines CL, Braune KF, Marco J, et al. A comparison of immediate angioplasty with thrombolytic therapy for acute myocardial infarction. N Engl J Med 1993; 328:673.

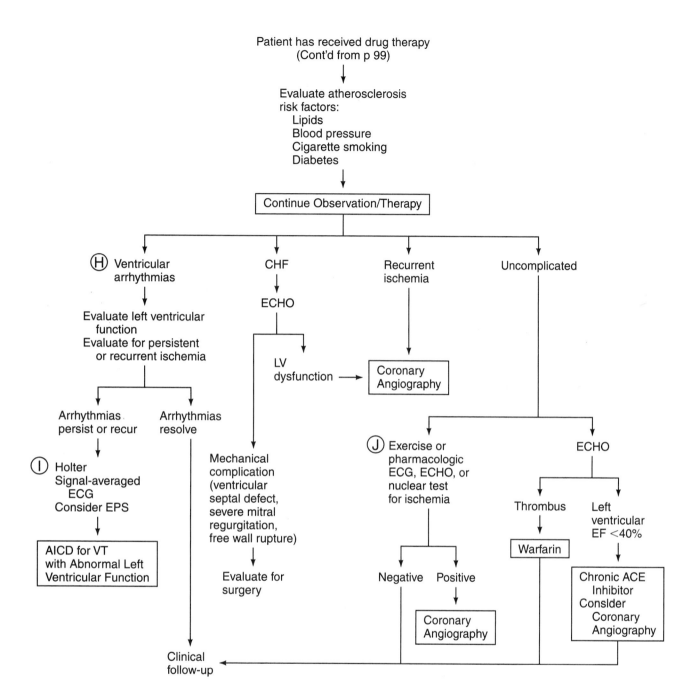

Patient has received drug therapy
(Cont'd from p 99)

Evaluate atherosclerosis
risk factors:
    Lipids
    Blood pressure
    Cigarette smoking
    Diabetes

Continue Observation/Therapy

(H) Ventricular arrhythmias

CHF

ECHO

Recurrent ischemia

Uncomplicated

Evaluate left ventricular function
Evaluate for persistent or recurrent ischemia

LV dysfunction → Coronary Angiography

Arrhythmias persist or recur

Arrhythmias resolve

(I) Holter
Signal-averaged ECG
Consider EPS

AICD for VT with Abnormal Left Ventricular Function

Mechanical complication (ventricular septal defect, severe mitral regurgitation, free wall rupture)

Evaluate for surgery

(J) Exercise or pharmacologic ECG, ECHO, or nuclear test for ischemia

ECHO

Thrombus

Left ventricular EF <40%

Warfarin

Negative   Positive

Coronary Angiography

Chronic ACE Inhibitor
Consider Coronary Angiography

Clinical follow-up

COUNSELING AFTER MYOCARDIAL INFARCTION

Susan McKenzie
Karl B. Kern

Counseling is an important aspect of care after a myocardial infarction (MI). Necessary components include educating the patient and determining the proper or optimal activity level.

A. Secondary prevention of coronary heart disease (CHD) through risk factor modification is an important beneficial strategy that complements both medical and surgical interventions in attempting to reduce the risk of further CHD events. The three most important controllable risk factors for CHD are hypertension, elevated serum cholesterol, and smoking. Successful control of hypertension and serum cholesterol is achieved through diet modification and pharmacologic management. Smoking cessation has been identified as the single most important lifestyle change to reduce morbidity and mortality after an MI. Other controllable risk factors are diabetes, obesity, and stress. Management of these factors by means of support groups and behavior modification also reduces the incidence of subsequent cardiac events. Education about risk factor modification should begin in inpatient cardiac rehabilitation and continue through all phases of outpatient rehabilitation. Patients should progress in activity from bed exercises with active and passive range of motion to sitting in a chair and performing activities of daily living and to walking in the halls of the hospital ward. Specific objectives of a cardiac rehabilitation program include (1) restoring individuals with cardiovascular disease to their optimal physiologic, psychosocial, and vocational status; (2) preventing progression or reversing the underlying atherosclerosis process in patients who have or are at high risk for CHD; and (3) reducing the risk of sudden death and reinfarction and alleviating angina pectoris in CHD patients.

B. During phase I (inpatient) cardiac rehabilitation or before phase II (outpatient) cardiac rehabilitation, risk stratification of MI patients is carried out on the basis of their prognosis for future CHD events and survival. The type and duration of supervision and frequency of monitoring in the rehabilitation setting is guided by the level of risk (low, moderate, or high). The patient's medical history, clinical course, physiologic variables, and test results assist in the risk stratification process.

C. Low-risk individuals (approximately 50% of all MI patients) include those with an uncomplicated hospital course, no evidence of myocardial ischemia after MI, functional capacity ≥7 METS, normal left ventricular function (LVEF > 50%), and absence of significant ventricular ectopy.

D. Intermediate- or moderate-risk patients include those with ST segment depression <2 mm, reversible thallium defects, moderate to good LVEF (35–49%), and stable angina pectoris.

E. High-risk patients include those with previous MI or infarct involving ≥35% of the left ventricle, LVEF <35% at rest, fall in exercise systolic blood pressure on exercise tolerance test, persistent or recurrent ischemic pain 24 hours or more after hospital admission, functional capacity <5 METS with hypotensive blood pressure response or positive ST depression at low levels of exercise, congestive heart failure in the hospital, >2 mm ST segment depression at peak heart rate ≤135 beats/min, or high-grade ventricular ectopy.

F. Symptom-limited exercise testing performed 3–6 weeks after MI helps determine functional capacity (resumption of physical activity including occupational work). If, on the exercise tolerance test, patients achieve a 9-MET level without symptoms, they can safely participate in home activity programs and return to work. If they experience cardiac abnormalities during the symptom-limited exercise test, continued attendance in a supervised rehabilitation program with intermittent monitoring is suggested. All post-MI patients should have eventual exercise goals of 30–45 minutes of exercise per day, 3–4 days per week at moderate intensities (3–7 METS), with an annual review by a cardiologist, including an exercise tolerance test.

References

American Association of Cardiovascular and Pulmonary Rehabilitation. Guidelines for cardiac rehabilitation programs. Middleton, WI: Human Kinetics, 1991.

DeBusk RF. Evaluation of patients after recent acute myocardial infarction. Ann Intern Med 1989; 110:485.

DeBusk RF, Miller NH, Superko HR, et al. A case-management system for coronary risk factor modification after acute myocardial infarction. Ann Intern Med 1994; 120:721.

Leon AS, Certo C, Comoss P, et al. Scientific evidence of the value of cardiac rehabilitation services with emphasis on patients following myocardial infarction—section I: exercise conditioning component. J Cardiopulm Rehabil 1990; 10:79.

Miller NH, Taylor CB, Davidson DM, et al. The efficacy of risk factor intervention and psychosocial aspects of cardiac rehabilitation. J Cardiopulm Rehabil 1990; 10:198.

Patient Ready for POST–MYOCARDIAL INFARCTION REHABILITATION

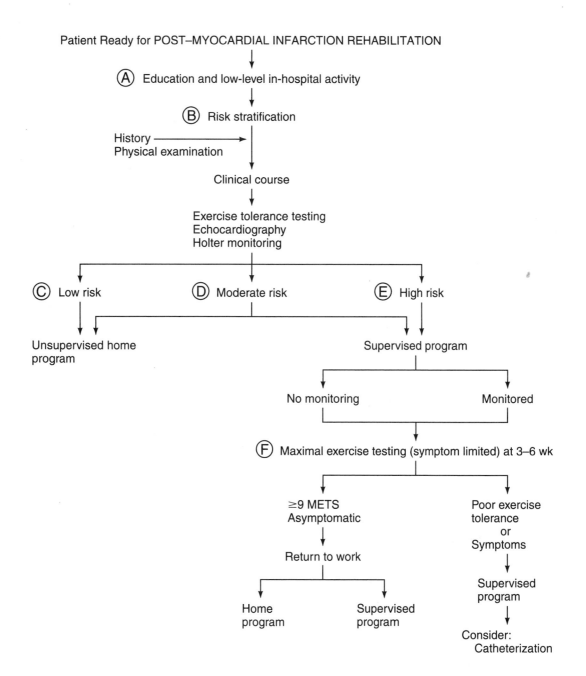

Ⓐ Education and low-level in-hospital activity

Ⓑ Risk stratification

History ──────→
Physical examination

Clinical course

Exercise tolerance testing
Echocardiography
Holter monitoring

Ⓒ Low risk   Ⓓ Moderate risk   Ⓔ High risk

Unsupervised home   Supervised program
program

No monitoring   Monitored

Ⓕ Maximal exercise testing (symptom limited) at 3–6 wk

≥9 METS   Poor exercise
Asymptomatic   tolerance
                                 or
                                 Symptoms
Return to work
                                 Supervised
                                 program
Home   Supervised
program   program   Consider:
                                 Catheterization

DERMATOLOGY

PIGMENTED LESIONS

Mark J. Scharf
Norman Levine

Skin color is determined mainly by the amount and distribution of melanin, a pigmented polymer produced by melanocytes. Hyperpigmentation is almost always the result of either production of too much melanin or abnormal distribution of pigment, although heavy metals or drug metabolites can change skin color.

A. Dermal melanosis/melanocytosis refers to a group of pigmentary skin conditions in which an increased number of melanocytes are producing melanin within the deeper levels of the dermis. The skin overlying these pigmented cells appears slate-blue to bluish-black. Mongolian spots are bluish macules presenting at or near birth that occur in 95% of black and 10% of white newborns. Of these lesions, 75% occur over the sacrum. They may be single or multiple and may be as large as 10 cm. They generally disappear by 5 years of age. Nevus of Ota is a form of dermal melanocytosis involving the distribution of the fifth cranial nerve. It is more common in Asians and also occurs in blacks. It is present at birth in 60% of those affected. Skin color is blue-gray to blue-brown. The sclera of the eye may also be involved.

B. Blue nevi are localized benign proliferations of melanocytes. They may be congenital or acquired. There are two types. Common blue nevi range in size from 2–10 mm. They present as small round to oval, smooth surfaced, well-defined papules with a bluish black pigmentation. Cellular blue nevi are less common and tend to be >1 cm. They are also bluish-black and may be mistaken for nodular melanoma. Rarely, cellular blue nevi can undergo malignant transformation.

C. When pigment derived from melanocytes is concentrated in the epidermis, the resulting skin color may range from tan to brown or even black. Freckles are an example of localized areas of increased pigment production caused by a normal concentration of melanocytes. They appear as small (2–5 mm) tan to brown macules on sun-exposed areas of skin and arise by age 2–4 years. They can be differentiated clinically from lentigos or nevi by the fact that they darken with sun exposure in the summer and fade in the winter. Café-au-lait spots present at birth as well-marginated tan macules. Six or more lesions >1.5 cm in diameter are diagnostic of neurofibromatosis (NF). In these patients, take a history for any personal or family history of NF. In patients suspected of having NF, do a slit-lamp examination of their eyes to look for Lisch nodules, which are pathognomonic for NF and are present in all cases by age 5. Lentigos ("liver spots") are well-demarcated tan to brown macules that may occur on any part of the skin, but particularly on sun-exposed areas of the face and dorsum of the hands. Unlike freckles, they do not fade over time. They are caused by an increased number of melanocytes with increased pigment production at the dermal-epidermal (DE) junction. Most lentigos are <5 mm. When lentigos are >5 mm and have irregular borders, perform a biopsy to determine whether the lesion is a lentigo maligna (LM). LMs are a form of melanoma in situ that can progress to invasive melanoma if not treated in time. If an LM is suspected, perform an incisional biopsy.

D. Congenital nevi are present from birth and range from 2 mm to >20 cm in diameter. They are typically deeply pigmented brown to black papules or plaques that may have verrucous surfaces and associated thick dark hairs. Giant congenital nevi (GCN) may involve an entire extremity or even large sections of the torso, scalp, or face. The risk of melanoma occurring in a GCN is estimated to be 5%. Although small and medium congenital nevi are associated with melanoma, the incidence of malignant transformation is far less than with GCNs; however, they should be followed with photographs and biopsied or excised if changes are seen.

E. Common acquired nevi (moles) appear during the first three decades of life and begin to regress after age 65. The average person has 40 nevi. Acquired nevi are divided into three categories depending on the localization of their melanocytes. In junctional nevi the melanocytes are present at the DE junction. These lesions are smooth bordered macules <5 mm with uniform color ranging from light to dark brown or even black. Compound nevi are raised well-demarcated symmetric papules or thin plaques. They range from light to dark brown; some have a stippled appearance. Melanocytes are present at the DE junction and within the dermis. Dermal nevi present as flesh-colored or pink papules. All melanocytes are found within dermis. Compound nevi may progress to dermal nevi as the melanocytes lose their ability to produce pigment and melanocytes are lost from the DE junction.

F. A number of acquired pigmented lesions can mimic nevi. The most common of these are seborrheic keratoses and dermatofibromas. Seborrheic keratoses (SKs) usually occur after age 35 and are well-defined, verrucous, usually hyperpigmented papules or plaques without surrounding pigment incontinence. They may become irritated by clothing or trauma, in which case they may show signs of inflammation or pruritus and require removal by cryotherapy, curettage, or shave excision. Occasionally, SKs may be misdiagnosed as melanomas because of their dark colors, and at times, melanomas may masquerade as SKs. When there is any doubt, a biopsy is indicated. Dermatofibromas are smooth,

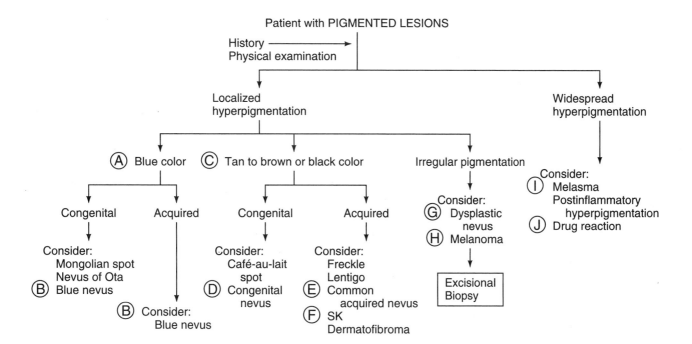

Patient with PIGMENTED LESIONS

History → Physical examination

Localized hyperpigmentation | Widespread hyperpigmentation

(A) Blue color | (C) Tan to brown or black color | Irregular pigmentation | Consider:
(I) Melasma
Postinflammatory hyperpigmentation
(J) Drug reaction

Congenital | Acquired | Congenital | Acquired | Consider:
(G) Dysplastic nevus
(H) Melanoma

Consider:
Mongolian spot
Nevus of Ota
(B) Blue nevus

(B) Consider:
Blue nevus

Consider:
Café-au-lait spot
(D) Congenital nevus

Consider:
Freckle
Lentigo
(E) Common acquired nevus
(F) SK
Dermatofibroma

Excisional Biopsy

brown or pink papules that often pucker in the center when compressed from the edges (the "dimple sign" of Fitzpatrick). Although their cause is unclear, they may arise after minor trauma such as an insect bite or razor cut. Becker's nevus is a uniformly tan to brown plaque that occurs primarily on the upper trunk and shoulders. It is more common in males than in females. These lesions usually present in adolescents and may be confused with large congenital nevi as they mature and acquire coarse dark hairs. They are a form of connective tissue nevus and present no malignant potential.

G. Dysplastic or atypical nevi are acquired nevi that are >5 mm in diameter and have irregular or variegate pigmentation with poorly defined or irregular borders. Some of these lesions may be precursors for melanomas. Patients with atypical nevi who have two or more first-degree relatives with dysplastic nevi and a history of melanoma have nearly a 100% chance of developing melanomas. Follow these patients carefully for any signs of change in their nevi. These changes can best be assessed when baseline high-quality photographs have been taken so that the current findings can be compared with previous images.

H. Melanomas are skin cancers arising from the malignant transformation of melanocytes. As discussed, they may arise from precursor lesions such as atypical nevi, congenital nevi, and LM. They may also arise de novo from melanocytes within the skin. Suspect melanoma if a pigmented lesion displays any combination of asymmetry, border irregularity, variegate colors (blues, browns, black, red, or white), or a diameter >5 mm. Other worrisome signs are pruritus, ulceration, bleeding, or change in color or size of the lesion.

I. Melasma is a form of hyperpigmentation characterized by mottled tan to brown macules coalescing into irregular patches on the face. The forehead, cheeks, and upper lip are often involved. Melasma is common in preg-

nancy, when it is called chloasma. The condition may be triggered by oral contraceptives. It may be idiopathic or familial and can also be seen in men. Postinflammatory hyperpigmentation is another form of localized macular hyperpigmentation that occurs after cutaneous trauma or inflammatory dermatoses. It is more common and may be more severe in darker skinned individuals.

J. Pigmentary abnormalities of the skin can have both exogenous and endogenous causes. A number of medications can cause hyperpigmentation. Minocycline, if given in sufficient quantities for prolonged periods, can produce a gray-brown discoloration in old acne scars or a pattern of more diffuse hyperpigmentation over the anterior legs or trunk. Phenothiazines may cause a blue-gray color, particularly in sun-exposed skin. Hydroxychloroquine may produce irregular gray patches on the legs. Patients taking amiodarone may develop a slate-gray hyperpigmentation on the face, particularly after long-term sun exposure. Exposure to heavy metals such as gold or silver may result in a diffuse bluish-gray cast to the skin. Systemic disorders such as Addison's disease, uremia, and hemochromatosis can cause distinctive generalized patterns of hyperpigmentation.

References

Arndt KA, Leboit PE, Robinson JK, Wintroub BU, eds. Cutaneous medicine and surgery. Philadelphia: WB Saunders, 1996.

Fitzpatrick TB, Eisen AZ, Wolff K, et al, eds. Dermatology in general medicine. 4th ed. New York: McGraw-Hill, 1993.

Swerdlow AJ, English JS, Qiao Z. The risk of melanoma in patients with congenital nevi: a cohort study. J Am Acad Dermatol 1995; 32:595.

Tucker MA, Halpern A, Holly EA, et al. Clinically recognized dysplastic nevi: a central risk factor for cutaneous melanoma. JAMA 1997; 277:1439.

Yohn J, Hoffman S, Norris D, Robinson W. Melanoma: diagnosis and treatment. Hosp Pract (Off Ed) 1994; 29:27.

LEG ULCER

Cynthia A. O'Neil

A. The cause of a leg ulcer usually can be determined by history and physical examination alone. It is therefore important to ask the patient about trauma and any history of diseases such as coronary artery disease, deep venous thrombosis, and diabetes mellitus. Inquire about symptoms of vasculitis, chronic inflammatory disorders, and neoplasms. The physical examination should focus on evidence of edema, varicosities, arterial insufficiency, neuropathy, and infection.

B. Arterial ulcers account for 5% of all leg ulcers. They result from impairment of blood flow and have multiple causes, including emboli, thrombi, arteriosclerosis, Buerger's disease, hypertension, vasospasm, vasculitis, and hematologic disorders. Patients complain of pain at rest that is exacerbated with leg elevation and relieved with dependency. The ulcers are characterized by a pale or eschar-covered base with minimal granulation tissue, usually occurring on the distal foot. Other important signs of arterial involvement are coolness of the extremities, decreased pulses and slow capillary refill, a palpable or audible bruit over the femoral artery, and decreased hair on the distal legs. If arterial pulses are not palpable, use a Doppler flowmeter to hear the pulsations over the dorsalis pedis and posterior tibial arteries and calculate the ankle/brachial index (ABI) of systolic pressure. If the index is <0.7, moderate to severe disease is present and arteriography should be considered.

C. Chronic venous insufficiency accounts for about 90% of all leg ulcers. Venous stasis results from a dysfunction of venous outflow, most commonly caused by defective valves (usually secondary to deep venous thromboses or a congenital defect). Patients have edema and, in contrast to those with arterial disease, have relatively little pain. On physical examination an ulcer with exudate and granulation tissue often is seen over the medial malleolus. Varicosities, brown hemosiderin pigment, and dermatitis support the diagnosis.

D. Neurotrophic ulcers are caused by the repeated trauma or pressure on weight-bearing areas where there is impaired cutaneous sensation. Diabetes mellitus accounts for most of these ulcers, but other causes include other forms of vascular disease (polyarteritis nodosa), lead/arsenic polyneuropathies, alcoholic polyneuropathy, sarcoidosis, leprosy, and syphilis.

E. Infection is another etiologic factor in leg ulcers. It occurs most commonly after primary inoculation of a pathogen, although dissemination from a primary focus elsewhere also is possible. Lesions are inflamed and purulent and may have draining sinuses. Perform a biopsy at the ulcer margin and send the tissue to be cultured for bacterial, fungal, mycobacterial, and viral pathogens.

F. Lack of response of an ulcer to therapy or rapid growth of a lesion that was previously stable should lead one to suspect neoplasm. An elevated ulcer edge with central crust or granulation tissue is characteristic of many tumors. A biopsy of the ulcer margin should be performed.

G. Traumatic ulcers are diagnosed by history. Some patients with self-induced disease may be unwilling to divulge the cause and may, in fact, be inappropriately unconcerned. These ulcers are characterized by bizarre shapes that have minimal surrounding erythema.

References

Burton CS III. Treatment of leg ulcers. Dermatol Clin 1993; 11:315.

Douglas WS, Simpson NB. Guidelines for the management of chronic venous leg ulceration. Br J Dermatol 1995; 132:446.

Krull EA. Chronic cutaneous ulcerations and impaired healing in the human skin. J Am Acad Dermatol 1995; 12:394.

Phillips TJ, Dover JS. Leg ulcers. J Am Acad Dermatol 1991; 25:965.

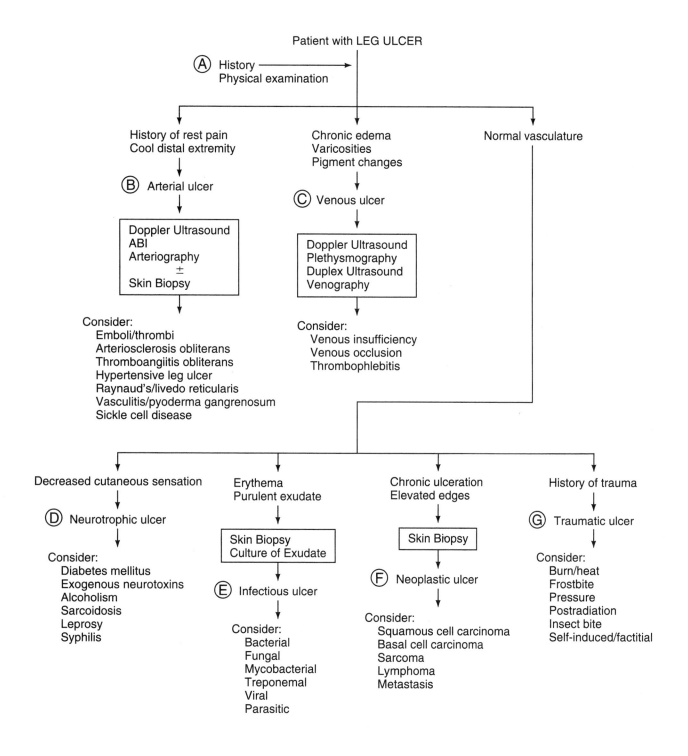

Patient with LEG ULCER

(A) History
Physical examination

History of rest pain
Cool distal extremity

(B) Arterial ulcer

Doppler Ultrasound
ABI
Arteriography
±
Skin Biopsy

Consider:
Emboli/thrombi
Arteriosclerosis obliterans
Thromboangiitis obliterans
Hypertensive leg ulcer
Raynaud's/livedo reticularis
Vasculitis/pyoderma gangrenosum
Sickle cell disease

Chronic edema
Varicosities
Pigment changes

(C) Venous ulcer

Doppler Ultrasound
Plethysmography
Duplex Ultrasound
Venography

Consider:
Venous insufficiency
Venous occlusion
Thrombophlebitis

Normal vasculature

Decreased cutaneous sensation

(D) Neurotrophic ulcer

Consider:
Diabetes mellitus
Exogenous neurotoxins
Alcoholism
Sarcoidosis
Leprosy
Syphilis

Erythema
Purulent exudate

Skin Biopsy
Culture of Exudate

(E) Infectious ulcer

Consider:
Bacterial
Fungal
Mycobacterial
Treponemal
Viral
Parasitic

Chronic ulceration
Elevated edges

Skin Biopsy

(F) Neoplastic ulcer

Consider:
Squamous cell carcinoma
Basal cell carcinoma
Sarcoma
Lymphoma
Metastasis

History of trauma

(G) Traumatic ulcer

Consider:
Burn/heat
Frostbite
Pressure
Postradiation
Insect bite
Self-induced/factitial

URTICARIA

Norman Levine

Urticaria is a vascular reaction of the skin characterized by evanescent edematous plaques (wheals, hives). Angioedema differs only in that the edema extends into the deep dermis and subcutaneous tissue. About 15% of the population develop this problem at some time in life. In about 60% of cases the lesions resolve in <6 weeks (acute urticaria); in the remaining patients the disease persists longer, usually in the form of recurrent episodes.

A. In about 25% of cases a definite cause can be uncovered, and in most of these patients the history and physical examination alone are sufficient to determine the cause.

B. The most common cause of acute urticaria is a drug reaction. The agents often implicated are sulfonamides, penicillin derivatives, barbiturates, diuretics, and antiinflammatory agents. Medications taken within 14 days of the onset of the urticaria are the most likely offenders. Certain foods such as nuts, shellfish, and eggs may produce urticaria in susceptible individuals. Focal infections such as sinusitis or genitourinary infections, and systemic infections such as viral hepatitis or infectious mononucleosis, occasionally produce urticaria. In rare instances, patients may develop localized wheals after direct contact with an offending agent (contact urticaria).

C. Certain chronic skin diseases have lesions that appear urticarial and must be differentiated from urticaria. Urticaria pigmentosa (mastocytosis) presents with stable brown papules that urticate when rubbed. The lesions of urticarial vasculitis are wheals that persist for several days and often have a violaceous color. These diagnoses can be confirmed by a skin biopsy.

D. Many cases of chronic urticaria are secondary to physical stimuli that produce hives in susceptible patients. Dermographism occurs in 5% of the population and consists of wheals that develop 1–3 minutes after skin stroking. Stimuli as innocuous as toweling after bathing or rubbing one's eyes can produce hives. Less commonly, patients develop wheals after cold, heat, water, or sun exposure. Patients with cholinergic urticaria develop 2- to 4-mm wheals within 2–20 minutes after general overheating of the body, such as occurs after vigorous exercise.

E. In patients with chronic urticaria that are not secondary to physical stimuli, a routine noninvasive laboratory screen is indicated. However, abnormal laboratory test results rarely uncover an occult cause of urticaria in the face of a normal history and physical examination.

F. In many patients an identifiable cause of chronic urticaria is never uncovered. In some of these there may be psychogenic influences that exacerbate the urticarial episodes. Others may have a genetic tendency that makes them more prone to hives from a variety of stimuli. Some cases of chronic urticaria are caused by an autoimmune phenomenon in which autoantibodies bind to IgE receptors on the surface of mast cells, resulting in mast cell activation and degranulation.

References

Arndt KA, Leboit PE, Robinson JK, Wintroub BU, eds. Cutaneous medicine and surgery. Philadelphia: WB Saunders, 1996.

Hirschmann JV, Lawlor F, English JSC, et al. Cholinergic urticaria: a clinical and histologic study. Arch Dermatol 1987; 123:462.

Jacobson KW, Branch CB, Nelson HS. Laboratory tests in chronic urticaria. JAMA 1980; 243:1644.

Kulp-Shorten CL, Callen JP. Urticaria, angioedema, and rheumatologic disease. Rheum Dis Clin North Am 1996; 22:95.

Mahmood T. Urticaria. Am Fam Physician 1995; 51:811.

Pollack CV Jr, Romano TJ. Outpatient management of acute urticaria: the role of prednisone. Ann Emerg Med 1995; 26:547.

Sveum RJ. Urticaria: the diagnostic challenge of hives. Postgrad Med 1996; 100:77.

Wong RC, Fairley JA, Ellis CN. Dermographism: a review. J Am Acad Dermatol 1984; 11:643.

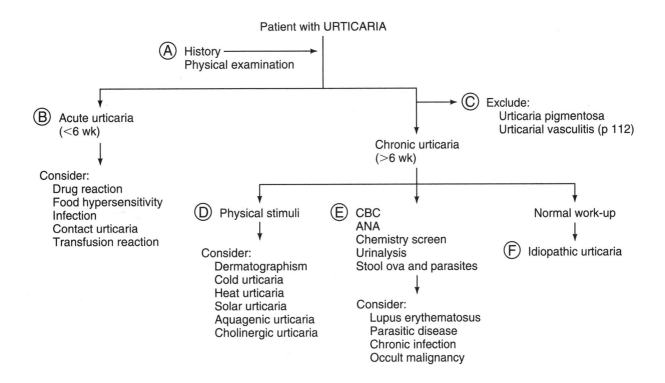

Patient with URTICARIA

(A) History ———→
Physical examination

(B) Acute urticaria
(<6 wk)
↓
Consider:
 Drug reaction
 Food hypersensitivity
 Infection
 Contact urticaria
 Transfusion reaction

(C) Exclude:
Urticaria pigmentosa
Urticarial vasculitis (p 112)

Chronic urticaria
(>6 wk)

(D) Physical stimuli
↓
Consider:
 Dermatographism
 Cold urticaria
 Heat urticaria
 Solar urticaria
 Aquagenic urticaria
 Cholinergic urticaria

(E) CBC
ANA
Chemistry screen
Urinalysis
Stool ova and parasites
↓
Consider:
 Lupus erythematosus
 Parasitic disease
 Chronic infection
 Occult malignancy

Normal work-up
↓
(F) Idiopathic urticaria

GENERALIZED PRURITUS

Norman Levine

Pruritus is an unpleasant sensation that provokes the desire to scratch. Regardless of the underlying cause, most patients have maximal itching at bedtime. There are many pruritic dermatoses, but relatively few of these cause generalized itching. Generalized pruritus can be divided into conditions in which there is an associated dermatosis and those in which pruritus is a symptom of a noncutaneous disease.

A. Physical examination alone is sufficient to diagnose most primary cutaneous pruritic diseases. In the absence of an obvious primary lesion, a medical history may uncover occult dermatoses. For example, xerotic (dry) skin often itches just after bathing. Scabies may affect multiple household members and can be a venereally transmitted condition. Atopic dermatitis often appears in successive generations and is associated with asthma and allergic rhinitis.

B. The two most common causes of generalized pruritus are xerosis and atopic dermatitis. Xerosis is most prominent on the anterior legs and lateral arms. The plaques have fine fissures that look like a cracked pot ("erythema craquele"). The lesions of atopic dermatitis are thickened (lichenified) and excoriated.

C. Diagnosis often can be confirmed by a skin biopsy. If scabies is suspected, examine the superficial contents of a burrow by performing a skin scraping.

D. In the absence of an obvious cutaneous cause of generalized pruritus, empirically treat for xerosis with moisturizers. If the pruritus persists, a laboratory work-up is indicated and should include a hemogram, serum chemistries, glucose tolerance test, thyroid function studies, urinalysis, and chest radiography.

E. Pruritus rarely predates the diagnosis of systemic malignancy except in Hodgkin's disease, where 6% of cases present with pruritus alone.

F. Polycythemia vera is associated with pruritus after quick temperature change (e.g., bathing). Itching occurs commonly in leukemia and rarely in iron deficiency states, even in the absence of other signs and symptoms.

G. Pruritus often is the first symptom of biliary cirrhosis and extrahepatic biliary obstruction. An elevated serum alkaline phosphatase level is characteristic.

H. The pruritus of diabetes mellitus occurs in <5% of patients and is not correlated with disease severity.

I. Hyperthyroidism may produce generalized pruritus that improves when the patient becomes euthyroid. Most cases of pruritus with hypothyroidism are secondary to xerosis.

J. Chronic renal failure commonly produces generalized pruritus in patients with BUN >50 mg/dl. Dialysis may produce paroxysms of intense itching. Phototherapy with ultraviolet B (UVB) may relieve itching in these patients.

K. Although psychogenic pruritus is a common cause of itching, consider it only after all other causes have been ruled out. If after a routine work-up there are no localizing signs of carcinoma, further evaluation usually is not indicated.

References

Bergasa NV, Jones EA. The pruritus of cholestasis. Semin Liver Dis 1993; 13:319.

Denman ST. A review of pruritus. J Am Acad Dermatol 1986; 14:375.

Greaves MW. New pathophysiological and clinical insights into pruritus. J Dermatol 1993; 29:735.

Kantor GR, Lookingbill DP. Generalized pruritus and systemic disease. J Am Acad Dermatol 1983; 9:375.

Levine N. "Winter itch": what's causing this rash? Geriatrics 1996; 51:20.

Lober CW. Pruritus and malignancy. Clin Dermatol 1993; 11:125.

Martin J. Pruritus. Int J Dermatol 1985; 24:634.

Patient with GENERALIZED PRURITUS

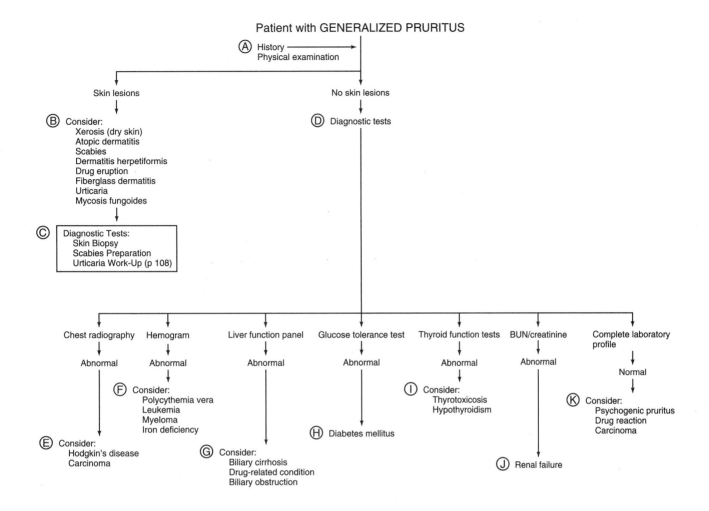

PALPABLE PURPURA

Norman Levine

Palpable purpura is a skin lesion that is purpuric and has substance. It can be a papule, vesicle, or pustule. These lesions are highly indicative of inflammatory destruction of cutaneous blood vessel walls (vasculitis). Immune-mediated mechanisms of damage often are operative. Many clinically distinct disorders fall under the general heading of vasculitis, but the pathologic processes are similar in most of them.

A. The presence of palpable purpura is considered septic vasculitis until proved otherwise. Therefore, rule out underlying causes of sepsis before doing any other work-up. Signs and symptoms of sepsis include fever, chills, mental status changes, tachycardia, tachypnea, and hypotension. In this clinical setting, several blood cultures and a skin biopsy of a purpuric lesion for light microscopy, bacterial smear, and culture are indicated.

B. Although there are few distinguishing clinical features of the skin lesions in septic vasculitis that would lead to the diagnosis of a specific infection, there occasionally are clues. In staphylococcal sepsis, showers of purpuric pustules appear. Gram stain reveals the offending organism. In gonococcemia, there are relatively few acral purpuric papules and vesicles that subsequently develop into pustules. Patients with meningococcemia have an explosive onset of hundreds of hemorrhagic macules and papules over the whole body. In Rocky Mountain spotted fever, palpable purpuric lesions occur after several days of illness, and only after the lesions have progressed from pink macules to red papules to purpuric papules.

C. In many cases, palpable purpura of the skin mirrors systemic vasculitides, most of which are immune mediated. Although laboratory abnormalities are common in systemic vasculitis, there are few abnormalities pathognomonic for given diseases. Therefore, the work-up includes measurements of organ function and immune status along with the history and physical examination.

D. Henoch-Schönlein purpura is a small vessel vasculitis, usually occurring in children, that involves the skin (palpable purpura), joints, kidneys, and GI tract. In 90% of cases this follows an upper respiratory infection and lasts for 7–14 days. There may be recurrences. Several chronic disorders are characterized by granuloma formation involving blood vessels that can produce palpable purpuric lesions. Wegener's granulomatosis is a disease involving the skin, kidneys, and upper respiratory tract. Allergic granulomatosis (Churg-Strauss syndrome) occurs in asthmatic patients who develop palpable purpura, hypertension, chronic pneumonitis, and a neuropathy. Polyarteritis nodosa is a vasculitis of small- and medium-sized arteries with involvement of the skin, kidneys, pulmonary and nervous system, and joints. The skin lesions may be purpuric papules, subcutaneous nodules, and/or cutaneous ulcerations along with livedo reticularis (p 114). Urticarial vasculitis is a multisystem disorder with recurrent crops of purpuric wheals lasting several days. Some of these patients have associated hypocomplementemia. This is differentiated from other forms of vasculitis by the relatively evanescent nature of the lesions and by the fact that the lesions appear more urticarial.

E. In many cases, palpable purpura (vasculitis) occurs in an otherwise clinically healthy patient. A limited laboratory work-up, including skin biopsy, is indicated to rule out occult immune complex diseases such as essential mixed cryoglobulinemia and hyperglobulinemic purpura, and purely cutaneous vasculitides such as erythema elevatum diutinum.

F. Hypersensitivity vasculitis does not have pathognomonic criteria but depends on a constellation of signs and symptoms. Most patients are >16 years of age and may have a history of intake of a medication that could be causative. They have palpable purpura and nonblanching red papules and macules, usually on the lower extremities.

References

Calabrese LH, Michel BA, Bloch DA, et al. The American College of Rheumatology 1990 criteria for the classification of hypersensitivity vasculitis. Arthritis Rheum 1990; 33:1108.

Eckstein E, Callen JP. Cutaneous leukocytoclastic vasculitis: clinical and laboratory features of 82 patients seen in private practice. Arch Dermatol 1984; 120:484.

Jorizzo JL, Solomon AR, Zanolli MD. Neutrophilic vascular reactions. J Am Acad Dermatol 1988; 19:983.

Lightfoot RW Jr, Michel BA, Bloch DA, et al. The American College of Rheumatology 1990 criteria for the classification of polyarteritis nodosa. Arthritis Rheum 1990; 33:1088.

Manders SM. Serious and life-threatening drug eruptions. Am Fam Physician 1995; 51:1805.

Mills JA, Michel BA, Bloch DA, et al. The American College of Rheumatology 1990 criteria for the classification of Henoch-Schönlein purpura. Arthritis Rheum 1990; 33:1114.

Tapson KM. Henoch-Schönlein purpura. Am Fam Physician 1993; 47:633.

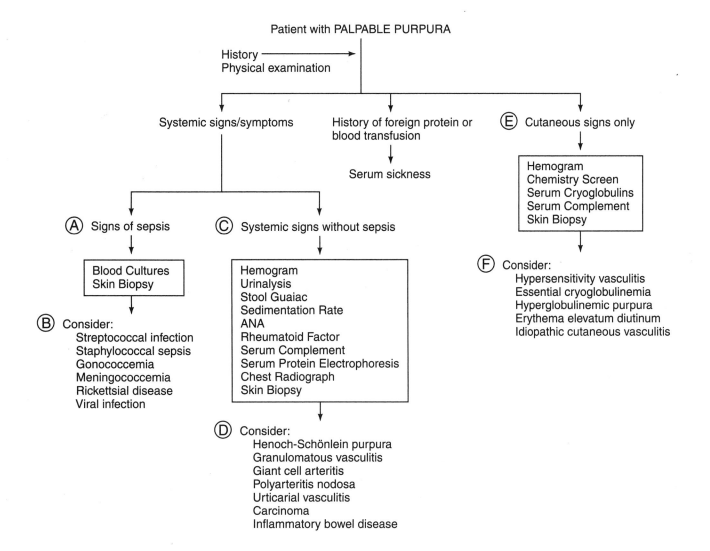

Patient with PALPABLE PURPURA

History
Physical examination

Systemic signs/symptoms

History of foreign protein or blood transfusion
Serum sickness

Ⓔ Cutaneous signs only

Hemogram
Chemistry Screen
Serum Cryoglobulins
Serum Complement
Skin Biopsy

Ⓕ Consider:
    Hypersensitivity vasculitis
    Essential cryoglobulinemia
    Hyperglobulinemic purpura
    Erythema elevatum diutinum
    Idiopathic cutaneous vasculitis

Ⓐ Signs of sepsis

Blood Cultures
Skin Biopsy

Ⓑ Consider:
    Streptococcal infection
    Staphylococcal sepsis
    Gonococcemia
    Meningococcemia
    Rickettsial disease
    Viral infection

Ⓒ Systemic signs without sepsis

Hemogram
Urinalysis
Stool Guaiac
Sedimentation Rate
ANA
Rheumatoid Factor
Serum Complement
Serum Protein Electrophoresis
Chest Radiograph
Skin Biopsy

Ⓓ Consider:
    Henoch-Schönlein purpura
    Granulomatous vasculitis
    Giant cell arteritis
    Polyarteritis nodosa
    Urticarial vasculitis
    Carcinoma
    Inflammatory bowel disease

LIVEDO RETICULARIS

Angela Murphy McGhee

Livedo reticularis is a netlike (reticulate) mottling of the skin encountered with some frequency in medical practice, in both pediatrics and adult medicine. It may represent a normal variant or may be a sign of a serious systemic disorder.

A. The age of the patient is important in evaluating the cause of livedo reticularis. If the livedo pattern is first observed in the adult, it is associated more often with underlying diseases than when seen in the child.

B. When the skin appears mottled upon exposure to cold but returns to normal when the body is warmed over minutes to hours, physiologic factors are operative.

C. In adults the pattern (symmetry versus asymmetry) and location (extremities, trunk, generalized) can help determine the cause of a livedo reticularis pattern. In general, symmetric involvement, especially of the extremities, usually is physiologic, whereas asymmetric, patchy, or truncal involvement often indicates pathologic change.

D. Long-standing livedo reticularis without ulcerations and no other signs or symptoms is the idiopathic variant, but this can be diagnosed only after other causes are excluded. However, in patients with abrupt-onset livedo without ulcerations, consider the rheumatologic diseases.

E. Fixed livedo accompanied by leg ulcerations represents a variant that usually occurs in women <40 years of age. It is the result of long-standing microvascular stasis. Although fixed, the livedo pattern is accentuated by the cold. Rarely, there is an associated arterial disease elsewhere, such as endarteritis obliterans or arteriosclerosis. The livedo pattern in these instances is widespread and the disease progressive. Rheumatic diseases with accompanying vasculitis should also be considered here. The work-up should include CBC, ESR, ANA, renal panel, and skin biopsy.

F. The clinical picture of fixed livedo in a discontinuous pattern, especially that of recent onset, suggests an underlying pathologic condition such as systemic lupus erythematosus (SLE), systemic vasculitis, malignancies, hypo- or hyperparathyroidism, infections (tuberculosis, syphilis), infectious or cholesterol emboli, pancreatitis, reactions to drugs (e.g., amantadine), and hematologic disorders (e.g., thrombocythemia).

References

Jacobs AH. Vascular malformations. In: Schachner LA, ed. Pediatric dermatology. 2nd ed. New York: Churchill Livingstone, 1995.

Kampe CE. Clinical syndromes associated with lupus anticoagulants. Semin Thromb Hemost 1994; 20:16.

Kontos HA. Vascular diseases of the limbs. In: Bennett JC, Plum F, eds. Cecil textbook of medicine. 20th ed. Philadelphia: WB Saunders, 1996:346.

Picascia DD, Pellegrini JR. Livedo reticularis. Cutis 1987; 39:429.

Young PC, Cuozzo DW, Seidman AJ, et al. Widespread livedo reticularis with painful ulcerations. Arch Dermatol 1995; 131:786.

Patient with LIVEDO RETICULARIS

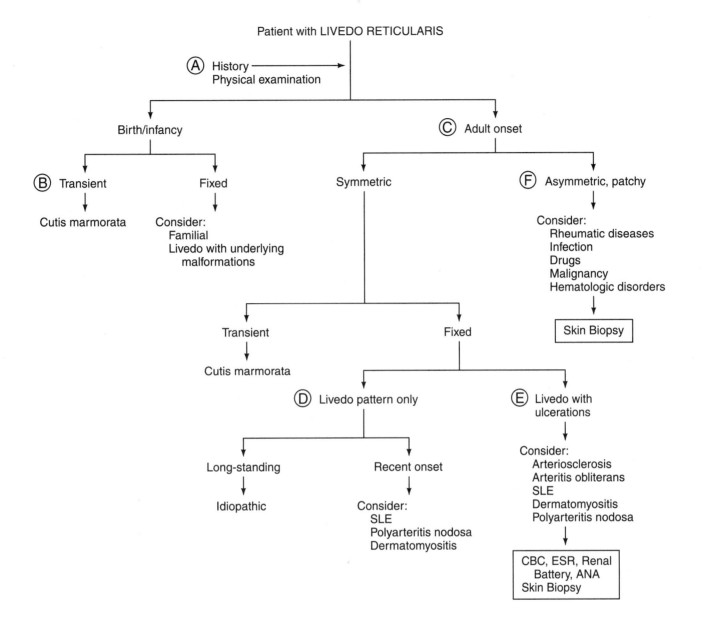

A. History
   Physical examination

Birth/infancy

B. Transient

Cutis marmorata

Fixed

Consider:
   Familial
   Livedo with underlying
      malformations

C. Adult onset

Symmetric

Transient

Cutis marmorata

Fixed

D. Livedo pattern only

Long-standing

Idiopathic

Recent onset

Consider:
   SLE
   Polyarteritis nodosa
   Dermatomyositis

E. Livedo with
   ulcerations

Consider:
   Arteriosclerosis
   Arteritis obliterans
   SLE
   Dermatomyositis
   Polyarteritis nodosa

CBC, ESR, Renal
   Battery, ANA
Skin Biopsy

F. Asymmetric, patchy

Consider:
   Rheumatic diseases
   Infection
   Drugs
   Malignancy
   Hematologic disorders

Skin Biopsy

ENDOCRINOLOGY

DYSLIPIDEMIA

Stephen P. Thomson
Thomas W. Boyden

Patient concerns about possible dyslipidemia often reflect their deeper concerns about risk of coronary artery disease (CAD). Patients may use cholesterol level as a simple estimate of their risk for CAD, excluding other risk factors, and focus on only the pharmacologic control of cholesterol to prevent CAD. Clinicians know that risk for CAD cannot be simplified to cholesterol alone. Therefore the approach to possible dyslipidemia usually includes identification of other risk factors and an acknowledgment that although cholesterol is important, it has limitations if used alone. Because of their concerns about preventing CAD, most patients need specific advice about dyslipidemia *combined* with information and treatment of other CAD risk factors (e.g., obesity, diabetes, hypertension, smoking, lack of estrogen).

A. There are no obvious "threshold" levels to define dyslipidemia. Complications associated with dyslipidemia increase as levels of LDL cholesterol (LDL-C) or triglycerides (TG) increase and HDL levels decrease. The National Cholesterol Education Program (NCEP) thresholds were derived from epidemiologic data and include a total cholesterol level of ≥200 mg/dl for the general population. For patients with CAD, drug treatment is considered for LDL-C ≥130 mg/dl. A clinically derived threshold for LDL-C of ≥125 mg/dl was noted in the recent secondary prevention CARE trial. It used pravastatin to lower cholesterol in patients after a myocardial infarction (MI). Only patients with an initial LDL-C ≥125 mg/dl benefited from drug treatment. Elevated levels of TG are not clearly an independent risk factor for CAD. However, TG ≥400 mg/dl may confer risk because they typically are associated with high cholesterol, low HDL, and other risk factors. Patients with TG levels ≥1000 mg/dl are at risk for pancreatitis.

B. In the history and physical examination, assess prior CAD and CAD risk factors: smoking, hypertension, diabetes, family history of CAD before age 60, abdominal obesity, lack of estrogen, and cerebrovascular or peripheral vascular disease. Also note the presence of palmar, tuberous, or tendinous xanthomas, which occur in familial dyslipidemia syndromes. Consider checking TSH, fasting glucose, liver blood tests, and urinary protein to find secondary causes of dyslipidemia: hypothyroidism, diabetes, chronic liver disease, or nephrotic syndrome.

C. Dyslipidemia syndromes account for <5% of patients with dyslipidemia. Consider these syndromes in patients with a personal or family history of CAD before age 40, cholesterol ≥300 mg/dl, TG ≥1000 mg/dl, pancreatitis, or xanthomas. These patients often require combination drug therapy and benefit from consultation with an endocrinologist. Familial hypercholesterolemia is an autosomal-dominant disorder caused by a mutation in the gene for the LDL receptor. Homozygotes ($1/10^6$) develop CAD in childhood. Heterozygotes (1/500) have premature CAD, often as young adults. They may have xanthomas, total cholesterol of 350–550 mg/dl, and normal TG levels. Combination therapy with a statin, niacin, and resin binders is usually required. Familial combined hyperlipidemia is a mixed group of genetic disorders that occurs in about 2% of adults. Cholesterol, TG, or both increase in young adults to above the 90th percentile. Hypertriglyceridemia can be familial or acquired and can respond to weight loss and avoidance of alcohol. Familial lipoprotein lipase deficiency is a rare autosomal-recessive disorder ($1/10^6$) that results in accumulation of chylomicrons, severe hypertriglyceridemia, xanthomas, and childhood pancreatitis. Dysbetalipoproteinemia causes increased cholesterol and TG levels, premature CAD, and pathognomonic palmar xanthomas (orange-yellow palmar creases).

(Continued on page 118)

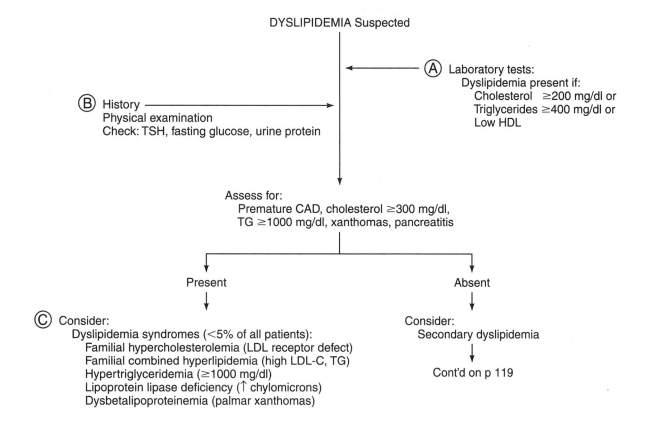

DYSLIPIDEMIA Suspected

Ⓐ Laboratory tests:
   Dyslipidemia present if:
      Cholesterol ≥200 mg/dl or
      Triglycerides ≥400 mg/dl or
      Low HDL

Ⓑ History
   Physical examination
   Check: TSH, fasting glucose, urine protein

Assess for:
   Premature CAD, cholesterol ≥300 mg/dl,
   TG ≥1000 mg/dl, xanthomas, pancreatitis

Present

Absent

Ⓒ Consider:
   Dyslipidemia syndromes (<5% of all patients):
      Familial hypercholesterolemia (LDL receptor defect)
      Familial combined hyperlipidemia (high LDL-C, TG)
      Hypertriglyceridemia (≥1000 mg/dl)
      Lipoprotein lipase deficiency (↑ chylomicrons)
      Dysbetalipoproteinemia (palmar xanthomas)

Consider:
   Secondary dyslipidemia

Cont'd on p 119

D. Secondary dyslipidemia commonly occurs with poorly controlled diabetes, hypothyroidism, or nephrotic syndrome. Rarer causes include chronic liver disease, renal failure, excessive alcohol consumption, and use of progestins, isotretinoin, or anabolic steroids. Antihypertensive agents rarely cause persistent, clinically significant changes in lipid levels. If lipids are still high after treating the underlying cause of secondary dyslipidemia, consider treating the persistent dyslipidemia.

E. In low-risk groups it is hard to prevent CAD events because they occur relatively infrequently, even without treatment. The costs and hazards of treatment may outweigh the benefits in patients at low risk for CAD. Because so many patients must be treated to avoid a CAD event, it could cost several million dollars per year of life saved. These patients should optimize their diet and exercise. Patients with severe increases in LDL-C levels or a dyslipidemia syndrome and few risk factors should still be treated because they are not in a low-risk group. Although the NCEP guidelines suggest screening people every 5 years after the age of 20, there have been no screening trials to demonstrate improved outcome. Long-term drug therapy in very low-risk groups could be hazardous.

F. In high-risk groups the CAD rate is similar to that for patients with known CAD, so the costs and hazards of treatment are outweighed by the benefits of lowering CAD events. In the West of Scotland trial, high-risk patients treated with pravastatin had a decrease in coronary death and nonfatal MI (5.5% vs. 7.9%, a relative risk reduction of 31%). Note that this study used a high-risk primary prevention group that had a CAD event rate of 1.6% per year, the same rate for patients with known CAD.

G. Consider lipid treatment for all patients with CAD. Optimize other treatments, such as aspirin, β blocker, angiotensin-converting enzyme (ACE) inhibitor, and Mediterranean diet. This diet uses monounsaturated fat (canola or olive oil), fruits, vegetables, and limited red meat and was used in the Lyon Heart Study. This study was stopped early because patients consuming this diet had a marked reduction in recurrent MI (relative risk reduction [RRR] 27%) and death (RRR 30%). Consider using insulin to treat diabetic patients because a randomized trial has shown that intensive treatment during and after an MI was associated with a reduction in 1 year mortality (18.6% vs. 26.1%, RRR 29%), especially if oral hypoglycemic agents were stopped (8.6% vs. 18%, RRR 52%). Dyslipidemia treatment in patients with CAD clearly decreases cardiovascular and overall mortality. Many physicians start with a statin drug because they are potent and well tolerated. For example, in the "4S" simvastatin trial, there was a reduction in mortality after 5.4 years of treatment (8% vs. 12%, RRR 30%). Niacin may also be used as an initial drug because it lowers LDL-C and TG, increases HDL, and has increased long-term survival (52% vs. 58.2%). Some patients may require the combination of a statin drug with niacin or a resin binder to lower LDL-C to <100 mg/dl. Patients with a poor prognosis may not benefit from pharmacologic lipid treatment because significant benefit typically requires years of treatment.

References

American College of Physicians. Guidelines for using serum cholesterol, high-density lipoprotein cholesterol, and triglyceride levels as screening tests for preventing coronary heart disease in adults. Ann Intern Med 1996; 124:515.

Canner PL, Berge KG, Wenger NK, et al. Fifteen year mortality in coronary drug project patients: long-term benefit with niacin. J Am Coll Cardiol 1986; 8:1245.

De Lorgeril M, Renaud S, Mamelle N, et al. Mediterranean alpha-linolenic acid-rich diet in secondary prevention of coronary heart disease. (The Lyon Diet Heart Study). Lancet 1994; 343:1454.

Garber AM, Browner WS, Hulley SB. Cholesterol screening in asymptomatic adults, revisited. Ann Intern Med 1996; 124:518.

Malmberg K, Ryden L, Efendic S, et al. Randomized trial of insulin-glucose infusion followed by subcutaneous insulin treatment in diabetic patients with acute myocardial infarction (DIGAMI Study): effect on mortality at 1 year. J Am Coll Cardiol 1995; 26:57.

Sacks FM, Pfeffer MA, Moye LA, et al. The effect of pravastatin on coronary events after myocardial infarction in patients with average cholesterol levels. N Engl J Med 1996; 335:1001.

Scandinavian Simvastatin Survival Study Group. Randomized trial of cholesterol lowering in 4444 patients with coronary heart disease: the Scandinavian Simvastatin Survival Study (4S). Lancet 1994; 344:1383.

Shepherd F, Cobbe SM, Ford I, et al. For West of Scotland Coronary Prevention Study Group. Prevention of coronary heart disease with pravastatin in men with hypercholesterolemia. N Engl J Med 1995; 333:1301.

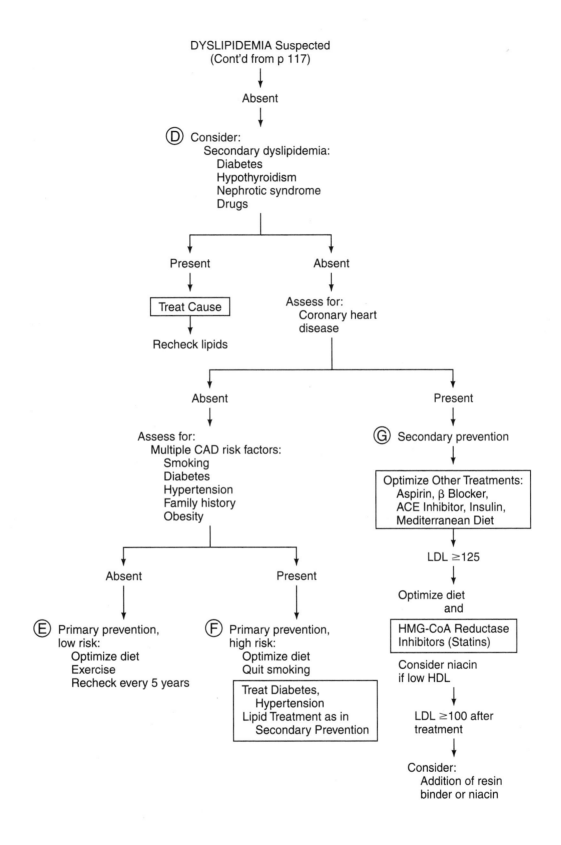

DYSLIPIDEMIA Suspected
(Cont'd from p 117)

↓

Absent

↓

(D) Consider:
    Secondary dyslipidemia:
        Diabetes
        Hypothyroidism
        Nephrotic syndrome
        Drugs

Present

Treat Cause

↓

Recheck lipids

Absent

Assess for:
    Coronary heart
    disease

Absent

Assess for:
    Multiple CAD risk factors:
        Smoking
        Diabetes
        Hypertension
        Family history
        Obesity

Absent

(E) Primary prevention,
low risk:
    Optimize diet
    Exercise
    Recheck every 5 years

Present

(F) Primary prevention,
high risk:
    Optimize diet
    Quit smoking

Treat Diabetes,
    Hypertension
Lipid Treatment as in
    Secondary Prevention

Present

(G) Secondary prevention

Optimize Other Treatments:
Aspirin, β Blocker,
ACE Inhibitor, Insulin,
Mediterranean Diet

LDL ≥125

Optimize diet
and

HMG-CoA Reductase
Inhibitors (Statins)

Consider niacin
if low HDL

↓

LDL ≥100 after
treatment

↓

Consider:
    Addition of resin
    binder or niacin

HYPOGLYCEMIA

Nancy A. Curosh

Hypoglycemia occurs when there is decreased glucose production, increased glucose use, or a combination of both. Normally, hypoglycemia is prevented by neural and hormonal mechanisms. As blood sugar falls, there is increased sympathetic activity and release of catecholamines, which prevents further uptake of glucose by insulin-dependent tissues and stimulates hepatic gluconeogenesis. Counter-regulatory hormones such as glucagon, cortisol, and growth hormone are also released, which stimulate gluconeogenesis and lipolysis. The symptoms of hypoglycemia may be nonspecific and depend on the rate of fall and the level of plasma glucose. The release of catecholamines may cause palpitations, sweating, anxiety, hunger, and tremulousness. If neuroglycopenia occurs, the patient may develop headache, confusion, light-headedness, aberrant behavior, dysarthria, visual symptoms, seizures, and coma, and death may occur.

A. Documentation of hypoglycemia may be difficult but is important because many patients have symptoms of hypoglycemia but few are actually hypoglycemic. Hypoglycemia cannot be defined by precise quantitative measures. In normal healthy individuals, the plasma glucose level at which counter-regulatory hormones are released may vary from 50–70 mg/dl. In diabetic patients who are chronically hyperglycemic, a rapid drop of blood glucose may provoke symptoms even if their plasma glucose is well within the normal range for nondiabetic patients. In fasting healthy males, plasma glucose may be as low as 55 mg/dl, and in females it may be even lower, but they remain asymptomatic. Therefore an arbitrary level of 50 mg/dl is used as a cutoff point to proceed with a detailed evaluation of hypoglycemia. A low glucose level must be documented in the laboratory using plasma or whole blood; fingersticks are inaccurate at low levels and are insufficient documentation of hypoglycemia. In addition to low blood sugar, the other conditions of Whipple's triad should be met: symptoms at the time of hypoglycemia and relief of symptoms with food. Relief should occur within minutes. If Whipple's triad is present, further investigation is warranted.

B. Often during a thorough history taking it is obvious that the hypoglycemia has exogenous causes, the most common being insulin or an oral hypoglycemic agent in diabetic patients. Alcohol can cause hypoglycemia, particularly in people who are drinking but not eating. If caloric intake is insufficient, glycogen stores are depleted. If alcohol then inhibits gluconeogenesis, hypoglycemia may occur. Other drugs such as propranolol, aspirin, pentamidine,and the antimalarials may precipitate hypoglycemia.

C. By means of a detailed history, patients usually can be divided into two categories: those whose symptoms occur while fasting and those whose symptoms occur after eating. Patients with fasting hypoglycemia tend to notice symptoms just before meals or early in the morning after an overnight fast. Fasting hypoglycemia often results from organic causes and requires thorough investigation. In some cases, documenting the hypoglycemia is difficult, especially if it occurs intermittently. In these cases the patient should be admitted for an observed fast. When symptoms develop, blood should be drawn. If the plasma glucose <50 mg/dl, further testing such as insulin and C-peptide levels should be analyzed simultaneously. Also give the patient glucose to document relief of symptoms. Most patients with fasting hypoglycemia develop symptoms within 24–48 hours, but some may take up to 72 hours. If no low plasma glucose levels were recorded during a 72-hour fast, fasting hypoglycemia is unlikely.

D. Insulinomas often are small and difficult to locate. Consult with the surgeon before localization procedures. Although a CT scan is fairly benign, other localization techniques are invasive and many surgeons prefer intraoperative ultrasonography.

E. The cosyntropin stimulation test is used when primary adrenal insufficiency is suspected. A plasma cortisol level is drawn at baseline. Cosyntropin (synthetic adrenocorticotropic hormone), 0.25 mg, is given IV or IM. A second plasma cortisol level is obtained at 60 minutes. Normal stimulation is >7 µg/dl above the baseline cortisol or an absolute value of >18 µg/dl. A normal response excludes the diagnosis of primary adrenal insufficiency.

F. The cause of fasting hypoglycemia with suppressed insulin levels often is obvious. Liver disease, renal disease, and malnutrition usually are severe before hypoglycemia occurs. Nonpancreatic tumors often are very large. Other causes such as adrenal insufficiency, growth hormone deficiency, and hypothyroidism may be subtle and require further testing.

G. Postprandial hypoglycemia usually produces symptoms 2–4 hours after a meal. These patients often complain of hunger, palpitations, and tremulousness, which are promptly relieved with food. Patients rarely develop symptoms of neuroglycopenia. A small subset of these patients have undergone GI surgery and have symptoms of hypoglycemia, but hypoglycemia is not the cause of the symptoms. However, most postprandial hypoglycemia is idiopathic. There is much controversy about the existence of this syndrome; this is reflected by its numerous names, including reactive, functional, idiopathic, and nonhypoglycemic hypoglycemia. Although commonly performed in the past, the oral glucose tolerance test usually is not indicated. Studies have shown that many healthy asymptomatic individuals have plasma glucose levels <50 mg/dl during an oral glucose tolerance test. Therefore this test has

Patient with SYMPTOMS OF HYPOGLYCEMIA

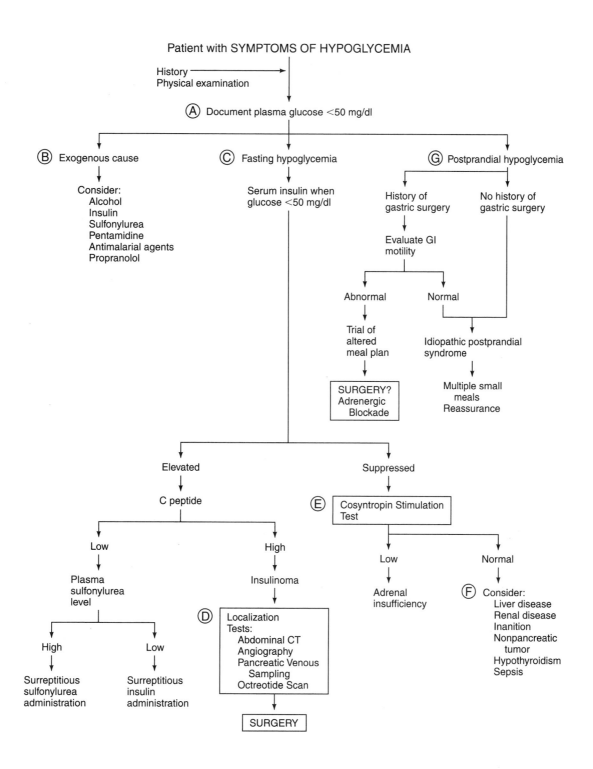

little meaning or diagnostic value. These patients are best treated with reassurance. They may try multiple small meals, but the high-protein, low-carbohydrate diet advocated in the past is not effective.

References

Comi RJ. Approach to acute hypoglycemia. Endocrinol Metab Clin North Am 1993; 22:247.

Comi RJ, Gorden P. Approach to hypoglycemia in adults. Compr Ther 1987; 13:38.

Malouf R, Brust JC. Hypoglycemia: causes, neurological manifestations, and outcome. Ann Neurol 1985; 17:421.

Service FJ. Hypoglycemias. J Clin Endocrinol Metab 1993; 76:269.

Service FJ. Hypoglycemia. Med Clin North Am 1995; 79:1.

Shamoon H. Hypoglycemia. In: Felig P, Baxter JD, Frohman LA, eds. Endocrinology and metabolism. 3rd ed. New York: McGraw-Hill, 1995.

HYPERGLYCEMIA

Philip R. Orlander
Thomas W. Boyden

Approximately 16 million Americans have diabetes mellitus, 50% of whom are undiagnosed. More than 90% have non–insulin-dependent diabetes mellitus (NIDDM), which is characterized by insufficient insulin secretion and marked insulin resistance. Criteria for the diagnosis of diabetes mellitus and other categories of glucose intolerance have been established by consensus of expert committees. A fasting serum glucose value ≥126 mg/dl (7 mmol/L) on several occasions, a 2-hour postprandial serum glucose >200 mg/dl (11.1 mmol/L), and/or random serum glucose values ≥200 mg/dl (11.1 mmol/L), along with classic symptoms of uncontrolled diabetes, establish the diagnosis of diabetes, and no further testing is needed. An oral glucose tolerance test is no longer recommended for nonpregnant adults. The intent is to simplify screening methods to detect the large number of undiagnosed patients in high-risk populations. All pregnant women should be screened for diabetes using separate specific criteria.

A. Mild hyperglycemia often is asymptomatic and discovered inadvertently. Pertinent findings in the history include symptoms of polyuria, polydipsia, polyphagia, visual changes, weight changes, intercurrent illnesses, and mental status changes. Risk factors for NIDDM include age >40 years, family history of diabetes, prior gestational diabetes, ethnicity (Hispanic-, African-, Asian-, and Native-American), obesity (especially abdominal), and sedentary lifestyle. Other disorders associated with insulin-resistant states include hypertension, hypertriglyceridemia, low HDL-cholesterol, hyperuricemia, ovarian hyperandrogenism, and premature atherosclerosis. Approximately 20% of newly diagnosed patients with NIDDM have evidence of end-organ damage on initial presentation (fundoscopic abnormalities, peripheral and autonomic neuropathy, erectile dysfunction, peripheral neuropathy, foot ulcers, peripheral vascular disease, or proteinuria).

B. Numerous medications may adversely affect carbohydrate tolerance. Glucocorticoids increase gluconeogenesis as well as impairing insulin action. Individuals at increased risk of NIDDM often develop persistent hyperglycemia even after withdrawal of these medications.

C. Excess antagonistic counter-regulatory hormones (glucagon, catecholamines, growth hormone, and cortisol) at times of illness may precipitate glucose intolerance. Gestational diabetes occurs only during pregnancy and resolves at delivery. Of those women with prior gestational diabetes, approximately 7% per year develop NIDDM. Many endocrine disorders are associated with abnormal glucose tolerance: Cushing's syndrome, acromegaly, hyperthyroidism, pheochromocytoma, glucagonoma, and somatostatinoma. Other disease states affecting the pancreas include acute and chronic pancreatitis (secondary to alcohol), hemochromatosis, cystic fibrosis, and trauma.

D. Diabetes mellitus is conventionally divided into two major clinical syndromes: insulin-dependent (IDDM, or type 1), which makes up <10% of diabetes, and non–insulin-dependent (NIDDM, or type 2), which makes up the remainder. There is a long list of rare secondary forms of diabetes: those previously mentioned as well as rare genetic conditions such as ataxia-telangiectasia and lipoatrophic syndromes. IDDM most commonly occurs in young, thin, generally Caucasian populations and typically presents with diabetic ketoacidosis (DKA). It is characterized by irreversible autoimmune destruction of the β cells and is highly associated with certain HLA haplotypes and the presence of islet cell antibodies at onset. Approximately 90% of individuals with NIDDM are obese. Both major clinical syndromes can occur at any age, although IDDM is more common in children and NIDDM is more common in adults. Specific genes have been identified in large family pedigrees that may be related to glucose intolerance.

E. Maturity-onset diabetes of the young (MODY) is a subset of NIDDM occurring in families with an autosomal-dominant form of inheritance, presenting at <30 years of age and associated with abnormalities in the glucose kinase gene. Many patients (especially African- and Hispanic-Americans) are not easily classified by these clinical criteria. Measurement of serum insulin concentrations is not useful clinically for managing the patient with diabetes. Acanthosis nigricans is a hyperpigmented skin lesion common in African- and Hispanic-Americans with impaired glucose tolerance or diabetes; it indicates hyperinsulinemia and insulin resistance. Rare extreme insulin-resistance syndromes may be associated with hyperandrogenism and defects in the insulin receptor (type A) or with autoimmune phenomenon and antibodies to the insulin receptor (type B).

(Continued on page 124)

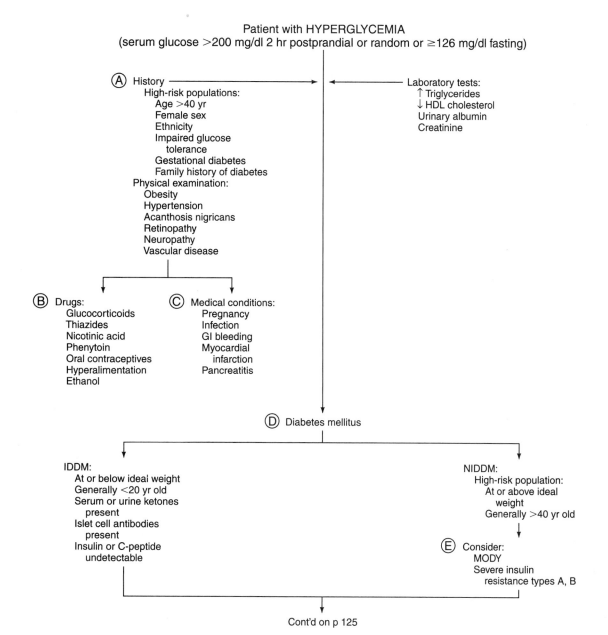

Patient with HYPERGLYCEMIA
(serum glucose >200 mg/dl 2 hr postprandial or random or ≥126 mg/dl fasting)

Ⓐ History
  High-risk populations:
    Age >40 yr
    Female sex
    Ethnicity
    Impaired glucose
      tolerance
    Gestational diabetes
    Family history of diabetes
  Physical examination:
    Obesity
    Hypertension
    Acanthosis nigricans
    Retinopathy
    Neuropathy
    Vascular disease

Laboratory tests:
  ↑ Triglycerides
  ↓ HDL cholesterol
  Urinary albumin
  Creatinine

Ⓑ Drugs:
  Glucocorticoids
  Thiazides
  Nicotinic acid
  Phenytoin
  Oral contraceptives
  Hyperalimentation
  Ethanol

Ⓒ Medical conditions:
  Pregnancy
  Infection
  GI bleeding
  Myocardial
    infarction
  Pancreatitis

Ⓓ Diabetes mellitus

IDDM:
  At or below ideal weight
  Generally <20 yr old
  Serum or urine ketones
    present
  Islet cell antibodies
    present
  Insulin or C-peptide
    undetectable

NIDDM:
  High-risk population:
    At or above ideal
      weight
    Generally >40 yr old

Ⓔ Consider:
  MODY
  Severe insulin
    resistance types A, B

Cont'd on p 125

F. The presence of serum ketone bodies indicates accelerated fatty acid oxidation as a result of severe insulin deficiency. Although DKA is a cardinal feature of IDDM, it occasionally is seen in patients with NIDDM who are subjected to severe stress (e.g., GI hemorrhage, myocardial infarction, sepsis). The differential diagnosis includes alcoholic ketoacidosis and starvation ketosis. Nonketotic hyperosmolar states typically occur in patients with NIDDM who are elderly with multiple medical problems.

G. Acutely ill patients require immediate IV fluid resuscitation and parenteral insulin during evaluation for an underlying illness (i.e., infection). Patients suspected of having IDDM require lifelong insulin therapy coordinated with a diet and exercise program to maintain ideal body weight. The initial therapy for obese patients with NIDDM is a weight-reducing diet and exercise regimen. The level of glycemic control, as assessed by measurement of glycohemoglobin, is strongly related to microvascular complications. Direct therapy toward obtaining the best possible glucose control. One or more oral medications, with or without insulin, may be needed to achieve euglycemia in selected individuals with NIDDM.

References

American Diabetes Association. Report of the Expert Committee on the Diagnosis and Classification of Diabetes. Diabetes Care 1997; 20:1183.

DeFronzo RA, Bonadonna RC, Ferraninni E. Pathogenesis of NIDDM. Diabetes Care 1992; 15:318.

DeFronzo RA, Ferraninni E. Insulin resistance. Diabetes Care 1991; 14:173.

Diabetes Control and Complications Trial Research Group. The effect of intensive treatment of diabetes on the development and progression of long-term complications in insulin-dependent diabetes mellitus. N Engl J Med 1993; 329:977.

Eisenbarth GS. Type I diabetes mellitus: a chronic autoimmune disease. N Engl J Med 1986; 314:1360.

Genuth S. Insulin use in NIDDM. Diabetes Care 1990; 13:1240.

Harris M. Diabetes in America. 2nd ed. Washington, DC: National Institutes of Health; 1995. NIH publication 95-1468.

Ohkuba Y, Kishikawa H, Araki E, et al. Intensive insulin therapy prevents the progression of diabetic microvascular complications in Japanese patients with non-insulin-dependent diabetes mellitus: a randomized prospective 6-year study. Diabetes Res Clin Pract 1995; 28:103.

Reaven GM, Lithell H, Landsberg L. Hypertension and associated metabolic abnormalities: the role of insulin resistance and the sympathoadrenal system. N Engl J Med 1996; 334:374.

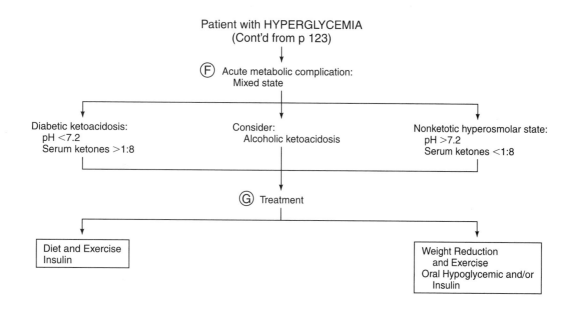

Patient with HYPERGLYCEMIA
(Cont'd from p 123)

(F) Acute metabolic complication:
Mixed state

Diabetic ketoacidosis:
  pH <7.2
  Serum ketones >1:8

Consider:
  Alcoholic ketoacidosis

Nonketotic hyperosmolar state:
  pH >7.2
  Serum ketones <1:8

(G) Treatment

Diet and Exercise
Insulin

Weight Reduction
  and Exercise
Oral Hypoglycemic and/or
  Insulin

HYPOCALCEMIA

Philip R. Orlander

A. Hypocalcemia may be seen in critically ill patients (sepsis) because of acquired defects in the parathyroid-vitamin D axis. Improved outcome is related to adequate replacement. The classic clinical signs of tetany may be associated with hypocalcemia, hypomagnesemia, hypokalemia, or alkalosis. Hypocalcemia enhances neuromuscular irritability, causing paresthesias, carpopedal spasm, and (if extreme) laryngeal spasm and seizures. ECG abnormalities occur with severe hypocalcemia. The severity of symptoms depends on the rate of decrease of the calcium. Chronic hypocalcemia may show only signs of latent tetany (Chvostek's or Trousseau's sign), but the long-term consequences are substantial (lenticular cataracts, basal ganglion calcification, poor integuments, intestinal malabsorption, pseudotumor cerebri, psychiatric manifestations, and abnormal cardiac function). Hypoalbuminemia is associated with lower serum calcium concentrations but normal ionized calcium levels. Simple correction formulas adjusting for the serum albumin generally suffice in estimating ionized calcium if a direct measurement is not readily available. In pancreatitis, hypocalcemia results from a combination of saponification of calcium salts and impairment of parathyroid hormone (PTH) secretion as a result of the hypomagnesemia caused by alcohol abuse. Although cancer is much more commonly associated with hypercalcemia, patients with extensive osteoblastic metastases from prostate or breast rarely may have hypocalcemia.

B. A low serum phosphate level generally indicates adequate parathyroid reserve. Direct attention to conditions that interfere with vitamin D metabolism, such as malabsorption states (sprue, short bowel, regional enteritis), hepatobiliary disease, anticonvulsant therapy, and vitamin D deficiency or resistance states. These conditions are associated with elevated PTH and alkaline phosphatase levels and low 25-hydroxyvitamin D levels. There may be evidence of metabolic bone disease.

C. A high serum phosphate level indicates PTH deficiency or resistance. Excessive phosphate intake or massive cell destruction (e.g., with chemotherapy or rhabdomyolysis) can substantially raise serum phosphate levels and thus lower serum calcium.

D. Renal insufficiency is a common cause of secondary hyperparathyroidism. Low 1,25-dihydroxyvitamin D levels are commonly found.

E. Pseudohypoparathyroidism is a rare inherited condition involving a generalized impairment in G regulatory protein signal transduction, resulting in target tissue resistance to PTH as well as other hormones. Afflicted individuals are short and often have cognitive handicaps and musculoskeletal abnormalities, including a short fourth metacarpal. Several subtypes of this disorder are described and distinguished by the response of urinary cyclic adenosine monophosphate (cAMP) concentration to exogenous PTH infusion.

F. Idiopathic hypoparathyroidism is a rare condition that may be isolated or associated with familial polyglandular endocrinopathy type 2 (mucocutaneous candidiasis, Addison's disease, hypoparathyroidism). It usually presents in childhood. Other rare causes of hypoparathyroidism include DiGeorge's syndrome, Wilson's disease, hemochromatosis, and granulomatous disease.

G. Head and neck surgery, primarily for thyroid or parathyroid diseases, and rarely radiation therapy, can result in transient or sometimes permanent PTH deficiency because of parathyroid ischemia. Autotransplantation of the parathyroids at the time of surgery has decreased the incidence of this complication.

H. Hypomagnesemia is most commonly found in patients with a history of heavy alcohol abuse, malabsorption, intestinal tract diseases, or primary renal tubular defects or in patients receiving prolonged nutritional therapy that may have been lacking in magnesium (hyperalimentation). Certain drugs and antibiotics (diuretics, aminoglycosides, cisplatin, amphotericin B) may cause a renal loss of magnesium.

I. Treatment includes adequate replacement of calcium, magnesium, and vitamin D. Administer IV calcium to symptomatic individuals. In conditions in which conversion of vitamin D to 1,25-vitamin D is perturbed (i.e., renal disease, vitamin D–resistant rickets), replacement with calcitriol or a similar metabolite (dihydrotachysterol) is desirable. In other circumstances, vitamin D_2 (ergocalciferol) is less expensive, although the risk of prolonged hypercalcemia is higher.

References

Ahonen P, Myllärniemi S, Sipilä I, Perheentupa J. Clinical variation of autoimmune polyendocrinopathy-candidiasis-ectodermal dystrophy (APECED) in a series of 68 patients. N Engl J Med 1990; 322:1829.

Faull CM, Welbury RR, Paul B, Kendall-Taylor P. Pseudohypoparathyroidism: its phenotypic variability and associated disorders in a large family. Q J Med 1991; 78:251.

Lebowitz MR, Moses AM. Hypocalcemia. Semin Nephrol 1992; 12:146.

Mundy GR. Calcium homeostasis: hypercalcemia and hypocalcemia. 2nd ed. London: Martin Dunitz, 1990.

Zaloga GP, Chernow B. The multifactorial basis of hypocalcemia during sepsis: studies of the parathyroid hormone-vitamin D axis. Ann Intern Med 1987; 107:36.

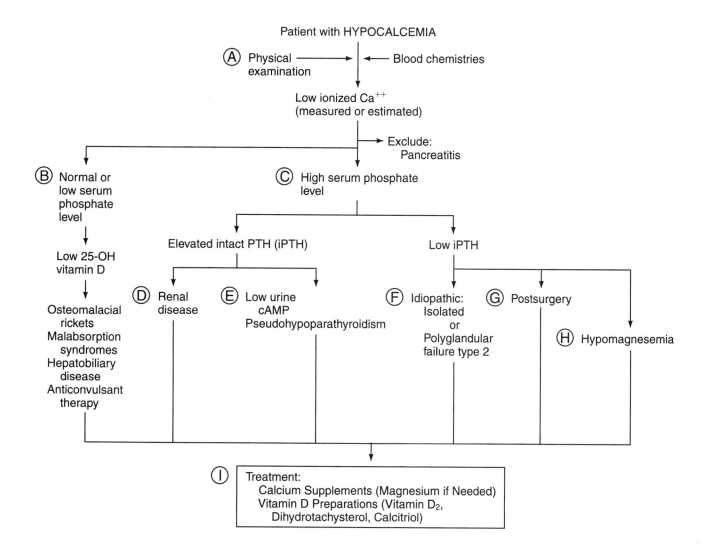

Patient with HYPOCALCEMIA

(A) Physical examination ⟶ ⟵ Blood chemistries

Low ionized Ca^{++}
(measured or estimated)

⟶ Exclude:
Pancreatitis

(B) Normal or low serum phosphate level

Low 25-OH vitamin D

Osteomalacial rickets
Malabsorption syndromes
Hepatobiliary disease
Anticonvulsant therapy

(C) High serum phosphate level

Elevated intact PTH (iPTH)

(D) Renal disease

(E) Low urine cAMP Pseudohypoparathyroidism

Low iPTH

(F) Idiopathic: Isolated or Polyglandular failure type 2

(G) Postsurgery

(H) Hypomagnesemia

(I) Treatment:
   Calcium Supplements (Magnesium if Needed)
   Vitamin D Preparations (Vitamin D_2, Dihydrotachysterol, Calcitriol)

HYPERCALCEMIA

Philip R. Orlander
Thomas W. Boyden

A. The clinical presentation of hypercalcemia ranges from severe dehydration, polyuria, and obtundation to a fortuitous discovery in an asymptomatic individual. Although there are many causes of hypercalcemia, the most likely diagnosis in an ambulatory population is hyperparathyroidism; malignancy is more common in a hospitalized population. Before initiating an extensive evaluation, establish that the patient has persistent hypercalcemia. An estimate of ionized calcium is useful in excluding dehydration or increased protein binding (i.e., multiple myeloma). A careful medication history is essential because several commonly used drugs can cause or exacerbate hypercalcemia (i.e., thiazide diuretics, calcium carbonate, vitamin A and D preparations, lithium, and antiestrogens in the treatment of breast carcinoma). Excessive use of calcium carbonate can result in a milk-alkali syndrome characterized by alkalosis, hypokalemia, hyperphosphatemia, hypercalcemia, and nephrocalcinosis. Strict immobilization may be associated with hypercalcemia only when there is concomitant accelerated bone resorption (i.e., children, severe trauma, or Paget's disease of bone). The physical examination will probably exclude several endocrine problems that may be associated with mild hypercalcemia (i.e., pheochromocytoma, Addison's disease, hyperthyroidism).

B. Multiphasic chemistry studies, CBC, and chest x-rays, although not diagnostic, may indicate the cause of the hypercalcemia. Hypercalcemia is seen in about 10–20% of patients with sarcoidosis and rarely in other granulomatous diseases. The hypercalcemia is caused by production of 1,25-dihydroxyvitamin D by the alveolar macrophages. Low serum phosphate, elevated chloride, low bicarbonate, and elevated serum alkaline phosphatase levels commonly are seen in hyperparathyroidism. Acute renal failure can cause hypercalcemia, especially when accompanied by rhabdomyolysis.

C. The immunoradiometric assay for intact parathyroid hormone (iPTH) demonstrates elevated levels in most cases of PTH-related hypercalcemia and should replace the former assays.

D. Non–PTH-related hypercalcemia may be caused by excess production or ingestion of vitamin D or by excess bone resorption. Hypercalcemia is common in individuals with many types of malignancy. In most cases cancer has already been diagnosed, but occasionally hypercalcemia is noted while the tumor is still occult. Although extensive bone metastases may cause hypercalcemia, more commonly a humoral factor has been implicated: PTH-related protein (PTH-rP) in squamous cell carcinomas of the head, neck, lung, and genitourinary tract; prostaglandins, cytokines, and lymphokines in other tumors. Levels of PTH-rP are elevated in most patients with humoral hypercalcemia of malignancy. Levels of 1,25-dihydroxyvitamin D generally are decreased in most cancers but may be elevated in patients with vitamin D intoxication, granulomatous disease, and rarely in hematologic malignancies. Obtain a detailed history, and perform a physical examination (including careful breast, rectal, and pelvic examinations) along with cancer-detecting studies (mammography, bone scan, serum protein electrophoresis, urinalysis, stool for occult blood) in patients with unexplained hypercalcemia and suppressed iPTH measurements.

E. Familial benign hypercalcemia (FBH) and neonatal hyperparathyroidism (NHPT) are rare disorders of calcium homeostasis that are associated with missense mutations of the calcium-sensing receptor. The condition is characterized by elevated serum magnesium, normal PTH, and very low urinary calcium levels. The heterozygous disease (FBH) has a benign course and does not respond well to parathyroid surgery, whereas the homozygous form (NHPT) is associated with severe hypercalcemia. It must be distinguished from other familial forms of hypercalcemia (multiple endocrine neoplasia [MEN] types 1 and 2).

F. Primary hyperparathyroidism is common in the elderly (prevalence 1/1000 with female predominance); >80% are caused by a single parathyroid adenoma. Most cases of hyperparathyroidism are discovered early, in routine blood chemistry studies, and it is now rare to see long-term complications such as osteitis fibrosa cystica, band keratopathy, or nephrocalcinosis. Surgery is indicated for those with evidence of osteitis fibrosa, reduced or falling cortical or trabecular bone mass, declining renal function, renal stones, mental status changes, pancreatitis, or serum calcium levels >12 mg/dl or in patients <50 years old. Removal of the adenoma is curative in >90% of patients. Preoperative evaluation (i.e., ultrasonography of the neck, nuclear medicine imaging, CT of the chest, venous sampling for iPTH) is useful only if the patient has undergone a previous unsuccessful neck exploration. Tertiary hyperparathyroidism may develop in patients with prolonged parathyroid stimulation (because of renal insufficiency) who receive a functioning renal transplant. Hyperplasia of all parathyroid glands is seen in MEN syndromes both 2a and 2b. Seek a family history, and exclude the possibility of accompanying neoplasias (pheochromocytoma, medullary thyroid carcinoma) before surgery. Parathyroid carcinoma is particularly rare and can be diagnosed with certainty only after metastases have been demonstrated.

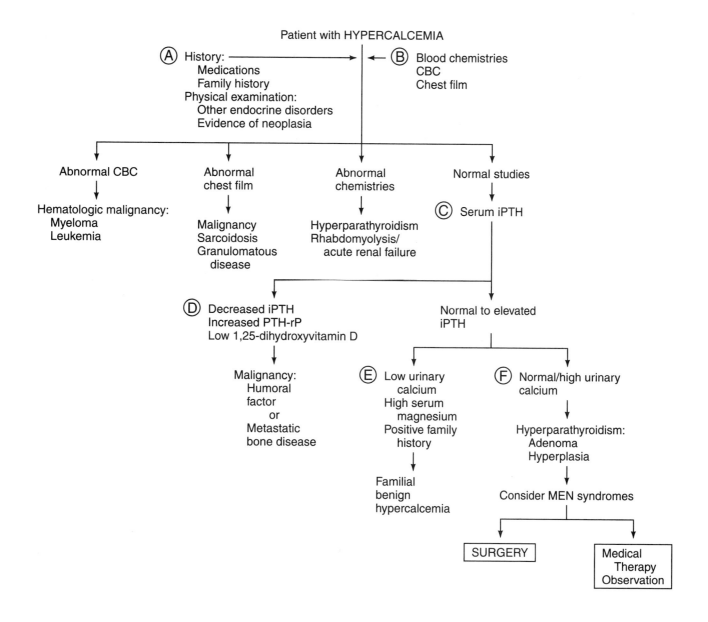

Patient with HYPERCALCEMIA

Ⓐ History: ———————→ ←— Ⓑ Blood chemistries
   Medications   CBC
   Family history   Chest film
   Physical examination:
      Other endocrine disorders
      Evidence of neoplasia

Abnormal CBC

Hematologic malignancy:
Myeloma
Leukemia

Abnormal chest film

Malignancy
Sarcoidosis
Granulomatous disease

Abnormal chemistries

Hyperparathyroidism
Rhabdomyolysis/ acute renal failure

Normal studies

Ⓒ Serum iPTH

Ⓓ Decreased iPTH
Increased PTH-rP
Low 1,25-dihydroxyvitamin D

Malignancy:
Humoral factor
or
Metastatic bone disease

Normal to elevated iPTH

Ⓔ Low urinary calcium
High serum magnesium
Positive family history

Familial benign hypercalcemia

Ⓕ Normal/high urinary calcium

Hyperparathyroidism:
Adenoma
Hyperplasia

Consider MEN syndromes

SURGERY

Medical Therapy Observation

References

Deftos LJ. Hypercalcemia: mechanisms, differential diagnosis, and remedies. Postgrad Med 1996; 100:119.
Nussbaum SR. Pathophysiology and management of severe hypercalcemia. Endocrinol Metab Clin North Am 1993; 2:343.

Pearce SH, Brown EM. Disorders of calcium ion sensing. J Clin Endocrinol Metab 1996; 81:2030.
Potts JT. Management of asymptomatic hyperparathyroidism. J Clin Endocrinol Metab 1990; 70:1489.
Stewart AF, Broadus AE. Parathyroid hormone related proteins: coming of age in the 1990's. J Clin Endocrinol Metab 1990; 71:1410.

TESTS OF THYROID FUNCTION

Julie I. Rifkin
Thomas W. Boyden

The modern clinical laboratory offers several tests of thyroid function. The physician must be aware of the diagnostic accuracy and limitations of these tests. Abnormal test results must be interpreted with good clinical judgment. Thyroid function tests are probably not cost-effective as routine screens for thyroid disease.

Sensitive Thyroid-Stimulating Hormone (sTSH): A very useful test. Immunometric assays for TSH were introduced in the early 1980s. These assays generally make it possible to distinguish hyperthyroid from euthyroid patients. The sTSH is elevated in hypothyroidism. The sTSH assay has less cross reactivity with luteinizing hormone (LH), follicle-stimulating hormone (FSH), and human chorionic gonadotropin (hCG). The normal range for an sTSH assay is about 0.4–6.2 μU/ml. The older nonsensitive radioimmunoassay (RIA) TSH assays have a range of 0–10 μU/ml.

Free Thyroxine Index (FTI): A useful calculation may soon be obsolete as new immunoassays for free thyroxine (FT_4) become available:

$$FTI = \text{total } T_4 \cdot \left[\frac{(RT_3U = (\text{Resin}T_3 \text{ uptake of patient})}{\text{mean normal } RT_3U} \right]$$

This calculation "corrects" the total T_4 for protein-binding abnormalities. The FTI has several limitations. It is misleading in patients with familial and congenital thyroxine-binding protein disorders. Most important, the FTI is falsely low in euthyroid patients who are acutely ill.

Free Thyroxine (FT_4): FT_4 is the amount of non–protein-bound circulating thyroxine (about 0.03%). It is a better indicator of thyroid status than total T_4. Previously, measurement of FT_4 was difficult and time-consuming (equilibrium dialysis). Two-step immunoassays are now available to measure FT_4 quickly and accurately and probably will replace the calculated FTI.

Triiodothyronine by RIA (T_3 RIA): Measures total T_3. Useful only in diagnosing T_3 toxicosis.

Thyroid Antimicrosomal (TMab) and Antithyroglobulin (TgAb) Antibodies: These antibodies may be elevated in Graves' disease and Hashimoto's thyroiditis. A patient may have Hashimoto's thyroiditis and no circulating antibodies. Positive antibodies also are found in portions of the general population and in patients with nonthyroidal illness.

24-Hour Radioactive Iodine Uptake (RAIU): Measures the thyroid's ability to take up iodine. The test uses a tracer amount of ^{123}I or ^{131}I given orally. A gamma scintillation counter is used to measure the radioactivity over the thyroid at 4–6 hours and 24 hours after the dose. Normal percentage uptake varies widely. By itself, this test is not a very accurate test of thyroid function.

Thyroid Imaging–Radionuclide Scan (^{123}I or ^{99m}Tc pertechnetate): Does not produce a picture like a CT or MRI scan. Can provide information about gland/lobe contour. Identifies thyroid nodules as "hot" (functioning), "cold" (nonfunctioning), or "warm." Cannot be used to diagnose a nodule as benign or malignant.

References

Bauer DC, Brown AN. Sensitive thyrotropin and free thyroxine testing in outpatients: are both necessary? Arch Intern Med 1996; 156:2333.

Behnia M, Gharib H. Primary care diagnosis of thyroid disease. Hosp Pract (Off Ed) 1996; 31:121.

Bethune JE. Interpretation of thyroid function tests. Dis Mon 1989; 35:543.

Kaye TB. Thyroid function tests: application of newer methods. Postgrad Med 1993; 94:81.

Klee GG, Hay ID. Sensitive thyrotropin assays: analytical and clinical performance criteria. Mayo Clin Proc 1988; 63:1123.

Santos ET, Mazzaferri EL. Thyroid function tests: guidelines for interpretation in common clinical disorders. Postgrad Med 1989; 85:333.

Surks MI, Chopra IJ, Mariash CN, et al. American Thyroid Association guidelines for use of laboratory tests in thyroid disorders. JAMA 1990; 263:1529.

HYPOTHYROIDISM

Stephen P. Thomson
Thomas W. Boyden

Suspect hypothyroidism in patients with fatigue, cold intolerance, hoarseness, dry skin, constipation, lower extremity edema, mental impairment, depression, menstrual irregularities, or weight gain. Elderly patients with hypothyroidism may have few, if any, specific complaints. The incidence of hypothyroidism increases with advancing age, and screening the elderly may be cost-effective. In the past, some patients with normal thyroid function were diagnosed with hypothyroidism and treated with thyroid hormone for weight gain, fatigue, poor energy, and other complaints, mainly because clinicians did not have accurate thyroid laboratory tests. Many of these patients could safely discontinue their "replacement" thyroid hormone therapy. Patients taking one of the old desiccated animal thyroid preparations, which contain variable amounts of T_4 and T_3 and usually are prescribed in grains, should be converted to L-thyroxine (T_4) therapy.

A. In the history ask about the previously mentioned signs and symptoms; use of lithium, amiodarone, propylthiouracil, methimazole or excessive iodine; and prior thyroid irradiation or surgery. Helpful physical examination findings include decreased heart rate, hoarseness, delayed relaxation phase of deep tendon reflexes, slow speech, cool dry skin, and goiter or nonpalpable gland. Serum thyroid-stimulating hormone (TSH) >20 mU/L confirms the diagnosis of hypothyroidism. Free T_4 (FT_4), rather than total T_4, commonly is obtained with the TSH to avoid the confounding effect of changes in serum thyroid-binding globulin.

B. Elevation of TSH >20 mU/L confirms the diagnosis of primary hypothyroidism. The most common cause in the United States is lymphocytic or Hashimoto's thyroiditis, a chronic autoimmune disease. Most patients have a firm, finely nodular or bosselated goiter. Serum antithyroidal antibodies (antimicrosomal or antithyroglobulin antibodies) often are elevated. However, these studies are discouraged because they add cost without changing the diagnosis or therapy and the abnormalities also occur in a small percentage of patients without hypothyroidism. The hypothyroid phase of postpartum thyroiditis is common, usually mild, and a transient cause of primary hypothyroidism; <5% develop permanent hypothyroidism. Hypothyroidism also can occur with use of lithium, amiodarone, or antithyroidal medications, with excess iodine ingestion, or after thyroidectomy or radiation treatment.

C. Replacement therapy with L-thyroxine is conveniently and accurately monitored with the serum TSH level. The pituitary typically requires 6–8 weeks to reach a new steady state after the start of therapy or a change in thyroxine dosage. Do not check TSH until the steady state has been reached. Some patients with severe hypothyroidism receiving adequate thyroxine replacement therapy may not normalize their TSH for up to 6 months. The usual replacement dosage of L-thyroxine is 0.05–0.2 mg/day with an average of 0.1–0.125 mg/day. When treating patients with thyroxine for replacement or suppression, keep TSH within the euthyroid range. Older patients may need less L-thyroxine. There has been some variation between different preparations of L-thyroxine, but recent data suggest bioequivalence. However, when switching brands of L-thyroxine, monitor TSH and adjust the dosage to keep TSH within the normal range.

D. Patients with a slightly raised serum TSH, a normal FT_4, and no clinical features of hypothyroidism have subclinical hypothyroidism. The prevalence of subclinical hypothyroidism is 4–17% and increases with age. Whether these patients benefit from treatment with L-thyroxine is controversial. Some endocrinologists favor screening and treatment for these patients because they may have subtle symptoms that improve with treatment. They also have a significant rate of progression to overt hypothyroidism (5–20% per year). Other common causes of slightly raised serum TSH include poor compliance with T_4 therapy and recovery from nonthyroidal illness (sick euthyroid, low T_3 syndrome).

E. Normal TSH and low FT_4 suggest the possibility of central hypothyroidism. However, the most common reason for these results is the use of salsalate, phenytoin, or carbamazepine. These medications interfere with current clinical tests and cause inaccurate low values for FT_4. More accurate testing in patients taking these medications shows that the FT_4 is normal. Use the history, physical examination, and TSH for the diagnosis of hypothyroidism in these patients. If hypothyroidism is suspected, discontinue medication for 2 weeks and measure serum TSH and FT_4. If the FT_4 is still low, evaluate the patient for central hypothyroidism. Secondary (pituitary) or tertiary (hypothalamic) hypothyroidism are rare causes of normal or low serum TSH and low FT_4. These patients should have a cranial MRI and an evaluation of the gonadal and adrenal axes.

References

Danese MD, Powe NR, Sawin CT, Ladenson PW. Screening for mild thyroid failure at the periodic health examination. JAMA 1996; 276:285.

Dong BJ, Hauck WW, Gambertoglio JG, et al. Bioequivalence of generic and brand-name Levothyroxine products in the treatment of hypothyroidism. JAMA 1997; 277:1205.

Lindsay RS, Toft AD. Hypothyroidism. Lancet 1997; 349:413.

Mandel SJ, Brent GA, Larsen PR. Levothyroxine therapy in patients with thyroid disease. Ann Intern Med 1993; 119:492.

Singer PA, Cooper DS, Levy EG, et al. Treatment guidelines for patients with hyperthyroidism and hypothyroidism. JAMA 1995; 273:806.

Surks MI, Defesi CR. Normal serum free thyroid hormone concentrations in patients treated with phenytoin of Carbamazepine: a paradox resolved. JAMA 1996; 275:1495.

Toft AD. Thyroxine therapy. N Engl J Med 1994; 331:174.

HYPOTHYROIDISM Suspected

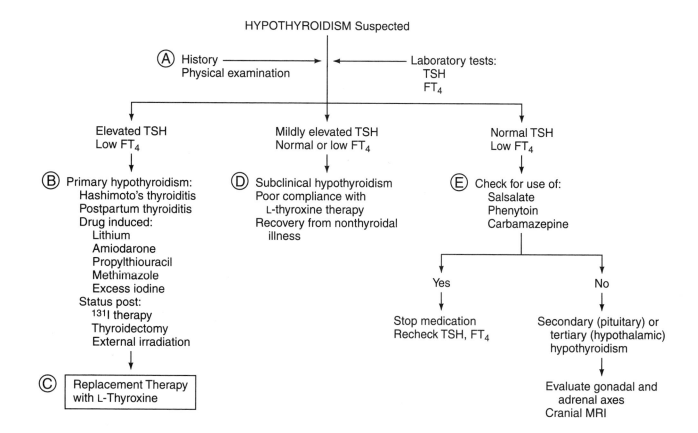

HYPERTHYROIDISM

Stephen P. Thomson
Thomas W. Boyden

Suspect hyperthyroidism in patients with palpitations, nervousness, fatigue, weight loss, or heat intolerance. These symptoms may be less pronounced or absent in older patients. Evaluate patients with atrial fibrillation for hyperthyroidism.

A. In the history ask about diplopia, eye dryness and irritation, neck tenderness, and the use of thyroid- or iodine-containing medications such as amiodarone. Helpful physical examination findings include increased heart rate, widened pulse pressure, fine tremor, and increased thyroid size and/or tenderness. Examine eyes for paresis of extraocular muscles, proptosis, erythema, or conjunctival edema. Completely suppressed "undetectable" thyroid-stimulating hormone (TSH) confirms the diagnosis of hyperthyroidism. Free T_4 (FT_4), rather than total T_4, commonly is obtained with the TSH to avoid the effect of changes in serum thyroid-binding globulin.

B. Radioactive iodine uptake (RAIU) is the main test used to separate causes of hyperthyroidism. An RAIU usually is done at 6 and 24 hours because occasionally a patient has an elevation only at one of these times. A low RAIU can occur in hyperthyroid patients recently exposed to excess iodine, such as IV contrast agents used for radiologic studies.

C. Elevated RAIU occurs in most patients with hyperthyroidism. A radioactive iodine scan seldom provides useful additional information and should be avoided to save costs. Graves' disease is the most common cause. It is an autoimmune disorder with antibodies that stimulate the TSH receptor to cause overproduction of thyroid hormones. Patients usually have a smooth, symmetric goiter, ophthalmopathy, and rarely pretibial myxedema. Multinodular goiters can develop enough autonomous function to become "toxic" and cause hyperthyroidism. They occur mainly in older adults. Solitary, large, functioning thyroid adenomas (toxic adenomas or Plummers' disease) can also cause hyperthyroidism. Rarely hyperthyroidism can occur in a previously hypothyroid patient with Hashimoto's chronic thyroiditis if they develop significant amounts of stimulatory antibodies.

D. Most patients in the United States with Graves' disease are treated with [131]I. Many endocrinologists favor a generous dose because it predictably induces a remission. Hypothyroidism also occurs sooner with a generous dose and can be treated quickly. Smaller doses may not induce a remission, and hypothyroidism may take years to develop. This increases the possibility of a second ^{131}I treatment and prolongs the period of close observation. Antithyroidal medication is the other common treatment. However, propylthiouracil or methimazole less predictably induces remission and is associated with agranulocytosis. Patients should promptly report signs of infection such as fever or sore throat. Some clinicians monitor blood counts during therapy. Surgical treatment rarely is used for Graves' disease.

E. Depressed RAIU most often occurs with one of several types of thyroiditis. Thyroiditis causes some destruction of the gland and release of excess thyroid hormone. This causes the hyperthyroidism and depressed RAIU. Ingestion of excess T_4 also depresses RAIU and is called *thyrotoxicosis factitia.*

F. Suppressed TSH and "normal" FT_4 occur because the FT_4 is elevated above the level that a patient usually maintains. Therefore, although an individual's FT_4 level may be within the overall normal range for a group of healthy people, it can be above the level that individual usually maintains and thus be high enough to suppress TSH and cause hyperthyroidism. Suppressed TSH and normal FT_4 also can occur in T_3 toxicosis, which is caused by excess secretion of T_3, the most active form of thyroid hormone. Measurement of serum T_3 can confirm the diagnosis.

G. Low, but not completely suppressed, TSH occurs when there is a slight excess of thyroid hormone. This is called *subclinical hyperthyroidism* because it typically is not associated with symptoms. However, recently it has been shown that these patients are at risk for developing atrial fibrillation. No clinical trials have examined the outcome of treatment for subclinical hyperthyroidism. However, some clinicians treat these patients to reduce the risk of atrial fibrillation if the subclinical hyperthyroidism persists.

H. TSH-secreting pituitary tumors are rare.

References

Franklyn JA. The management of hyperthyroidism. N Engl J Med 1994; 330:1731.

Klein I, Becker DV, Levey GS. Treatment of hyperthyroid disease. Ann Intern Med 1994; 121:281.

Sawin CT, Geller A, Wolf PA, et al. Low serum thyrotropin concentrations as a risk factor for atrial fibrillation in older persons. N Engl J Med 1994; 331:1249.

Singer PA, Cooper DS, Levy EG, et al. Treatment guidelines for patients with hyperthyroidism and hypothyroidism. JAMA 1995; 273:806.

Tajiri J, Noguchi S, Marakami T, et al. Anti-thyroid drug induced agranulocytosis: the usefulness of routine white blood cell counting. Arch Intern Med 1990; 150:621.

HYPERTHYROIDISM Suspected

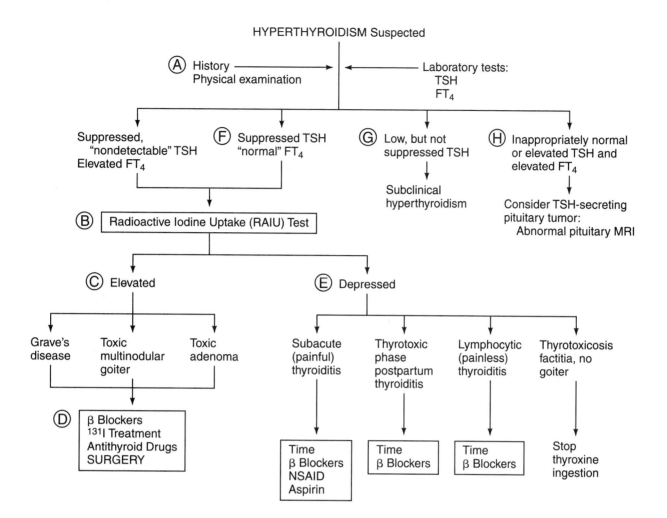

Ⓐ History ⟶ ⟵ Laboratory tests:
Physical examination
TSH
FT_4

Suppressed, "nondetectable" TSH Elevated FT_4

Ⓕ Suppressed TSH "normal" FT_4

Ⓖ Low, but not suppressed TSH
↓
Subclinical hyperthyroidism

Ⓗ Inappropriately normal or elevated TSH and elevated FT_4
↓
Consider TSH-secreting pituitary tumor:
Abnormal pituitary MRI

Ⓑ Radioactive Iodine Uptake (RAIU) Test

Ⓒ Elevated

Grave's disease

Toxic multinodular goiter

Toxic adenoma

Ⓓ β Blockers
131I Treatment
Antithyroid Drugs
SURGERY

Ⓔ Depressed

Subacute (painful) thyroiditis

Thyrotoxic phase postpartum thyroiditis

Lymphocytic (painless) thyroiditis

Thyrotoxicosis factitia, no goiter

Time
β Blockers
NSAID
Aspirin

Time
β Blockers

Time
β Blockers

Stop thyroxine ingestion

GOITER

Stephen P. Thomson
Thomas W. Boyden

Patients with goiters usually are euthyroid but can have significant hyper- or hypothyroidism, compressive symptoms of dysphagia or sensations of choking, and concerns about cancer and the appearance of the goiter. Common types of goiter include multinodular goiter (MNG) and those associated with hypo- (Hashimoto's thyroiditis) or hyperthyroidism (Graves' disease). Less commonly, goiters are produced by consumption of goitrogens. Lithium commonly induces a modest goiter. Rarer goitrogens include kelp, the antithyroidal medications propylthiouracil and methimazole, and cassava root, rutabaga, and turnips in association with an iodine-deficient diet. Excess iodine, including iodine-containing medications (amiodarone), occasionally can cause significant goiters. Iodine treatment during pregnancy has been associated with goiter in newborns. Endemic goiter has essentially disappeared in the United States because of adequate iodine intake, but about 200 million people around the world have it. Medullary carcinoma of the thyroid is a rare cause of goiter. It occurs sporadically and as part of multiple endocrine neoplasia (MEN) type 2. Other rare causes of goiter include acromegaly, subacute thyroiditis, systemic lupus, erythematosus, metastases, and thyroid hemorrhage.

A. Physical examination of the thyroid starts with careful visual inspection while the patient is swallowing. Often the outline of the entire goiter can be seen because the thyroid gland moves with swallowing. Next, palpate the entire gland during repeated swallows to characterize the goiter as diffuse or nodular, and identify any dominant nodules. Obvious dominant nodules should have a fine needle aspiration (see p 138). If the inferior border of the goiter is not easily palpable, try palpation with the patient supine and the neck moderately extended. If the inferior border is still not palpable, the patient may have a substernal goiter.

B. Measure serum concentrations of thyroid-stimulating hormone (TSH) and free T_4 (FT_4). If the TSH is completely suppressed ("undetectable"), the patient is hyperthyroid. If the TSH is >20 μU/ml, the patient is hypothyroid. If the TSH is normal, the patient typically is euthyroid. If the TSH is low but not completely suppressed, the thyroid gland is producing a slight excess of thyroid hormone. This typically occurs in patients with MNGs that develop autonomously functioning nodules and cause subclinical hyperthyroidism. Some of these patients may develop frank hyperthyroidism, but most remain with goiters that are autonomously functioning.

C. Hypothyroidism with goiter usually is caused by the autoimmune disease lymphocytic or Hashimoto's thyroiditis. Autoantibodies destroy parts of the thyroid. The goiters typically are modest in size, 2–3 times normal, and slightly nodular (bosselated) and firmer than normal thyroid tissue because there are areas of fibrosis and active follicles. Treat with T_4 replacement.

D. Euthyroid patients with goiters usually are older adults with MNG. One theory on the formation of MNG (simple or nonimmunologic goiters) is that there is underproduction of thyroid hormone with a compensatory increase in TSH that stimulates goiter formation. Therefore a common, but not universally accepted, therapy is T_4 suppression to remove the TSH stimulation. However, T_4 therapy in older adults must be administered cautiously, starting at a low dosage, perhaps 0.05 mg/day, and keeping TSH within the normal range while increasing the dosage. MNG can slowly develop autonomous functioning nodules that produce enough hormone to cause hyperthyroidism in combination with exogenous T_4. Therefore patients should be aware of the symptoms of hyperthyroidism and have TSH monitored at least every year after achieving a steady dose of T_4. Substernal and large goiters may respond to T_4 suppression or radioactive ^{131}I, so surgical treatment for goiter rarely is necessary. Large substernal goiters can cause superior venocaval syndrome, and some patients have signs of obstruction if they raise their arms above their head (Pemberton's sign). Occasionally surgery is done because of patients' concern about appearance.

E. Hyperthyroid patients with diffuse goiters usually have autoimmune Graves' disease. Thyroid-stimulating antibodies typically cause a diffuse enlargement of the entire gland. A unilateral asymmetric goiter associated with hyperthyroidism can occur in patients with a large functioning adenoma (Plummer's disease). Treatment of hyperthyroidism usually decreases the size of these goiters (see p 134).

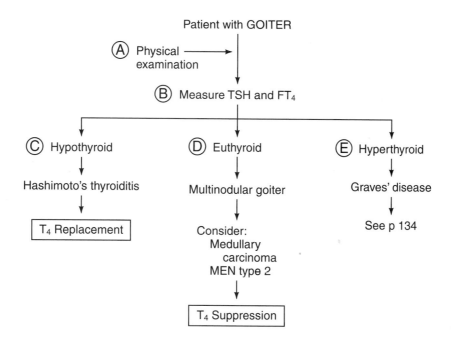

Patient with GOITER

(A) Physical examination

(B) Measure TSH and FT₄

(C) Hypothyroid

Hashimoto's thyroiditis

T₄ Replacement

(D) Euthyroid

Multinodular goiter

Consider:
Medullary
carcinoma
MEN type 2

T₄ Suppression

(E) Hyperthyroid

Graves' disease

See p 134

References

Berghout A, Wiersinga WM, Drexhage HA, et al. Comparison of placebo with L-thyroxine alone or with carbimazole for treatment of sporadic non-toxic goitre. Lancet ii 1990; 336:193.

Hurley DL, Gharib H. Thyroid nodular disease: is it toxic or nontoxic, malignant or benign? Geriatrics 1995; 50:24.

Hurley DL, Gharib H. Evaluation and management of multinodular goiter. Otolaryngol Clin North Am 1996; 29:527.

Kay TW, d'Emden MC, Andrews JT, Martin FI. Treatment of non-toxic multinodular goiter with radioactive iodine. Am J Med 1988; 84:19.

Siminoski K. Does this patient have a goiter? JAMA 1995; 273:813.

THYROID NODULE

Julie I. Rifkin
Thomas W. Boyden

Thyroid nodules can be found in approximately 4% of the adult U.S. population. They occur four times more often in females. Most thyroid nodules are benign. Conditions that may present as a thyroid nodule include thyroid cysts, parathyroid and thyroglossal duct cysts, a focal area of thyroiditis, a dominant portion of a multinodular gland, agenesis of a thyroid lobe, benign adenoma, and thyroid malignancies. Thyroid cysts usually are benign, but aspirated fluid should always be sent for cytologic analysis. Suspicion of thyroid malignancy is increased in a patient with a recent enlargement of a nodule, hoarseness or dysphagia, or a family history of medullary thyroid cancer (measure serum calcitonin). Suspicion of malignancy is heightened in young adults, men, and persons with a history of exposure to ionizing radiation.

A. Thin needle aspiration (TNA) or fine needle aspiration biopsy (FNAB) of thyroid nodules has been in use for more than 40 years. It is an outpatient procedure that causes little discomfort to the patient and provides a cytologic tissue diagnosis.

B. Results of TNA are accurate about 96% of the time when reviewed by an experienced cytopathologist. A study with a 6-month follow-up found no significant difference in nodule size between thyroxine- and placebo-treated patients. Suppressive therapy with L-thyroxine is used by many endocrinologists for patients with benign thyroid nodules, although there is controversy about the success of this therapy. A nodule that enlarges on suppressive therapy requires repeat biopsy.

C. Exogenous L-thyroxine given in replacement doses (0.05–0.2 mg/day) is given to suppress the thyroid's production of endogenous T_4 and T_3. This therapy is used in the euthyroid patient with a thyroid nodule. While the patient is receiving suppressive therapy, the sensitive thyroid-stimulating hormone (sTSH) should not fall below the normal range. During management of patients who have been treated for thyroid malignancy, however, more aggressive TSH suppression may be desirable because growth of these neoplasms often is TSH dependent.

D. According to the Third National Cancer Survey, thyroid cancer accounts for 0.004% per year of cancer cases. The most common form of thyroid cancer is papillary carcinoma. With proper management, most of these patients are cured. Poor prognostic factors include age >40 years, male gender, primary lesion >4 cm, and extent of local invasion (node status does not correlate with outcome). The surgical procedure for treatment depends on the histologic type of the malignancy, the size of the primary tumor, and the extent of local disease. Pre- and postoperative serum thyroglobulin measurements are helpful. Postoperative ^{131}I therapy is useful in selected patients with papillary/follicular cancers after surgical management.

E. About 85% of follicular neoplasms are benign and 15% are malignant. Most of these lesions are identified as "cold" on thyroid scans, but some may be "hot."

References

Boigon M, Moyer D. Solitary thyroid nodules: separating benign from malignant conditions. Postgrad Med 1995; 98:73.

Gharib H. Current evaluation of thyroid nodules. Trends Endocrinol Metab 1994; 5:365.

Gharib H, Goellner JR. Fine-needle aspiration biopsy of the thyroid. Endocr Pract 1995; 1:410.

Giuffrida D, Gharib H. Controversies in the management of cold, hot, and occult thyroid nodules. Am J Med 1995; 99:642.

Mainini E, Martinelli I, Morandi G, et al. Levothyroxine suppressive therapy for solitary thyroid nodule. J Endocr Invest 1995; 18:796.

Mazzaferri EC. Management of a solitary thyroid nodule. N Engl J Med 1993; 328:553.

Tan GH, Gharib H, Reading CC. Solitary thyroid nodule: comparison between palpation and ultrasonography. Arch Intern Med 1995; 155:2418.

Woeber KA. Cost-effective evaluation of the patient with a thyroid nodule. Surg Clin North Am 1995; 75:357.

Patient with PALPABLE THYROID NODULE

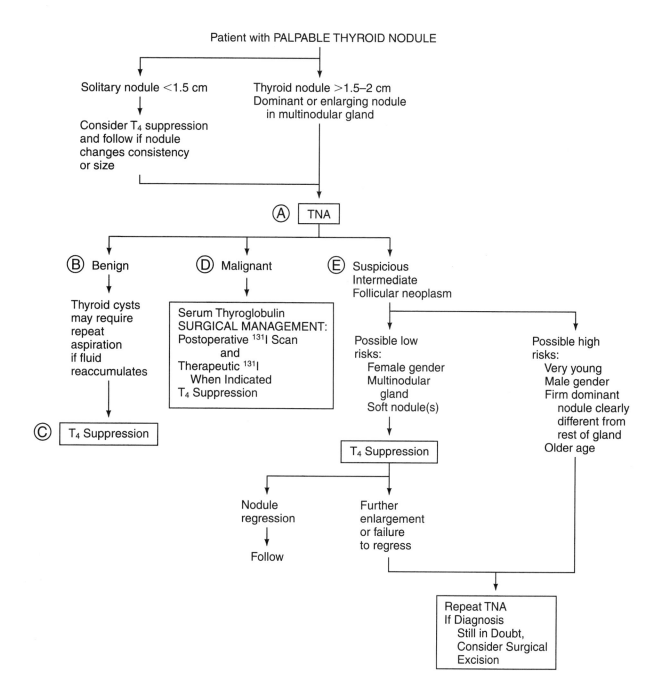

Solitary nodule <1.5 cm

Consider T$_4$ suppression
and follow if nodule
changes consistency
or size

Thyroid nodule >1.5–2 cm
Dominant or enlarging nodule
in multinodular gland

Ⓐ TNA

Ⓑ Benign

Thyroid cysts
may require
repeat
aspiration
if fluid
reaccumulates

Ⓒ T$_4$ Suppression

Ⓓ Malignant

Serum Thyroglobulin
SURGICAL MANAGEMENT:
Postoperative ^{131}I Scan
and
Therapeutic ^{131}I
When Indicated
T$_4$ Suppression

Ⓔ Suspicious
Intermediate
Follicular neoplasm

Possible low
risks:
Female gender
Multinodular
gland
Soft nodule(s)

Possible high
risks:
Very young
Male gender
Firm dominant
nodule clearly
different from
rest of gland
Older age

T$_4$ Suppression

Nodule
regression

Follow

Further
enlargement
or failure
to regress

Repeat TNA
If Diagnosis
Still in Doubt,
Consider Surgical
Excision

PAINFUL THYROID

Nancy A. Curosh

Any condition that causes rapid growth of the thyroid may cause pain because the thyroid is an encapsulated gland. Pain may be confined to the thyroid gland itself but often radiates to the ears, jaw, or chest. Subacute thyroiditis is the classic disease causing severe thyroid pain. Acute suppurative thyroiditis and radiation thyroiditis are rare conditions that often are obvious on presentation. Hemorrhage into a cyst can be painful; it usually is suspected at physical examination and from its sudden onset. Common conditions that can cause very enlarged thyroids such as Graves' disease, Hashimoto's thyroiditis, and cancer may cause mild thyroid tenderness or pressure but rarely cause pain because they develop less rapidly. Other nonthyroidal illnesses may cause neck pain, but the thyroid itself is not swollen or painful.

A. Rarely, treatment of hyperthyroidism with ^{131}I therapy can cause a painful thyroid clinically resembling subacute thyroiditis. Pain and swelling of the thyroid develops within 1–2 weeks of treatment and usually resolves within 3–4 weeks.

B. Acute suppurative thyroiditis is an inflammatory disease caused by bacterial, fungal, or parasitic infection of the thyroid. Since the discovery of antibiotics, this disease has become extremely rare. The thyroid itself is relatively resistant to infection, probably because of its complete encapsulation, rich blood supply and lymphatic drainage, and high iodide content. Acute suppurative thyroiditis usually is preceded by an infection elsewhere in the body, most commonly an upper respiratory infection or pharyngitis. Many patients have a history of pre-existing thyroid disease. Patients often appear septic with fever, chills, tachycardia, and a painful swollen neck. Sore throat and dysphagia commonly occur. Laboratory evaluation reveals leukocytosis, but thyroid function tests and radioactive iodine uptake (RAIU) are normal. Fine needle aspiration (FNA) should be performed to identify the offending organism so that proper antibiotic therapy can be instituted. Surgical incision and drainage sometimes are required.

C. The RAIU test helps differentiate the types of hyperthyroidism. The patient ingests a small amount of radioactive iodine, and the percentage of iodine that is taken up by the thyroid gland at 24 hours is determined. In Graves' disease, in which the thyroid is actively producing thyroid hormone, the uptake is increased. In subacute thyroiditis the uptake is decreased as the gland is damaged and unable to trap iodine and make thyroid hormone. The patient may be hyperthyroid because of leakage of preformed hormone.

D. Subacute thyroiditis is a spontaneously remitting inflammatory disease of the thyroid that is most likely caused by a viral infection. Infiltration of inflammatory cells leads to rapid thyroid swelling and pain. Because the thyroid gland is damaged, there is leakage of preformed thyroid hormone into the circulation, causing hyperthyroidism. However, because the gland is damaged, it temporarily cannot take up iodine and make more thyroid hormone. This results in the low RAIU, which can help clarify the diagnosis. In most cases the diagnosis is obvious when the patient has rapid onset of a swollen tender thyroid gland without evidence of sepsis. In some cases, however, it may be difficult to differentiate subacute from acute thyroiditis because fever and pain are common to both. Subacute thyroiditis also may be preceded by an upper respiratory infection. If one is in doubt clinically, some tests can be helpful. In subacute thyroiditis the WBC count is normal, and as mentioned, the patient usually is hyperthyroid with a low RAIU. A fine needle biopsy can confirm the diagnosis in difficult cases, but this rarely is necessary. Subacute thyroiditis is treated with salicylates for their anti-inflammatory action. In severe cases corticosteroids may be needed. β Blockers can be used during the initial hyperthyroid phase to decrease symptoms of hyperthyroidism. As the gland recovers, a transient hypothyroid phase may occur, but most people ultimately become euthyroid. Rarely, malignancies of the thyroid have presented with symptoms that mimic subacute thyroiditis. Therefore, if a patient fails to respond to the usual treatment, a biopsy should be performed to investigate for cancer.

E. Occasionally a patient has pain from a single thyroid nodule in an otherwise normal gland, or one prominent nodule in a multinodular gland. FNA should be performed. Possible causes include hemorrhage into a cyst, localized subacute thyroiditis, or (rarely) cancer.

F. A diffusely painful goiter in a euthyroid or hypothyroid patient probably is a result of thyroid carcinoma or acute onset of Hashimoto's thyroiditis. Any condition that is suspicious for cancer, such as a rapidly growing gland or the development of hoarseness, should be investigated with a biopsy. Hashimoto's or chronic lymphocytic thyroiditis is an autoimmune disease that rarely causes thyroid pain. High titers of microsomal antibodies or thyroglobulin antibodies are often seen in Hashimoto's thyroiditis but are not specific. Caution is necessary because malignancies, especially lymphomas, may develop in patients with chronic lymphocytic thyroiditis. Therefore if cancer seems unlikely and the presumptive diagnosis is Hashimoto's thyroiditis, a trial of thyroid hormone suppression and observation is indicated. However, a biopsy must be performed if the gland continues to enlarge.

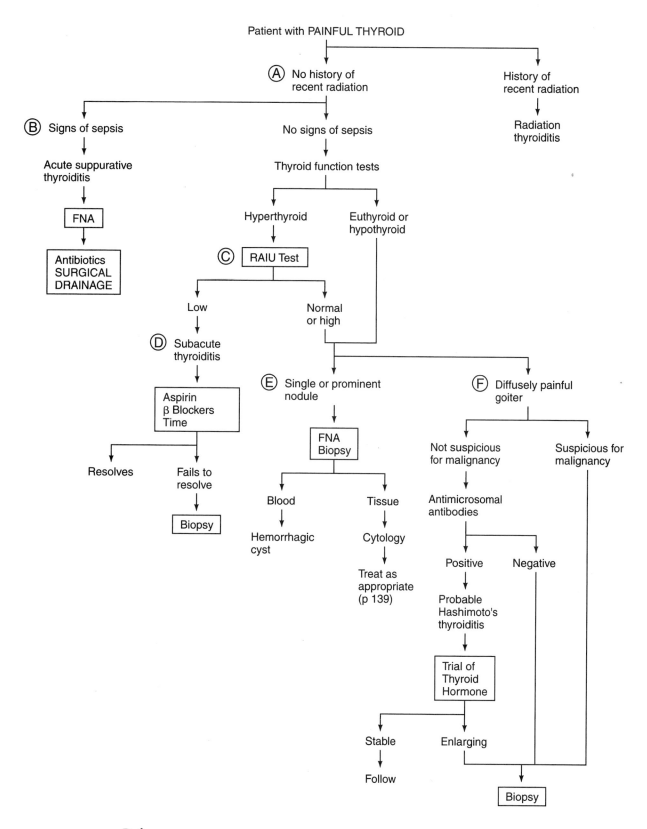

Patient with PAINFUL THYROID

(A) No history of recent radiation | History of recent radiation → Radiation thyroiditis

(B) Signs of sepsis → Acute suppurative thyroiditis → FNA → Antibiotics SURGICAL DRAINAGE

No signs of sepsis → Thyroid function tests

Hyperthyroid → (C) RAIU Test

Euthyroid or hypothyroid

Low → (D) Subacute thyroiditis → Aspirin β Blockers Time → Resolves / Fails to resolve → Biopsy

Normal or high

(E) Single or prominent nodule → FNA Biopsy → Blood → Hemorrhagic cyst / Tissue → Cytology → Treat as appropriate (p 139)

(F) Diffusely painful goiter

Not suspicious for malignancy → Antimicrosomal antibodies → Positive → Probable Hashimoto's thyroiditis → Trial of Thyroid Hormone → Stable → Follow / Enlarging → Biopsy

Negative → Biopsy

Suspicious for malignancy → Biopsy

References

Farwell AP, Braverman LE. Inflammatory thyroid disorders. Otolaryngol Clin North Am 1996; 29:541.

Hamburger JI. The various presentations of thyroiditis: diagnostic considerations. Ann Intern Med 1986; 104:219.

Hay ID. Thyroiditis: a clinical update. Mayo Clin Proc 1985; 60:836.

Rosen IB, Strawbridge HG, Walfish PG, Bain J. Malignant pseudothyroiditis: a new clinical entity. Am J Surg 1978; 136:445.

Szabo SM, Allen DB. Thyroiditis: differentiation of acute suppurative and subacute. Clin Pediatr 1989; 28:171.

Volpe R. The management of subacute (DeQuervain) thyroiditis. Thyroid 1993; 3:253.

THYROID FUNCTION TESTS IN NONTHYROIDAL ILLNESS

Julie I. Rifkin

In hospitalized patients the incidence of true hypo- or hyperthyroidism is <1%. Clinical signs of thyroid disease may be masked in acutely ill patients. Conversely, some signs of severe illness mimic changes seen in thyroid diseases. Serum T_3 radioimmunoassay (RIA) usually is decreased in patients with nonthyroidal illness. The thyroid-stimulating hormone (TSH) response to thyrotropin-releasing hormone (TRH) also usually is normal. It may be difficult to identify acutely ill patients with hypothalamic or pituitary disease. An sTSH above 20 μU/ml and low free T_4 (FT_4) are good evidence for primary thyroid failure.

A. The free thyroxine index (FTI) often is misleading because of drug-induced or disease-related binding protein abnormalities. The FT_4 is the preferred test for assessing the thyroxine level in this setting.

B. Up to 50% of acutely ill patients have a decrease in total T_4 and/or T_3. Both FT_4 and sTSH usually are normal. These findings provide good evidence that the patient is euthyroid.

C. During the acute phase of an illness, especially an acute psychiatric illness, a few patients have elevation of total T_4 and FT_4 and a normal sTSH. These patients also may display a flat response to TRH stimulation. Because these abnormalities resolve after a few weeks, take great care in diagnosing an acutely psychotic patient as hyperthyroid. T_3 RIA usually is normal in these patients. Rarely, propranolol dosages >320 mg/day, amiodarone, heparin, furosemide, and acute alcoholic hepatitis may all produce elevations of FT_4 with normal sTSH levels. In these situations, if there are no compelling clinical findings to indicate hyperthyroidism, it is best to simply repeat the tests in 2–3 weeks.

D. Patients with nephrotic syndrome may have mildly depressed FT_4 and normal sTSH. Glucocorticoids in stress doses acutely inhibit TSH secretion, and a small decrement in both sTSH and FT_4 may be observed. Dopamine infusions also cause acute suppression of TSH. In a truly hypothyroid patient receiving a dopamine infusion and/or stress doses of glucocorticoids, the TSH may be suppressed into the normal range.

E. Elevation of sTSH with normal FT_4 is found in patients recovering from a nonthyroidal illness. sTSH usually is <20 μU/ml, but rebound of up to 30 μU/ml may occur in patients recovering from severe sepsis. Slight elevations of TSH commonly are found in patients with chronic renal failure. Although the pathophysiology is unknown, these patients have a blunted TSH response to TRH.

References

Burmeister LA. Reverse T_3 does not reliably differentiate hypothyroid sick syndrome from euthyroid sick syndrome. Thyroid 1995; 5:435.

Cavaliere RR. The effects of nonthyroid disease and drugs on thyroid function tests. Med Clin North Am 1991; 75:27.

Docter R, Krenning EP, deJong M, Henneman G. The sick euthyroid syndrome: changes in thyroid hormone serum parameters and hormone metabolism (review). Clin Endocrinol 1993; 39:499.

Faber J, Kirkegaena C, Rasmassen B, et al. Pituitary-thyroid axis in critical illness. J Clin Endocrinol Metab 1987; 65:315.

Lim S, Fang V, Katz A, et al. Thyroid dysfunction in chronic renal failure: a study of the pituitary-thyroid axis and peripheral turnover kinetics of thyroxine and triiodothyronine. J Clin Invest 1977; 60:522.

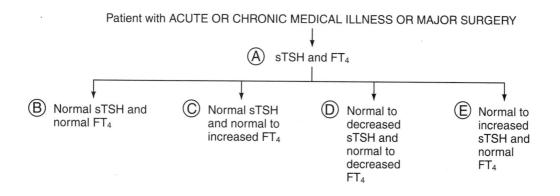

Patient with ACUTE OR CHRONIC MEDICAL ILLNESS OR MAJOR SURGERY

(A) sTSH and FT$_4$

(B) Normal sTSH and normal FT$_4$

(C) Normal sTSH and normal to increased FT$_4$

(D) Normal to decreased sTSH and normal to decreased FT$_4$

(E) Normal to increased sTSH and normal FT$_4$

ADRENAL MASS

Nancy A. Curosh

Abdominal CT has become common, detecting incidental adrenal masses with increased frequency. The incidence has been estimated at 1–10% of patients having a high-resolution abdominal CT scan. In most cases the patient is asymptomatic. Autopsy series have found macroscopic adrenal nodules in 2–9% of patients. The history and physical examination may suggest a cause (evidence of adrenal hormone excess, discovery of a primary carcinoma that may have metastasized to the adrenal), and this should be pursued vigorously. Otherwise, complete diagnostic testing for every adrenal mass is not cost-effective.

A. The likelihood of a pheochromocytoma in an incidentally discovered adrenal mass is low. However, because it is a potentially lethal condition that can have grave consequences if not diagnosed preoperatively, a high index of suspicion is necessary. Most patients with a pheochromocytoma have symptoms. The classic triad is headache, diaphoresis, and palpitations; the presence of two or more of these greatly increases the likelihood that the disease is present. New-onset hypertension; labile or severe hypertension; family history of multiple endocrine neoplasia (MEN) type 2A or type 2B; severe pressor responses to surgery, pregnancy, or anesthesia; and paradoxical responses to antihypertensive medications are all warning signs. Other symptoms occasionally seen with pheochromocytomas include pallor, paroxysms, anxiety, chest pain, weakness, and nausea.

B. In patients who are hypertensive at the time of sampling, a negative urine screening test makes a pheochromocytoma unlikely. In normotensive or intermittently hypertensive patients, repeat testing may be necessary. The choice of screening and confirmation tests may depend on which assays are available. Usually the best screening tests are 24-hour urine collections for metanephrines or free catecholamines. Many medications and foods interfere with these assays, so it is essential to understand which assays are performed by a particular laboratory to prepare the patient adequately for collection and interpret the results correctly. In general, high-performance liquid chromatography methods are the most sensitive and reliable. The plasma norepinephrine level can also be a helpful diagnostic test, if available. For this test, strict guidelines must be followed in the collection and handling of the blood to avoid false-positive results.

C. MRI, meta-iodobenzylguanidine (MIBG), and selective venous sampling are all tests available to help localize a pheochromocytoma. If a pheochromocytoma is seen on CT, these tests usually are unnecessary. In some cases, especially in MEN syndromes, there may be multiple pheochromocytomas. If this is suspected, one of these additional tests may be useful.

D. Signs of female virilization include male-pattern baldness, deepening of the voice, clitoromegaly, increased strength, and increased libido. Male feminization may include decreased body hair, loss of muscle strength and mass, gynecomastia, and decreased libido.

E. Adrenal carcinomas are rare and have a poor prognosis. Abdominal pain and a palpable mass often are present at the time of diagnosis. Hypokalemia is commonly seen. Excessive glucocorticoid, androgen, and mineralocorticoid hypersecretion has a rapid onset, and therefore the usual clinical features of hormonal excess may not have time to develop fully. Surgical resection is the treatment of choice if possible. Although surgical cure is rare because of frequent metastases, it at least reduces the tumor mass and the amount of steroid hypersecretion. Medical therapies include mitotane (*o, p*'-DDD), metyrapone, and aminoglutethimide.

F. Patients with Cushing's syndrome often have weight gain with truncal obesity, proximal muscle weakness, spontaneous ecchymoses, striae, and alterations in reproductive function (oligomenorrhea or amenorrhea in females; decreased libido or impotence in males). Hypertension is common.

G. Aldosterone-secreting tumors are rare, and the confirmatory tests are complicated and time-consuming. If the patient is not hypertensive and does not spontaneously have hypokalemia, it is not cost-effective to pursue this etiology. Serum potassium levels should be obtained with the patient on a normal- to high-sodium diet and off any potassium-altering medications.

References

Cook DM, Loriaux DL. The incidental adrenal mass. Endocrinologist 1996; 6:1.

Copeland PM. The incidentally discovered adrenal mass. Ann Intern Med 1983; 98:940.

Gross MD, Shapiro B. Clinically silent adrenal masses. J Clin Endocrinol Metab 1993; 77:4.

Gross MD, Shapiro B, Bouffard JA, et al. Distinguishing benign from malignant euadrenal masses. Ann Intern Med 1988; 109:613.

Ross NS, Aron DC. Hormonal evaluation of the patient with an incidentally discovered adrenal mass. N Engl J Med 1990; 323:1401.

Stein PP, Black HR. A simplified diagnostic approach to pheochromocytoma: a review of the literature and report of one institution's experience. Medicine 1990; 70:46.

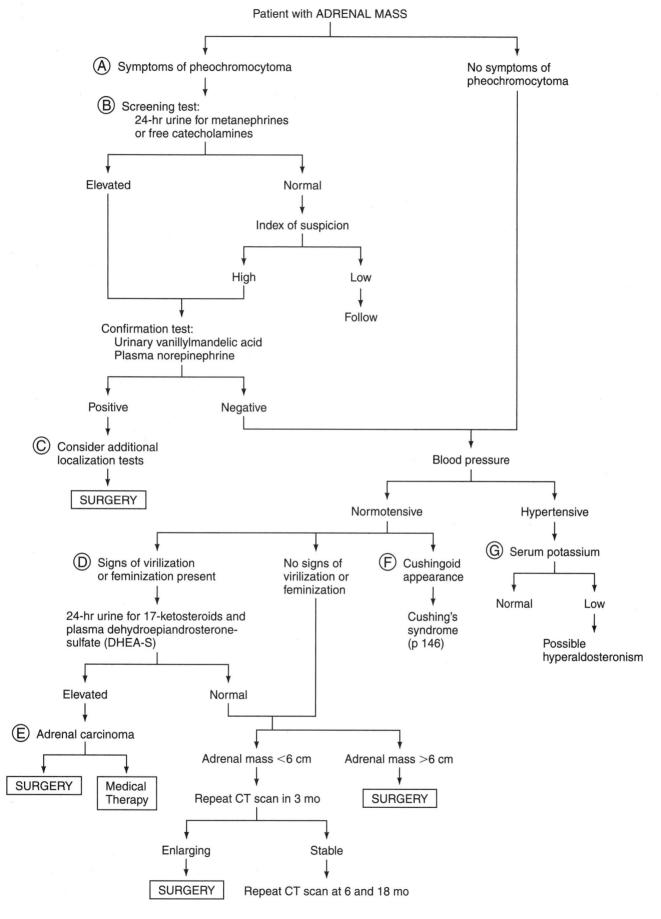

Patient with ADRENAL MASS

Ⓐ Symptoms of pheochromocytoma

No symptoms of pheochromocytoma

Ⓑ Screening test:
24-hr urine for metanephrines
or free catecholamines

Elevated

Normal

Index of suspicion

High

Low

Follow

Confirmation test:
Urinary vanillylmandelic acid
Plasma norepinephrine

Positive

Negative

Ⓒ Consider additional
localization tests

SURGERY

Blood pressure

Normotensive

Hypertensive

Ⓓ Signs of virilization
or feminization present

No signs of
virilization or
feminization

Ⓕ Cushingoid
appearance

Ⓖ Serum potassium

24-hr urine for 17-ketosteroids and
plasma dehydroepiandrosterone-
sulfate (DHEA-S)

Cushing's
syndrome
(p 146)

Normal

Low

Possible
hyperaldosteronism

Elevated

Normal

Ⓔ Adrenal carcinoma

Adrenal mass <6 cm

Adrenal mass >6 cm

SURGERY

Medical
Therapy

Repeat CT scan in 3 mo

SURGERY

Enlarging

Stable

SURGERY

Repeat CT scan at 6 and 18 mo

CUSHING'S SYNDROME

Nancy A. Curosh

Cushing's syndrome is caused by a chronic increase in circulating glucocorticoids. The most common cause is exogenous use of glucocorticoids in the treatment of other illnesses. Endogenous Cushing's syndrome can be caused by several different pathophysiologic mechanisms that all cause the adrenal glands to overproduce glucocorticoids. About 80% of cases of endogenous Cushing's syndrome result from Cushing's disease, which is caused by excessive pituitary secretion of adrenocorticotropic hormone (ACTH). Ectopic ACTH-producing tumors and adrenal adenomas each occur about 10% of the time. Rare causes include adrenal carcinoma, bilateral nodular adrenal hyperplasia, and corticotropin-releasing hormone (CRH)-secreting tumors. Cushing's disease is more common in females than in males, but the other forms of Cushing's syndrome have an equal sex frequency. The clinical signs and symptoms of Cushing's syndrome are protean and are modified by the amount and duration of cortisol excess. Common manifestations include central obesity, hypertension, thin skin with easy bruising, purple striae, hirsutism, oligomenorrhea in females or decreased libido in males, proximal muscle weakness, osteoporosis, glucose intolerance, and depression or psychosis. It often is difficult to distinguish Cushing's syndrome from Cushingoid obesity because many symptoms are common to both. The following may be seen with Cushing's syndrome but usually are not seen with Cushingoid obesity: objective weakness, striae >1 cm in diameter, hypokalemia, spontaneous bruising, and osteoporosis.

A. Urinary free cortisol confirms the diagnosis of cortisol excess. Low-dose dexamethasone suppression tests are made to rule out Cushing's syndrome; an abnormal test result does not establish the diagnosis. There are two low-dose suppression tests. In the overnight dexamethasone suppression test, 1 mg dexamethasone is given orally at midnight. A plasma cortisol level is drawn at 8 AM. If the cortisol is <5 µg/dl, Cushing's syndrome is excluded. The Liddle low-dose test is performed by giving 0.5 mg dexamethasone every 6 hours for 2 days. Plasma cortisol, urinary 17-hydroxycorticosteroid, or urine-free cortisol is obtained each day. Cushing's syndrome is excluded if suppression occurs.

B. Suppression may not occur if the patient failed to take the dexamethasone, was taking medication(s) that may have interfered with the test (estrogen, dilantin, phenobarbital, rifampin), or was under stress. Depressed patients often have elevated cortisol production rates and fail to suppress with low-dose dexamethasone. However, they do not have the stigmata of Cushing's syndrome. Occasionally alcoholics appear floridly Cushingoid and may fail to suppress during the low-dose test. These manifestations usually disappear within days of abstinence. The cortisol response to an insulin tolerance test may be useful in differentiating true Cushing's syndrome, where cortisol does not rise with hypoglycemia, from the depressed or alcoholic patient, where a normal cortisol increase occurs. This test may be dangerous and warrants adequate precautions. CRH stimulation test may be helpful in selected cases.

C. High-dose dexamethasone suppression testing can be done by two methods. The traditional Liddle test consists of 2 mg dexamethasone every 6 hours for 2–3 days. Plasma cortisol, urinary 17-hydroxycorticosteroid, or urine-free cortisol levels are obtained at baseline and each day. A 50% reduction from baseline indicates pituitary disease. The alternative test is an 8-mg overnight dexamethasone suppression test. Cushing's disease responds to suppression, resulting in an 8 AM plasma cortisol <50% of baseline.

D. The plasma ACTH level is helpful in differentiating ectopic tumors, where ACTH is high, from adrenal tumors, where it is suppressed. Strict guidelines for collection times and handling of the specimen must be adhered to for an accurate test. Localization procedures usually aid in the diagnosis.

E. Most patients with ectopic ACTH have known malignancies. Oat cell carcinoma is the most common; others include bronchial adenomas or carcinoids, pheochromocytomas, thymic carcinoids, pancreatic islet cell tumors, and medullary carcinomas of the thyroid. In some cases, because of rapid progression of the disease, the classic characteristics of Cushing's syndrome may not be present. Spontaneous hypokalemia may be a diagnostic clue. Several cases have been reported in which the malignant tumor secretes CRH instead of ACTH.

F. Cushing's disease usually is caused by very small pituitary adenomas. If these are seen on CT or MRI, this may help confirm the diagnosis. In most cases, however, the scans are normal. Additional confirmatory tests can be performed as deemed necessary. These include bilateral inferior petrosal sinus catheterization or exaggerated responses to metyrapone, ACTH, or CRH. Cushing's disease is best treated with transsphenoidal pituitary surgery, preferably by a neurosurgeon with extensive personal experience. Bilateral adrenalectomy is an alternative choice, but 10–15% of patients may develop Nelson's syndrome: hyperpigmentation and increasing size of the pituitary tumor, which may invade locally.

References

Carpenter PC. Diagnostic evaluation of Cushing's syndrome. Endocrinol Metab Clin North Am 1988; 17:445.
Felicetta JV. Cushing's syndrome: how to pinpoint and treat the underlying cause. Postgrad Med 1989; 86:79.

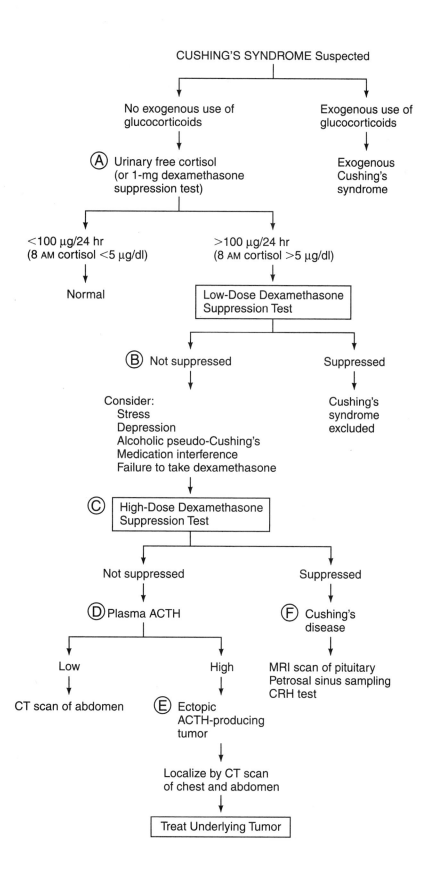

CUSHING'S SYNDROME Suspected

No exogenous use of glucocorticoids

Exogenous use of glucocorticoids

(A) Urinary free cortisol (or 1-mg dexamethasone suppression test)

Exogenous Cushing's syndrome

<100 µg/24 hr (8 AM cortisol <5 µg/dl)

>100 µg/24 hr (8 AM cortisol >5 µg/dl)

Normal

Low-Dose Dexamethasone Suppression Test

(B) Not suppressed

Suppressed

Consider:
  Stress
  Depression
  Alcoholic pseudo-Cushing's
  Medication interference
  Failure to take dexamethasone

Cushing's syndrome excluded

(C) High-Dose Dexamethasone Suppression Test

Not suppressed

Suppressed

(D) Plasma ACTH

(F) Cushing's disease

Low

High

MRI scan of pituitary
Petrosal sinus sampling
CRH test

CT scan of abdomen

(E) Ectopic ACTH-producing tumor

Localize by CT scan of chest and abdomen

Treat Underlying Tumor

Findling JW. Differential diagnosis of Cushing's syndrome. Endocrinologist 1997; 7(Suppl 1):1.

Flack MR, Oldfield EH, Cutler GB, et al. Urine free cortisol in the high dose dexamethasone suppression test for the differential diagnosis of the Cushing syndrome. Ann Intern Med 1992; 116:211.

Kaye TB, Crapo L. The Cushing syndrome: an update on diagnostic tests. Ann Intern Med 1990; 112:434.

PITUITARY TUMOR

Philip R. Orlander

A. Suspect a pituitary tumor if there is evidence of either hormonal excess or deficiency or if symptoms suggest compression of surrounding brain structures. Symptoms of hypopituitarism may be gradual in onset and nonspecific: malaise, weakness, weight loss, anorexia, nausea, menstrual irregularities, depression, hair loss, and polyuria. Specific hormonal deficiencies may have a more characteristic presentation (e.g., hypothyroidism). Incidental abnormalities of the pituitary may be noted during an evaluation for head injury or other common neurologic complaints. Consider pituitary abnormalities in women with complaints of infertility. Pituitary adenomas that are completely within the sella turcica (<1 cm) are considered microadenomas and primarily present with hormone excess syndromes. Macroadenomas may expand in a suprasellar direction, causing neuroanatomic manifestations such as headache, bitemporal hemianopsia, cranial nerve abnormalities, CSF rhinorrhea, and hypothalamic dysregulation. Formal visual field tests should be performed by an ophthalmologist. In patients with abrupt onset of severe headache, change in mental status, and evidence of a hormone deficiency, consider the rare syndrome of pituitary apoplexy with hemorrhage into a macroadenoma.

B. Prolactinomas are the most common pituitary tumors. They generally present as microadenomas in women with symptoms of infertility, menstrual irregularities, or galactorrhea, whereas men have larger lesions accompanied by impotence and symptoms of mass effect. The differential diagnosis of hyperprolactinemia includes numerous medications (e.g., phenothiazines, narcotics, estrogens, reserpine), hypothyroidism, renal disease, cirrhosis, chest wall or breast disease, pregnancy, and hypothalamic disease affecting the pituitary stalk. The clinical suspicion of acromegaly can be confirmed with an elevated serum growth hormone (GH) level that does not suppress normally after an oral 100-g glucose load or an elevated serum insulin-like growth factor level (IGF-I). The diagnosis of pituitary-dependent Cushing's disease requires consistent evidence of hypercortisolism (elevated urinary-free cortisol and inadequate suppression after dexamethasone; see p 146). Rare thyrotropin (TSH)-secreting tumors can produce hyperthyroidism. Gonadotrophin-secreting tumors generally are large and primarily present with neurologic complaints.

C. For patients with borderline morning cortisol levels (<18 μg/dl), perform a cortrosyn stimulation test. A cortisol level is drawn before and after cortrosyn. Any value >18 mg/dl is considered adequate. Lower values require further evaluation. The posterior pituitary can be evaluated with a water deprivation test. Most pituitary lesions do not cause hypopituitarism. Primary empty sella is a defect in the diaphragm of the sella and rarely is associated with any hormone abnormality. Large pituitary adenomas, craniopharyngiomas, and other tumors and infiltrating diseases of the hypothalamus and pituitary can be associated with panhypopituitarism (anterior and posterior pituitary). Diabetes insipidus may be the presenting complaint. Patients with untreated primary hypothyroidism or gonadal failure (Turner's or Klinefelter's syndrome) may be found to have an enlarged sella.

D. MRI of the pituitary has replaced older techniques such as lateral skull radiography and tomography of the sella, but fine-cut CT imaging of the pituitary is still useful if MRI is unavailable. The optic chiasm and pituitary stalk are easily demonstrated. In a high percentage of patients with Cushing's disease, there is no detectable lesion in the pituitary on MRI. Autopsy studies demonstrate that pituitary microadenomas are common, and abnormal scans in the absence of hormonal abnormality or mass effect may not require therapy.

E. Rapid responses to medical therapy with marked tumor shrinkage have been noted in patients with prolactinomas and, less often, in those with acromegaly. Unfortunately, tumor re-expansion generally is seen after discontinuation of treatment, and maintenance therapy usually is necessary. Replacement of all target organ hormones is essential in patients with pituitary deficiency. Desmopressin (DDAVP) is the treatment of choice for diabetes insipidus. Most pituitary lesions can be reached by a transsphenoidal approach. Macroadenomas may require additional radiation therapy, and the risk of hypopituitarism is high.

References

Grinspoon SK, Biller BM. Laboratory assessment of adrenal insufficiency. J Clin Endocrinol Metab 1994; 79:923.

Molitch ME. Evaluation and treatment of the patient with a pituitary incidentaloma. J Clin Endocrinol Metab 1995; 80:3.

Rolih CA, Ober KP. Pituitary apoplexy. Endocrinol Metab Clin North Am 1993; 22:291.

Tsigos C, Chrousos GP. Differential diagnosis and management of Cushing's syndrome. Annu Rev Med 1996; 47:443.

Wen PY, Loeffler JS. Advances in the diagnosis and management of pituitary tumors. Curr Opin Oncol 1995; 7:56.

PITUITARY TUMOR Suspected

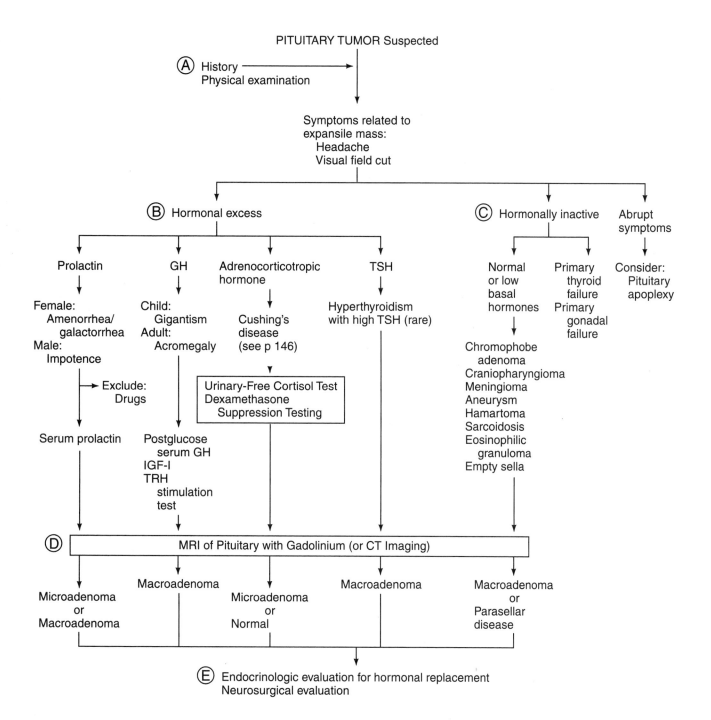

HIRSUTISM

Nancy A. Curosh

Hirsutism is the presence of excessive coarse terminal hair in a male-pattern growth distribution such as on the face, chest, abdomen, lower back, and thighs. This is caused by increased androgen production or action. Hirsutism must be distinguished from hypertrichosis, which is an excess of thin vellus hair in a nonsexual hair distribution. The amount of vellus hair highly depends on patients' racial and family background. An increase in vellus hair can also be caused by some metabolic disorders such as anorexia nervosa, porphyria cutanea tarda, and hypothyroidism.

A. Certain drugs, including phenytoin, anabolic steroids, diazoxide, minoxidil, and cyclosporine, may cause hirsutism. Virilization is not present except in some cases of anabolic steroid use.

B. Signs of virilization include male-pattern baldness, deepening of the voice, clitoromegaly, increasing strength, loss of breast tissue, and increasing libido. Benign causes of hirsutism often begin gradually around the time of puberty. Hirsutism that has a rapid onset or that begins in childhood or after menopause is compatible with an ovarian or adrenal tumor.

C. Dehydroepiandrosterone sulfate (DHEA-S) levels >700 μg/dl usually are a result of an adrenal tumor. These are rare and about half are palpable at the time of diagnosis. If an abdominal CT scan does not show a tumor, adrenal hyperplasia should be considered because this rarely can show very elevated DHEA-S levels.

D. The virilizing forms of congenital adrenal hyperplasia are the 11-hydroxylase, 21-hydroxylase, and 3β-hydroxysteroid dehydrogenase deficiencies. By far the most common is the 21-hydroxylase–deficient form. The classic forms usually are discovered in childhood, but the attenuated or late-onset forms may first be discovered in adulthood during investigation of hirsutism or virilization. In these patients the early-morning 17-hydroxyprogesterone level usually is elevated. The exact deficiency can be discovered by measuring specific precursor-to-product ratios. In mild cases, adrenocorticotropic hormone (ACTH) stimulation may be needed to exaggerate these differences. If the patient has only mild hirsutism, it may not be cost efficient to elucidate the exact cause. These patients usually respond to the same treatment as is given to idiopathic hirsutism.

E. If the onset of the hirsutism is gradual, usually beginning around the time of puberty, and if there is no evidence of virilization, a careful menstrual history is helpful. Patients who have irregular menses must be investigated for hypothyroidism and prolactinomas.

If these are excluded, the most likely diagnosis is polycystic ovarian disease. This classically consists of obesity, anovulation, and hyperandrogenemia, but the clinical presentation varies widely. The anovulation may be expressed as oligomenorrhea, amenorrhea, dysfunctional uterine bleeding, or infertility. The hyperandrogenemia may be asymptomatic or may present as hirsutism or acne. Obesity is seen in fewer than half of the patients. Ovarian size can be determined by pelvic examination or ultrasonography, but is not always a helpful parameter for diagnosis. Classically, polycystic ovaries are 2–5 times enlarged with 20 or more follicles, but this does not occur in all patients. Many patients have normal ovarian structures. Polycystic ovarian disease appears primarily to be a functional rather than anatomic abnormality. It usually is associated with a strong family history and may be inherited in an autosomal-dominant pattern. Testosterone often is moderately elevated. The luteinizing hormone/follicle-stimulating hormone ratio (LH/FSH) is >2 in 80% of cases. However, in most circumstances the diagnosis can be achieved without these laboratory values.

F. If the menses are regular, polycystic ovarian disease is still possible but less likely, and the aforementioned laboratory tests may be helpful. If polycystic ovarian disease seems improbable, the diagnosis of idiopathic hirsutism is made. *Idiopathic hirsutism* is the term used to describe patients with hirsutism for which a distinct cause cannot be found. Most patients have regular menses, but irregular menses may occur. Intensive study may disclose a cause in many of these women, but this is not cost-effective and would most likely not change the therapeutic options.

G. Treatment of hirsutism caused by polycystic ovarian disease or idiopathic hirsutism often is the same. Options include mechanical treatments (e.g., bleaching, shaving, or electrolysis) or drug therapy (e.g., low-dose glucocorticoids, oral contraceptives, or antiandrogens).

References

Barnes R, Rosenfield RL. The polycystic ovary syndrome: pathogenesis and treatment. Ann Intern Med 1989; 110:386.

Ehrmann DA, Rosenfield RL. An endocrinologic approach to the patient with hirsutism. J Clin Endocrinol Metab 1990; 71:1.

Rittmaster RS. Medical treatment of androgen-dependent hirsutism. J Clin Endocrinol Metab 1995; 80:9.

Rittmaster RS, Loriaux DL. Hirsutism. Ann Intern Med 1987; 106:95.

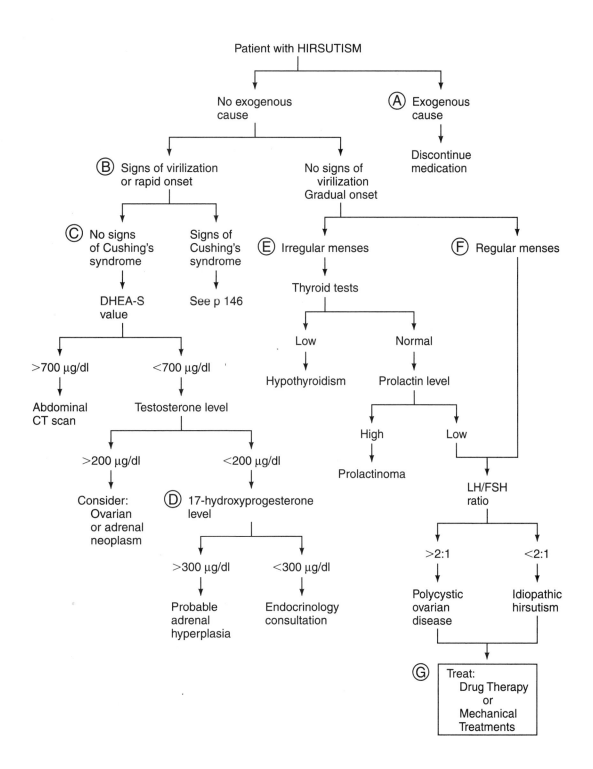

Patient with HIRSUTISM

No exogenous cause

Ⓐ Exogenous cause

Discontinue medication

Ⓑ Signs of virilization or rapid onset

No signs of virilization Gradual onset

Ⓒ No signs of Cushing's syndrome

Signs of Cushing's syndrome

DHEA-S value

See p 146

>700 µg/dl

<700 µg/dl

Abdominal CT scan

Testosterone level

>200 µg/dl

<200 µg/dl

Consider: Ovarian or adrenal neoplasm

Ⓓ 17-hydroxyprogesterone level

>300 µg/dl

<300 µg/dl

Probable adrenal hyperplasia

Endocrinology consultation

Ⓔ Irregular menses

Thyroid tests

Low

Normal

Hypothyroidism

Prolactin level

High

Low

Prolactinoma

Ⓕ Regular menses

LH/FSH ratio

>2:1

<2:1

Polycystic ovarian disease

Idiopathic hirsutism

Ⓖ Treat:
Drug Therapy
or
Mechanical
Treatments

GYNECOMASTIA

Nancy A. Curosh
Thomas W. Boyden

Gynecomastia is a glandular enlargement of the male breast with a simultaneous increase in surrounding connective tissue. The breasts are sensitive to hormonal influences, and gynecomastia can occur as a result of an excess of stimulatory hormones such as estrogens, a decrease in inhibitory hormones such as androgens, or an imbalance between stimulatory and inhibitory hormones. Gynecomastia is not a rare finding when careful examination is performed. Often, the patient is unaware of its presence, but it is sometimes quite painful.

A. Numerous drugs have been associated with gynecomastia (Table 1), and their mechanisms of action vary. Estrogens directly stimulate the breasts. Androgens are converted to estrogens. Cytotoxic agents damage the testes, causing primary hypogonadism. Cimetidine blocks androgen receptors. Alcohol lowers serum testosterone levels and may increase estrogen levels because of augmented peripheral conversion of androgens to estrogen. Some drugs increase prolactin levels and cause a hypogonadal state. In many drugs the mechanism of action is unknown.

B. After World War II many former prisoners of war developed gynecomastia after they were renourished. This also has been observed in patients recovering from any prolonged illness in which they had lost considerable weight. This refeeding gynecomastia usually resolves in months to 2 years.

C. Gynecomastia can occur in a wide range of illnesses. Patients with liver disease, especially cirrhosis, develop gynecomastia because of an estrogen excess; there is increased production of estrogen from circulating precursors, and elevated levels of sex hormone–binding globulin decrease free testosterone. Hyperthyroidism also causes gynecomastia because of increased estrogen levels. Adrenal diseases can cause gynecomastia because cortisol excess inhibits testosterone production. Prolactin excess also works through this mechanism. Patients with chronic renal disease often develop gynecomastia soon after beginning hemodialysis, probably because of a refeeding phenomenon caused by their improved well-being and appetite. Patients receiving dialysis also often have low serum testosterone,

elevated luteinizing hormone (LH), an increased estrogen/androgen ratio, and mildly increased prolactin. Pulmonary and cardiac diseases and AIDS are other illnesses sometimes associated with gynecomastia.

D. Carefully perform a breast examination to distinguish gynecomastia from a breast carcinoma. Gynecomastia relates to subareolar glandular tissue. To be sure it is glandular and not adipose tissue, compare the tissue with the adipose tissue of the anterior axillary fold. Gynecomastia often is asymptomatic and may be unilateral. Fixed, indurated, irregular, or firm areas suggest breast carcinoma. Mammography or ultrasonography may be useful in this situation, but if any doubt remains, biopsy is indicated.

E. A normal adult testis measures 3.5–5.5 cm in length and 2.1–3.2 cm in width. With a Prader orchidometer, the volume should be 20–30 ml. Eunuchoidal proportions are present if the arm span is >2 cm longer than the patient's height and the floor-to-pubis length is 2 cm greater than the pubis-to-crown distance. Eunuchoidal proportions often are seen in patients who were hypogonadal before puberty.

F. Gynecomastia is common at certain stages in life. Neonates often have gynecomastia because of high levels of estrogen in the placental-fetal circulation. During puberty gynecomastia can be found in 40–60% of boys. This may be because of an increase in plasma estrogens compared with androgens. Likewise, gynecomastia is common in men >65 years of age, probably because of varying degrees of testicular failure. If these patients are asymptomatic, observation may be all that is necessary.

G. A low testosterone level with a high LH level indicates testicular failure. Klinefelter's syndrome is a male genetic disorder in which there is an extra X chromosome. Patients have a eunuchoidal appearance and small testes. Of patients with Klinefelter's syndrome, 85% have gynecomastia. It is important to differentiate Klinefelter's syndrome from other causes of testicular failure such as trauma, orchitis, and damage from radiation or chemotherapy. Unlike most other conditions causing gynecomastia, Klinefelter's syndrome is associated with an increased incidence of breast cancer, and therefore closer observation is needed. If suspected, Klinefelter's syndrome can be confirmed by a buccal smear or chromosomal karyotyping.

H. A serum β–human chorionic gonadotropin (β-hCG) radioimmunoassay is recommended because urinary pregnancy tests, which also measure hCG, are not sufficiently sensitive. Elevated hCG indicates a tumor. A variety of malignant testicular tissues produce hCG, and

TABLE 1 Some Drugs Associated with Gynecomastia

Alcohol	Ketoconazole
Androgens	Marijuana
Calcium channel blockers	Methyldopa
Cimetidine	Phenytoin
Cytotoxic drugs	Reserpine
Digitalis	Spironolactone
Estrogens	Tricyclic antidepressants
Isoniazid	

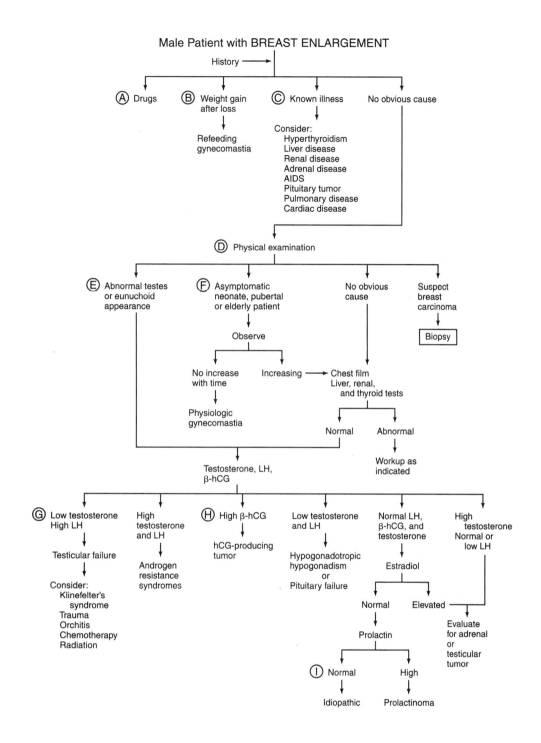

Male Patient with BREAST ENLARGEMENT

History →

Ⓐ Drugs Ⓑ Weight gain after loss Ⓒ Known illness No obvious cause

Refeeding gynecomastia

Consider:
  Hyperthyroidism
  Liver disease
  Renal disease
  Adrenal disease
  AIDS
  Pituitary tumor
  Pulmonary disease
  Cardiac disease

Ⓓ Physical examination

Ⓔ Abnormal testes or eunuchoid appearance   Ⓕ Asymptomatic neonate, pubertal or elderly patient   No obvious cause   Suspect breast carcinoma

Biopsy

Observe

No increase with time   Increasing →   Chest film Liver, renal, and thyroid tests

Physiologic gynecomastia

Normal   Abnormal

Workup as indicated

Testosterone, LH, β-hCG

Ⓖ Low testosterone High LH   High testosterone and LH   Ⓗ High β-hCG   Low testosterone and LH   Normal LH, β-hCG, and testosterone   High testosterone Normal or low LH

Testicular failure

Consider:
  Klinefelter's syndrome
  Trauma
  Orchitis
  Chemotherapy
  Radiation

Androgen resistance syndromes

hCG-producing tumor

Hypogonadotropic hypogonadism or Pituitary failure

Estradiol

Normal   Elevated

Evaluate for adrenal or testicular tumor

Prolactin

Ⓘ Normal   High

Idiopathic   Prolactinoma

these may be suggested by an asymmetrically enlarged testis. However, nontesticular tumors such as some pulmonary, gastric, and pancreatic tumors may also secrete hCG. A careful search must be made to locate these tumors.

I. In a significant number of patients, no definitive cause of gynecomastia is found after thorough investigation. These patients should receive periodic follow-up.

References

Carlson HE. Gynecomastia. N Engl J Med 1980; 303:795.
Couderc LJ, Clauvel JP. HIV-infection-induced gynecomastia. Ann Intern Med 1987; 107:257.
Glass AR. Gynecomastia. Endocrinol Metab Clin North Am 1994; 23:825.

GASTROENTEROLOGY

ACUTE ABDOMINAL PAIN

Steven Palley

Evaluation of acute abdominal pain remains difficult in clinical medicine. The internist addressing the patient with acute abdominal pain ideally should eliminate medical causes and recognize the proper setting for surgical consultation. There should be a low threshold for involving surgical expertise. History and physical examination are critical in evaluation. Admission for evaluation is common and should be considered for acute pain without obvious surgical indication that persists for 6 hours.

A. A careful history can narrow the differential diagnosis. Age and sex are important considerations. Mesenteric adenitis occurs in younger persons, whereas vascular and neoplastic disease occurs in the elderly. In a sexually active female, consider ectopic pregnancy or pelvic inflammatory disease. Medical history can reveal previous peptic ulcer disease, gallstones, diverticular disease, inflammatory bowel disease, and abdominal surgery. Medication history can disclose corticosteroids or immunosuppressants. Coexisting medical conditions such as diabetes mellitus can affect the presentation. The onset and character of the pain is important. A sudden onset of intense, localized, "somatic" pain suggests peritonitis, as in perforation of bowel. Crescendo-decrescendo "visceral" pain or colic is more characteristic of bowel, cystic duct, or ureteral obstruction. An evolving pain pattern, visceral at first and later somatic, may suggest appendicitis, cholecystitis, or strangulated bowel. Disproportionate pain compared with a lesser physical finding occurs with ischemia. Characteristic radiation patterns are noted with cholecystitis (scapula), pancreatitis (back), and appendicitis (right lower quadrant).

B. Observe the patient before the examination. Visceral pain usually causes restlessness; parietal pain increases with movement. Auscultate the abdomen for bruits, rubs, and bowel sounds. Palpation should begin away from the site of pain. Involuntary guarding or rebound tenderness, especially with light percussion, implies peritonitis. Deeper palpation can be used to search for organomegaly or masses. Perform rectal and pelvic examinations.

C. A hemodynamically unstable patient with possible intra-abdominal hemorrhage may require immediate laparotomy. The acutely ill patient with hypotension, high fever, leukocytosis, and a suggestive physical examination (involuntary guarding, rigidity, increasing severe tenderness) should also undergo immediate surgical evaluation. Suspected bowel ischemia with acidosis, fever, and evidence of hypovolemia also should be evaluated surgically, as should the patient with evidence of perforation by plain radiography, contrast study, or paracentesis. Resuscitation is critical both before and during further evaluation, including possible ventilatory support, IV access and fluids, nasogastric suction, oxygen, and urinary output monitoring, as well as frequent checks on vital signs and preliminary laboratory tests. Ideally, important medical causes of acute pain can be ruled out before surgery with urinalysis, electrocardiography, and abdominal films.

D. The more stable patient should be observed closely. Medical causes of acute abdominal pain can be ruled out, although the list can be extensive. The more common causes are acute pneumonitis, especially lower lobe; pyelonephritis; and mesenteric adenitis. Collagen vascular disease can cause perforation. Multiple metabolic disorders, including diabetic ketoacidosis, Addisonian crisis, uremia, and acute intermittent porphyria, can lead to abdominal pain. A history of chronic liver disease with ascites may suggest spontaneous bacterial peritonitis.

E. Certain patients may present with a discrepancy between severity of disease and physical findings. These include patients who are elderly, malnourished, obese, immunosuppressed, or taking steroids; early postoperative patients; those with mental status changes; and paraplegics.

F. Laboratory evaluation should include hemoglobin/hematocrit, WBC count, differential, electrolytes, blood gases, amylase, liver tests, coagulation times, and urinalysis. Supine and upright abdominal films may suggest obstruction, ischemia, perforation, biliary calculi, or intra-abdominal abscess. Angiography is useful for suspected hemorrhage or ischemia. Contrast studies are useful for suspected perforation. Ultrasonography and CT imaging can demonstrate pancreatitis, cholecystitis, abscess, retroperitoneal mass, or dilated biliary tree.

G. Close observation may disclose an evolutionary pattern to the abdominal pain syndrome. If acute pain persists >6 hours, obtain a surgical consultation if this has not already been requested.

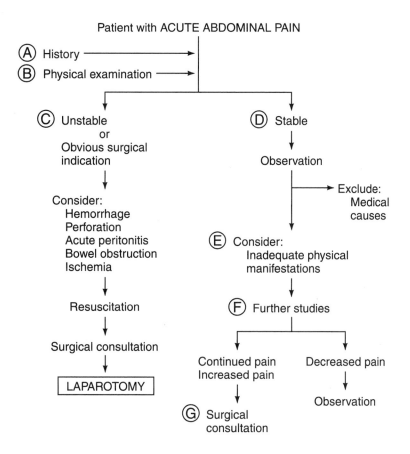

Patient with ACUTE ABDOMINAL PAIN

(A) History

(B) Physical examination

(C) Unstable
or
Obvious surgical
indication

Consider:
    Hemorrhage
    Perforation
    Acute peritonitis
    Bowel obstruction
    Ischemia

Resuscitation

Surgical consultation

LAPAROTOMY

(D) Stable

Observation

Exclude:
    Medical
    causes

(E) Consider:
    Inadequate physical
    manifestations

(F) Further studies

Continued pain
Increased pain

Decreased pain

Observation

(G) Surgical
consultation

References

Boey JH. Acute abdomen. In: Way LW, ed. Current surgical diagnosis and treatment. Norwalk, CT: Appleton & Lange, 1988:393.

Fulenwider JT, McGarity WC. Evaluation of acute abdominal pain in adults. In: Conn R, ed. Current diagnosis 7. Philadelphia: WB Saunders, 1985:31.

Silen W. Abdominal pain. In: Fauci AS, Braunwald E, Isselbacher KJ, et al, eds. Harrison's principles of internal medicine. 14th ed. New York: McGraw-Hill, 1997:65.

Thomson JH, Jones PF. Active observation in acute abdominal pain. Am J Surg 1986; 2:522.

CHRONIC ABDOMINAL PAIN

Lee J. Hixson

A. Postprandial pain suggests peptic ulceration, pancreatitis, biliary obstruction, partial small bowel obstruction, irritable bowel syndrome (IBS), lactose intolerance, or chronic mesenteric insufficiency. Pain that is diminished by bending forward suggests pancreatic cancer, chronic pancreatitis, or an abdominal aortic aneurysm. Most patients with chronic recurrent abdominal pain are, after exhaustive evaluation, labeled with a "functional" disorder such as IBS or nonulcer dyspepsia.

B. Screening laboratory tests should generally include a CBC with differential, liver biochemistries (bilirubin, transaminases, alkaline phosphatase), and amylase. Additional appropriate tests commonly include a full chemistry panel, urinalysis, stool analysis (microscopic for leukocytes, ova, and parasites), and abdominal radiography to detect conditions such as stones, bowel obstruction, visceral displacement or enlargement, and calcification.

C. Pain originating in the abdominal wall is superficial and exacerbated by movement or touch. It often is attributed to costochondritis when localized to the upper abdomen over the xiphoid or costal margin. Pain associated with recently healed lesions may indicate nerve entrapment or regeneration with neuroma formation. Radicular pain across the abdomen may also be worse with movement and be caused by irritation of the spinal nerve root from disc and vertebral body disease, a meningeal tumor, tabes dorsalis secondary to syphilis or diabetes, or postherpetic neuralgia. Abdominal wall and radicular pain usually can be obliterated by blocking the intercostal or paravertebral nerves.

D. If pain has a pelvic source, consider ovarian and uterine cysts and tumors, chronic pelvic inflammatory disease, and endometriosis.

E. The following metabolic disorders may be associated with abdominal pain: porphyria, hyper- and hypothyroidism, adrenal insufficiency, hypercalcemia, familial Mediterranean fever, hereditary angioedema, diabetic neuropathy, and carcinoid syndrome.

F. Chronic narcotic use may result in the narcotic bowel syndrome with pain presumably secondary to bowel spasm. Dilantin, NSAIDs, and other agents also may be associated with chronic abdominal pain.

G. "Functional" pain is a diagnosis of exclusion. The pain may be severe, well localized, or diffuse, and rarely awakens the patient from sleep. IBS is classically associated with altered bowel habits, constipation alternating with diarrhea. Pain relief with defecation, mucus in the stool, and a sensation of incomplete evacuation are typical.

H. Chronic mesenteric ischemia is an uncommon clinical diagnosis characterized by postprandial pain and weight loss. Mesenteric vasculitis usually is associated with signs and symptoms of concurrent involvement in other organ systems outside the abdomen.

I. Pain originating from the liver results from distension of the hepatic capsule, which may be secondary to hepatic congestion, inflammation, infiltration, or tumor/cyst growth.

J. Colonic tumors and diverticulosis usually are not painful but may become so with bowel perforation or obstruction. Diverticulosis may be associated with marked hypertrophy and thickening of the bowel wall, which on occasion may produce left lower quadrant pain with constipation.

References

Drossman DA. Chronic functional abdominal pain. In: Feldman M, Scharschmidt BF, Sleisenger MH, eds. Gastrointestinal and liver disease. 6th ed. Philadelphia: WB Saunders, 1998:90.

Glasgow RE, Mulvihill SJ. Abdominal pain, including the acute abdomen. In: Feldman M, Scharschmidt BF, Sleisenger MH, eds. Gastrointestinal and liver disease. 6th ed. Philadelphia: WB Saunders, 1998:80.

Phillips SF. The diverse spectrum of irritable bowel syndrome. Hosp Pract (Off Ed) 1995; 30:69.

Patient with CHRONIC ABDOMINAL PAIN

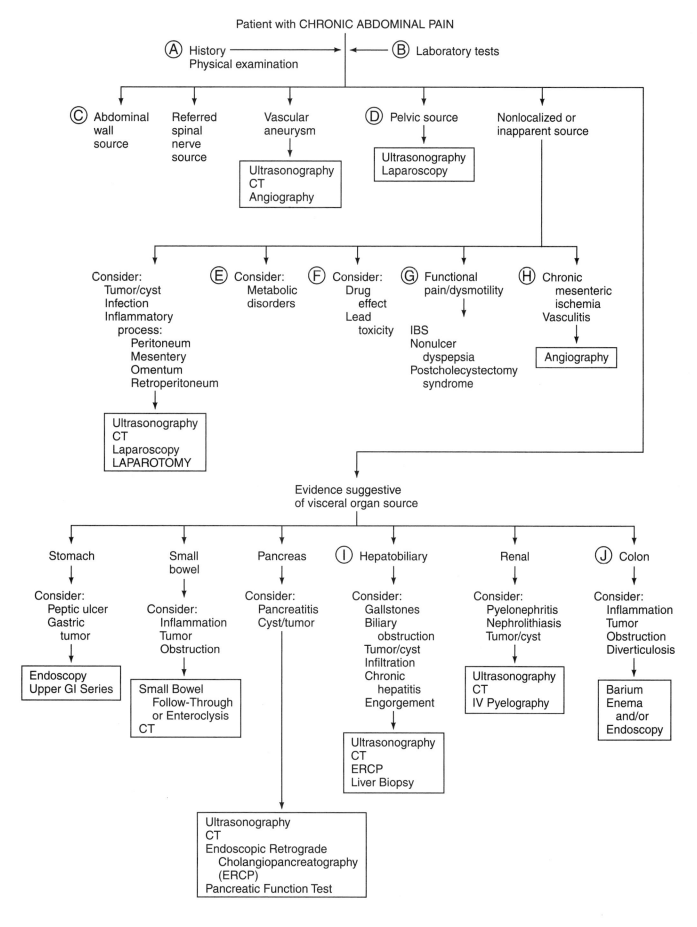

(A) History
Physical examination

(B) Laboratory tests

(C) Abdominal wall source

Referred spinal nerve source

Vascular aneurysm

Ultrasonography
CT
Angiography

(D) Pelvic source

Ultrasonography
Laparoscopy

Nonlocalized or inapparent source

Consider:
Tumor/cyst
Infection
Inflammatory
process:
Peritoneum
Mesentery
Omentum
Retroperitoneum

Ultrasonography
CT
Laparoscopy
LAPAROTOMY

(E) Consider:
Metabolic disorders

(F) Consider:
Drug effect
Lead toxicity

(G) Functional pain/dysmotility

IBS
Nonulcer
dyspepsia
Postcholecystectomy
syndrome

(H) Chronic mesenteric ischemia
Vasculitis

Angiography

Evidence suggestive of visceral organ source

Stomach

Consider:
Peptic ulcer
Gastric tumor

Endoscopy
Upper GI Series

Small bowel

Consider:
Inflammation
Tumor
Obstruction

Small Bowel
Follow-Through
or Enteroclysis
CT

Pancreas

Consider:
Pancreatitis
Cyst/tumor

Ultrasonography
CT
Endoscopic Retrograde
Cholangiopancreatography
(ERCP)
Pancreatic Function Test

(I) Hepatobiliary

Consider:
Gallstones
Biliary obstruction
Tumor/cyst
Infiltration
Chronic hepatitis
Engorgement

Ultrasonography
CT
ERCP
Liver Biopsy

Renal

Consider:
Pyelonephritis
Nephrolithiasis
Tumor/cyst

Ultrasonography
CT
IV Pyelography

(J) Colon

Consider:
Inflammation
Tumor
Obstruction
Diverticulosis

Barium
Enema
and/or
Endoscopy

NAUSEA AND VOMITING

Steven Palley

Although a common symptom, nausea is difficult to define precisely. Vomiting is a complex, well-coordinated act with neurologic pathways that are described, at least in part. Vomiting needs to be distinguished from regurgitation in which gastric or esophageal contents are returned to the pharynx by pressure differentials. Regurgitation can occur with gastroesophageal reflux disease, esophageal stricture, achalasia, Zenker's diverticulum, and rumination syndrome.

A. The history may reveal the possibility of pregnancy, a family history of similar disorder, drug intake, or psychiatric abnormality. The characteristics of the vomiting episode are relatively nonspecific. A large volume of emesis or emesis of food ingested >12 hours previously suggests organic causes. A succussion splash, skin changes or Raynaud's phenomenon, orthostatic hypotension, or neurologic finding may suggest the cause. A plain abdominal film is inexpensive and easy and may contribute valuable information.

B. Nausea and vomiting of acute onset (<1 week) should prompt a different work-up from that of a long-standing complaint. Historical considerations are important. A careful drug history may disclose opiates, anticholinergics, β agonists, erythromycin, or chemotherapeutics. Consider drug toxicity such as from digoxin. Acute vestibular causes such as motion sickness and acute labyrinthitis are possible. Viral gastroenteritis is a common cause. Visceral pain syndromes causing acute nausea include myocardial infarction, pancreatitis, and renal and biliary colic.

C. Chronic nausea and vomiting is commonly related to structural lesions affecting the upper GI tract. Rule out pregnancy in appropriate patients. Perform upper endoscopy to evaluate mucosal lesions, peptic ulcer disease, a deformed pylorus, or other gastric outlet obstruction. If the examination is unhelpful or there is a suggestion of an extrinsic process, perform an upper GI contrast study. Extrinsic lesions should be further evaluated with ultrasonography or abdominal CT.

D. If the above examinations are negative, perform a thorough neurologic and vestibular evaluation. Psychiatric screening can be useful. Further evaluation for collagen vascular disease or endocrine disorder should be considered. If the above evaluations are unhelpful, offer a therapeutic trial with a promotility agent such as metoclopramide.

E. If the therapeutic trial is unsuccessful, further evaluation is warranted. Perform a radionuclide gastric emptying study, and evaluate solid and liquid emptying. This may document a gastric emptying disorder but unfortunately cannot determine the cause. This may suffice in the appropriate setting, such as long-standing diabetes mellitus, autonomic insufficiency, or progressive systemic sclerosis.

F. In severe, persistent, unexplained nausea and vomiting, further evaluation may be warranted. The patient should show evidence of functional impairment or nutritional deficit. Evaluation at a specialized gastric motility center can determine the type of motility disorder and may suggest a specific intervention such as antrectomy for distal gastric motility disorder. Exploratory laparotomy with full-thickness small bowel biopsy can sometimes yield a diagnosis.

References

Feldman M. Nausea and vomiting. In: Sleisenger MH, Fordtran JS, eds. Gastrointestinal disease. 4th ed. Philadelphia: WB Saunders, 1989:222.

Hanson JS, McCallum RW. The diagnosis and management of nausea and vomiting: a review. Am J Gastroenterol 1985; 80:210.

Herrstadt J. New perspectives in antiemetic treatment. Support Care Cancer 1996; 4:416.

Lichter I. Nausea and vomiting in patients with cancer. Hematol Oncol Clin North Am 1996; 10:207.

Malagelada JR, Camilleri M. Unexplained vomiting: a diagnostic challenge. Ann Intern Med 1984; 101:211.

Patient with NAUSEA AND VOMITING

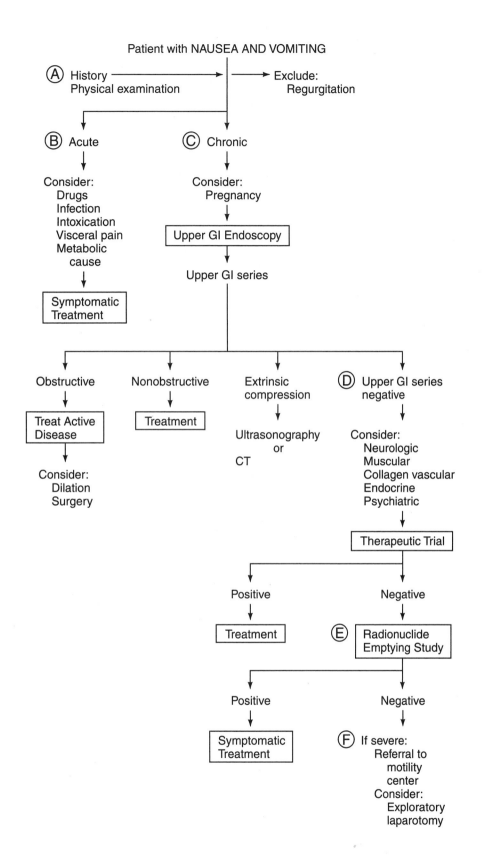

Ⓐ History ──────────→ ──→ Exclude:
   Physical examination   Regurgitation

Ⓑ Acute   Ⓒ Chronic

Consider: Consider:
   Drugs   Pregnancy
   Infection
   Intoxication   ┌─────────────────────┐
   Visceral pain   │ Upper GI Endoscopy │
   Metabolic   └─────────────────────┘
     cause
                      Upper GI series
┌──────────────┐
│ Symptomatic │
│ Treatment   │
└──────────────┘

Obstructive   Nonobstructive   Extrinsic   Ⓓ Upper GI series
                                       compression   negative
┌──────────────┐   ┌──────────────┐
│ Treat Active │   │ Treatment   │   Ultrasonography   Consider:
│ Disease   │   └──────────────┘   or   Neurologic
└──────────────┘   CT   Muscular
                                                            Collagen vascular
Consider: Endocrine
   Dilation   Psychiatric
   Surgery
                                                      ┌──────────────────┐
                                                      │ Therapeutic Trial│
                                                      └──────────────────┘

                                    Positive   Negative

                              ┌──────────────┐   Ⓔ ┌──────────────────┐
                              │ Treatment   │   │ Radionuclide   │
                              └──────────────┘   │ Emptying Study   │
                                                          └──────────────────┘

                                    Positive   Negative

                              ┌──────────────┐   Ⓕ If severe:
                              │ Symptomatic │   Referral to
                              │ Treatment   │   motility
                              └──────────────┘   center
                                                          Consider:
                                                            Exploratory
                                                            laparotomy

ANOREXIA

M. Angelo Trujillo

A. Anorexia (loss of appetite) often is clinically difficult to differentiate from weight loss without an effect of appetite. However, the diagnostic considerations and work-up usually are the same for both clinical problems. Perform a careful history and physical examination, including medication history, social history, and psychological screening examination. The causes of anorexia and weight loss may be divided into five major groups: (1) medical conditions, (2) psychological conditions, (3) social factors, (4) age-related factors, and (5) anorexia nervosa and related eating disorders.

B. A medication profile on patients with anorexia is of utmost importance because it can identify an easily treated cause. The medications listed are commonly associated with anorexia, especially in elderly patients.

C. Perform a head CT or MRI scan in patients who have anorexia with suspected CNS disease. Symptoms of visual disturbance, headaches, or signs of increased intracranial pressure (e.g., papilledema or cranial nerve involvement) should alert one to a potential CNS cause. Consider CNS tumors, especially hypothalamic tumors.

D. Several GI disorders can cause anorexia and/or weight loss. Malabsorption syndromes can mimic eating disorders (e.g., parasitic diseases, inflammatory bowel disease, celiac sprue, pancreatic insufficiency). Laboratory findings that can help differentiate organic disease from eating disorders are leukocytosis, steatorrhea, fever, hematochezia, and histologic or radiographic findings typical of certain GI disease states. Malignancy involving the GI tract can cause weight loss by several mechanisms: oral cavity pain or swallowing difficulty, esophageal obstruction or motility problems, gastric outlet obstruction, bowel obstruction, biliary disease, pancreatitis, and abdominal pain. Distant metastases of GI malignancies also can produce anorexia or weight loss by several mechanisms.

E. Social and cultural factors play an important role in the attitudes and behaviors of eating and body image. These factors are important components in the complex etiology of eating disorders. Other factors, such as difficulty with food acquisition and social isolation, can be important in some patients, especially the elderly.

F. Dementia and depression may cause significant weight loss. These are more commonly seen in the elderly and are important considerations because these disorders are potentially treatable. All cases of depression should be treated and reversible causes for dementia sought. Alcoholism is a common cause of anorexia or weight loss. Obtain a careful alcohol and drug abuse history in all cases.

G. Normal physiologic changes in the elderly may cause anorexia and weight loss. Hypogeusia (diminished sense of taste) and decreased olfactory function may result in food being less desirable. Visual and hearing problems may interfere with the usual mealtime socialization and may cause social isolation. Visual disorders and other physical disabilities may interfere with food preparation.

H. Anorexia nervosa and bulimia nervosa are eating disorders that affect 1–4% of women and are rarely found in men. These disorders usually are diagnosed in the second or third decades, but reports of diagnosis in older persons are increasing. Anorexia nervosa and bulimia nervosa result from complex interactions of physiologic, psychological, and sociocultural dysfunction. Diagnostic criteria for these eating disorders used by most authors are those found in the DSM-IV of the American Psychiatric Association. Patient history reveals intense fear of fatness, disturbed perception of body image, and an obsessional desire to lose weight. Patients with bulimia nervosa classically have binge eating commonly associated with self-induced vomiting, abuse of cathartics or diuretics, and fear of loss of control over eating. Treatment of these disorders is complex and should follow a team approach, with a primary care physician managing medical care and coordinating treatment by psychiatric/psychological and nutritional consultants. Many medical complications may result from eating disorders; treatment of these should have priority. See the chapter "Eating Disorders" for more detail.

References

Bo-Linn GW. Obesity, anorexia nervosa, bulimia, and other eating disorders. In: Sleisenger MH, Fordtran JS, eds. Gastrointestinal disease. 4th ed. Philadelphia: WB Saunders, 1989:173.

Comerci GD. Medical complications of anorexia nervosa and bulimia nervosa. Med Clin North Am 1990; 74:1293.

Morley JE. Anorexia in older patients: its meaning and management. Geriatrics 1990; 45:59.

Olsen-Noll EG, Bosworth MF. Anorexia and weight loss in the elderly. Postgrad Med 1989; 15:140.

Patient with ANOREXIA

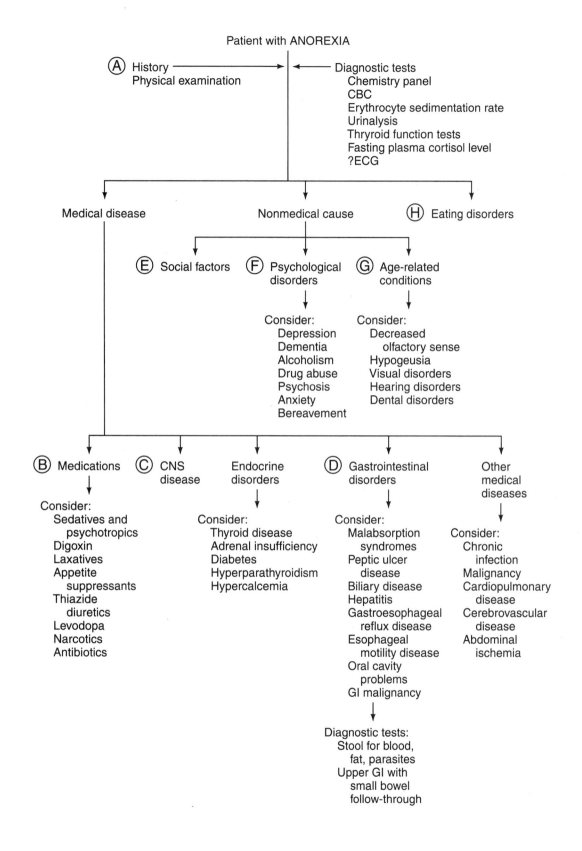

(A) History ——————→ ←——— Diagnostic tests
Physical examination   Chemistry panel
        CBC
        Erythrocyte sedimentation rate
        Urinalysis
        Thryroid function tests
        Fasting plasma cortisol level
        ?ECG

Medical disease   Nonmedical cause   (H) Eating disorders

(E) Social factors   (F) Psychological disorders   (G) Age-related conditions

Consider:
  Depression
  Dementia
  Alcoholism
  Drug abuse
  Psychosis
  Anxiety
  Bereavement

Consider:
  Decreased
    olfactory sense
  Hypogeusia
  Visual disorders
  Hearing disorders
  Dental disorders

(B) Medications   (C) CNS disease   Endocrine disorders   (D) Gastrointestinal disorders   Other medical diseases

Consider:
  Sedatives and
    psychotropics
  Digoxin
  Laxatives
  Appetite
    suppressants
  Thiazide
    diuretics
  Levodopa
  Narcotics
  Antibiotics

Consider:
  Thyroid disease
  Adrenal insufficiency
  Diabetes
  Hyperparathyroidism
  Hypercalcemia

Consider:
  Malabsorption
    syndromes
  Peptic ulcer
    disease
  Biliary disease
  Hepatitis
  Gastroesophageal
    reflux disease
  Esophageal
    motility disease
  Oral cavity
    problems
  GI malignancy

Consider:
  Chronic
    infection
  Malignancy
  Cardiopulmonary
    disease
  Cerebrovascular
    disease
  Abdominal
    ischemia

Diagnostic tests:
  Stool for blood,
    fat, parasites
  Upper GI with
    small bowel
    follow-through

DYSPHAGIA

Philip E. Jaffe

A. Dysphagia consists of a sense that there is impairment in the act of swallowing. It can result from (1) abnormalities in preparing and delivering the food bolus from the mouth to the esophagus (transfer dysphagia), (2) structural abnormalities of the esophagus (rings, webs, strictures, tumor masses, infection, or inflammation) or of adjacent structures (mediastinal masses or enlargement of the left atrium), or (3) motility abnormalities of the esophagus (achalasia, esophageal spasm, nutcracker esophagus, nonspecific motility disorders). Depending on the characteristics of the symptoms (dysphagia to solids, mechanical obstruction versus liquids, motility disorder), chronicity of complaints, and the patient's age, one may suspect a specific cause. However, esophagogastroduodenoscopy (EGD) should be performed in virtually all patients with this complaint. In rare cases when there is a compelling temporal relationship to a recent cerebrovascular accident (CVA) or progressive neurologic disease (amyotrophic lateral sclerosis, Parkinson's disease, myasthenia gravis) and a history suggestive of transfer dysphagia, or if the patient has scleroderma, the work-up may begin with barium esophagography. Because of the relative insensitivity of barium esophagography in detecting mucosal abnormalities, including early esophageal cancers, esophagoscopy is the preferred means of initial evaluation. This is especially true in immunocompromised patients in whom fungal or viral esophagitis is suspected.

B. When an etiology is determined on EGD, a specific treatment plan usually is undertaken. Dilate strictures, rings and webs using either rubber or plastic bougies or balloon catheters through an endoscope. Concurrent antireflux measures and antiacid treatment in the case of peptic strictures are imperative. Occasionally severe reflux disease may cause dysphagia without anatomic obstruction. There are many options in treating esophageal cancer, including dilation, chemotherapy, surgery, radiation therapy, laser, tumor probe, alcohol injection, and stenting. Their application depends on the extent and location of disease as well as the condition of the patient.

C. With a normal EGD, a motility disturbance of the esophagus should be suspected. Here again history usually is helpful, but esophageal manometry is needed to differentiate achalasia from the other motility disorders because the treatment differs radically. If the history suggests transfer dysphagia, cine or video esophagography should precede manometry. A barium esophagram with the use of barium-impregnated marshmallows or cookies may detect subtle strictures and/or rings missed by endoscopy.

D. Abnormalities in the preparation and passage of the food bolus from the tongue to the pharynx and then into the esophagus (transfer dysphagia) are most commonly seen with acute CVAs or progressive neurologic disorders (see section A). The dysfunction may slowly resolve over weeks after a CVA, and temporary nasogastric feeding supplementation may be necessary. In many cases the abnormality persists and endoscopic or surgical gastrostomy offers the best palliation. For patients who have progressive neurologic disorders with transfer dysphagia, referral to a speech pathologist who works with them to determine the optimal consistency of foods and ideal head and neck positioning to facilitate swallowing is useful. However, many patients ultimately require a gastrostomy.

E. Abnormalities in esophageal peristalsis and lower esophageal sphincter (LES) pressure and coordination with peristalsis are known as motility disorders. Measurement of the esophageal intraluminal pressures via manometry may define (1) achalasia—aperistalsis of the esophageal body and incomplete LES relations; (2) diffuse esophageal spasm—intermittent, simultaneous contraction in >10% of swallows; (3) nutcracker esophagus—high-amplitude esophageal contractions; and (4) nonspecific motility disorder—nontransmitted, triple-peaked or simultaneous contractions or low-amplitude contractions that do not fit into other defined disturbances. The association of chest pain with liquid dysphagia often suggests a motility disorder and is often a more disturbing symptom to the patient. The use of edrophonium during manometry may precipitate these symptoms and manometric findings. Treatment of achalasia usually requires fluoroscopically guided balloon dilation. Good results are seen in 60–95% of patients; the procedure is complicated by perforation in 2–4%. Surgical myotomy is now generally reserved for those who fail balloon dilation. Botulinum toxin injection into the LES has recently been shown to offer safe and effective short-term response and is growing in popularity. Other measures, including serial bougienage, nitrates, and calcium channel blockers, are effective but offer only temporary relief of symptoms. For patients with diffuse esophageal spasm, nutcracker esophagus, or nonspecific motility disorders, drugs that decrease esophageal contractility (nitrate or calcium channel blockers) may be of value.

F. If esophagoscopy and manometry are normal and symptoms persist, consider an extrinsic esophageal mass or adjacent structure partially obstructing the esophagus. In this case barium esophagography may be superior to esophagoscopy. Mediastinal tumors, left atrial enlargement, and osteophytes from cervical degenerative joint disease are the most common causes.

G. In a significant number of patients the evaluation yields no diagnosis. It is important to be sure the patient truly has dysphagia because some may misinterpret the sense that something is constantly stuck in the upper neck

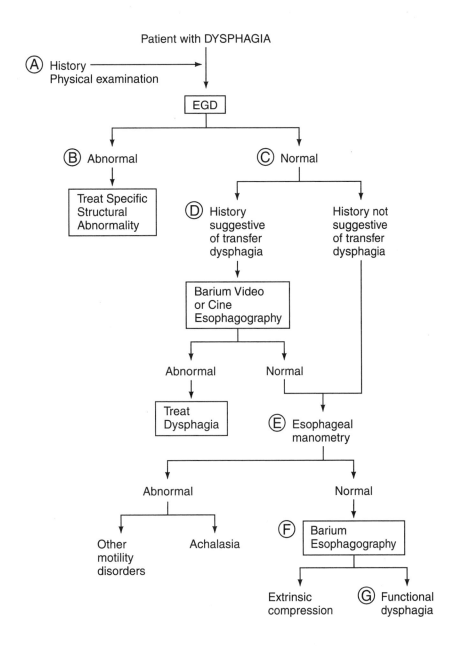

Patient with DYSPHAGIA

(A) History
Physical examination

EGD

(B) Abnormal → Treat Specific Structural Abnormality

(C) Normal

(D) History suggestive of transfer dysphagia

History not suggestive of transfer dysphagia

Barium Video or Cine Esophagography

Abnormal → Treat Dysphagia

Normal

(E) Esophageal manometry

Abnormal → Other motility disorders / Achalasia

Normal

(F) Barium Esophagography → Extrinsic compression / (G) Functional dysphagia

region ("globus") as dysphagia. In the remaining patients the symptoms may be related to emotional or psychiatric disorders or may be part of a more complex functional GI disorder (e.g., anorexia nervosa).

References

Bonavina L, DeMeester TR, McChesney L, et al. Drug-induced esophageal strictures. Ann Surg 1987; 206:173.

Clouse RE, Lustman PJ. Psychiatric illness and contraction abnormalities of the esophagus. N Engl J Med 1983; 309:1337.

Gelfand M, Botoman V. Esophageal motility disorders: a clinical overview. Am J Gastroenterol 1987; 82:181.

Patterson DJ, Graham DY, Smith JL, et al. Natural history of benign esophageal strictures treated by dilatation. Gastroenterology 1983; 85:346.

Rothstein R. A systematic approach to the patient with dysphagia. Hosp Pract (Off Ed) 1997; 32:169.

Trate D, Parkman H, Fisher R. Dysphagia: evaluation, diagnosis, and treatment. Prim Care 1996; 23:417.

Triadafilopoulous G. Nonobstructive dysphagia in reflux esophagitis. Am J Gastroenterol 1989; 84:614.

HEARTBURN

Richard E. Sampliner

A. Heartburn is the leading symptom of gastroesophageal reflux disease (GERD). It is a substernal sensation of burning that radiates orad and usually reflects the presence of acid in the esophagus.

B. Lifestyle modifications that can ameliorate the symptom of heartburn include losing weight, elevating the head of the bed, avoiding tight clothing around the waist, avoiding eating 3 hours before reclining, and avoiding foods and medications that decrease the lower esophageal sphincter pressure. When lifestyle modifications are accompanied by conventional dose twice-daily H_2-receptor antagonist (H_2RA) therapy, most patients have resolution of symptoms.

C. Step-down treatment indicates the need to define the lowest level of therapy that will provide symptom relief. This may include only lifestyle modifications or perhaps these plus a nocturnal dose of H_2RA.

D. The alarm symptoms and signs of GERD include dysphagia (difficulty swallowing), weight loss, and anemia. These findings warrant immediate endoscopy to look for complications that need prompt attention, such as esophageal stricture, esophageal ulcer, and cancer.

E. Upper GI endoscopy plays an essential role in the evaluation of patients with heartburn. It helps identify the subgroup of patients with erosive esophagitis who will ultimately develop the inflammatory complications of GERD. The 40–50% of patients with chronic reflux symptoms who have erosive esophagitis are subject to the complications of esophageal ulcer, esophageal stricture, and ultimately Barrett's esophagus—a metaplastic change in the esophageal epithelium that can proceed to adenocarcinoma of the esophagus.

F. In patients lacking endoscopic esophagitis in whom the diagnosis of GERD needs to be confirmed, the next step is 24-hour pH monitoring to document abnormal esophageal acid exposure.

G. More intensive medical therapy involves increasing the dosage of H_2RA, adding measures such as promotility agents or mucosal defense agents, or using a proton pump inhibitor.

H. Patients with erosive esophagitis commonly require maintenance with proton pump inhibitor therapy.

I. Surgery is a viable option for patients who either have failed medical therapy or choose surgery instead of a long-term medical regimen. The procedure of fundoplication has been standardized sufficiently and has a high enough success rate to be an acceptable therapeutic option. Laparoscopic fundoplication is now an effective approach.

References

Hetzel DJ, Dent J, Reed WD, et al. Healing and relapse of severe peptic esophagitis after treatment with omeprazole. Gastroenterology 1988; 95:903.

Pope CE 2nd. Acid-reflux disorders. N Engl J Med 1994; 331:656.

Richter JE, Castell DO. Gastroesophageal reflux: pathogenesis, diagnosis, and therapy. Ann Intern Med 1982; 97:93.

Schindlbeck NE, Heinrich C, Konig A, et al. Optimal thresholds, sensitivity, and specificity of long-term pH-metry for the detection of gastroesophageal reflux disease. Gastroenterology 1987; 93:85.

Sontag SJ. The medical management of reflux esophagitis: role of antacids and acid inhibition. Gastroenterol Clin North Am 1990; 19:683.

Weinberg DS, Kadish SL. The diagnosis and management of gastroesophageal reflux disease. Med Clin North Am 1996; 80:411.

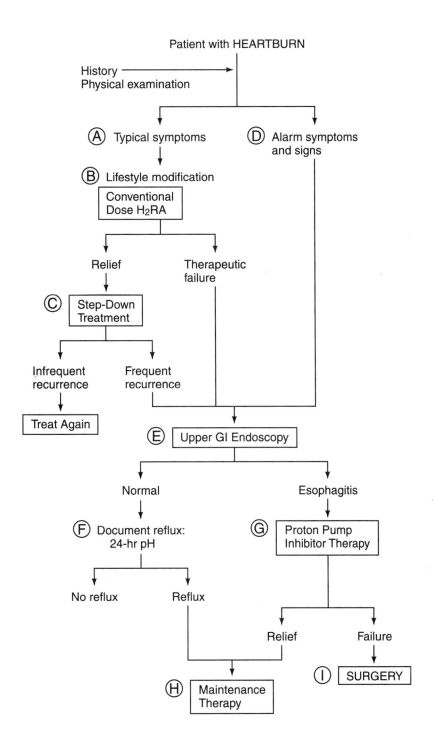

NONCARDIAC CHEST PAIN

M. Brian Fennerty

A. Chest pain causes anxiety because of the possibility of cardiac disease. Coronary disease should be excluded before investigating esophageal causes of chest pain. Although microvascular angina is possible with normal coronary arteries, this probably is unusual. More than 600,000 patients a year undergo cardiac catheterization, and one-third have normal coronary arteries. Thus, >150,000 patients per year may require evaluation for noncardiac chest pain. Esophageal disorders may cause cardiac-type chest pain in up to 50% of these patients. Associated symptoms of dysphagia, odynophagia, or heartburn are suggestive of an esophageal source but are often absent.

B. Endoscopy is used initially to exclude structural or mucosal abnormalities such as erosive esophagitis, esophageal strictures/tumors, achalasia, hiatal hernia, and gastric ulcers. Although the diagnostic yield is low, this remains an important test for excluding complicated esophageal disease.

C. Of patients with normal coronary arteries and cardiac chest pain, 35–50% have gastroesophageal reflux disease (GERD). This may or may not be manifested by erosive esophagitis. Therefore, a normal endoscopic result does not exclude reflux, and reflux may cause cardiac-type chest pain without symptoms of dysphagia or heartburn. In addition, acid perfusion of the esophagus not only lowers the threshold for myocardial ischemia but may induce this condition. The most sensitive test for documenting GERD is 24-hour ambulatory pH monitoring, which allows correlation of chest pain events with reflux events. Another commonly used "diagnostic" test is a 2- to 4-week therapeutic trial with a proton pump inhibitor (omeprazole or lansoprazole) at a high dosage. Resolution of chest pain implies that it was caused by acid (e.g., reflux), and appropriate therapy can then be prescribed. An etiologic association can be assumed if cardiac-type chest pain is temporally related to reflux. Unfortunately, pH monitoring is not widely available.

D. Motility disorders of the esophagus account for cardiac-type chest pain in 5–38% of patients evaluated in noncardiac chest pain series. Manometry measures the pressure and function of the lower esophageal sphincter and the motility of the esophageal body. Most motility abnormalities are intermittent and may be missed during manometry. In addition, the motility abnormality rarely is accompanied by chest pain during the study. Nutcracker esophagus is the most common motility disorder diagnosed in patients with chest pain (up to 30%), followed by nonspecific motility disorders (20–30%), diffuse esophageal spasm (5–10%), and achalasia (2–3%). Unless chest pain occurs with the observed motility disturbance, causation cannot be assumed.

E. If motility testing is nonspecific or nondiagnostic, provocative testing may be done. Provocative testing is based on the hypothesis that the esophagus is hypersensitive to normal or physiologic stimuli and that chest pain is simply an altered or heightened perception of these stimuli. Most patients with noncardiac chest pain have personality traits similar to those of patients with irritable bowel syndrome (i.e., they are anxious, depressed, hypochondriacal, and neurotic), and one-third meet diagnostic criteria for panic disorder. Provocative tests include perfusing the distal esophagus with acid (Bernstein test), IV infusion of a cholinergic agent (Tensilar), or inflation of a balloon in the esophagus (balloon distension). Reproduction of cardiac-type pain is diagnostic of an esophageal source of the pain.

References

Browning TH. Diagnosis of chest pain of esophageal origin: a guideline of the Patient Care Committee of the American Gastrointestinal Organization. Dig Dis Sci 1990; 35:289.

Cannon RO, Cattau LE, Yokshe PN, et al. Coronary flow reserve, esophageal motility, and chest pain in patients with angiographically normal coronary arteries. Am J Med 1990; 88:217.

Just RJ, Castell DO. Chest pain of undetermined origin. Gastrointest Endosc Clin N Am 1994; 4:731.

Katz PO, Dalton CB, Richter JE, et al. Esophageal testing of patients with noncardiac chest pain or dysphagia: results of three years' experience with 1161 patients. Ann Intern Med 1987; 106:593.

Lieberman D. Noncardiac chest pain: there's often an esophageal cause. Postgrad Med 1989; 86:207.

Richter JE, Bradley LA, Castell DO. Esophageal chest pain: current controversies in pathogenesis, diagnosis and therapy. Ann Intern Med 1989; 100:66.

Voskuil JH, Cramer MJ, Breumelhof R, et al. Prevalence of esophageal disorders in patients with chest pain newly referred to the cardiologist. Chest 1996; 109:1210.

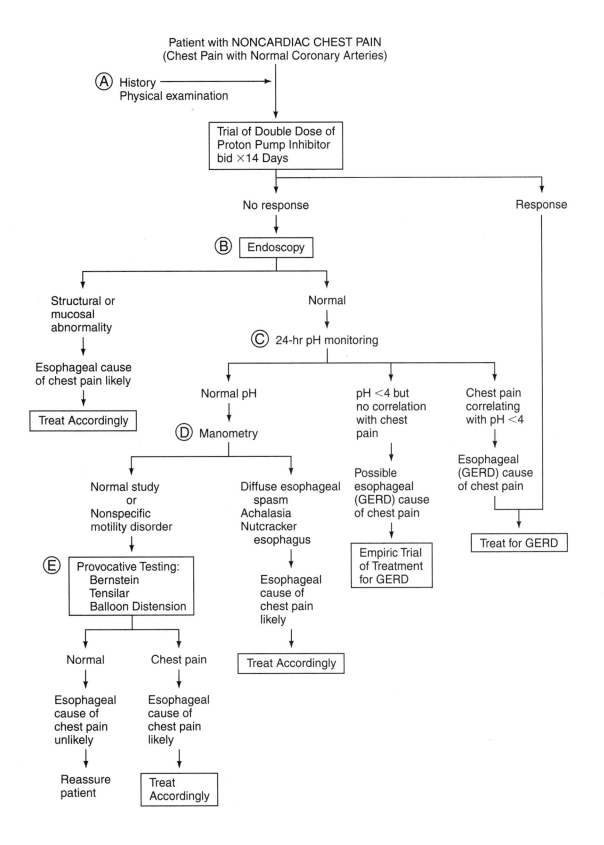

Patient with NONCARDIAC CHEST PAIN
(Chest Pain with Normal Coronary Arteries)

(A) History
Physical examination

Trial of Double Dose of
Proton Pump Inhibitor
bid ×14 Days

No response

Response

(B) Endoscopy

Structural or
mucosal
abnormality

Esophageal cause
of chest pain likely

Treat Accordingly

Normal

(C) 24-hr pH monitoring

Normal pH

(D) Manometry

Normal study
or
Nonspecific
motility disorder

(E) Provocative Testing:
Bernstein
Tensilar
Balloon Distension

Normal

Esophageal
cause of
chest pain
unlikely

Reassure
patient

Chest pain

Esophageal
cause of
chest pain
likely

Treat
Accordingly

Diffuse esophageal
spasm
Achalasia
Nutcracker
esophagus

Esophageal
cause of
chest pain
likely

Treat Accordingly

pH <4 but
no correlation
with chest
pain

Possible
esophageal
(GERD) cause
of chest pain

Empiric Trial
of Treatment
for GERD

Chest pain
correlating
with pH <4

Esophageal
(GERD) cause
of chest pain

Treat for GERD

BELCHING

Gregory L. Eastwood

A. *Belching, burping,* and *eructation* have roughly the same meaning and refer to the passage of gas from the stomach or esophagus through the mouth. In some patients, belching is the only symptom. In others, belching may be accompanied by abdominal discomfort, chest pain, or the passage of excess flatus. All people swallow air in variable amounts, and all people belch from time to time.

B. Most patients who complain of belching swallow excess amounts of air. In fact, they may unwittingly take air into the esophagus before each belch that then is eructated. This practice may be associated with psychological stress or is thought by some patients to relieve other abdominal symptoms. Some patients may improve simply by being made aware of the cause of belching and reassurance that they are otherwise well. Avoidance of gum chewing and carbonated beverages also is helpful.

C. Occasionally, belching is a sign of organic disease. If the gastric outlet is obstructed partially by peptic disease or carcinoma, swallowed air cannot pass into the bowel and eructation may develop, sometimes accompanied by abdominal pain and vomiting. For unexplained reasons, patients who have symptomatic gallstones may complain of belching. Finally, belching of feculent-smelling gas may indicate prolonged gastric stasis or a gastrocolic fistula that has developed from a carcinoma of the stomach or transverse colon.

D. Upper GI x-ray series or upper GI endoscopy are used to evaluate the stomach for partial gastric outlet obstruction and in rare cases may indicate a gastrocolic fistula complicating a gastric carcinoma. In general, because gastric outlet obstruction or a carcinoma that is large enough to erode into the colon is likely to be diagnosed by an upper GI x-ray series, that study is the appropriate first step in the diagnostic evaluation of belching. However, in some patients with peptic disease who have a small ulcer or have erosions and gastritis, the upper GI x-ray series may be nondiagnostic. In these patients, an upper GI endoscopy may be necessary to confirm the diagnosis.

E. The diagnosis of gallstones and gallbladder disease usually is made by ultrasonography of the upper abdomen. If ultrasound examination is nondiagnostic and the suspicion of gallbladder disease remains, a scan using technetium 99m-dimethylphenylcarbamylmethyl-iminodiacetic acid (HIDA) with determination of ejection fraction during stimulated gallbladder emptying may be indicated. Oral cholecystography is performed rarely.

F. Perform a barium enema if the patient belches foul-smelling gas and if the question of a gastrocolic fistula remains after a nondiagnostic upper GI x-ray series or endoscopy.

References

Eastwood GL, Avunduk C. Intestinal gas and bloating. In: Manual of gastroenterology. Diagnosis and therapy. 2nd ed. Boston: Little, Brown, 1994:221.

Perman JA, Montes RG. Approach to the patient with gas and bloating. In: Yamada T, ed. Textbook of gastroenterology. 2nd ed. Philadelphia: JB Lippincott, 1995:772.

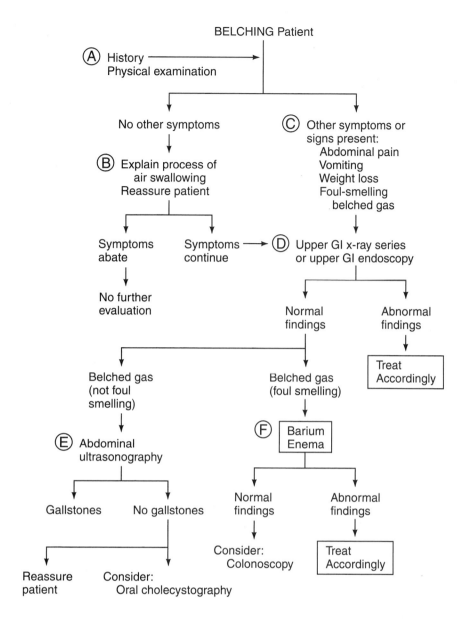

BELCHING Patient

Ⓐ History ──────────→
Physical examination

No other symptoms

Ⓒ Other symptoms or
signs present:
  Abdominal pain
  Vomiting
  Weight loss
  Foul-smelling
    belched gas

Ⓑ Explain process of
air swallowing
Reassure patient

Symptoms   Symptoms ──→ Ⓓ Upper GI x-ray series
abate   continue   or upper GI endoscopy

No further
evaluation

Normal   Abnormal
findings   findings

Treat
Accordingly

Belched gas   Belched gas
(not foul   (foul smelling)
smelling)

Ⓔ Abdominal   Ⓕ Barium
ultrasonography   Enema

Gallstones   No gallstones   Normal   Abnormal
                               findings   findings

Reassure   Consider: Consider: Treat
patient   Oral cholecystography Colonoscopy Accordingly

DYSPEPSIA

Lee J. Hixson

Dyspepsia may be defined as episodic or persistent upper abdominal symptoms, often related to eating, which are attributed to disorders of the proximal digestive tract. Symptoms may include upper abdominal discomfort, postprandial fullness, early satiety, anorexia, belching, bloating, and nausea with or without vomiting. Overall, ≤25% of dyspeptic patients harbor a peptic ulcer and <1% have cancer. In ≥50% of patients there remains no pathologic diagnosis after a complete evaluation describing functional, nonulcer, or essential dyspepsia.

A. Consider eosinophilic gastroenteritis, Crohn's disease, sarcoidosis, and infections (syphilis and mycobacteria). Much debate centers on whether *Helicobacter pylori* colonization may cause dyspepsia when not associated with ulceration. Recent evidence suggests screening for and treating *H. pylori* to at least benefit those with ulcers.

B. Functional dyspeptic symptoms often overlap with those of irritable bowel syndrome and are commonly associated with features suggestive of psychiatric disease. Historical risk factors suggesting an "organic" process include dysphagia, weight loss, GI bleeding, onset of symptoms after age 50, male sex, active smoking, previous ulcer history, pain that interrupts sleep, and vomiting.

C. Lactose intolerance secondary to acquired lactase deficiency may cause dyspepsia without diarrhea. Specific food allergy is rare.

D. Disruption of normal motility within the proximal GI tract may result in dysphagia, regurgitation, nausea, vomiting, and abdominal pain. Intrinsic disease of smooth muscle and the enteric and/or autonomic nervous systems, drug effect, metabolic and electrolyte derangements, and paraneoplastic syndromes may impair normal gut motility.

E. Examination should assess for GI blood loss, jaundice, an abdominal mass, presence of succussion splash over the stomach (suggestive of retained fluid), organomegaly, and signs of malabsorption.

F. Screening laboratory tests should include CBC, general (including liver) biochemistries, and amylase. Additional studies may include stool inspection with suspected malabsorption or parasitosis, abdominal radiography (for obstruction, mass effect, calcification), and ECG.

G. An empiric trial of *H. pylori* therapy for presumed peptic disease often is warranted before radiographic or endoscopic testing if the clinical scenario suggests an uncomplicated course. Response of symptoms to antisecretory therapy is not specific for peptic disease because functional dyspepsia or gastroesophageal reflux disease may also be ameliorated. Persistent symptoms after 3–4 weeks or recurrence after completion of therapy warrants a more aggressive diagnostic evaluation. Endoscopy is more sensitive than radiography in detecting a mucosal process and allows procurement of mucosal biopsies.

H. Perform manometry of the proximal GI tract by placing a multiport catheter connected with pressure transducers into the appropriate viscus lumen, and recording pressure fluctuation over time as a reflection of periodic peristaltic contractions. Dysmotility may be characterized by lack of or disorganized peristalsis, abnormal contraction configuration, and abnormal motor response to stimuli.

References

Axon AT. Chronic dyspepsia: who needs endoscopy? Gastroenterology 1997; 112:1376.

Ofman JJ, Erchason J, Fullerton S, et al. Management strategies for *Helicobacter pylori*-seropositive patients with dyspepsia: clinical and economic consequences. Ann Intern Med 1997; 126:280.

Talley NJ, Phillips SF. Non-ulcer dyspepsia: potential causes and pathophysiology. Ann Intern Med 1988; 108:865.

Talley NJ, Silverstein MD, Agreus L, et al. AGA technical review: evaluation of dyspepsia. Gastroenterology 1998; 114:582.

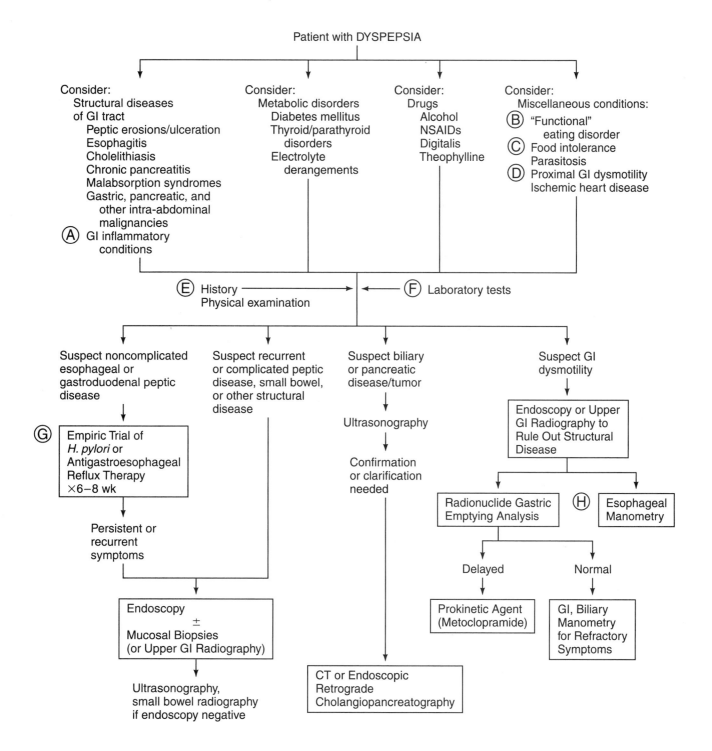

Patient with DYSPEPSIA

Consider:
Structural diseases
of GI tract
Peptic erosions/ulceration
Esophagitis
Cholelithiasis
Chronic pancreatitis
Malabsorption syndromes
Gastric, pancreatic, and
other intra-abdominal
malignancies
Ⓐ GI inflammatory
conditions

Consider:
Metabolic disorders
Diabetes mellitus
Thyroid/parathyroid
disorders
Electrolyte
derangements

Consider:
Drugs
Alcohol
NSAIDs
Digitalis
Theophylline

Consider:
Miscellaneous conditions:
Ⓑ "Functional"
eating disorder
Ⓒ Food intolerance
Parasitosis
Ⓓ Proximal GI dysmotility
Ischemic heart disease

Ⓔ History
Physical examination

Ⓕ Laboratory tests

Suspect noncomplicated
esophageal or
gastroduodenal peptic
disease

Suspect recurrent
or complicated peptic
disease, small bowel,
or other structural
disease

Suspect biliary
or pancreatic
disease/tumor

Ultrasonography

Confirmation
or clarification
needed

Suspect GI
dysmotility

Endoscopy or Upper
GI Radiography to
Rule Out Structural
Disease

Ⓖ Empiric Trial of
H. pylori or
Antigastroesophageal
Reflux Therapy
×6–8 wk

Persistent or
recurrent
symptoms

Radionuclide Gastric
Emptying Analysis

Ⓗ Esophageal
Manometry

Delayed

Normal

Endoscopy
±
Mucosal Biopsies
(or Upper GI Radiography)

Prokinetic Agent
(Metoclopramide)

GI, Biliary
Manometry
for Refractory
Symptoms

Ultrasonography,
small bowel radiography
if endoscopy negative

CT or Endoscopic
Retrograde
Cholangiopancreatography

JAUNDICE

Richard E. Sampliner

A. Clinical evaluation of jaundice consists of history, physical examination, and laboratory tests focused on highlighting medication exposures and diseases that may cause impaired bile flow. The diagnosis may be apparent in a patient taking a medication known to cause a cholestatic drug reaction. In contrast, some patients may have many factors that could lead to jaundice. A complete battery of liver tests, including aminotransferases, alkaline phosphatase, albumin, globulin, and prothrombin time, may point the way toward a clinical diagnosis. An "obstructive" pattern with elevated bilirubin, markedly elevated alkaline phosphatase, and moderately elevated aminotransferase levels may suggest obstruction but also can be seen with infiltrative liver disease. These overlapping patterns in laboratory tests necessitate a more elaborate work-up as detailed in the decision tree.

B. An inadequate ultrasound study may result from patient obesity or excess abdominal gas. It also is necessary to calibrate the local ultrasonography, because ultrasound is a more operator-dependent imaging technique than CT. If the ultrasound study is technically inadequate or equivocal, abdominal CT may help clarify the issue.

C. When the clinical evaluation suggests an intrahepatic process, the inciting agent (alcohol or a medication) should be discontinued. If within the next 2 weeks there is an appropriate resolution of laboratory abnormalities, the work-up may be complete. However, if there is no resolution, a liver biopsy is essential to define the cause of jaundice.

D. When extrahepatic obstruction is suspected on the basis of the clinical evaluation, and even if an imaging procedure reveals a nondilated biliary system, direct visualization of the common bile duct is essential. As many as 10% of patients in whom jaundice is diagnosed have a nondilated system despite documented extrahepatic obstruction.

E. Percutaneous transhepatic cholangiography (PTC) is used if endoscopic retrograde cholangiopancreatography (ERCP) has been unsuccessful in demonstrating the biliary tree. ERCP is the first procedure used because it affords an opportunity to visualize the pancreatic duct and has a lower risk in a patient with ascites or coagulopathy.

F. Therapy proceeds on the basis of the ductal abnormality defined by direct visualization. The former distinction of "medical" and "surgical" jaundice no longer exists. With the possibility of intervening by means of therapeutic endoscopy or therapeutic radiology, what was formerly possible only by surgery can now be accomplished by nonsurgical techniques. Malignant obstruction can be bypassed by placement of either a retrograde or a percutaneous stent. The common bile duct can be cleared of gallstones by means of retrograde sphincterotomy.

References

Bergman J, VanderMey S, Rauws E, et al. Long-term follow-up after endoscopic sphincterotomy for bile duct stones in patients younger than 60 years of age. Gastrointest Endosc 1996; 44:643.

Frank BV. Clinical evaluation of jaundice. JAMA 1989; 262:3031.

Hawes RH, Cotten PB, Vallon AG. Follow-up 6–11 years after duodenoscopic sphincterotomy for stones in patients with prior cholecystectomy. Gastroenterology 1990; 98:1008.

Lai EC, Mok TP, Tan ES, et al. Endoscopic biliary drainage for severe acute cholangitis. N Engl J Med 1992; 326:1582.

O'Connor KW, Snodgrass PJ, Swonder JE, et al. A blinded prospective study comparing four current non-invasive approaches in the differential diagnosis of medical vs. surgical jaundice. Gastroenterology 1983; 84:1498.

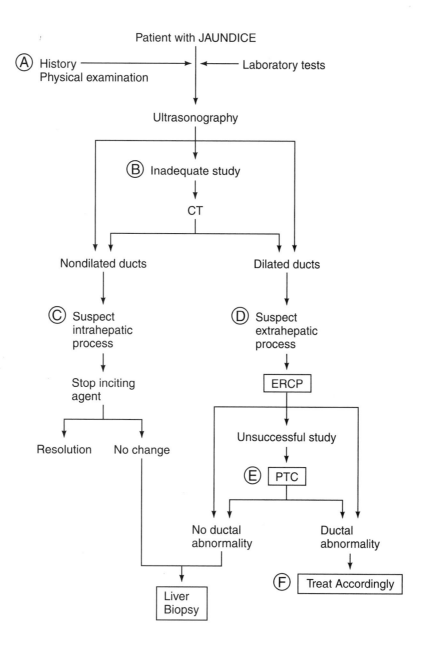

Patient with JAUNDICE

Ⓐ History ——————→   ←—————— Laboratory tests
Physical examination

Ultrasonography

Ⓑ Inadequate study

CT

Nondilated ducts   Dilated ducts

Ⓒ Suspect   Ⓓ Suspect
intrahepatic   extrahepatic
process   process

Stop inciting   ERCP
agent

Resolution   No change   Unsuccessful study

                                    Ⓔ PTC

                        No ductal   Ductal
                        abnormality   abnormality

                        Liver   Ⓕ Treat Accordingly
                        Biopsy

ASCITES

Richard E. Sampliner

A. Perform paracentesis in any patient with ascites. A good reason needs to be found *not* to perform a paracentesis. New ascites should be evaluated diagnostically to determine the cause. In a patient with decompensated liver disease who has been hospitalized with ascites, a paracentesis is essential to rule out spontaneous bacterial peritonitis. The database obtained at the time of paracentesis includes WBC count, differential, total protein, albumin, culture, sensitivity, and amylase. The serum-ascites albumin gradient should be calculated; that is, the albumin level in the ascites is subtracted from that in the serum.

B. When the serum albumin minus the ascites albumin is <1.1, this represents low-gradient ascites. This implies an exudative process from something other than just portal hypertension.

C. If a specific diagnosis is not evident after the results of culture and cytology, abdominal CT is appropriate to seek intra-abdominal malignancy or abscess. The final possible evaluation short of an exploratory laparotomy is laparoscopy, which can examine and sample the peritoneal and hepatic surfaces for potential malignant or infectious processes.

D. High-gradient ascites (serum albumin minus ascites albumin >1.1) indicates portal hypertension.

E. Once ascites due to portal hypertension has been established, therapy can be initiated. Its aggressiveness needs to be tempered by the patient's renal function, electrolyte balance, and level of encephalopathy. A stable patient can be treated vigorously with diuretics or large-volume paracentesis as long as careful daily monitoring is performed. Follow-up should include observation of weight, peripheral edema, mental status, volume compensation, electrolytes, and renal function.

F. An absolute polymorphonuclear (PMN) count >250 is the most sensitive rapid way of detecting spontaneous bacterial peritonitis. Because of the high frequency of spontaneous bacterial peritonitis in patients hospitalized with cirrhosis and ascites, it is essential to evaluate ascites and treat early with appropriate antibiotics.

G. The only way to recognize the pancreas as the source of ascites is to determine the amylase level. The ascitic amylase usually is a multiple of the serum amylase in a pancreatic process. Chronic pancreatic ascites may present clinically very similarly to decompensated liver disease.

References

Mauer K, Manzione NC. Usefulness of serum-ascites albumin difference in separating transudative from exudative ascites. Dig Dis Sci 1988; 33:1208.

Pockros PJ, Reynolds TB. Rapid diuresis in patients with ascites from chronic liver disease: the importance of peripheral edema. Gastroenterology 1986; 90:1827.

Quintero E, Gines P, Arroyo V, et al. Paracentesis vs. diuretics in the treatment of cirrhotics with tense ascites. Lancet 1985; i:611.

Runyan BA. Care of patients with ascites. N Engl J Med 1994; 330:337.

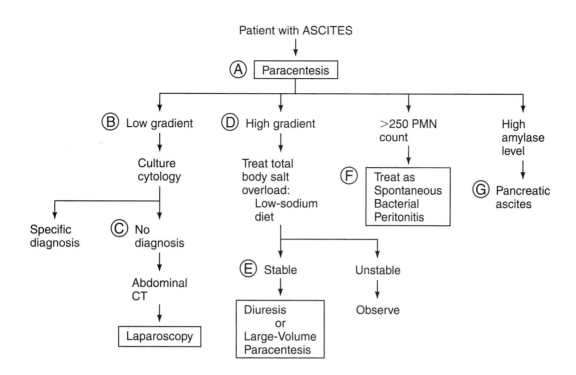

BILIARY COLIC

Philip E. Jaffe

Biliary colic is abdominal pain caused by sudden obstruction of the cystic or common bile duct (CBD). This generally occurs in the right upper quadrant (RUQ) or epigastrium, lasts 15 minutes to 4 hours, comes on suddenly, and may be severe, requiring narcotics for pain relief. Gallstone disease is by far the most common cause, although biliary parasites, clots, or tumor may cause a similar picture. The pain may be confused with peptic ulcer disease, pancreatitis, urinary calculi, diverticulitis, or functional bowel disease.

A. The initial history taking should attempt to elicit the location, duration, and character of pain as described above. Nausea and vomiting often are associated with pain. There usually is a history of less severe episodes. An association with fatty meals often is touted as a reliable sign but has not been proved. Murphy's sign (involuntary cessation of inspiration while the RUQ is being palpated secondary to pain) is seen commonly with cholecystitis but is not specific. RUQ tenderness is common, and peritoneal signs may be elicited with more severe attacks. The WBC count generally is normal or mildly elevated. Bilirubin or aminotransferase levels are mildly elevated in many patients but normal in nearly 60%. Evaluate serum amylase and urinalysis to exclude pancreatitis (with or without biliary disease) and nephrolithiasis.

B. Abdominal ultrasonography detects gallstones with about 95% sensitivity. It is less valuable in detecting CBD stones (15–25% sensitivity) and CBD reveals CBD dilation in about three fourths of patients with CBD obstruction. Other causes of abdominal pain that may mimic biliary colic (e.g., pancreatitis and nephrolithiasis) may also be detected.

C. Occasionally, patients with a history consistent with biliary colic but no gallstones on ultrasound study may be found to have gallstones on oral cholecystography. This technique, combined with administration of cholecystokinin, also gives information about the contractile function of the gallbladder. However, oral cholecystography has limited value in centers with high-quality ultrasonography.

D. The absence of gallstones should suggest another cause such as peptic ulcer disease, functional bowel disease, or sphincter of Oddi dysfunction. Upper GI endoscopy is a safe and reliable test to exclude ulcer disease and should be performed in the right clinical setting. If liver tests are abnormal, this may be bypassed and direct evaluation of the biliary tract with endoscopic retrograde cholangiopancreatography (ERCP) and/or biliary manometry performed.

E. A history compatible with biliary colic along with elevated bilirubin and/or alkaline phosphatase levels and no detectable gallbladder disease suggests possible CBD pathology. Perform ERCP in these patients to exclude choledocholithiasis, tumors, parasites, and biliary dyskinesia. Order delayed images of the bile ducts in patients in whom no anatomic obstruction is seen on ERCP. Persistence of contrast in the bile ducts at 45 minutes suggests sphincter of Oddi dysfunction, and sphincterotomy is warranted in the proper clinical setting. Biliary manometry, where available, is useful in defining specific sphincter of Oddi disorders that may be responsive to sphincterotomy.

F. When gallstones are detected on ultrasonography, consider CBD stones. Markedly elevated alkaline phosphatase and/or bilirubin levels or a dilated CBD are suggestive, and ERCP should be performed where available. Alternatively, if an open cholecystectomy is planned and the patient is a good surgical candidate, perform intraoperative cholangiography to evaluate this. If a laparoscopic cholecystectomy is planned and if choledocholithiasis is suspected, perform ERCP preoperatively. In centers where highly experienced biliary endoscopists are available and laparoscopic cholecystectomy is planned, consider proceeding with laparoscopic cholecystectomy and intraoperative cholangiography. If choledocholithiasis is found, the patient can undergo postoperative ERCP with stone extraction.

G. If there is nothing to suggest CBD pathology, treatment should be aimed at removing the gallbladder stones. In otherwise healthy patients, cholecystectomy (either open or laparoscopic) is now a relatively safe procedure. In the elderly or infirm, alternatives include oral dissolution therapy, shock wave lithotripsy, or the use of direct dissolution agents (e.g., methyl-tert-butyl ether) in centers where these techniques are available. Of patients who have undergone sphincterotomy for removal of CBD stones and who have cholelithiasis, about 10% go on to require cholecystectomy for subsequent cholecystitis. Therefore, for patients in this unique situation who have multiple comorbid conditions that may limit their life expectancy and increase the hazards of cholecystectomy, observation without cholecystectomy or gallstone dissolution is a reasonable alternative.

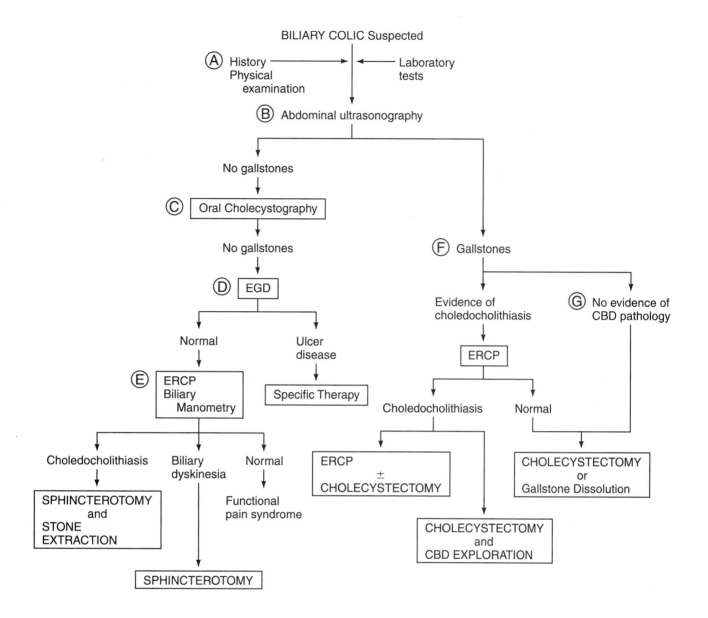

References

Anclaux M, et al. Prospective study of clinical and biological features of symptomatic choledocholithiasis. Dig Dis Sci 1986; 31:449.

Davidson B, et al. Endoscopic sphincterotomy for common bile duct calculi in patients with gall bladders in situ considered unfit for surgery. Gut 1988; 29:114.

Einstein D, et al. Insensitivity of sonography in the detection of choledocholithiasis. AJR Am J Roentgenol 1984; 142:725.

Geenen J, et al. The efficacy of endoscopic sphincterotomy after cholecystectomy in patients with sphincter of Oddi dysfunction. N Engl J Med 1989; 320:82.

Jaffe P. Gallstones. Who are good candidates for nonsurgical treatment? Postgrad Med 1993; 94:45.

Marton K, Doubilet P. How to image the gallbladder in suspected cholecystitis. Ann Intern Med 1988; 109:722.

Patankar R, Ozmen N, Bailey I, Johnson C. Gallbladder motility, gallstones, and the surgeon. Dig Dis Sci 1995; 40:2323.

GASTROINTESTINAL BLEEDING

Gregory L. Eastwood

The principles of acute management of active GI bleeding are the same in almost all patients, although diagnostic tests vary depending on the presumed site of bleeding (Table 1). In an emergency (i.e., active bleeding), the usual orderly sequence of history taking, physical examination, diagnostic evaluation, and treatment is altered to meet immediate demands. In patients who are acutely ill, prompt resuscitative measures may be necessary.

A. Melena, or black stool, may develop with as little as 50 ml of blood loss per day. Although melena usually signifies bleeding from the upper GI tract, it can result from a source as low as the proximal colon. Brisker rates of bleeding may appear as red blood per rectum (hematochezia) or vomiting of blood (hematemesis). Hematemesis of either frank red blood or "coffee-ground" material usually signifies an upper GI tract source but can result from swallowed blood from the respiratory tract. Hematochezia usually is a sign of lower GI tract bleeding, although it may result from profuse upper GI bleeding (e.g., from esophageal varices or an eroded artery in the base of an ulcer).

Advanced age worsens the prognosis. The patient's age also makes some diagnoses more or less likely. The differential diagnosis of acute lower GI bleeding in patients >60 years of age includes ischemic colitis, colon carcinoma, arteriovenous malformation, and diverticulosis; none of these is a serious consideration in a 25-year-old patient. Bleeding from inflammatory bowel disease or a Meckel's diverticulum is more likely in a child or young adult.

Recent ingestion of aspirin, other NSAIDs, or alcohol predisposes patients to gastric mucosal injury. Aspirin also interferes with platelet adhesion, so bleeding lesions in patients who take aspirin are less likely to clot.

The number of associated medical conditions is directly related to increasing risk of death in acute GI bleeding. Patients with liver disease are at risk for esophageal varices. Although upper GI bleeding in patients with esophageal varices is most likely to be from the varices, other sources must be considered.

Bleeding from a Mallory-Weiss mucosal tear at the esophagogastric junction traditionally is associated with repeated vomiting or retching before the onset of hematemesis. However, such a history is obtained in fewer than one third of patients. The diagnosis must be made by endoscopy. Patients with an aortoenteric fistula typically have massive hematemesis or hematochezia. The bleeding may stop abruptly; if it recurs, it often is fatal. Most fistulas occur in patients who have had aortic grafts, developing between the graft on the aorta and the adjacent portion of the GI tract. They also may develop between unoperated aneurysms and the GI tract. Promptly arrange upper endoscopy for any older patient with massive GI bleeding that stops abruptly, particularly if there is a history of aneurysm or aneurysm repair. Endoscopy rarely identifies the fistula, but if it identifies no other source of bleeding, consider emergency surgery.

CT of the abdomen may show a leaking aneurysm or fistula and thus helps in the decision of whether to operate. Nonocclusive ischemic vascular disease of the bowel typically occurs in patients >60 years of age who have a cardiovascular condition (e.g., congestive heart failure, arrhythmia) that predisposes them to a transient reduction in bowel perfusion. Also, aortic aneurysm repair places a patient at risk for ischemic colitis because of interruption of inferior mesenteric artery blood flow in the absence of adequate collateral circulation. Patients with ischemic colitis characteristically have an abrupt onset of moderate lower abdominal pain with bloody stool. In most patients the course is self-limited, with spontaneous recovery in several days. A few patients develop bowel infarction and peritonitis and require surgical intervention.

GI bleeding may develop from the acute effects of irradiation on the gut or may occur months to years after irradiation. The latter is a form of ischemic colitis that is accelerated by the perivascular inflammation that results from the effects of irradiation.

B. Cardiac output and BP fall and pulse rate increases in response to acute blood loss. Under conditions of severe volume loss, postural compensation of BP and pulse are inadequate. If pulse rate increases >20 beats/min and systolic BP drops >10 mm Hg when the patient stands,

TABLE 1 Diagnostic Considerations in GI Bleeding

Upper GI Bleeding	Lower GI Bleeding
Nose or pharyngeal bleeding	Hemorrhoids
Hemoptysis	Anal fissure
Esophageal rupture (Boerhaave's syndrome)	Inflammatory bowel disease (Crohn's disease, ulcerative colitis)
Esophagogastric mucosal tear (Mallory-Weiss syndrome)	Neoplasm (carcinoma or polyps)
Inflammation and erosions (esophagitis, gastritis, duodenitis)	Ischemic enteritis or colitis
Peptic ulcer of esophagus, stomach, or duodenum or surgical anastomosis	Angiodysplasia
	Diverticulosis
Dieulafoy's lesion (ruptured mucosal artery)	Antibiotic-associated colitis
Varices of esophagus, stomach, or duodenum	Radiation colitis
	Amyloidosis
Neoplasm (carcinoma, lymphoma, leiomyosarcoma, polyps)	Meckel's diverticulum
	Vascular-enteric fistula
Hemobilia	Brisk bleeding from an upper GI source
Vascular-enteric fistula (usually from aortic aneurysm or graft)	

(Continued on page 180)

Patient with GASTROINTESTINAL BLEEDING

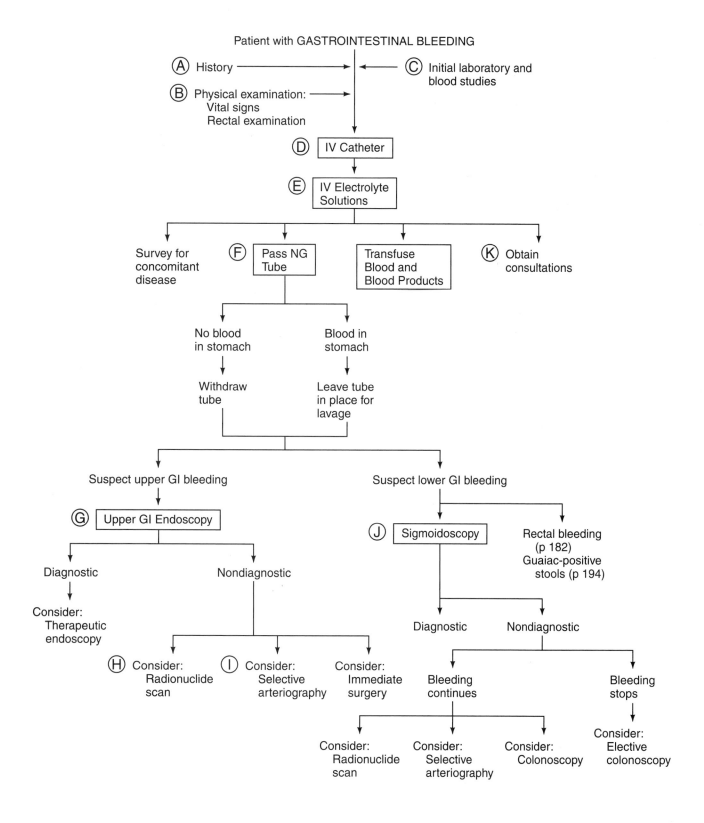

Ⓐ History

Ⓒ Initial laboratory and blood studies

Ⓑ Physical examination:
Vital signs
Rectal examination

Ⓓ IV Catheter

Ⓔ IV Electrolyte Solutions

Survey for concomitant disease

Ⓕ Pass NG Tube

Transfuse Blood and Blood Products

Ⓚ Obtain consultations

No blood in stomach

Blood in stomach

Withdraw tube

Leave tube in place for lavage

Suspect upper GI bleeding

Suspect lower GI bleeding

Ⓖ Upper GI Endoscopy

Ⓙ Sigmoidoscopy

Rectal bleeding (p 182)
Guaiac-positive stools (p 194)

Diagnostic

Nondiagnostic

Diagnostic

Nondiagnostic

Consider: Therapeutic endoscopy

Ⓗ Consider: Radionuclide scan

Ⓘ Consider: Selective arteriography

Consider: Immediate surgery

Bleeding continues

Bleeding stops

Consider: Radionuclide scan

Consider: Selective arteriography

Consider: Colonoscopy

Consider: Elective colonoscopy

blood loss is probably >1 L. However, age, cardiovascular status, and rate of blood loss influence the development of these postural signs. Blood loss and peripheral vasoconstriction may result in coolness of the extremities and pallor of the conjunctivae, mucous membranes, nailbeds, and palmar creases. Rectal examination provides direct access to the GI tract and should not be omitted, even when upper GI bleeding appears obvious. As indicated, red blood per rectum usually signifies lower GI bleeding, whereas melena may indicate an upper GI source. If the patient has vomited blood or coffee-ground material yet the stool is brown or even negative for occult blood, the bleeding may have been brief. Occult blood in the stool can be detected with as little as 15 ml of blood loss per day. Stools may remain positive for occult blood for nearly 2 weeks after an acute loss of ≥1000 ml of blood from an upper GI source.

C. Initial laboratory studies should include CBC, electrolytes, BUN, creatinine, glucose, calcium, phosphate, magnesium, and blood typing. Blood gases should be monitored in severely ill patients. Hemoglobin and hematocrit usually are low and may be related to blood loss. However, some patients bleed so rapidly that the blood volume has insufficient time to equilibrate, and hemoglobin and hematocrit are normal or only slightly reduced. In acutely bleeding patients, changes in BP and pulse and direct evidence of continued bleeding via nasogastric (NG) tube or per rectum are better indicators of the need to administer electrolyte solutions and replace blood. Assess clotting status by means of platelet count, prothrombin time, and partial thromboplastin time. Prompt correction of any clotting defect is crucial. Extensive blood transfusion dilutes platelets and clotting factors, especially factors V and VII. This can be treated by infusion of platelets and fresh frozen plasma as needed. Many patients who bleed while taking therapeutic anticoagulants do so from a clinically significant lesion. Therefore, it is important to evaluate these patients for GI pathology in addition to correcting the clotting status. An elevation in WBC count can be associated with acute GI bleeding but usually is not >15,000/mm^3. Do not attribute leukocytosis to acute blood loss without first considering sources of infection. Elevated BUN in a patient whose BUN has recently been normal or whose creatinine is normal suggests an upper GI source if the site of bleeding is not initially apparent. The rise in BUN can result from digestion of blood in the small intestine and absorption of nitrogenous products. However, hypovolemia from acute blood loss of either upper or lower GI origin also can raise BUN. In patients with marginal liver function, the increased protein load from blood in the gut may induce or aggravate hepatic encephalopathy. Therefore, gastric lavage and control of bleeding are of particular importance in these patients.

D. Promptly insert a large-bore IV catheter into a peripheral vein. In a profusely bleeding patient, two or more IV catheters may be needed to provide adequate blood replacement. In an acute emergency in which a peripheral vein is not available, establish venous access via a jugular, subclavian, or femoral vein. A central venous pressure or Swan-Ganz catheter may be needed to evaluate the effects of volume replacement and the need for continued infusion of blood, particularly in elderly patients or those with cardiovascular disease.

E. Rapidly infuse normal saline until blood is available for transfusion. In actively bleeding patients who have excess body sodium (e.g., those with ascites or peripheral edema), restoration of hemodynamic stability should take precedence over other considerations. Therefore, if blood is not yet available for transfusion, infuse saline without regard to the sodium balance. If bleeding is less severe, infuse hypotonic sodium solutions until blood arrives.

F. Pass an NG tube in patients with a history of melena or hematemesis. Blood from an esophageal or gastric source will pool in the stomach, and in >90% of bleeding duodenal ulcers, the blood refluxes back across the pyloric channel into the stomach. If the aspirate is clear or clears promptly with lavage, the NG tube may be removed. If there is a large amount of blood or retained material, lavage the stomach with a large-bore sump tube (20–24 Fr). Removal of gastric contents facilitates subsequent endoscopy and decompresses the stomach. Because the NG tube is uncomfortable for the patient, predisposes him or her to gastroesophageal reflux and pulmonary aspiration, and may irritate the esophageal and gastric mucosa, remove it when it is no longer fulfilling a purpose.

G. Endoscopic diagnosis of a specific bleeding site may dictate a specific treatment regimen. Furthermore, identification of the so-called stigmata of recent hemorrhage (SRH) within an ulcer crater has prognostic and therapeutic implications. SRH include a protruding visible vessel, an adherent clot, a black eschar, and actual oozing or spurting of blood. Patients with SRH are more likely to have uncontrolled or recurrent bleeding and to require therapeutic endoscopy or surgery. The treatment of bleeding lesions through the endoscope has become widely available through a variety of methods, including thermal electrocoagulation, laser photocoagulation, injection of ethanol or hypertonic solutions, and injection sclerosis of esophageal varices.

H. Scanning the abdomen after IV injection of sulfur colloid or ^{99}Tc-labeled RBCs may indicate the bleeding site. A positive scan may lead to more definitive diagnostic or therapeutic procedures. The radionuclide scan appears to be more sensitive than selective arteriography in detecting active bleeding because a positive scan requires a lower rate of bleeding (0.1 ml/min vs. 0.5–1.0 ml/min). However, the radionuclide scan is less specific than arteriography in locating the site of bleeding.

I. Selective arteriography of the celiac axis, the superior or inferior mesenteric artery, or their branches can be diagnostic and therapeutic. A focal extravasation of dye usually indicates an arterial bleeding source. A diffuse blush in the stomach area may be found in hemorrhagic gastritis. During the venous phase of the study, esophageal, gastric, or intestinal varices may be seen, although actual variceal bleeding cannot be detected. Angiodysplastic lesions and vascular tumors can be suspected by their angiographic appearance. Bleeding from arterial lesions may be controlled by injecting autologous clot or small pieces of gel foam. Variceal bleeding has been treated by infusion of vasopressin, 0.1–0.5 U/min, into the superior mesenteric artery to diminish mesenteric blood flow and reduce portal venous pressure. Venous infusion of nitroglycerin should be given simultaneously with vasopressin in patients at risk for ischemic cardiovascular disease.

J. Sigmoidoscopy using either a rigid or flexible instrument should be performed early in the evaluation of acute lower GI bleeding. The role of emergency colonoscopy is somewhat controversial because the diagnostic value of the procedure is limited by blood and stool. Cleanse the colon with osmotically balanced electrolyte solution, administered orally or by NG tube; this enhances the diagnostic capability of colonoscopy.

K. The management of acute GI bleeding involves a team of health care workers. Specific diagnostic studies usually require the skills of a gastroenterologist or a radiologist. The surgeon, when consulted early, may offer valuable assistance in managing the patient and is in a better position to make a decision regarding operative intervention should the need arise later.

References

Bornman PC, Theodorou NA, Shuttleworth RD, et al. Importance of hypovolaemic shock and endoscopic signs in predicting recurrent haemorrhage from peptic ulceration: a prospective evaluation. BMJ 1985; 291:245.

Jiranek GC, Kozarek RA. A cost-effective approach to the patient with peptic ulcer bleeding. Surg Clin North Am 1996; 76:83.

Jutabha R, Jensen DM. Management of upper gastrointestinal bleeding in the patient with chronic liver disease. Med Clin North Am 1996; 80:1035.

Navarro VJ, Garcia-Tsao G. Variceal hemorrhage. Crit Care Clin 1995; 11:391.

Savides TJ, Jensen DM. Endoscopic therapy for severe gastrointestinal bleeding. Adv Intern Med 1995; 40:243.

Steer ML, Silen W. Diagnostic procedures in gastrointestinal hemorrhage. N Engl J Med 1983; 309:646.

Steffes BC, O'Leary JP. Primary aortoduodenal fistula: a case report and review of the literature. Am Surg 1980; 46:121.

Talbot-Stern JK. Gastrointestinal bleeding. Emerg Med Clin North Am 1996; 14:173.

Wara P. Endoscopic prediction of major rebleeding. A prospective study of stigmata of hemorrhage in bleeding ulcer. Gastroenterology 1985; 88:1209.

RECTAL BLEEDING

Steven Palley

Visible blood per rectum is called *hematochezia*. It can present as blood on toilet tissue, blood-streaked stool, bright red blood, or maroon liquid stool.

A. The primary assessment determines bleeding severity. Rapid blood loss is suggested by hemodynamic alterations. Resting tachycardia (rate >100) or systolic hypotension (systolic blood pressure <100) suggest a 20–30% decrease in blood volume. Orthostatic hypotension suggests a 10–20% decrease. Hematocrit determination is misleading in the face of acute bleeding. Significant history includes peptic ulcer disease, vascular grafts, inflammatory bowel disease, weight loss or change of stool caliber, hemorrhoidal disease, or acute diarrheal illness. Physical examination may disclose an abdominal or rectal mass or hemorrhoids. Always perform anoscopy with the initial assessment.

B. In the absence of evidence of severe bleeding, the work-up can proceed electively. If there is a history of hematochezia but no active bleeding, further evaluation is influenced by the risk of colorectal carcinoma. A patient <40 years of age without a family history of colorectal carcinoma, previous colorectal neoplasm, or long-standing ulcerative colitis should undergo sigmoidoscopy and possibly air-contrast barium enema if negative. Older patients should undergo colonoscopy.

C. A patient with evidence of active bleeding should undergo urgent sigmoidoscopy in an attempt to identify the bleeding source while it is still active. Distal lesions such as anorectal disease (hemorrhoids, anal fissure), left-sided neoplasia, rectal ulceration, ulcerative proctitis, or infectious colitis can be visualized. Identification of an active bleeding site precludes need for further evaluation. If no active bleeding site is noted, prepare the patient for colonoscopy. A negative colonoscopic examination may lead to further evaluation depending on bleeding severity.

D. The differential diagnosis for severe rectal bleeding is similar to that for milder bleeding. However, upper GI sources must be included and can account for about 10% of severe hematochezia. The distribution of diagnoses varies with the method of evaluation in various series. In a colonoscopic series, bleeding angiodysplasia was diagnosed in 30%, diverticular bleeding in 17%, and neoplasm in 11%.

E. Patients thought to have severe bleeding should be resuscitated in an ICU. Adequate IV access is essential. Place a nasogastric tube, and perform aspiration in all patients. Further evaluation depends on patient stability. The rare patient who cannot be stabilized should be rushed for emergent laparotomy. If the situation permits, perform preoperative or intraoperative angiography.

F. Patients who can be stabilized should undergo a limited sigmoidoscopy with retroflexion examinations of the anorectal region. If these are negative, the patient should receive a rapid bowel prep (purge) and then undergo colonoscopy. In most instances upper endoscopy should precede colonoscopy. If the bleeding obscures the field or if colonoscopy is negative, perform a tagged RBC scan, with angiography if positive.

G. A negative evaluation may be followed with small bowel enteroclysis study. Although its yield is small, it can be as high as 20% if it follows adequate upper and lower GI evaluation.

H. Finally, if all previous evaluation is nondiagnostic and the patient has repeated episodes of severe hematochezia, consider provocative testing. Administer anticoagulants, thrombolytics, or vasodilators, with angiographic and surgical backup, to encourage bleeding with immediate diagnosis and treatment.

References

Helfand M, Marton KI, Zimmer-Gembeck MJ, Sox HC Jr. History of visible rectal bleeding in a primary care population: initial assessment and 10-year follow-up. JAMA 1997; 277:44.

Jensen DM, Machicado GA. Diagnosis and treatment of severe hematochezia. Gastroenterology 1988; 95:1569.

Koval G, Benner KG, Rösch J, Kozak BE. Aggressive angiographic diagnosis in acute lower gastrointestinal hemorrhage. Dig Dis Sci 1987; 32:248.

Rex DK, Lappas JC, Maglinte DD, et al. Enteroclysis in the evaluation of suspected small intestinal bleeding. Gastroenterology 1989; 97:58.

Schrock TR. Colonoscopic diagnosis and treatment of lower gastrointestinal bleeding. Surg Clin North Am 1989; 69:1309.

Patient with RECTAL BLEEDING

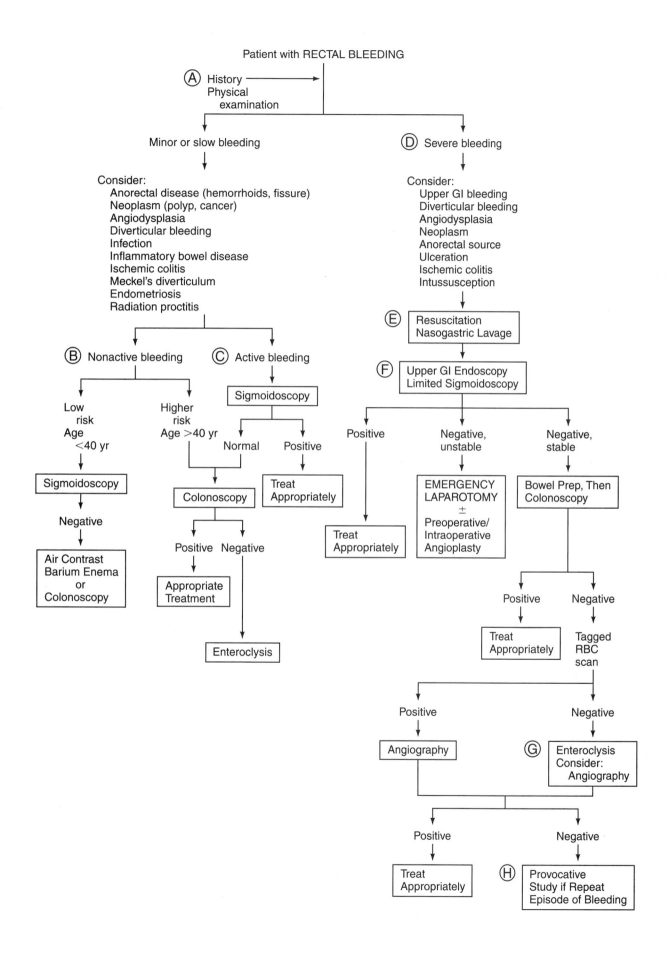

Ⓐ History ⟶
Physical
examination

Minor or slow bleeding

Consider:
    Anorectal disease (hemorrhoids, fissure)
    Neoplasm (polyp, cancer)
    Angiodysplasia
    Diverticular bleeding
    Infection
    Inflammatory bowel disease
    Ischemic colitis
    Meckel's diverticulum
    Endometriosis
    Radiation proctitis

Ⓑ Nonactive bleeding   Ⓒ Active bleeding

Low risk Age <40 yr   Higher risk Age >40 yr

Sigmoidoscopy

Sigmoidoscopy   Normal   Positive

Negative

Air Contrast Barium Enema or Colonoscopy

Colonoscopy

Treat Appropriately

Positive   Negative

Appropriate Treatment

Enteroclysis

Ⓓ **Severe bleeding**

Consider:
    Upper GI bleeding
    Diverticular bleeding
    Angiodysplasia
    Neoplasm
    Anorectal source
    Ulceration
    Ischemic colitis
    Intussusception

Ⓔ Resuscitation Nasogastric Lavage

Ⓕ Upper GI Endoscopy Limited Sigmoidoscopy

Positive   Negative, unstable   Negative, stable

Treat Appropriately

EMERGENCY LAPAROTOMY ± Preoperative/ Intraoperative Angioplasty

Bowel Prep, Then Colonoscopy

Positive   Negative

Treat Appropriately   Tagged RBC scan

Positive   Negative

Angiography   Ⓖ Enteroclysis Consider: Angiography

Positive   Negative

Treat Appropriately   Ⓗ Provocative Study if Repeat Episode of Bleeding

ACUTE DIARRHEA

M. Brian Fennerty

A. Diarrhea is one of the most common complaints resulting in visits to a physician. The history and physical (including rectal examination) are critical in determining who needs further diagnostic evaluation and in selecting appropriate therapy. Important questions to ask are duration of illness, volume of stool, presence of blood or pus in stool, and symptoms of systemic illness such as fever, anorexia, weight loss, and volume depletion. Most patients should not undergo further evaluation at this time but be treated symptomatically. However, the presence of systemic symptoms dictates that the stool be more closely evaluated for evidence of invasive infection or inflammatory bowel disease (IBD).

B. The simplest test that can be performed in the office to evaluate inflammatory changes of the bowel mucosa is to inspect by microscopy a fecal sample for WBCs/RBCs. The presence of either of these implies infection with invasive organisms and/or IBD.

C. To evaluate infection by an invasive bacterial organism, a stool culture is necessary. Most clinical laboratories routinely test for *Shigella, Salmonella,* and *Campylobacter* spp. If travel or other historical features suggest other pathogens, more specific testing for *Amoeba, Yersinia* spp., or *Clostridium difficile,* and others may be necessary. In certain clinical situations, testing for *Escherichia coli* may be prudent. In patients with HIV disease, testing for unusual pathogens (e.g., cryptosporidia, mycobacteria) may be necessary.

D. In patients who have WBCs/RBCs in the stool and a negative culture, or those without inflammatory cells but continued diarrhea, perform flexible sigmoidoscopy to evaluate for IBD, which may be present even if the mucosa is grossly normal appearing. Therefore, a biopsy is helpful in detecting minimal mucosal changes. In addition, the histologic appearance in the setting of gross inflammatory changes can help differentiate acute infectious self-limited colitis from IBD. Generally perform a biopsy irrespective of gross findings.

E. In patients with negative cultures and sigmoidoscopy but continued diarrhea, further evaluation may be required.

References

Fedorak R. Antidiarrheal therapy. Dig Dis Sci 1987; 32:195.
Harris JC, DuPont HL, Hornick RB. Fecal leukocytes in diarrheal illness. Ann Intern Med 1972; 76:697.
Plotkin G. Gastroenteritis: etiology, pathophysiology and clinical manifestations. Medicine 1979; 58:95.
Slutsker L, Ries AA, Greene KD, et al. *Escherichia coli* O157:H7 diarrhea in the United States: clinical and epidemiologic features. Ann Intern Med 1997; 126:505.

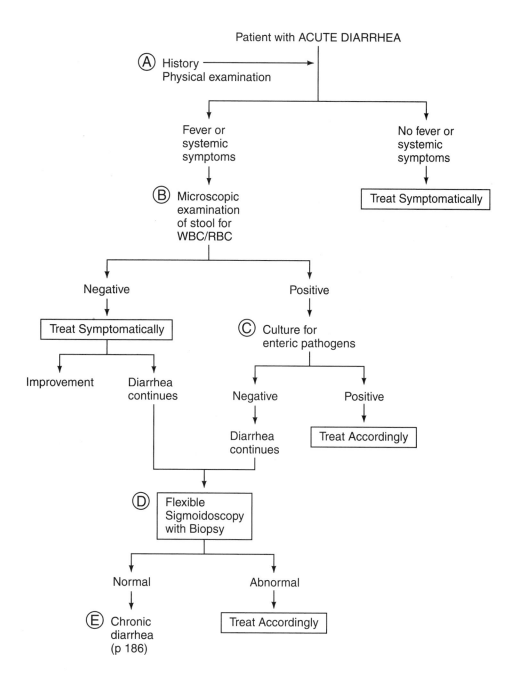

Patient with ACUTE DIARRHEA

(A) History
Physical examination

Fever or systemic symptoms

No fever or systemic symptoms

Treat Symptomatically

(B) Microscopic examination of stool for WBC/RBC

Negative

Treat Symptomatically

Improvement

Diarrhea continues

Positive

(C) Culture for enteric pathogens

Negative

Diarrhea continues

Positive

Treat Accordingly

(D) Flexible Sigmoidoscopy with Biopsy

Normal

(E) Chronic diarrhea (p 186)

Abnormal

Treat Accordingly

CHRONIC DIARRHEA

Lee J. Hixson

Diarrhea is an increase in stool weight and liquidity. Normal stool weight for a western diet is <200 g/day. Chronicity is diarrhea lasting >3 weeks.

A. Most intestinal bacterial infections resolve spontaneously within 1–2 weeks, although symptoms occasionally persist for 2–3 months. Giardiasis and amebiasis may result in chronic symptoms, as can most helminthic infestations. Infectious diarrhea in the setting of AIDS is most commonly secondary to usual enteric pathogens but also includes cryptosporidosis, microsporidosis, and *Mycobacterium avium-intracellulare*. Bacterial overgrowth within the small intestine, usually secondary to disorders that promote intestinal stasis or recirculation of enteric contents, causes diarrhea by several potential mechanisms.

B. Hydroxylated fatty acids and bile acids that are not absorbed by the small intestine stimulate electrolyte and H_2O secretion by the colonic mucosa. Malabsorbed carbohydrates exert an osmotic force within the bowel lumen, leading to excessive fecal H_2O losses.

C. Irritable bowel syndrome (IBS) is classically characterized by alternating diarrhea and constipation, although a subset of patients have mainly loose stools. Fecal output in IBS has been reported to range up to 400 g/day.

D. A variety of commonly used drugs, including ethanol, antihypertensive agents, H_2-receptor antagonists, antacids, and digoxin, can cause diarrhea. Surreptitious laxative and diuretic abuse accounts for a significant percentage of patients with chronic diarrhea of unknown cause. Fecal impaction may present with frequent small-volume, liquid stools secondary to an "overflow" secretory response by the colon attributed to high intraluminal hydrostatic pressure.

E. Bloody diarrhea suggests inflammatory bowel disease (IBD), ischemia, radiation damage, or certain infections (cholera, giardiasis, and cryptosporidiosis do not cause bleeding). Additional historical features to note are recent foreign travel (increased risk of infectious diarrhea), sexual exposure (gay bowel syndrome), drug history including recent antibiotic use (increased risk of *Clostridium difficile* infection), surgical history (for dumping syndrome, and ileal resection that promotes bile acid and fat malabsorption), and a history of associated arthritis (suggestive of IBD, certain bacterial infections, and Whipple's disease, and after intestinal bypass surgery).

F. Examine a wet mount of fresh stool and saline for ova, parasites, and meat fibers. Multiple samples may need to be examined to detect parasitosis. Fecal leukocytes, indicative of intestinal inflammation, are best seen with methylene blue, Wright, or Gram stains. Excessive stool fat is determined with a Sudan stain. A low fecal pH suggests carbohydrate malabsorption. A fecal osmotic gap (serum Osm − 2 × {fecal [Na] + [K]}) >150 confirms that an unmeasured osmotic agent is present. Stool water that turns red after alkalinization confirms the presence of phenolphthalein, a stimulant laxative.

G. Inspection of the rectal and left colon mucosa often detects changes secondary to inflammatory disorders. Despite normal-appearing mucosa at sigmoidoscopy, mucosal biopsies may suggest Crohn's disease and microscopic and collagenous colitis.

H. Colonoscopy is more sensitive than barium enema in detecting mucosal disease and allows procurement of mucosal biopsies. The terminal ileum may also be inspected in most patients.

I. An imaging study of the abdomen may demonstrate evidence suggestive of an inflammatory or neoplastic process involving the intestines, mesentery, and other abdominal viscera that may promote diarrhea.

J. Chronic secretory diarrhea may be associated with a variety of endocrine tumors, including gastrinomas and vipomas (usually arising in the pancreas), medullary thyroid carcinoma, carcinoid syndrome, and pheochromocytoma. Hyperthyroidism typically is associated with hyperdefecation without increased stool liquidity.

References

Donowitz M, Kokke FT, Saidi R. Evaluation of patients with chronic diarrhea. N Engl J Med 1995; 332:725.

Framm SR, Soave R. Agents of diarrhea. Med Clin North Am 1997; 81:427.

Kirsh M. Bacterial overgrowth. Am J Gastroenterol 1990; 85:231.

Morris AI, Turnberg LA. Surreptitious laxative abuse. Gastroenterology 1979; 77:780.

Read NW, Krejs GH, Read MG, et al. Chronic diarrhea of unknown origin. Gastroenterology 1980; 78:264.

Shian YF, Feldman GM, Resnick MA, Coff PM. Stool electrolyte and osmolality measurements in the evaluation of diarrheal disorders. Ann Intern Med 1985; 102:773.

Patient with CHRONIC DIARRHEA

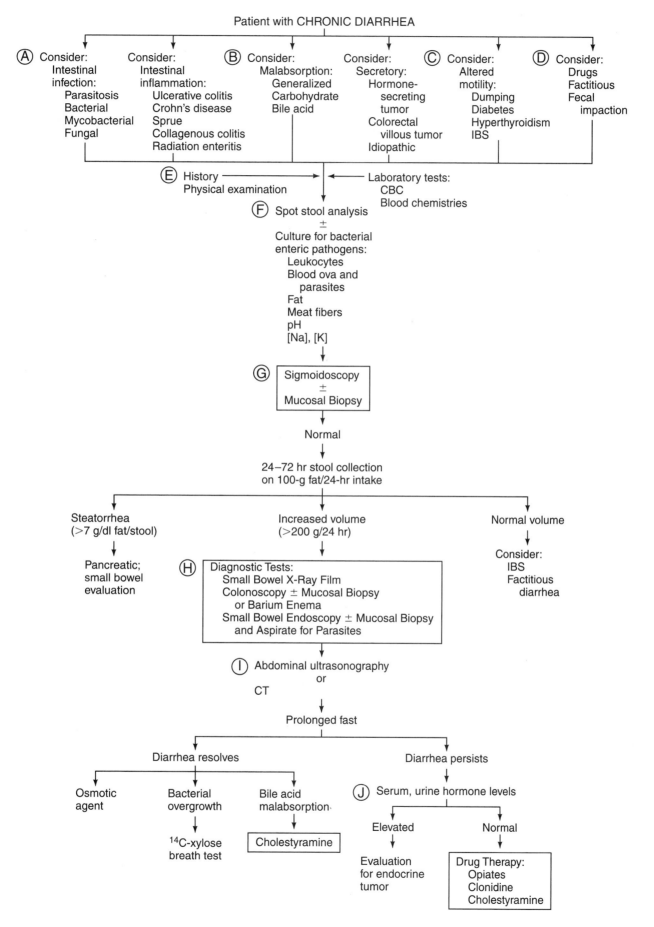

A Consider:
Intestinal infection:
  Parasitosis
  Bacterial
  Mycobacterial
  Fungal

Consider:
Intestinal inflammation:
  Ulcerative colitis
  Crohn's disease
  Sprue
  Collagenous colitis
  Radiation enteritis

B Consider:
Malabsorption:
  Generalized
  Carbohydrate
  Bile acid

Consider:
Secretory:
  Hormone-secreting tumor
  Colorectal villous tumor
  Idiopathic

C Consider:
Altered motility:
  Dumping
  Diabetes
  Hyperthyroidism
  IBS

D Consider:
Drugs
Factitious
Fecal impaction

E History
Physical examination

Laboratory tests:
  CBC
  Blood chemistries

F Spot stool analysis
±
Culture for bacterial enteric pathogens:
  Leukocytes
  Blood ova and parasites
  Fat
  Meat fibers
  pH
  [Na], [K]

G Sigmoidoscopy
±
Mucosal Biopsy

Normal

24–72 hr stool collection on 100-g fat/24-hr intake

Steatorrhea
(>7 g/dl fat/stool)

Pancreatic; small bowel evaluation

Increased volume
(>200 g/24 hr)

H Diagnostic Tests:
  Small Bowel X-Ray Film
  Colonoscopy ± Mucosal Biopsy or Barium Enema
  Small Bowel Endoscopy ± Mucosal Biopsy and Aspirate for Parasites

Normal volume

Consider:
  IBS
  Factitious diarrhea

I Abdominal ultrasonography
or
CT

Prolonged fast

Diarrhea resolves

Osmotic agent

Bacterial overgrowth

14C-xylose breath test

Bile acid malabsorption

Cholestyramine

Diarrhea persists

J Serum, urine hormone levels

Elevated

Evaluation for endocrine tumor

Normal

Drug Therapy:
  Opiates
  Clonidine
  Cholestyramine

CONSTIPATION

Philip E. Jaffe

A. In Western society, adults average three bowel movements per week. There is significant variation in normals, and stool frequency varies depending on age, sex, diet, culture, and geography. Direct the history toward defining the character, chronicity, and severity of patients' complaints. New onset of decreased stool frequency in older patients requires exclusion of an obstructing colonic lesion by flexible sigmoidoscopy and barium enema, unless there is rectal bleeding or a strong family history of colorectal neoplasia suggesting colonoscopy as the initial study. In patients with more chronic complaints and in younger age groups, Hirschsprung's disease, irritable bowel syndrome (IBS), colorectal motility disorders, and anorectal processes (fissures, abscesses, thrombosed hemorrhoids) are more common. The use of medications, including antidepressants, calcium channel blockers, sedatives, opiate analgesics, aluminum antacids, and oral iron supplements, should be discontinued. Evaluate for systemic diseases, including diabetes mellitus, multiple sclerosis, and scleroderma or CREST syndrome. Perform a physical examination, including rectal examination and anoscopy, in all patients. Look for physical signs of hypothyroidism, hypercalcemia, Parkinson's disease, and autonomic neuropathy. Check serum Ca^{++} and thyroid-stimulating hormone (TSH) levels. In many cases simple dietary changes and discontinuation of offending medications cause symptoms to abate; however, persistent symptoms warrant exclusion of an obstructing colorectal mass.

B. Flexible sigmoidoscopy and barium enema exclude an obstructing colorectal lesion in most patients. If Hemoccult-positive stools or rectal bleeding accompany complaints of constipation, colonoscopy is indicated as the initial diagnostic procedure. The finding of a neoplastic polyp on flexible sigmoidoscopy also warrants colonoscopy because of the greater frequency of finding proximal colonic polyps and/or cancer.

C. The finding of an obstructing colonic mass, usually adenocarcinoma, generally requires surgical intervention to prevent complete obstruction. In selected cases when there is metastatic disease or the patient is a poor surgical candidate, effective palliation with laser photocoagulation via endoscopy or the placement of expandable metal stents may be achieved.

D. Anorectal disorders, including fissures, thrombosed hemorrhoids, and perirectal abscesses may lead to constipation by causing avoidance of defecation because of pain. This in turn may worsen the underlying condition. Conservative measures, including stool-bulking agents, local anesthetics, and sitz baths, are preferred unless symptoms persist or an abscess develops, requiring surgery.

E. In patients with chronic constipation and normal imaging studies of the colon and rectum, a radiopaque marker study confirms a transit problem and helps define the cause. The number of markers present in each segment of the large bowel on any given day after ingestion of markers is determined by radiography and compared with normals. Often marker evacuation is normal and the "constipation" is either misinterpreted or misrepresented by the patient. The finding of normal marker transit may encourage a concerned patient by presenting objective evidence that the problem is one of perception. Those with persistence of markers in the rectosigmoid region should be evaluated for an anorectal motility disorder as described in section H. Those who have persistence of markers throughout the colon are said to have colonic inertia. Bulking agents and osmotic agents are advocated in this condition.

F. A significant percentage of patients complaining of constipation have normal colonic transit times as measured by marker studies. In some the feeling of constipation may reflect their expectations relative to their upbringing or cultural norms; most probably have a variant of IBS. Empiric treatment generally begins with a bulking agent, a high-fiber diet, and increased fluid intake. Some patients also require osmotic agents such as lactulose or milk of magnesia. Avoid chronic use of stimulant or irritant laxatives because this may precipitate the development of colonic hypomotility and dilation (cathartic colon).

G. The finding of colonic dilation on barium enema suggests the possibility of neurologic impairment of the colon (e.g., Hirschsprung's disease), an anorectal motility disorder, chronic cathartic use, or colonic pseudo-obstruction. Rectal biopsy in children is useful in diagnosing Hirschsprung's disease (absence of neurons in the rectum). The finding of melanosis coli, either endoscopically or by biopsy, is diagnostic of chronic abuse of anthraquinone laxatives (e.g., cascara or senna).

H. Anorectal motility studies using catheters that measure pressures within the rectum and across the anal sphincter are useful in excluding Hirschsprung's disease or anorectal motility disorders in patients with colonic dilation and no clear cause on biopsy. In addition, if significant numbers of markers remain in the rectosigmoid when transit is measured, an anorectal motility study is indicated. Specific treatment for anorectal motility disorders depends on the specific cause but includes biofeedback training, bulking agents, and occasionally surgery.

I. When further anatomic definition of the anorectal abnormality is required, perform defecography using barium paste or other synthetic radiopaque substances

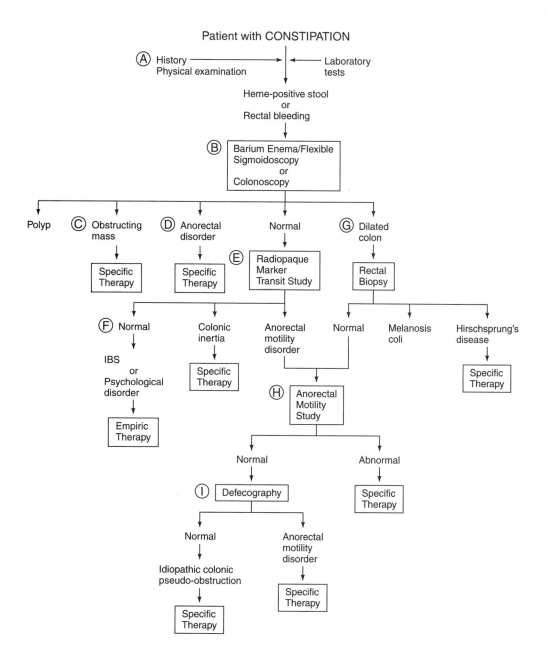

Patient with CONSTIPATION

A History — Physical examination → ← Laboratory tests

Heme-positive stool
or
Rectal bleeding

B Barium Enema/Flexible
Sigmoidoscopy
or
Colonoscopy

Polyp

C Obstructing mass → Specific Therapy

D Anorectal disorder → Specific Therapy

E Radiopaque Marker Transit Study

Normal

G Dilated colon → Rectal Biopsy

F Normal → IBS or Psychological disorder → Empiric Therapy

Colonic inertia → Specific Therapy

Anorectal motility disorder

Normal

Melanosis coli

Hirschsprung's disease → Specific Therapy

H Anorectal Motility Study

Normal

Abnormal → Specific Therapy

I Defecography

Normal → Idiopathic colonic pseudo-obstruction → Specific Therapy

Anorectal motility disorder → Specific Therapy

that simulate the characteristics of stool. By doing so, abnormalities in the perineal descent during defecation and complications of chronic constipation and straining, including rectal prolapse and rectocele, may be detected. Those with chronic constipation and colonic dilation with normal anatomic studies, biopsy, and anorectal motility are said to have chronic idiopathic colonic pseudo-obstruction. In the past this often was treated by colectomy and ileostomy. However, up to 50% have subsequent small bowel obstruction, and surgery is now considered only after a long therapeutic trial of more conservative measures.

References

Rao S. Manometric evaluation of constipation. Part I. Gastroenterologist 1996; 4:145.

Read N, Timms J. Defecation and the pathophysiology of constipation. Clin Gastroenterol 1986; 15:937.

Reynolds JC, Ouyang A, Lee CA, et al. Chronic severe constipation: prospective motility studies in 25 consecutive patients. Gastroenterology 1987; 92:414.

Romero Y, Evans J, Fleming K, Phillips S. Constipation and fecal incontinence in the elderly population. Mayo Clin Proc 1996; 71:81.

Sagar P, Pemberton JH. Anorectal and pelvic floor function: relevance of continence, incontinence, and constipation. Gastroenterol Clin North Am 1996; 25:163.

Schuster M. Evaluation and treatment of constipation. Pract Gastroenterol 1986; 10:15.

IRRITABLE BOWEL SYNDROME

William P. Johnson

Irritable bowel syndrome (IBS) is a common symptom complex arising from the interactions among the digestive system, the psyche, and luminal factors. A wide anatomic spectrum of the digestive tract, including the esophagus, gastroduodenal region, biliary tract, or intestine, may be affected; however, the term *IBS* is confined to symptoms presumed to arise from the small bowel and colon.

A. Apply the Rome diagnostic criteria for IBS (Table 1).

B. To avoid unnecessary, costly, or potentially dangerous investigations in patients with suspected IBS, the diagnostic strategy should be evidence based. A limited series of initial investigations is needed to exclude organic, structural, metabolic, or infectious diseases. These include CBC; renal panel; ESR; fecal occult blood testing; stool examination for ova, parasites, and enteric pathogens; and flexible sigmoidoscopy. In patients with colorectal cancer risk factors, consider barium enema or colonoscopy.

C. Once organic, structural, or biochemical disorders are excluded, stress the negative results of these tests and reassure the patient of these normal findings. Next assess which symptom is predominant. Symptoms may be classified as constipation, diarrhea, and pain/gas/bloat type.

D. A more detailed dietary history may help identify factors that are aggravating or even causing symptoms.

Common offenders are the nonabsorbable oligosaccharides, fructose, sorbitol, and lactose. Because lactose intolerance often is overdiagnosed, perform a lactose-hydrogen breath test before imposing a lactose-exclusion diet. For patients with the pain/gas/bloat syndrome, a plain film of the abdomen made during an acute bout provides reassurance that there is no mechanical obstruction. Therapeutic trials often are useful, depending on the symptom subgroup, including diet, exercise, relaxation therapy, stool softeners, osmotic laxatives, antimotility agents, low-dose tricyclic antidepressants, and antispasmodics.

E. In patients with constipation-type IBS consider pelvic floor dysfunction and colonic inertia. Delayed colonic transit is adequately assessed with the radiopaque marker method. Treatment includes biofeedback, prokinetic drugs, and surgery. Prognosis is guarded, so be conservative.

F. In patients with predominant diarrhea, repeat stool studies for infectious agents; these infestations are eminently treatable. Small bowel transit is methodologically flawed and cannot be recommended at this time outside of a research study. Some patients have bile acid malabsorption secondary to idiopathic bile acid catharsis. The most widely accepted method to demonstrate this condition is the selenium-75 homocholic acid taurine test. If this is unavailable, a therapeutic trial with cholestyramine, 4 g every 6 hours, is reasonable, although this strategy has an appreciable false-negative and false-positive rate.

G. Exclude small bowel mucosal disease or obstruction by barium follow-through examination. GI manometry and balloon distension tests cannot be recommended unless done by a laboratory that routinely performs these studies. This group may have visceral hyper-responsiveness and may be helped by agents that suppress visceral afferent function (e.g., 5-hydroxytryptamine antagonists).

TABLE 1   Rome Diagnostic Criteria for Irritable Bowel Syndrome

At least 3 months of continuous or recurrent symptoms of
  Abdominal pain or discomfort that is
    Relieved with defecation *and/or*
    Associated with a change in frequency of stool *and/or*
    Associated with a change in consistency of stool
                    and
  Two or more of the following, on at least one-fourth of
    occasions or days:
      Altered stool frequency
      Altered stool form
      Altered stool passage
      Passage of mucus
      Bloating or feeling of abdominal distension

References

Camilleri M, Prather CM. The irritable bowel syndrome: mechanisms and a practical approach to management. Ann Intern Med 1992; 116:1001.

Drossman DA. Diagnosing and treating patients with refractory functional gastrointestinal disorders. Ann Intern Med 1995; 123:688.

Drossman DA, Thompson WG. The irritable bowel syndrome: review and a graduated multicomponent treatment approach. Ann Intern Med 1992; 166:1009.

Patient with ABDOMINAL PAIN WITH/WITHOUT ALTERED BOWEL MOTILITY

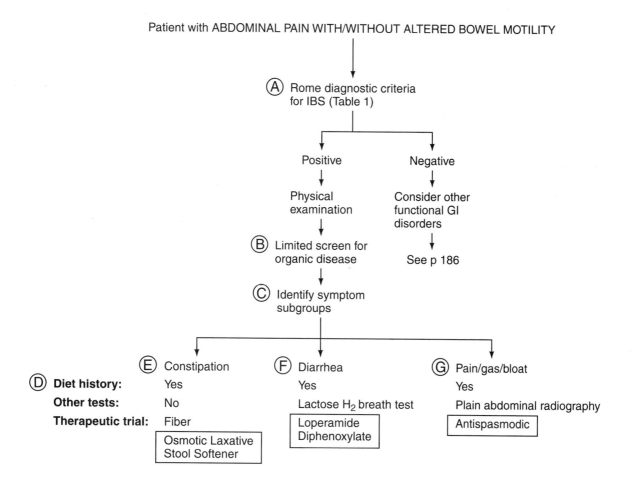

ANORECTAL PAIN

M. Angelo Trujillo

A. Anorectal pain has several potential causes, including local and nonlocal disease processes. A careful history and physical examination, including neurologic, anoscopic, and pelvic examinations, are important in the search for a cause, which may range from an easily treated condition to a life-threatening one. Important considerations in the history are associated symptoms and reported signs (e.g., fever, rectal bleeding, vaginal discharge, hematuria, neurologic dysfunction). Also note rapid onset of symptoms, sexual practices, and any history of inflammatory bowel disease.

B. Careful inspection, along with digital and anoscopic examinations, reveals most local causes of anorectal pain, but further evaluation with proctosigmoidoscopy may be necessary. This also provides a means for obtaining biopsy specimens for culture and histology. Rectal bleeding, mucus discharge, diarrhea, and anorectal pain suggest proctitis from infection or other inflammatory causes.

C. A pelvic examination and consideration of pelvic ultrasonography or CT scan are important in the diagnosis of conditions that may cause referred pain to the anus and rectum. Most of these conditions have a common pathway of irritation of the pudendal nerves that supply sensory innervation to the anus and rectum. Cervical and vaginal cultures plus urinalysis with culture are necessary when considering pelvic inflammatory disease, prostatitis, or nephrolithiasis. Consider IV pyelography if the clinical picture is otherwise consistent with nephrolithiasis.

D. The diagnosis of proctalgia fugax rests on the history and the exclusion of other pelvic or anorectal abnormality. It is a benign condition of unknown cause characterized by paroxysmal anorectal pain of varying severity and sudden onset. Coccygodynia consists of throbbing or aching pain in the coccygeal region. Organic causes include fracture of the coccyx and traumatic arthritis of the sacrococcygeal joint. A functional coccygodynia also exists. Coccygeal tenderness associated with spasm of surrounding muscles are common findings on physical examination. Tension myalgia of the pelvic floor describes a syndrome of chronic vague discomfort in the rectum, pelvis, or lower back in patients without any other definable cause of pain. Pain typically is constant. Some authorities believe that the pain may be related to poor posture, generalized deconditioning, and possible psychological disorders. Chronic idiopathic anal pain has features that overlap with the other chronic pain syndromes.

E. There are several neurologic causes of anorectal pain. Associated neurologic signs and symptoms, pain characteristics, onset of pain, and spinal pathology are important factors in considering a neurologic cause for rectal pain. After a careful neurologic examination the procedures listed will be helpful in diagnosis of a specific neurologic disorder. Formal neurology consultation is recommended.

F. Pain may originate in sacral spinal cord segments or sacral nerve roots. Neoplasm, abscess, or inflammatory processes of the conus medullaris may present with pain. Associated loss of bowel or bladder function often occurs.

G. Entrapment of the sacral nerve roots of the cauda equina may occur secondary to inflammatory reactions in the CSF, or they may be compressed by tumor, abscess, or lumbosacral disc herniation.

H. The sacral plexus is located against the posterior pelvic wall. The plexus may be compressed by tumor or enlarged lymph nodes. Consider CT or MRI of the sacral spine and pelvis.

I. Spinal subarachnoid hemorrhage is a rare cause of rectal pain. This is most commonly the result of vascular malformation rupture, but it may also be associated with trauma, anticoagulant therapy, blood dyscrasias, or tumor. Ependymoma is the most common tumor associated with spinal subarachnoid hemorrhage. In patients with sudden onset of rectal pain associated with back pain, headache, stiff neck, and fever, consider spinal subarachnoid hemorrhage.

References

Harper MB, Pope JB. Office procedures: flexible sigmoidoscopy. Prim Care 1997; 24:341.

Lieberman DA. Common anorectal disorders. Ann Intern Med 1984; 101:837.

Peery WH. Proctalgia fugax: a clinical enigma. South Med J 1988; 81:621.

Rappaport B, Emsellem HA, Shesser R, et al. An unusual case of proctalgia. Ann Emerg Med 1990; 19:201.

Schrock TR. Examination of the anorectum, rigid sigmoidoscopy, flexible sigmoidoscopy, and disease of the anorectum. In: Sleisenger MH, Fordtran JS, eds. Gastrointestinal Disease. 4th ed. Philadelphia: WB Saunders, 1989:1570.

Patient with ANORECTAL PAIN

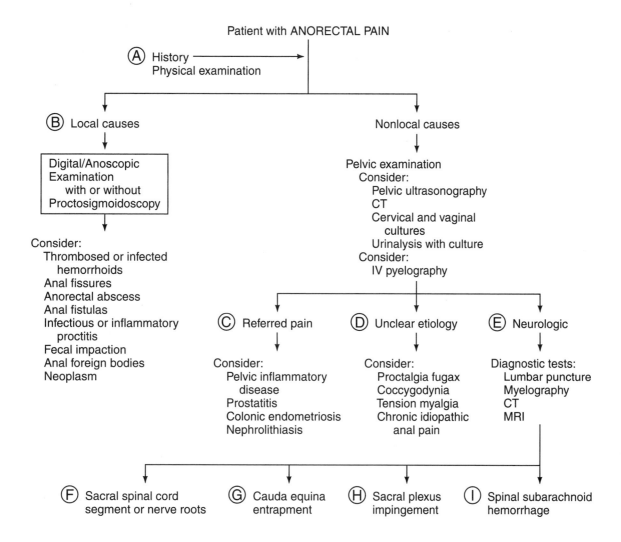

GUAIAC-POSITIVE STOOLS

M. Brian Fennerty

Colon cancer will affect 6% of us during our lifetime. Each year in the United States, there are more than 140,000 new cases and 60,000 deaths from colorectal carcinoma. Accumulating evidence suggests that screening patients for colorectal neoplasia may either prevent colorectal cancer by detecting individuals with colon polyps that may evolve into carcinoma, or allow detection of colorectal cancer at a presymptomatic earlier stage, making curative therapy more likely. At present this screening strategy consists of (1) testing stool for the presence of hemoglobin, most commonly using guaiac-impregnated cards; and (2) directly observing the distal colon by sigmoidoscopic examinations.

A. The clinical use of a positive Hemoccult test obtained at the time of digital rectal examination has not been adequately validated. Despite the absence of data regarding accuracy in detecting neoplastic disease, this is a widely accepted and practiced clinical test. It has been estimated that false-positive rates up to 25% occur with fecal occult blood testing (FOBT) on digital rectal examination. Until the specificity of FOBT by digital rectal examination is clarified, it is recommended that patients undergo FOBT only on spontaneously evacuated stools.

B. Patients should be sent home with guaiac cards and educated about diet and medicines while providing stool samples. Any one of six samples testing positive should be further evaluated. The test is positive in 4–6% of asymptomatic patients tested, but only 5–10% of these have colorectal cancer and 20–30% have colon polyps; therefore, 60–75% are false-positive results. In addition, 30–50% of patients with proven colon cancer have a false-negative test. Therefore, a positive test results in further evaluation in many patients without disease, and a negative test does not exclude disease.

C. For evaluating a patient with a positive FOBT, two strategies are available: (1) flexible sigmoidoscopy and air-contrast barium enema or (2) colonoscopy. With the first strategy, any positive finding (e.g., polyp or cancer) necessitates colonoscopy. In addition, the first strategy alone misses 10% of cancers and 20% of large polyps. Therefore, colonoscopy is the preferred means of evaluation when available. It also may provide the most cost-effective strategy under certain conditions.

D. If symptoms dictate or if there is iron deficiency, a normal colonoscopy indicates that a further search for

GI blood loss from the upper gut is indicated. Esophagogastroduodenoscopy (EGD) should be performed to evaluate the presence of upper GI structural lesions (ulcer, inflammation, tumors, arteriovenous malformations [AVMs]).

E. Although small bowel tumors, or Crohn's disease of the small bowel, unusually present with heme-positive stools, a negative endoscopic examination of colon and upper GI tract should prompt evaluation of the small bowel, preferably by enteroclysis or, if this is not available, a small bowel follow-through. However, neither of these tests detects small mucosal lesions such as AVM or small tumors.

F. If stools remain guaiac positive, consider invasive studies such as angiography or small bowel enteroscopy, which is now widely available. These may permit visualization of small vascular lesions or tumors undetectable by other means.

G. If a colon cancer or large "cherry"-red polyp is found, this may be presumed to be the cause of bleeding and may be treated endoscopically or surgically. Similarly, the presence of mucosal inflammation (i.e., colitis) is also presumably the source. However, the presence of AVMs or diverticula is not sufficient to exclude either proximal source.

References

Barry MJ, Mulley AG, Richter JM. Effect of workup strategy on the cost-effectiveness of fecal occult blood screening for colorectal cancer. Gastroenterology 1987; 93:301.

Fleisher DE, Goldberg SB, Browning TH, et al. Detection and surveillance of colorectal cancer. JAMA 1989; 261:580.

Knight KK, Fielding JE, Battista R. Occult blood screening for colorectal cancer. JAMA 1989; 261:587.

Levin B, Bond JH. Colorectal cancer screening: recommendations of the U.S. Preventive Task Force. Gastroenterology 1996; 111:1381.

Read TE, Read JD, Butterly LF. Importance of adenomas 5 mm or less in diameter that are detected by sigmoidoscopy. N Engl J Med 1997; 336:8.

Patient with GUAIAC-POSITIVE STOOLS

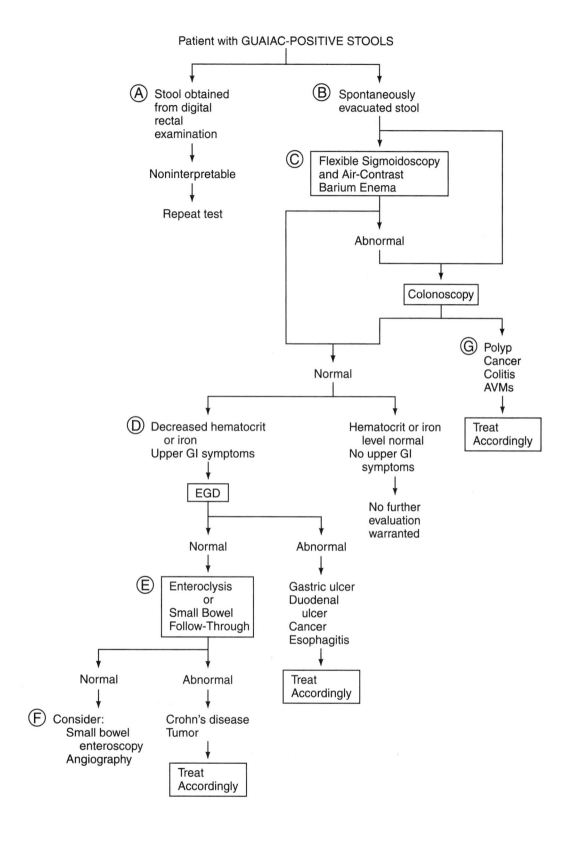

(A) Stool obtained from digital rectal examination

→ Noninterpretable

→ Repeat test

(B) Spontaneously evacuated stool

(C) Flexible Sigmoidoscopy and Air-Contrast Barium Enema

Abnormal

Colonoscopy

(G) Polyp
Cancer
Colitis
AVMs

Treat Accordingly

Normal

(D) Decreased hematocrit or iron
Upper GI symptoms

EGD

Normal

Abnormal

Hematocrit or iron level normal
No upper GI symptoms

No further evaluation warranted

(E) Enteroclysis or Small Bowel Follow-Through

Gastric ulcer
Duodenal ulcer
Cancer
Esophagitis

Treat Accordingly

Normal

Abnormal

(F) Consider:
Small bowel enteroscopy
Angiography

Crohn's disease
Tumor

Treat Accordingly

FLATULENCE

Gregory L. Eastwood

A. Flatulence is the passage of excess intestinal gas per rectum or the feeling that excessive gas is in the abdomen. Many patients complain of bloating, meaning that the abdomen becomes uncomfortably distended, usually after eating. Often, bloating is attributed to excessive intestinal gas. However, the perception that the passage of flatus or the amount of intestinal gas is excessive may be inaccurate because it may not actually be due to an abnormal amount of intestinal gas. Patients who complain of excessive flatus or of abdominal pain from gas sometimes have disorders of gut motility and a heightened pain response to intestinal gas, rather than excess intestinal gas. Some patients who complain of abdominal pain and bloating do have demonstrable disorders, such as peptic disease, gallbladder disease, Crohn's disease, or recurrent bowel obstruction. If, in addition to complaints of gaseousness, the patient has loss of weight, localized abdominal pain, vomiting, or blood in the stool, the suspicion of an organic GI disorder is increased.

B. Bacterial action on dietary substrates produces gas. Some patients can identify certain foods that aggravate the symptoms. A common offender is lactose, which causes excess intestinal gas production, cramps, and diarrhea in lactase-deficient individuals. Elimination of milk and milk products, legumes, cabbage, and similar foods may be effective in alleviating symptoms.

C. Perform sigmoidoscopy and a barium enema to look for anorectal disease and colonic disorders. Reflux into the terminal ileum may identify Crohn's disease.

D. Upper GI and small bowel x-ray series may identify Crohn's disease of the small intestine, recurrent small bowel obstruction, or other disorders of the upper GI tract. Ultrasonography of the abdomen and pelvis may identify gallstones or an extraintestinal mass.

E. High-fiber bulking agents or so-called antispasmodics, such as dicyclomine, may be useful in patients who have no demonstrable treatable disorder or in whom a specific food has not been implicated. However, bulking agents, because they contain nondigestible substrates, may cause increased flatus. In some patients, stress reduction therapy may be helpful.

References

Eastwood GL, Avunduk C. Intestinal gas and bloating. In: Manual of gastroenterology. Diagnosis and therapy. 2nd ed. Boston: Little, Brown, 1994:221.

Lasser RB, Bond JH, Levitt MD. The role of intestinal gas in functional abdominal pain. N Engl J Med 1975; 293:524.

Perman JA, Montes RG. Approach to the patient with gas and bloating. In: Yamada T, ed. Textbook of gastroenterology. 2nd ed. Philadelphia: JB Lippincott, 1995:772.

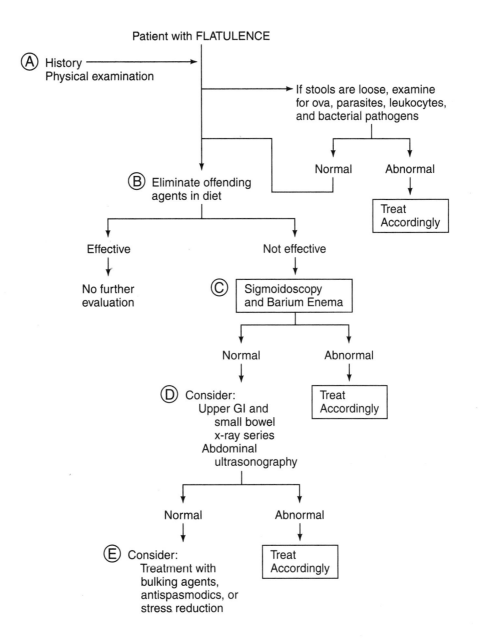

FECAL INCONTINENCE

Philip E. Jaffe

A. A history of rectal trauma, surgery, or infections often provides clues to the cause of incontinence. A temporal relation to systemic neuromuscular conditions, cerebrovascular accidents, or diabetes is also helpful. Diarrhea or tenesmus and urgency may suggest inflammatory proctitis. On physical examination, exclude perirectal disease, including fissures, hemorrhoids, abscesses, and prolapse. Perform a thorough digital examination and try to define sphincter laxity, puborectalis integrity, and the presence of masses. This also excludes rectal impaction, a common cause of incontinence in the elderly.

B. Perform proctoscopy with a flexible endoscope to exclude a distal rectal mass or proctitis. However, it is unusual for these to cause incontinence as an isolated symptom. The finding of ulcerative proctitis warrants a full colonoscopic examination to determine the extent and better define the cause.

C. Anorectal manometry with a balloon-tipped, water-infused catheter defines resting and squeeze sphincter pressures, the threshold for rectal sensation to distension, and the threshold for internal sphincter relaxation on rectal distension. It also occasionally helps determine abnormalities in rectal compliance. Higher than normal sensory thresholds are common in diabetic patients with incontinence and may respond to bulking agents, opioid antidiarrheal agents, and biofeedback when available. Those with traumatic disruption of the anal sphincter (e.g., through a childbirth injury or after hemorrhoidal surgery) should be considered for possible surgical repair if conservative measures fail and low pressures are documented manometrically.

D. When available, defecography can define abnormalities in the anorectal angle during defecation. This often correlates with weakness of the puborectalis and pelvic floor, and in selected patients may respond to surgical repair when conservative measures fail.

E. Diseases of the rectum, including inflammatory proctitis, ischemia, and radiation proctitis, can lead to decreased rectal compliance and incontinence. Infusion of saline into the rectum and simultaneous measurement of rectal pressure associated with leakage can define this condition. If the condition is severe enough and refractory to opioids, fecal diversion with a colostomy may be the only alternative in selected patients.

References

Sager P, Pemberton J. The assessment and treatment of anorectal incontinence. Adv Surg 1996; 30:1.

Schiller L. Fecal Incontinence. Clin Gastroenterol 1986; 15:687.

Schiller L, Santa Ana CA, Schmulen AC, et al. Pathogenesis of fecal incontinence in diabetes mellitus. N Engl J Med 1982; 307:1666.

Wald A. Fecal incontinence: effects of non-surgical treatment. Postgrad Med 1986; 80:123.

Wald A. Disorders of defecation and fecal incontinence. Cleve Clin J Med 1989; 56:491.

Whitehead W. Functional anorectal disease. Semin Gastroenterol 1996; 4:230.

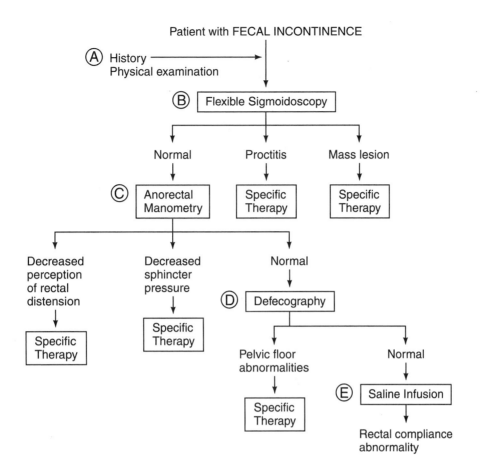

Patient with FECAL INCONTINENCE

(A) History
Physical examination

(B) Flexible Sigmoidoscopy

Normal — (C) Anorectal Manometry

Proctitis — Specific Therapy

Mass lesion — Specific Therapy

Decreased perception of rectal distension — Specific Therapy

Decreased sphincter pressure — Specific Therapy

Normal — (D) Defecography

Pelvic floor abnormalities — Specific Therapy

Normal — (E) Saline Infusion — Rectal compliance abnormality

ASYMPTOMATIC INCREASED TRANSAMINASES

Steven Palley

The increase in asymptomatic patients being evaluated for increased transaminase (TA) levels is related to the proliferation of automated chemistry panel use and the use of alanine aminotransferase (ALT) as a surrogate marker at blood donation centers.

A. Historical considerations are important. Patients with clear histories of ethanol intake should be asked to refrain from drinking alcohol and have a repeat blood test in 2–3 months. Many prescription drugs and some over-the-counter drugs can lead to elevated TA levels and should also be stopped as a trial. Look for a history of exposure to other hepatotoxins. Obesity, hyperlipidemia, and diabetes mellitus can lead to hepatic steatosis and TA elevation. A history of exposure to viral agents should include any IV drug abuse, transfusion, and homosexual contacts. Also assess HIV risk. Asymptomatic HIV-positive patients require no further work-up for elevated TA levels. A family history of hemochromatosis and Wilson's disease may be sought.

B. Physical examination may reveal evidence consistent with chronic liver disease, including spider angiomas, palmar erythema, hepatomegaly, or splenomegaly. Ethanol abuse is indicated by enlarged parotids. Obesity suggests a diagnosis of fatty liver.

C. The first evaluation should be a repeat TA determination along with a liver test panel, including alkaline phosphatase, total bilirubin, prothrombin time, and albumin and globulin levels as well as glucose and lipids. A cholestatic picture should prompt abdominal ultrasonography. Progressive elevation of TA levels requires further evaluation. An elevated aspartate aminotransferase (AST)/ALT ratio (>2–3 : 1) suggests alcoholic liver disease, and the patient should be questioned further.

D. The intensity of follow-up depends on the level of TA elevation. Follow low-level elevations (less than twofold) at 2- to 3-month intervals. Moderate-range elevations should lead to an etiologic battery of laboratory tests and repeat enzymes at 1- to 2-month intervals. The etiologic panel includes iron-binding capacity and ferritin for hemochromatosis, ceruloplasmin for Wilson's disease, α_1-antitrypsin levels, antinuclear antibodies (ANA) and antismooth muscle antibody for autoimmune chronic active hepatitis, and viral serology for hepatitis B and C. Follow higher elevations closely with enzyme levels every 2–4 weeks, and order an etiologic battery. A progressive rise in or unexplained etiology of TA should prompt early liver biopsy.

E. At 6 months, if TA levels have decreased to normal, resolving hepatitis is the likely diagnosis and liver biopsy is unnecessary. Repeat laboratory tests every 6–12 months. Persistent low-grade elevations (<2× normal) should prompt an etiologic panel, if not already done, and a liver biopsy should be considered. Higher elevations at this time should lead to a liver biopsy to establish histologic diagnosis. When pre- and postbiopsy diagnoses are compared, biopsy can change treatment in about 10% of patients and changes the diagnosis in a higher percentage.

References

Friedman LS, Dienstag JL, Watkins E, et al. Evaluation of blood donors with elevated serum alanine aminotransferase levels. Ann Intern Med 1987; 107:137.

Hultcrantz R, Glaumann H, Lindberg G, Nilsson LH. Liver investigation in 149 asymptomatic patients with moderately elevated activities of serum aminotransferases. Scand J Gastroenterol 1986; 21:109.

Neuschwander-Tetri BA. Common blood tests for liver disease. Which ones are most useful? Postgrad Med 1995; 98:49.

Sampliner RE, Beluk D, Harrow EJ, Rivers S. The persistence and significance of elevated alanine aminotransferase levels in blood donors. Transfusion 1985; 25:102.

Sherman KE. Alanine aminotransferase in clinical practice. Arch Intern Med 1991; 151:260.

Van Ness MM, Diehl AM. Is liver biopsy useful in the evaluation of patients with chronically elevated liver enzymes? Ann Intern Med 1989; 111:473.

Patient with ASYMPTOMATIC INCREASED TRANSAMINASE LEVEL

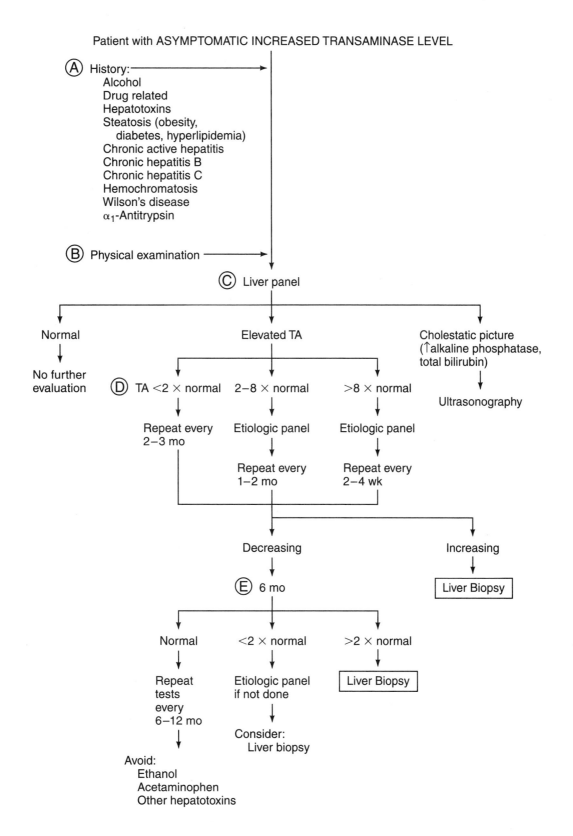

Ⓐ History:
    Alcohol
    Drug related
    Hepatotoxins
    Steatosis (obesity,
       diabetes, hyperlipidemia)
    Chronic active hepatitis
    Chronic hepatitis B
    Chronic hepatitis C
    Hemochromatosis
    Wilson's disease
    α_1-Antitrypsin

Ⓑ Physical examination

Ⓒ Liver panel

Normal → No further evaluation

Elevated TA

Ⓓ TA <2 × normal → Repeat every 2–3 mo

2–8 × normal → Etiologic panel → Repeat every 1–2 mo

>8 × normal → Etiologic panel → Repeat every 2–4 wk

Cholestatic picture (↑alkaline phosphatase, total bilirubin) → Ultrasonography

Decreasing

Increasing → Liver Biopsy

Ⓔ 6 mo

Normal → Repeat tests every 6–12 mo → Avoid: Ethanol, Acetaminophen, Other hepatotoxins

<2 × normal → Etiologic panel if not done → Consider: Liver biopsy

>2 × normal → Liver Biopsy

ELEVATED SERUM IRON

M. Brian Fennerty

A. Hemochromatosis is an inherited autosomal-recessive disorder characterized by excessive GI absorption of iron and progressive iron deposition in parenchymal organs. The gene frequency in the population is 0.06%. Clinical characteristics include lethargy, weight loss, increased skin pigmentation, loss of libido, abdominal pain, joint pain, diabetes, hepatomegaly, testicular atrophy, and arthropathy. Asymptomatic hemochromatosis patients with increased serum iron must be differentiated from patients with iron overload secondary to alcoholic liver disease, hemolytic anemias, and medicinal iron. The family history may indicate liver disease.

B. The serum iron is a poor screening test to detect idiopathic hemochromatosis (IHC) because false-positive results occur in those ingesting iron, alcoholic patients, and heterozygotes of the hemochromatosis allele. However, calculating the transferrin saturation from the serum iron and the iron-binding capacity proves to have a sensitivity >90% (for saturation >60%). Unfortunately as many as 24% of people (many heterozygotes) with normal iron stores also have saturation in this range. The serum ferritin reflects total body iron, and an increase in ferritin usually reflects increased body stores. When combined, increased transferrin saturation and elevated ferritin have a sensitivity of 94%.

C. The diagnosis of IHC requires direct documentation of excess iron in the liver. In addition, quantifying the amount of iron and liver damage has important treatment and prognostic implications. Hepatic iron concentrations in normals are 300–800 μg/g dry weight. In those with hemochromatosis, the hepatic iron concentration usually is >10,000 μg/g dry weight. Presymptomatic patients with hemochromatosis occasionally may have iron concentrations that overlap with those with alcoholic liver disease. The recent identification of a candidate gene for hereditary hemochromatosis may soon result in the ability to accurately diagnose the disease through a genetic screening test.

D. To differentiate alcoholic siderosis from hemochromatosis, Bassett et al. compared hepatic iron concentration in predominantly young homozygous hemochromatosis patients with that in patients with alcoholic liver disease. Hepatic iron index (HII) was calculated by converting micrograms of dry weight to micromoles (μg/56 = μmols) and then dividing by the patient's age. This group discovered that all homozygous patients had an HII >2.0, and all patients with alcoholic liver disease and heterozygotes had an HII <2.0. This value appears to be the most discriminating test available to diagnose IHC.

References

Bassett ML, Halliday JW, Powell LW. Genetic hemochromatosis. Semin Liver Dis 1984; 4:217.

Bassett ML, Halliday JW, Powell LW. Value of hepatic iron measurements in early hemochromatosis and determination of the critical iron level associated with fibrosis. Hepatology 1986; 6:24.

Bonkovsky HL, Ponka P, Bacon BR, et al. An update on iron metabolism: summary of the Fifth International Conference on Disorders of Iron Metabolism. Hepatology 1996; 24:718.

Dadone MM, Kushner JP, Edwards CQ, et al. Hereditary hemochromatosis: analysis of laboratory expression of the disease by gene type in 18 pedigrees. Am J Clin Pathol 1982; 78:196.

Edwards CQ, Griffen LM, Goldgar D, et al. Prevalence of hemochromatosis among 11,065 presumably healthy blood donors. N Engl J Med 1988; 318:1355.

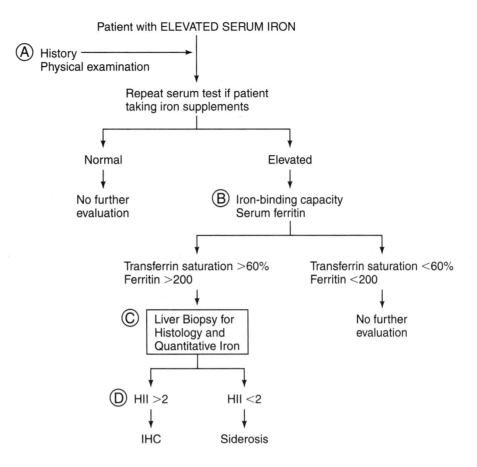

Patient with ELEVATED SERUM IRON

Ⓐ History
Physical examination

Repeat serum test if patient
taking iron supplements

Normal

No further
evaluation

Elevated

Ⓑ Iron-binding capacity
Serum ferritin

Transferrin saturation >60%
Ferritin >200

Ⓒ Liver Biopsy for
Histology and
Quantitative Iron

Ⓓ HII >2

IHC

HII <2

Siderosis

Transferrin saturation <60%
Ferritin <200

No further
evaluation

ELEVATED SERUM AMYLASE

M. Angelo Trujillo

A. Amylase is an enzyme with a 55,000-dalton molecular weight that hydrolyses starch. The pancreas and salivary glands contain very high concentrations of amylase. Amylase also is produced by a number of other organs in lower concentrations. Approximately 35–45% of normal serum amylase is of pancreatic origin. Amylase has a serum half-life of 1–2 hours. Approximately 20% of circulating amylase is excreted in the urine; the remainder is catabolized at an unknown site. Increased serum amylase is most commonly caused by pancreatitis, but hyperamylasemia may be associated with several other nonpancreatic or nonabdominal disorders with similar clinical presentations.

B. In acute pancreatitis serum amylase rises within 24–48 hours of the acute onset of pancreatitis. Levels return to normal within 3–5 days in most cases. A normal serum amylase level occasionally is seen in acute pancreatitis. This may represent early pancreatitis, after a transient rise and fall of amylase, extensive pancreatic necrosis with inability to produce amylase, or cases of acute exacerbation of chronic pancreatitis in which the gland cannot produce amylase. Serum amylase also may be normal when pancreatitis is associated with hypertriglyceridemia. In this case, a urinary amylase measurement usually shows a marked elevation. Cholelithiasis, ethanol, and idiopathic causes are responsible for about 90% of all cases of acute pancreatitis. Commonly used drugs known to cause pancreatitis include ethanol, hydrochlorothiazide, furosemide, sulfonamides, tetracyclines, estrogens, valproate, and azathioprine. A serum amylase level >3 times the upper limit of normal is consistent with pancreatitis. Other abdominal processes usually do not cause amylase levels >2–2.5 times the upper limit of normal, with the exception of salivary gland disease and gut perforation or infarction.

C. In acute pancreatitis with persistent elevated serum amylase levels, complications of acute pancreatitis as listed should be considered. Abdominal CT is useful in identifying pseudocysts, abscesses, ascites, and some tumors. Consider endoscopic retrograde cholangiopancreatography (ERCP) in pancreatitis of biliary origin or idiopathic pancreatitis.

D. In a patient with epigastric pain and elevated serum amylase, rule out causes other than acute pancreatitis. In cases of perforated peptic ulcer, peritoneal absorption of upper GI contents results in elevated serum amylase. The patient usually has a more abrupt onset of pain and more peritoneal irritation. Several other nonpancreatic conditions listed also present with more pronounced signs of peritonitis, and most need surgical intervention.

E. The elevation of serum amylase in renal insufficiency usually is modest, seldom >2 times the upper limit of normal. Macroamylasemia is a condition in which the major portion of serum amylase is bound to IgA. These macromolecular aggregates cannot undergo glomerular filtration, so the urine amylase level is low or normal. The amylase/creatinine clearance ratio (ACR) is calculated as follows:

$$ACR = \frac{A\ (urine) \times CR\ (serum)}{A\ (serum) \times CR\ (urine)} \times 100$$

where A = amylase concentration and CR = creatinine concentration. In macroamylasemia, the ACR is abnormally low (usually <0.2%).

F. After the common causes have been considered, more obscure causes should be sought. Isoamylase or lipase measurements may be helpful. Elevated serum amylase secondary to lung disease or certain tumors is commonly of the salivary or s-isoenzyme.

References

Jensen DM, Rayse VL, Newell J, et al. Use of amylase isoenzymes in laboratory evaluation of hyperamylasemia. Dig Dis Sci 1987; 32:561.

Ranson JH. Diagnostic standards for acute pancreatitis. World J Surg 1997; 21:136.

Salt WB, Schenker S. Amylase—its significance: a review of the literature. Medicine 1976; 55:269.

Soergel KH. Acute pancreatitis. In: Sleisenger MH, Fordtram JS, eds. Gastrointestinal disease. 4th ed. Philadelphia: WB Saunders, 1989:1814.

Tietz NW, Huang WY, Rauh DF, Shuey DF. Laboratory tests in the differential diagnosis of hyperamylasemia. Clin Chem 1986; 32:301.

Toskes PP. Biochemical tests in pancreatic disease. Curr Opin Gastro 1991; 7:709.

Patient with ELEVATED SERUM AMYLASE

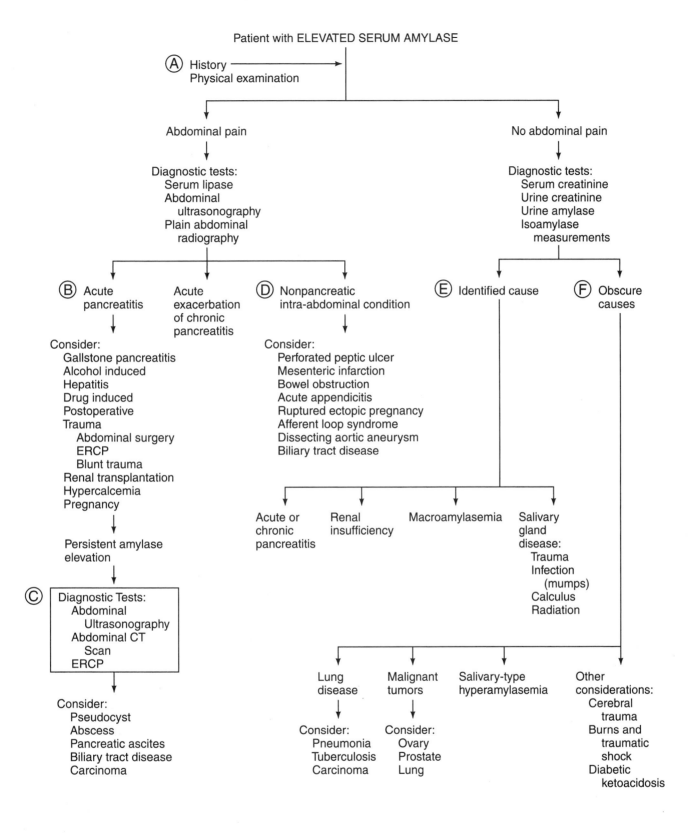

HEMATOLOGY/ONCOLOGY

ANEMIA

Raymond Taetle

A. The general evaluation of anemia includes an initial evaluation of volume status. If clinical signs of intravascular volume depletion such as orthostatic hypotension are present, RBC and plasma loss may have occurred. Correct intravascular volume by appropriate blood and other product support before evaluating the patient for anemia.

B. Begin evaluation of the pathophysiology of anemia by assessing effective RBC production. The normal steady-state reticulocyte production is approximately 50,000/mm^3/day (1% of 5 million), and the maximum production is approximately 400,000/mm^3. Under extreme stress, reticulocytes may be released from the marrow a day early, and even higher levels of apparent production are achieved. These figures may be used to interpret whether RBC production is increased or decreased.

C. Increased RBC production in an anemic patient is presumptive evidence of increased RBC destruction (hemolysis). The hemolysis may be intravascular or predominantly extravascular. In either case, haptoglobin, the major plasma heme-binding protein, may be depressed. In intravascular hemolysis, free hemoglobin (Hb) may be present in plasma, and Fe in renal tubule cells (urinary hemosiderin). Indirect bilirubin and lactate dehydrogenase may also be elevated. The Coombs' test is used to distinguish immune and nonimmune hemolysis. A positive, direct Coombs' test indicates antibody or complement on the RBC cell surface. Only certain IgG isotypes react with macrophage Fc receptors; therefore, a positive Coombs' test may be present without causing increased RBC destruction. Autoimmune antibodies have maximal binding at either 37° C (warm antibodies, usually IgG) or 4° C (cold antibodies, usually IgM).

D. If the spleen is palpable and thus clinically enlarged, hypersplenism cannot be definitively ruled out as a cause of RBC destruction. This can occur secondary to processes that themselves lead to anemia, such as the ineffective erythropoiesis accompanying thalassemia, and hemolysis from an abnormal Hb, such as sickle cell/C disease.

E. If hypersplenism is unlikely, hemolysis may be due to mechanical trauma, congenital enzyme, or Hb defects within the RBC. Microangiopathic hemolytic anemia (MAHA) results from RBC trauma from fibrin strands in small vessels (thrombotic thrombocytopenic purpura, hemolytic uremic syndrome, disseminated intravascular coagulation [DIC]), or more rarely, prosthetic heart valves. Enzymatic defects can be drug dependent, such as G6PD deficiency, or constitutive, such as pyruvate kinase deficiency. Abnormal Hbs (sickle hemoglobin) and membrane defects (hereditary spherocytosis) also cause hemolysis. Acquired causes of hemolysis include the excess complement sensitivity acquired in paroxysmal nocturnal hemoglobinuria (PNH) and infections such as malaria.

(Continued on page 208)

Patient with ANEMIA (DECREASED RBC MASS)

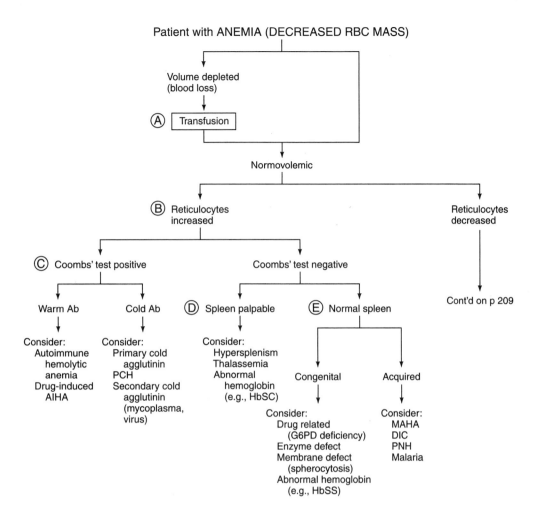

Volume depleted
(blood loss)

Ⓐ Transfusion

Normovolemic

Ⓑ Reticulocytes
increased

Reticulocytes
decreased

Ⓒ Coombs' test positive

Coombs' test negative

Cont'd on p 209

Warm Ab

Cold Ab

Ⓓ Spleen palpable

Ⓔ Normal spleen

Consider:
Autoimmune
hemolytic
anemia
Drug-induced
AIHA

Consider:
Primary cold
agglutinin
PCH
Secondary cold
agglutinin
(mycoplasma,
virus)

Consider:
Hypersplenism
Thalassemia
Abnormal
hemoglobin
(e.g., HbSC)

Congenital

Acquired

Consider:
Drug related
(G6PD deficiency)
Enzyme defect
Membrane defect
(spherocytosis)
Abnormal hemoglobin
(e.g., HbSS)

Consider:
MAHA
DIC
PNH
Malaria

F. When RBC production is decreased or normal in the face of anemia (normal production with a reduced RBC mass constitutes depressed production), guidance as to the origin of the anemia may be provided by RBC size obtained through automated cell counting. Microcytic anemias generally involve processes in which Hb or heme synthesis is impaired. Thalassemia minor is a common cause of microcytic anemia. Major thalassemias cause more severe anemia and often are accompanied by organomegaly and/or skeletal abnormalities caused by marrow expansion. Anemia of chronic disease is the most common anemia in hospitalized patients, can be mildly microcytic (MCV ≥75), and shows reduced serum Fe, reduced total iron-binding capacity (TIBC), and increased serum ferritin. In contrast, Fe deficiency is the most common outpatient anemia and is characterized by reduced serum Fe, *increased* TIBC, and *reduced* serum ferritin.

G. In normocytic anemias, consider anemia of chronic disease in appropriate clinical settings when the aforementioned laboratory findings are present. If anemia of chronic disease is absent, order a bone marrow aspiration and biopsy to rule out a marrow defect in RBC production due to aplasia, processes replacing the marrow (myelophthisic anemia), lympho- or myeloproliferative disorders, or malnutrition. Protein calorie malnutrition causes anemia in disorders such as anorexia nervosa. Other metabolic disorders also cause severe anemia, including uremia. The primary defect in uremic patients is a relative lack of the erythroid-stimulating hormone erythropoietin (EPO), which is now substantially corrected by EPO administration. The Fe status of these patients depends on their transfusion and medication histories.

H. Macrocytic anemias are due to either vitamin deficiencies or primary processes involving the marrow. Liver disease also can cause macrocytosis because of excess RBC membrane lipid, but it is not associated with vitamin deficiency. Vitamin B_{12} deficiency may be due to pernicious anemia or secondary to other causes of B_{12} malabsorption, but it is almost never due to dietary deficiency. In recent years, many early cases of B_{12} deficiency are detected by serum B_{12} assays and confirmatory tests (increased serum methylmalonic acid or homocysteine). Folate deficiency usually is due to dietary deficiency or diet in combination with ethanol ingestion. Some drugs also impair folate absorption (phenytoin) or metabolism (trimethoprim).

I. When folate and B_{12} levels are normal, macrocytic anemias often are due to myelodysplasia or to unusual congenital dyserythropoietic anemias (types 1, 2, or 3) diagnosed by bone marrow examination.

References

Dallman PR. Biochemical basis for the manifestations of iron deficiency. Ann Rev Nutr 1986; 6:13.

Doll DC, Weiss RB. Neoplasia and the erythron. J Clin Oncol 1985; 3:429.

Guyatt GH, Oxman AD, Ali M, et al. Tests for determination of iron-deficiency anemia: a meta-analysis. Laboratory diagnosis of iron-deficiency anemia: an overview. J Gen Intern Med 1992; 7:145.

Saxena S, Rabinowitz AP, Johnson C, Shulman IA. Iron-deficiency anemia: a medically treatable chronic anemia as a model for transfusion overuse. Am J Med 1993; 94:120.

Sears DA. Anemia of chronic disease. Med Clin North Am 1992; 76:567.

Thompson CE, Damon LE, Ries CA, Linker CA. Thrombotic microangiopathies in the 1980s: clinical features, response to treatment, and the impact of the human immunodeficiency virus epidemic. Blood 1992; 80:1890.

Van Wyck DB. Iron management during recombinant human erythropoietin therapy. Am J Kidney Dis 1989; 14:9.

Yip R, Dallman PR. The roles of inflammation and iron deficiency as causes of anemia. Am J Clin Nutr 1988; 48:1295.

Patient with ANEMIA (DECREASED RBC MASS)
(Cont'd from p 207)

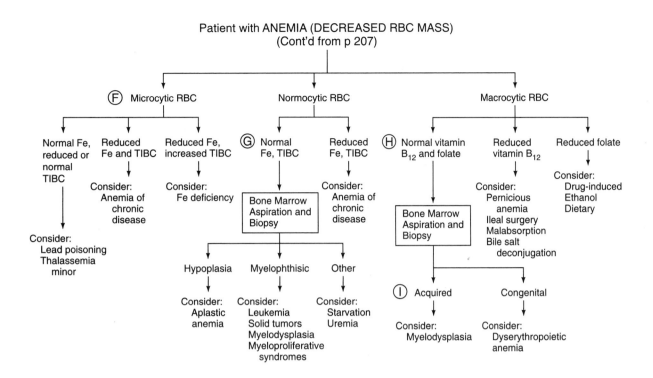

209

POLYCYTHEMIA

Raymond Taetle

A. Increased plasma hemoglobin (Hb) or hematocrit (Hct) does not necessarily reflect an elevated total body RBC mass. If repeat determinations confirm an increased plasma Hb, measure RBC mass and plasma volume using radiolabeled RBC and albumin. In the absence of frank volume contraction, a patient with very high Hct ($\geq$60%) nearly always has an elevated RBC mass.

B. Increased RBC mass indicates "true" polycythemia. An increase in plasma Hb attributed to a normal or high normal RBC mass and reduced plasma volume is termed *spurious* polycythemia. In the past, many cases of spurious polycythemia resulted from treatment with diuretics for hypertension. Although such patients do not have an expanded RBC mass, the decreased ratio of plasma to RBC in blood results in unfavorable whole blood rheology. Spurious polycythemia may be associated with a high incidence of morbid arterial thrombotic events. Discontinue diuretics and substitute other forms of treatment, or evaluate the patient to delineate other possible causes of the decreased plasma volume.

C. If the RBC mass is elevated, test ABGs for Hb O_2 saturation. When saturation is <90%, hypoxia may cause increased erythropoietin (EPO) production and secondary polycythemia. In some patients, hypoxia occurring only at night is revealed by sleep studies, and this is sufficient to elevate EPO levels and cause polycythemia. Nighttime blood gas or oximeter readings may clarify this problem. Regardless of the cause, elevation of Hb levels to above normal generally is considered to result in unfavorable rheology and O_2 delivery. Provide supplemental O_2 if indicated to lower the EPO stimulus. Right-to-left cardiac shunts can also cause decreased blood O_2 content and polycythemia but usually present in childhood.

D. When plasma EPO levels are increased in the absence of hypoxia, consider localized hypoxia within the kidney or impaired O_2 delivery. Renal cysts and tumors can compress intrarenal vessels and cause local hypoxia, leading to increased renal elaboration of EPO. Ultrasonography or CT of the kidneys usually is diagnostic, but in some patients arteriography is necessary. Certain rare tumors (e.g., hepatomas, cerebellar hemangiomas) can produce ectopic EPO. Rarely, uterine fibromas have also been associated with this finding. Secondary polycythemia can occur with normal EPO levels in chronic hypoxia or decreased oxyhemoglobin desaturation. During the initial response to hypoxia EPO levels are elevated, but once steady-state erythrocytosis is achieved, the EPO levels required to maintain an elevated Hb level may fall within the normal assay range.

E. Abnormal Hb levels that result in reduced O_2 unloading in tissues also cause tissue hypoxia and increased EPO production. The most common cause is probably increased carboxyhemoglobin levels from CO in cigarette smoke. Carboxyhemoglobin levels $\geq$6% can elevate EPO production and increase Hb levels. Unusual congenital Hbs may also release O_2 poorly and cause polycythemia. Both result in a shift in the oxyhemoglobin dissociation curve and an increased O_2 concentration at which 50% O_2 delivery (P-50) occurs.

F. Patients with normal plasma EPO levels and increased RBC mass have autonomous erythropoiesis, usually polycythemia vera (PV). In some cases this diagnosis remains unconfirmed because patients lack other evidence of PV. Such cases have recently been termed *pure erythrocytosis* and usually are managed by phlebotomy. The Polycythemia Vera Study Group (PVSG) proposed criteria for the diagnosis of PV. In concept, these criteria are clinical findings indicating the presence of a multilineage myeloproliferative disorder. A normal arterial O_2 saturation is assumed because, in the presence of hypoxia, increased erythropoiesis cannot be definitively said to be autonomous. An increased RBC mass also is required. If these findings are noted in a patient with a palpable spleen (major criteria), the diagnosis of PV is established. If a palpable spleen is absent, an increased RBC mass in the presence of persistently increased leukocyte alkaline phosphatase (LAP), platelet, or WBC counts or evidence of increased WBC turnover is accepted. Both the elevated vitamin B_{12} level and elevated B_{12}-binding capacity (transcobalamin) result from increased WBC membrane turnover and are thus indirect indices of increased WBC proliferation. The major criteria of increased RBC mass and two of these minor criteria are considered diagnostic. However, some patients with PV do not meet such criteria. Some present after GI bleeding and may have initially reduced Hb levels. Others lack the full diagnostic criteria but require therapy because of the unfavorable rheologic effects of polycythemia. Presenting symptoms of polycythemia are nonspecific and reflect increased blood viscosity. These include headaches, plethora, and fatigue. Occasional patients have major thrombotic events such as stroke or myocardial infarction or bleeding manifestations. Such patients should not undergo surgery until polycythemia has been corrected. For reasons that have not been fully elucidated, polycythemia per se results in a bleeding diathesis. Platelet dysfunction may exacerbate this problem in PV but is often normal at initial presentation.

G. PV is managed with phlebotomy to reduce Hb levels to normal. Patients treated with phlebotomy alone show an increased incidence of thrombotic events early in their disease. The addition of alkylating agents or ^{32}P to phlebotomy reduces thrombotic events but results in increased late transformation to acute leukemia. In recent years the antimetabolite hydroxyurea has been used instead of alkylating agents. No randomized trials examined effects of hydroxyurea on the natural history of PV, but retrospective studies suggest it does not increase leukemia transformation. Recently, a new

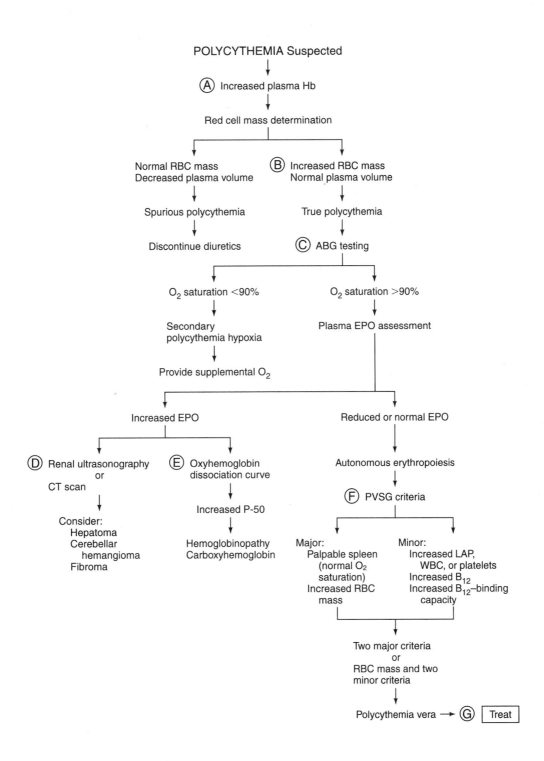

POLYCYTHEMIA Suspected

Ⓐ Increased plasma Hb

Red cell mass determination

Normal RBC mass
Decreased plasma volume

Ⓑ Increased RBC mass
Normal plasma volume

Spurious polycythemia

True polycythemia

Discontinue diuretics

Ⓒ ABG testing

O_2 saturation <90%

O_2 saturation >90%

Secondary
polycythemia hypoxia

Plasma EPO assessment

Provide supplemental O_2

Increased EPO

Reduced or normal EPO

Ⓓ Renal ultrasonography
or
CT scan

Ⓔ Oxyhemoglobin
dissociation curve

Autonomous erythropoiesis

Increased P-50

Ⓕ PVSG criteria

Consider:
Hepatoma
Cerebellar
hemangioma
Fibroma

Hemoglobinopathy
Carboxyhemoglobin

Major:
Palpable spleen
(normal O_2
saturation)
Increased RBC
mass

Minor:
Increased LAP,
WBC, or platelets
Increased B_{12}
Increased B_{12}–binding
capacity

Two major criteria
or
RBC mass and two
minor criteria

Polycythemia vera → Ⓖ Treat

agent with profound effects on platelet production, anegrelide, has been used to control elevated platelet counts in PV and other myeloproliferative disorders, but experience with this agent is limited.

References

Kaplan ME, Mack K, Goldberg JD, et al. Long-term management of polycythemia vera with hydroxyurea: a progress report. Semin Hematol 1986; 23:167.

Nissenson AR, Nimer SD, Walcott DL. Recombinant human erythropoietin and renal anemia: molecular biology, clinical efficacy, and nervous system effects. Ann Intern Med 1991; 114:402.

Polycythemia vera. Semin Hematol 34(1), 1997.

Prchal JF, Prchal JF. Evolving understanding of the cellular defect in polycythemia vera: implications for its clinical diagnosis and molecular pathophysiology. Blood 1994; 83:1.

Wasserman LR. Polycythemia Vera Study Group: a historical perspective. Semin Hematol 1986; 23:183.

LEUKOCYTOSIS

Robert M. Rifkin

Increases in the number of circulating leukocytes may represent either a primary disorder of WBC production or a secondary response to an underlying disease. Leukocytosis is defined by age-adjusted population normal values. Abnormal elevations in the mature neutrophil count (neutrophilia) are the most common cause of leukocytosis.

A. Neutrophilia is best defined as an elevation in the absolute neutrophil count by >2 standard deviations above the mean value for normal individuals. Neutrophil counts follow a diurnal variation, with peak counts occurring late in the afternoon. However, this variation is not enough to produce neutrophilia.

B. Initially, exclude laboratory error as the cause of neutrophilia. With the advent of electronic blood cell counting, human error has virtually been eliminated. Blood counts that do not make sense in the context of clinical history should be repeated. Always evaluate a peripheral blood smear. Factitious leukocytosis must result from blood sampling problems (inadequate anticoagulant). In this instance the WBC count is rarely increased by >10% and is accompanied by a spurious thrombocytopenia. In cryoglobulinemia a temperature-independent increase in the WBC and platelet count occurs when various sizes of precipitated cryoglobulin particles begin to clump.

C. Begin the evaluation of neutrophilia with a thorough history and physical examination to search for an underlying disease state. Neutrophilia commonly results from an acute or chronic inflammatory process. A bone marrow examination rarely provides useful information except in patients in whom direct marrow invasion is suspected. Bone marrow biopsy and culture may be helpful when chronic infections (fungal or mycobacterial) are suspected. In the asymptomatic patient with very mild neutrophilia, remember that the WBC in 2.5% of the general population must be >2 standard deviations above the mean. Because the regulation of the neutrophil count is genetically controlled, examination of siblings and family members is often helpful in these difficult cases.

D. Neutrophilia is best classified as acute or chronic. In normal individuals the neutrophil count varies directly with the serum cortisol level; both levels peak late in the afternoon. Neutrophil counts also rise slightly after meals, with postural changes, and with emotional stimuli. These physiologic changes are not sufficient to cause a significant change in the total WBC count.

E. Acute neutrophilia may result from a wide variety of physical and emotional stimuli, including cold, heat, exercise, seizures, pain, labor, surgery, panic, and rage. Many localized and systemic bacterial, mycotic, and viral infections may result in acute neutrophilia. Inflammation and tissue necrosis from burns, electric shocks, gout, collagen vascular disease, and activation of complement often are responsible for rises in the neutrophil count. Finally, the colony-stimulating factors (G-CSF and GM-CSF) also elicit a striking acute neutrophilia.

F. Chronic neutrophilia may result from a persistence of any of the infections that cause acute neutrophilia; it most commonly results from cigarette smoking. Long-standing inflammatory conditions, including rheumatoid arthritis, gout, vasculitis, myositis, colitis, dermatitis, peridontitis, and drug reactions, can produce puzzling chronic neutrophilia. Nonhematologic malignancies often are associated with chronic neutrophilia. These include carcinomas of the lung, stomach, breast, kidney, liver, pancreas, and uterus. Lymphomas (Hodgkin's disease and non-Hodgkin's lymphoma), brain tumors, melanoma, and myeloma are rare causes of neutrophilia. Benign hematologic disorders may also cause chronic neutrophilia. These include rebound from agranulocytosis or therapy for megaloblastic anemia, chronic hemolysis, asplenia, and chronic idiopathic leukocytosis. Malignant hematologic disorders such as chronic myelogenous leukemia (CML) and other myeloproliferative disorders must also be considered as causes of chronic neutrophilia. The leukocyte alkaline phosphatase (LAP) score is elevated in infectious causes of neutrophilia, variable in myeloproliferative states, and depressed in CML. Down syndrome and familial hyperleukocytosis are rare causes of chronic neutrophilia. Neutrophilia in response to drugs is uncommon except for the well-documented effects of epinephrine, catecholamines, and glucocorticosteroids. Lithium salts also cause sustained neutrophilia. Neutrophilia has also been reported with ranitidine and quinidine therapy. Specific therapy to reduce only the neutrophilia count generally is not suggested.

References

Coates T, Baehner R. Leukocytosis and leukopenia. In: Hoffman R, Benz EJ, Shattil SJ, et al, eds. Hematology: basic principles and practice. 2nd ed. New York: Churchill Livingstone, 1995:769.

Dale DC. Neutrophilia. In: Beutler E, Lichtman MA, Coller BS, Kipps TJ, eds. Williams hematology. 5th ed. New York: McGraw-Hill, 1995:824.

Jandl JH. Granulocytes. In: Jandl JH. Blood: textbook of hematology. 2nd ed. Boston: Little, Brown, 1996:615.

Lieschke GJ, Burgess AW. Granulocyte colony-stimulating factor and granulocyte-macrophage colony-stimulating factor. N Engl J Med 1992; 327:28, 328:99.

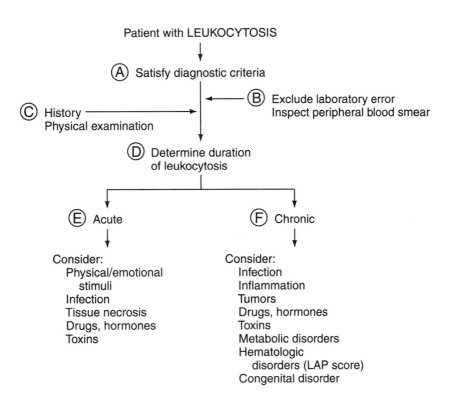

Patient with LEUKOCYTOSIS

(A) Satisfy diagnostic criteria

(B) Exclude laboratory error
Inspect peripheral blood smear

(C) History
Physical examination

(D) Determine duration
of leukocytosis

(E) Acute

Consider:
Physical/emotional
stimuli
Infection
Tissue necrosis
Drugs, hormones
Toxins

(F) Chronic

Consider:
Infection
Inflammation
Tumors
Drugs, hormones
Toxins
Metabolic disorders
Hematologic
disorders (LAP score)
Congenital disorder

LEUKOPENIA

William H. Kreisle
Manuel Modiano

In adults leukopenia is a total WBC count <3700 cells/mm^3. Most cases are due to absolute neutropenia (<2500 cells/mm^3); rare cases are secondary to absolute lymphopenia (<1000 cells/mm^3).

A. Initial evaluation should include a thorough history and physical examination. Give special attention to the use of drugs and the presence of adenopathy, splenomegaly, ecchymoses, petechiae, and signs of infection. CBC, differential, and platelet counts are essential to determine absolute neutrophil and lymphocyte counts and to rule out any accompanying anemia or thrombocytopenia. The blood smear provides important information concerning RBC and WBC morphology. The results of these tests often lead to specific diagnoses.

B. Neutropenic patients usually have signs and symptoms of infection that often are life threatening. Fever in the absence of localizing signs of infection is common. After obtaining cultures, start broad-spectrum antibiotics immediately.

C. Isolated neutropenia and pancytopenia can occur with many commonly used noncytotoxic drugs (e.g., quinidine, penicillins, sulfonamides, phenothiazines, diuretics), alkylating agents, antimetabolites, and other neoplastic agents. If physical examination and laboratory tests are negative for a neoplastic or hematologic disorder, stop the drug and observe the patient with frequent blood counts. Order a bone marrow biopsy and aspirate if the neutropenia fails to resolve in 5–7 days or if blood counts continue to decline.

D. Disorders leading to splenomegaly with splenic sequestration can cause neutropenia, but there usually is associated thrombocytopenia. Differential diagnosis includes cirrhosis, sarcoidosis, glycogen storage diseases, and other uncommon conditions.

E. If the bone marrow result is unremarkable and there is no evidence of splenomegaly or an autoimmune disorder, consider rare chronic neutropenic states. Observe the patient with serial blood counts to document the neutropenic pattern.

F. Most cases of neutropenia are associated with anemia and/or thrombocytopenia. Unless a drug is strongly suspected as the cause, order a bone marrow biopsy and aspirate to rule out a primary hematologic disorder that requires prompt treatment.

G. If the only bone marrow abnormality is the absence of mature granulocytes, this suggests maturation arrest or autoimmune destruction. Perform a work-up for an autoimmune disorder. If available, an antineutrophil antibody assay may be helpful.

H. Infections that can cause neutropenia with anemia and/or thrombocytopenia include viruses (Epstein-Barr, cytomegalovirus, HIV, hepatitis, measles); bacteria (severe gram-negative and gram-positive organisms); *Mycobacterium,* typhoid fever, malaria; and fungi. Bone marrow should be cultured as part of an extensive work-up for infection.

I. Lymphopenia without associated neutropenia is uncommon. Most cases are secondary to drugs (e.g., steroids), radiation injury, or renal failure. Some viral infections, particularly HIV, can also cause absolute lymphopenia.

References

Athens JW. Neutropenia. In Lee GR, Bithell TC, Foerster J, et al, eds. Wintrobe's clinical hematology. 9th ed. Philadelphia: Lea & Febiger, 1993:1589.

Dale DC. Neutrophil disorders: benign, quantitative abnormalities of neutrophils. In: Williams WJ, ed. Hematology. 4th ed. New York: McGraw-Hill, 1990:807.

Logue GL, Schimm DS. Autoimmune granulocytopenia. Annu Rev Med 1980; 31:191.

Murphy MF, Metcalf P, Waters AH, et al. Incidence and mechanism of neutropenia and thrombocytopenia in patients with human immunodeficiency virus infection. Br J Haematol 1987; 66:337.

Vincent PC. Drug-induced aplastic anemia and agranulocytosis. Incidence and mechanisms. Drugs 1986; 31:52.

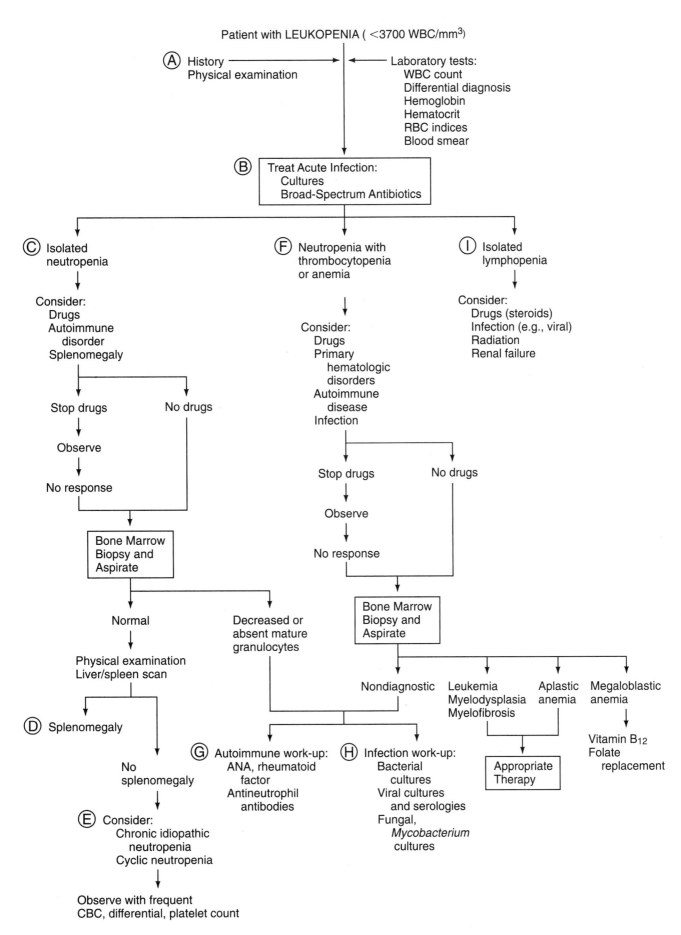

Patient with LEUKOPENIA (<3700 WBC/mm³)

(A) History
Physical examination

Laboratory tests:
  WBC count
  Differential diagnosis
  Hemoglobin
  Hematocrit
  RBC indices
  Blood smear

(B) Treat Acute Infection:
  Cultures
  Broad-Spectrum Antibiotics

(C) Isolated neutropenia

Consider:
Drugs
Autoimmune
  disorder
Splenomegaly

Stop drugs

No drugs

Observe

No response

Bone Marrow
Biopsy and
Aspirate

Normal

Decreased or
absent mature
granulocytes

Physical examination
Liver/spleen scan

(D) Splenomegaly

No
splenomegaly

(E) Consider:
Chronic idiopathic
  neutropenia
Cyclic neutropenia

Observe with frequent
CBC, differential, platelet count

(F) Neutropenia with
thrombocytopenia
or anemia

Consider:
Drugs
Primary
  hematologic
  disorders
Autoimmune
  disease
Infection

Stop drugs

No drugs

Observe

No response

Bone Marrow
Biopsy and
Aspirate

Nondiagnostic

(G) Autoimmune work-up:
ANA, rheumatoid
  factor
Antineutrophil
  antibodies

(H) Infection work-up:
Bacterial
  cultures
Viral cultures
  and serologies
Fungal,
  Mycobacterium
  cultures

Leukemia
Myelodysplasia
Myelofibrosis

Aplastic
anemia

Megaloblastic
anemia

Appropriate
Therapy

Vitamin B₁₂
Folate
replacement

(I) Isolated
lymphopenia

Consider:
Drugs (steroids)
Infection (e.g., viral)
Radiation
Renal failure

DISSEMINATED INTRAVASCULAR COAGULATION

Raymond Taetle

A. A wide variety of diseases, infections, and circulatory abnormalities initiate diffuse clotting within vessels. In many cases this occurs through tissue factor activation of the extrinsic clotting pathway, but other mechanisms are possible. These reactions share a common pathophysiology resulting from continuous clotting activation, consumption of clotting factors and platelets, and lysis of the generated fibrin. The clinical manifestations of DIC vary from diffuse hemorrhagic diathesis to clotting, depending on the balance between clot generation, consumption, and clot lysis. A complex syndrome involving both DIC and increased fibrinolysis occurs consistently in acute promyelocytic leukemia (APL; FAB class M3). This algorithm considers the evaluation of acute DIC resulting in a diffuse hemorrhagic diathesis (more than three bleeding sites). However, clotting within vessels is extremely important in the pathogenesis of this syndrome. Even in acute DIC, when most clinical manifestations are due to hemorrhage, substantial organ damage may occur from microvascular thrombosis. In settings such as advanced metastatic adenocarcinoma, patients may have veno-occlusive or, more rarely, arterial occlusive disease. This chronic DIC (Trousseau's syndrome) results from slow, continuous activation of clotting, presumably from tissue factor elaboration by tumor with relatively reduced fibrinolysis. Classically, these patients have migratory superficial thrombophlebitis but have varying degrees of thrombocytopenia and circulating fibrin split products (FDP) in plasma. However, excess bleeding may occur when patients are challenged by surgery or ulcer disease. This chronic form of DIC may be accompanied by microangiopathic hemolytic anemia (MAHA). In contrast to the situation displayed in the algorithm, such patients may have short prothrombin (PT) and partial thromboplastin times (PTT). This finding results from activated clotting factors in plasma causing rapid activation of clotting in vitro. It may be difficult to obtain blood from such patients because clotting occurs before calcium chelation can render plasma unclottable.

B. Most patients with DIC are seen in the setting of diffuse bleeding from venipuncture and other sites. Initial screening tests consist of PT, PTT, and platelets. If these tests are normal, bleeding must result from excessive activation of plasmin clot lysis or from platelet dysfunction. Deficiencies of α_2-antiplasmin can cause a lifelong hemorrhagic diathesis. Acquired cases of selective α_2-antiplasmin deficiency have been described. In the future, other acquired deficiencies of fibrinolysis will be documented. Platelet abnormalities are indicated by an abnormal bleeding time and/or abnormal platelet in vitro function.

C. A dramatic, isolated increase in PT sufficient to cause diffuse bleeding indicates an abnormality in the extrinsic pathway. Perform a quick screen for the presence of inhibitors by mixing patient plasma 1:1 with normal, pooled plasma and repeating the test. Correction (usually to within 1.5 seconds) indicates clotting factor deficiency. Failure to correct the PT suggests an acquired inhibitor of coagulation. Such inhibitors are uncommonly detected by the PT, but large quantities of heparin can cause this finding. Much more common are factor deficiencies from liver disease or vitamin K deficiency. In these cases, a 1:1 mix PT should be normal or near normal. Less commonly, surreptitious ingestion of warfarin or previously undetected congenital clotting factor deficiencies may be found.

D. The differential diagnosis for a prolonged PTT is similar, except that this test is much more sensitive to the presence of inhibitors. The most common source of this finding is heparin administration. However, acquired inhibitors of coagulation factors such as factor VIII can cause severe bleeding. The PTT is generally less affected by liver disease and vitamin K deficiency than the PT. Patients with varying degrees of hereditary factor deficiencies, including hemophilia, can have an increased PTT for the first time as adults.

E. Decreased platelets alone can cause severe bleeding, usually mucocutaneous. Myelophthisic processes or aplasia cause severe thrombocytopenia but usually are obvious from other blood findings. Examine the peripheral blood smear for fragmented RBC (MAHA) to rule out thrombotic thrombocytopenic purpura (TTP) or hemolytic uremic syndrome (HUS). MAHA also may occur in DIC but is accompanied by prolonged clotting times and increased FDP, findings absent in TTP. A normal peripheral smear and short clotting times suggest chronic DIC. A normal smear or one with large platelets suggests immune thrombocytopenia, which can be confirmed by assays for specific antiplatelet antibodies.

F. When both PT and PTT are significantly prolonged *and* the platelet count is depressed, DIC is suggested. When the platelet count is normal, consider a primary abnormality in fibrinogen function or amount, liver disease, or vitamin K deficiency.

G. DIC is confirmed by detecting products of fibrin degradation in plasma. The continuous fibrin generation results in secondary activation of plasmin and the generation of FDP. These tests include immunologic assays for FDP and assays for fibrin that has been cross-linked by factor XIII and then subject to plasmin lysis. These D-D dimer fragments are highly specific for clot lysis and correlate closely with other FDP measurements. A dramatic disparity between D-D dimer and other FDP assays suggests the rare syndrome of primary fibrinolysis due to plasminogen activation. Because of clotting factor consumption during DIC, factor VIII

DISSEMINATED INTRAVASCULAR COAGULATION Suspected

(A) Diffuse hemorrhagic diathesis

```
(B) Normal          (C) Increased PT      (D) Increased PTT     (E) Decreased
    PT, PTT,                                                        platelets
    platelets             1:1 PT                1:1 PTT
                                                                    Blood smear
    Clot lysis        Normal    Abnormal    Normal    Abnormal
                                                                 MAHA    RBC normal
    Consider:         Factor    Inhibitor   Factor    Inhibitor
    Fibrinolysis      assays                assays                TTP    Consider:
    abnormality                                                   HUS    Chronic DIC
    Platelet          Factor    Consider:   Factor    Consider:
    abnormality       deficiency Heparin    deficiency Heparin          Platelet
                                antibody               antibody         antibody
                      Consider:  to clotting Consider:  to clotting
                      Vitamin K  factor      Vitamin K  factor            ITP
                      deficiency             deficiency
                      Warfarin
                      ingestion
                      Liver disease
```

(F) Increased PT, PTT

Platelet count

```
        Decreased                    Normal

(G) FDP                      (H) Fibrinogen,
    Fibrinogen,                  thrombin time
    thrombin time                FDP

        DIC                      Consider:
                                 Abnormal fibrinogen
                                 Primary fibrinolysis
                                 Snake bite
                                 Severe liver disease
                                 Vitamin K deficiency
                                 Warfarin ingestion
```

levels usually are depressed and may be used as a confirmatory test. However, factor VIII is an acute-phase reactant and may be near normal in early DIC. Consumption and clotting factor destruction also consumes anticoagulant proteins, such as antithrombin (AT) III and protein C. ATIII levels may be useful as a confirmatory test for DIC but usually are not required. Transfusions of ATIII have been reported to ameliorate clinical manifestations of DIC, but experience is limited. Treatment of DIC is directed at eliminating the underlying process. Without correction of the inciting process, other interventions are unlikely to affect patient outcome.

H. When the PT and PTT are abnormal and platelet counts are normal, assess fibrinogen levels and thrombin time. Reduced levels of factors V, VII, X and fibrinogen, with normal factor VIII levels, suggests severe liver disease. Rarely, plasmin is activated without initiation of clotting. This "primary fibrinolysis" may be seen in patients with liver disease and some cancers. Fibrinogen and fibrin are consumed and FDP thus generated, but other clotting factor levels are normal. However, because clotting is not initiated, fibrin is not cross-linked, and the D-D dimer assay should be normal. Certain snake venoms also contain materials that lyse fibrinogen without

initiating DIC (DIC can also occur with some snake envenomation).

References

Bick RL. Disseminated intravascular coagulation: objective criteria for diagnosis and management. Med Clin North Am 1994; 78:511.

Carr JM, McKinney M, McDonagh J. Diagnosis of disseminated intravascular coagulation: role of D-dimer. Am J Clin Pathol 1989; 91:280.

Dombret H, Scrobohaci ML, Dhorra P, et al. Coagulation disorders associated with acute promyelocytic leukemia: corrective effect of all-*trans* retinoic acid treatment. Leukemia 7:2–9, 1993.

Hathaway WE, Goodnight SH Jr. Disorders of hemostasis and thrombosis: a clinical guide. New York: McGraw-Hill, 1993:219.

Pinzon R, Drewinko B, Trujillo JM, et al. Pancreatic carcinoma and Trousseau's syndrome: experience at a large cancer center. J Clin Oncol 1986; 4:509.

Wilde JT, Kitchen S, Kinsey S, et al. Plasma D-dimer levels and their relationship to serum fibrinogen/fibrin degradation products in hypercoagulable states. Br J Haematol 1989; 71:65.

DEEP VENOUS THROMBOSIS

Guillermo Gonzalez-Osete
Manuel Modiano

Deep venous thrombosis (DVT) is caused by intravascular deposits of predominantly fibrin, RBCs, platelets, and WBC components, accumulating in a vein and producing obstruction to venous outflow and/or vessel wall inflammation. The clinical manifestations depend on the severity of these inflammatory processes. Often the initial sign is a pulmonary embolus (PE).

A. Detailed history taking should look for previous episodes and for inherited disorders of protein C and S deficiency, antithrombin (AT) III deficiency, or an abnormal factor V (factor V_{LEIDEN}). With such deficiencies there is a strong family history of recurrent DVT or PE that presents at an early age; >80% of patients with protein C deficiency have had an episode of DVT or PE by age 40. Patients with ATIII deficiency have a similar presentation and also may have a history of failure to be anticoagulated with heparin. Obtain a complete drug and medication history, including use of estrogen or oral contraceptives. A history of frequent abortions with a prolonged partial thromboplastin time (PTT) should make one suspect a lupus anticoagulant. This also is present in some collagen vascular diseases such as systemic lupus erythematosus (p 452). Surgery that requires >30 minutes and certain surgical procedures (orthopedics; those involving trauma to lower limbs, e.g., knee surgery; urologic; gynecologic) are associated with increased incidence of DVT. Other risk factors are trauma, pregnancy, puerperium, congestive heart failure (CHF), myocardial infarction, cerebrovascular accidents, extremity paralysis, malignancy (especially of prostate or pancreas), obesity, varicose veins, immobilization, use of estrogens, and age. All of these may increase the risk of DVT by stasis and/or increased activation of coagulation.

B. Pain is present in approximately 50% of patients with DVT. Swelling and tenderness to compression also are found in 75% of patients. The clinical diagnosis of DVT is not accurate. Thrombosis does not always produce complete obstruction or inflammation. In 30% of patients who have pain and swelling, there is proven DVT. The classic Homan sign (discomfort in the calf muscles on forced dorsiflexion of the foot) is not sensitive. It is noted in 33% of patients with positive venography and 50% with negative venography. Unilateral swelling associated with discoloration is an important sign that should alert one to the diagnosis.

C. The differential diagnosis includes ruptured Baker's cyst, muscle tear, cramp, hematoma, arthritis, bone disease, varicose veins, and postphlebitic syndrome. If no cause is apparent, consider noninvasive screening.

D. When the history and physical examination suggest DVT, ancillary tests such as noninvasive impedance plethysmography (IPG) and duplex ultrasound or invasive tests such as ^{125}I and contrast xvenography will corroborate the diagnosis. Laboratory tests should include platelet count, prothrombin time (PT), and PTT.

E. Noninvasive diagnostic tests available are IPG and duplex ultrasonography (D-US). IPG is good for detecting proximal vein thrombosis and/or recurrent DVT but is insensitive for detecting nonobstructive proximal thrombosis and calf vein thrombosis. Its sensitivity is 83–93%; its specificity is 83–90%. It must be repeated serially to increase its sensitivity. False-positive results may occur with CHF, postoperative leg swelling, excessive leg tension, or external compression. D-US (sensitivity, 95%; specificity, 98%) is the ideal method of screening patients with suspected DVT. It is good for detecting proximal but not calf vein thrombosis. Calf vein thrombosis usually requires no treatment other than bed rest and elevation of the extremity. In 20–30% of cases, however, the thrombus may extend into the popliteal vein, and full anticoagulation is required because of the increased incidence of PE. Extension into the popliteal system often is missed on initial noninvasive tests but may be seen if the examination is repeated after 3–5 days.

F. ^{125}I with fibrinogen detects fibrin accretion to a thrombus and will be positive with active ongoing clotting. It detects calf vein thrombosis in 90% of cases and proximal vein thrombosis in 60–80%. Fibrinogen carries with it the risks of using any blood product, including allergic reactions and transmittal of infections. It is contraindicated in iodine allergy, pregnancy, and lactation. The combined approach of ^{125}I and IPG was positive in 81 of 86 patients with positive venograms; both tests were negative in 104 of 114 patients who had a negative venogram. This is a useful approach if DVT is suspected clinically and ^{125}I is inconclusive. Venography is the gold standard but is invasive, is not always available, and may not visualize the deep venous system. It may itself cause a DVT.

G. If the diagnosis is confirmed, begin treatment. Standard treatment includes IV or SC heparin, oral anticoagulants, bed rest, and extremity elevation. Patients with protein C deficiency may have skin necrosis and increased sensitivity to warfarin. Start therapy with IV heparin bolus, 5000 U, followed by continuous infusion of heparin, approximately 1000 U/hr or 800–10,000 U SC heparin every 6–8 hours. Monitor activated PTT at 6 hours and thereafter until stabilized at 1.5–2 times control values. Obtain a baseline platelet count and monitor every 3 days while the patient is taking heparin. Begin warfarin sodium on the first day by instituting the estimated daily maintenance dose (5–10 mg). Maintain INR at 2.0–3.0. It usually takes 72–96 hours for the INR to reach this

DEEP VENOUS THROMBOSIS Suspected

(A) History ──────────────→

(B) Physical examination ──────→
    Pain
    Swelling
    Homan's sign:
        Sensitivity 8–10%
        False-positive rate 11–12%

(C) History and physical examination where low probability for DVT

Consider:
    Ruptured Baker's cyst
    Muscle tear
    Hematoma
    Arthritis
    Bone disease
    Varicosities

(D) History and physical examination suspicious for DVT

(E) Noninvasive tests

IPG   D-US

Negative → Repeat tests → Negative / Positive → Therapy

Positive

(F) Invasive tests

125I with Fibrinogen

Negative → IPG or D-US → Positive / Negative

Positive → Calf vein → Follow-up: IPG D-US → Positive → Standard Therapy / Negative → Bed rest Elevation

Venography → Positive → Standard Therapy / Negative

(G) Standard Therapy:
    Bed Rest
    Warfarin
    Heparin

---

range, and heparin should be continued until the INR is at this level. Treatment should last at least 12 weeks.

References

Hommes DW, Bura A, Mazzolai L, et al. Subcutaneous heparin compared with continuous intravenous heparin administration in the initial treatment of deep vein thrombosis: a meta-analysis. Ann Intern Med 1992; 116:279.

Hull R, Raskob G, Pineo G, et al. A comparison of subcutaneous low-molecular-weight heparin with warfarin sodium for prophylaxis against deep-vein thrombosis after hip or knee implantation. N Engl J Med 1993; 329:1370.

Hull RD, Raskob GE, Rosenbloom D, et al. Heparin for 5 days as compared with 10 days in the initial treatment of proximal venous thrombosis. N Engl J Med 1990; 322:1260.

Hyers T, Hull RD, Weg J. Antithrombotic therapy for venous thromboembolic disease. Chest 1989; 95:37s.

Lensing AWA, Hirsh J, Buller HR. Diagnosis of venous thrombosis. In: Colman RW, Hirsh J, Marder VJ, Salzman EW, eds. Hemostasis and thrombosis. 3rd ed. Philadelphia: JB Lippincott, 1994.

Pini M, Pattachini C, Quintavalla R, et al. Subcutaneous vs. intravenous heparin in the treatment of deep venous thrombosis—a randomized clinical trial. Thromb Haemost 1990; 64:222.

Salzman EW, Hirsh J. The epidemiology, pathogenesis, and natural history of venous thrombosis. In: Colman RW, Hirsh J, Marder VJ, Salzman EW, eds. Hemostasis and thrombosis. 3rd ed. Philadelphia: JB Lippincott, 1994.

White R, McGahan JP, Daschbach M, Hartling RP. Diagnosis of deep vein thrombosis using duplex ultrasound. Ann Intern Med 1989; 111:297.

COAGULATION ABNORMALITIES

Manuel Modiano

A. Blood coagulation represents conversion of the soluble plasma protein fibrinogen into an insoluble fibrillar polymer, fibrin. It is the result of complex serial reactions involving procoagulant proteins that circulate in plasma as inert precursors until converted sequentially by specific chain reactions to their active forms. Factors are numbered not by the order in which they become activated, but by the order in which they were discovered. The prothrombin time measures the extrinsic and common pathways of coagulation, including factors VII, X, V, II, and I. The partial thromboplastin time (PTT) measures the intrinsic and common pathways of coagulation, including factors XII, XI, IX, VIII, X, V, II, and I. The thrombin time measures the time it takes to convert fibrinogen to fibrin, the last stage of the common pathway.

B. When confronted with a prolonged PT or PTT, first take a careful history, including previous bleeding or bruising, spontaneously or after surgery or trauma. A family history of bleeding and a complete list of medications being taken (prescription or not) are essential. Confirm that platelets are normal by count and bleeding time (if they are not, see p 224).

C. Patients with a history of bleeding disorders often know the etiologic factors and corrective measures taken in the past. If so, correct the situation as before (if possible, check with patients' regular physician for dosage and type of factor correction) or refer them to a hematologist.

D. When the cause is unknown or when there is no history of bleeding, first confirm the abnormality of the coagulation times, especially if there has been no previous bleeding with trauma or major surgery. Again, a detailed history, including medications, and a full physical examination are essential.

E. When coagulation tests do not correct mixing studies, it usually is because an inhibitor or anticoagulant is present. A correction denotes a deficiency of one or more coagulation factors. Inhibitors are either antibodies directed to specific factors (e.g., factor VIII or factor IX antobody) or an antiphospholipid antibody (lupuslike antibody) directed to phospholipid. Inhibition can also occur from a drug such as heparin or protamine, but it is usually known when these substances are present.

(Continued on page 222)

Patient with ABNORMAL COAGULATION TESTS

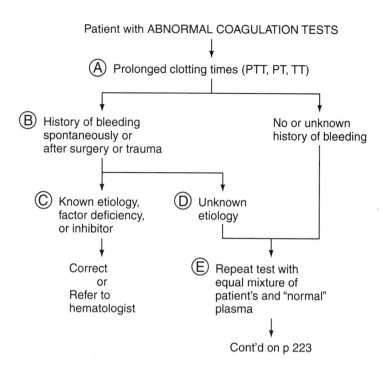

Ⓐ Prolonged clotting times (PTT, PT, TT)

Ⓑ History of bleeding spontaneously or after surgery or trauma

No or unknown history of bleeding

Ⓒ Known etiology, factor deficiency, or inhibitor

Ⓓ Unknown etiology

Correct
or
Refer to
hematologist

Ⓔ Repeat test with equal mixture of patient's and "normal" plasma

Cont'd on p 223

F. An isolated prolonged PT that corrects with mixing suggests a factor VII deficiency, and this factor can then be measured directly. If no correction on mixing with normal plasma, there is likely an inhibitor present, most likely a lupuslike inhibitor; however, a specific factor antibody could also be present. Specific assays for a lupuslike inhibitor are available.

G. An isolated prolonged PTT that corrects with mixing suggests one or more factor deficiencies (VIII, IX, XI, or XII). An inherited deficiency is often of a single factor, whereas multiple-factor deficiencies are usually acquired (e.g., liver disease). No correction suggests a lupus or specific inhibitor. Factor VIII deficiency (classic hemophilia A) is an X-linked inherited disorder that affects only males clinically; females are carriers. It is the most common severe coagulation disorder. Coordinate treatment with an experienced hematologist, but emergency replacement can be done with FFP, cryoprecipitate, or factor VIII concentrates. Von Willebrand's disease is the most common and most heterogeneous of heritable defects of coagulation. It arises from a qualitative or quantitative deficiency of the adhesive glycoprotein, von Willebrand factor (vWF) that is required for platelet adhesion. It serves as a carrier protein for factor VIII and stabilizes factor VIII in the plasma. vWF is an autosomal-dominant disorder with its gene located on chromosome 12. Last, factor IX deficiency (hemophilia B) is an X-linked disorder that is indistinguishable from factor VIII disease clinically, but it is treated with FFP or with factor IX concentrates.

H. A prolonged thrombin time (TT) is often caused by small amounts of heparin that many patients receive in the hospital; therefore a Reptilase Time (RT) may be done to exclude heparin. Reptilase is a thrombinlike enzyme from a particular snake venom that is not inhibited by heparin. If both the TT and RT are prolonged, the abnormality is from a low fibrinogen or the presence of fibrinogen degradation products (FDPs), a paraprotein, or an abnormal fibrinogen molecule, all of which can be measured directly.

I. When both the PT and PTT are prolonged, the same reasoning can be applied as discussed for each individual test, except that multiple factors in multiple pathways may be deficient (inhibitor mix corrects) or may be inhibited (inhibitor mix does not correct). Again, specific factors can be assayed directly and potential causes considered as indicated in the decision tree.

References

Ey FS, Goodnight SH. Bleeding disorders in cancer. Semin Oncol 1990; 17:187.

Jandl JH. Disorders of coagulation. In: Blood: textbook of hematology. 2nd ed. Philadelphia: Lippincott-Raven, 1996.

Levine M, Hirsh J. The diagnosis and treatment of thrombosis in the cancer patient. Semin Oncol 1990; 17:160.

Patterson WP. Coagulation and cancer: an overview. Semin Oncol 1990; 17:137.

Patterson WP, Caldwell CW, Doll DC. Hyperviscosity syndromes and coagulopathies. Semin Oncol 1990; 17:210.

Patterson WP, Ringenberg QS. The pathophysiology of thrombosis in cancer. Semin Oncol 1990; 17:140.

Rapaport S. Preoperative hemostatic evaluation: which tests, if any? Blood 1983; 61:229.

Schaffer AI. The hypercoagulable states. Ann Intern Med 1985; 102:814.

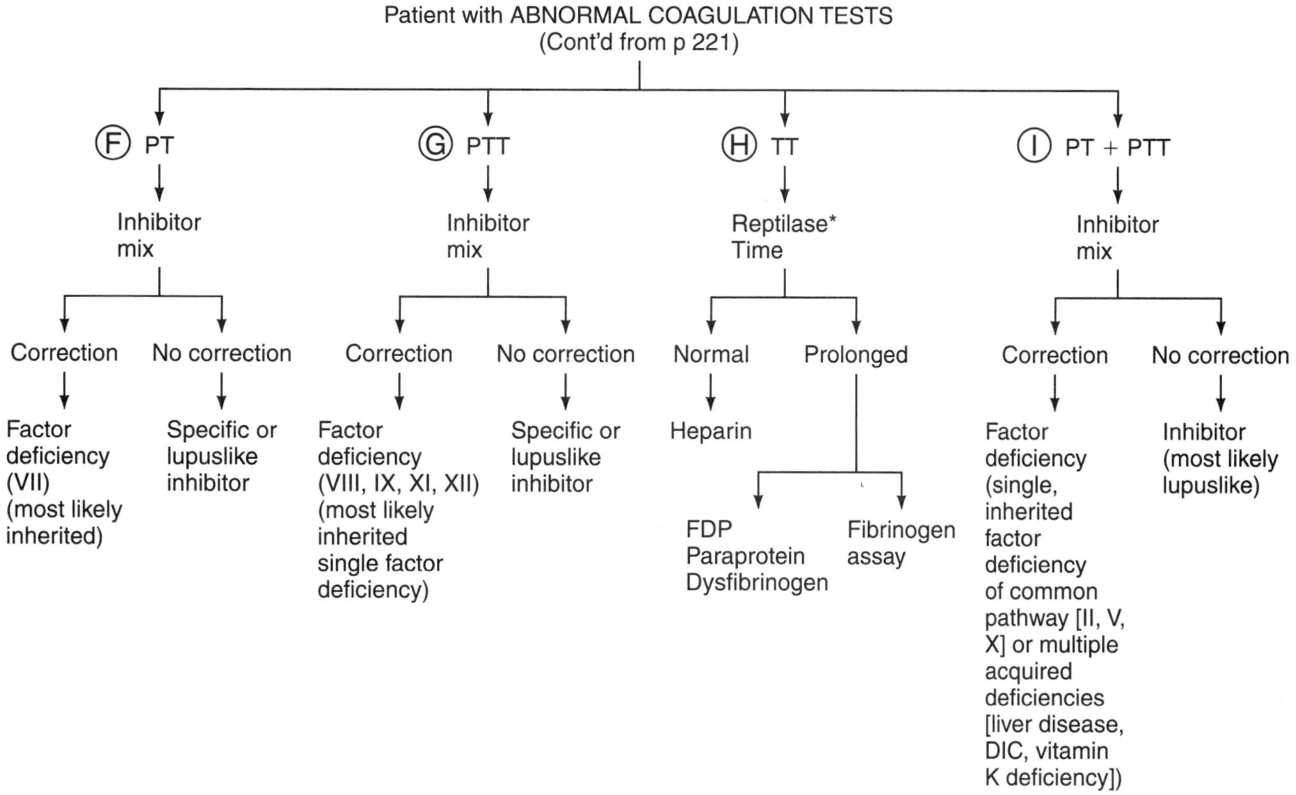

Patient with ABNORMAL COAGULATION TESTS
(Cont'd from p 221)

(F) PT

Inhibitor mix

Correction
↓
Factor deficiency (VII) (most likely inherited)

No correction
↓
Specific or lupuslike inhibitor

(G) PTT

Inhibitor mix

Correction
↓
Factor deficiency (VIII, IX, XI, XII) (most likely inherited single factor deficiency)

No correction
↓
Specific or lupuslike inhibitor

(H) TT

Reptilase* Time

Normal
↓
Heparin

Prolonged
↓

FDP
Paraprotein
Dysfibrinogen

Fibrinogen assay

(I) PT + PTT

Inhibitor mix

Correction
↓
Factor deficiency (single, inherited factor deficiency of common pathway [II, V, X] or multiple acquired deficiencies [liver disease, DIC, vitamin K deficiency])

No correction
↓
Inhibitor (most likely lupuslike)

TRANSFUSION THERAPY: PLATELETS

June Clements

Platelet concentrates (PCs) are obtained either from a unit of whole blood (random-donor unit, RDP) or by apheresis (single-donor apheresis unit, SDP). One SDP provides about the same number of platelets as seven RDPs. Platelets are appropriate for transfusion in situations of significant bleeding with a dangerously low platelet count. The risk of serious hemorrhage is low with a platelet count >20,000/µl. Some authors do not advocate transfusion until counts are <15,000 or even 10,000/µl. Platelet counts of 60,000–70,000/µl may be necessary for biopsy and/or surgery.

The dosage of PCs depends on the patient's size and clinical disorder. In adults, one RDP should increase the platelet count by 5000–10,000/µl. The dose is one RDP per 10 kg body weight, or one SDP. A 1-hour post-transfusion platelet count is important to assess the response. The following formula provides a corrected count increment:

$$\frac{\text{Absolute platelet count increment} \times \text{Body surface area (m}^2)}{\text{No. of platelets transfused} \times 10^{11}}$$

A poor response to transfused platelets may be due to alloimmunization, infection, sepsis, drugs, or splenomegaly. Repeated platelet transfusions may necessitate SDPs, which reduce exposure to platelet antigens and decrease the rate of alloimmunization. Previous transfusions and pregnancy may stimulate HLA and antiplatelet antibodies, in which case HLA-matched platelets may be necessary. Leukocyte filters seem to decrease HLA immunization. ABO-incompatible platelets may have a shortened blood survival. It is worth trying ABO-compatible PC for type O patients whose counts are refractory to unselected PC.

A. With spontaneous or excessive bleeding and a normal platelet count, suspect functional platelet disorder or factor deficiency. Use appropriate laboratory tests to differentiate between these two. If abnormal platelet function is suspected, examine a blood smear to assess platelet morphology. This may aid in the diagnosis of a hereditary platelet disorder. In such disorders, transfuse filtered SDP to decrease alloimmunization. Platelet transfusions are ineffective in uremic patients.

B. Platelet transfusions often are necessary to control bleeding in patients with decreased platelet production. Start with a dose of one RDP per 10 kg. In patients who may require long-term treatment, such as patients with aplastic anemia or leukemia, and transplantation patients, use SDP units with leukocyte filters to decrease alloimmunization.

C. Transfused platelets usually have a short survival in patients with increased platelet destruction. Treat the underlying cause of the thrombocytopenia. However, with life-threatening bleeding or anticipated surgery, give platelet transfusions. Begin with one RDP per 10 kg or one SDP and follow up according to clinical and platelet response. Do not give PCs in thrombotic thrombocytopenic purpura (TTP) and hemolytic uremic syndrome (HUS).

References

Bishop JF, McGrath K, Wolf MM, et al. Clinical factors influencing the efficacy of pooled platelet transfusions. Blood 1988; 71:383.

Bolan CD, Alving BM. Pharmacologic agents in management of bleeding disorders. Transfusion 1990; 30:541.

George JM, Shattil SJ. The clinical importance of acquired abnormalities of platelet function. N Engl J Med 1991; 324:27.

Harker LA, Malposs TW, Branson HE, et al. Mechanism of abnormal bleeding in patients undergoing cardiopulmonary bypass: acquired transient platelet dysfunction associated with selective alpha-granule release. Blood 1980; 56:824.

Kaplan BS, Proesmans W. Hemolytic uremic syndrome of childhood and its variants. Semin Hematol 1987; 24:148.

Webb IJ, Anderson KC. Transfusion support in acute leukemias. Semin Oncol 1997; 24:141.

Welborn JL, Emrick P, Acevedo M. Rapid improvement of thrombotic thrombocytopenic purpura with vincristine and plasmapheresis. Am J Hematol 1990; 35:18.

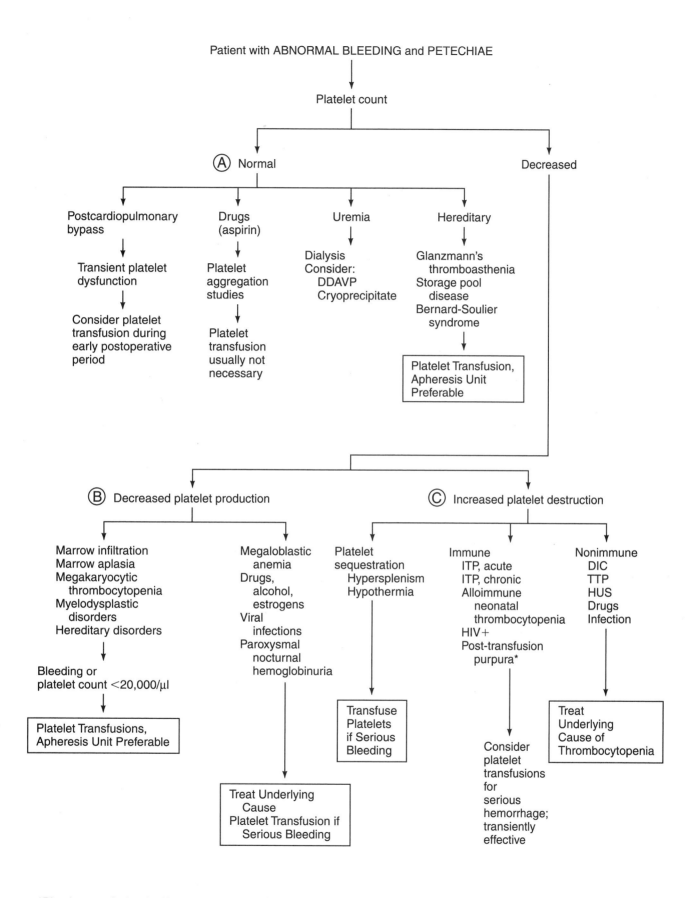

Patient with ABNORMAL BLEEDING and PETECHIAE

Platelet count

A Normal

Decreased

Postcardiopulmonary bypass

Transient platelet dysfunction

Consider platelet transfusion during early postoperative period

Drugs (aspirin)

Platelet aggregation studies

Platelet transfusion usually not necessary

Uremia

Dialysis Consider: DDAVP Cryoprecipitate

Hereditary

Glanzmann's thromboasthenia Storage pool disease Bernard-Soulier syndrome

Platelet Transfusion, Apheresis Unit Preferable

B Decreased platelet production

Marrow infiltration
Marrow aplasia
Megakaryocytic thrombocytopenia
Myelodysplastic disorders
Hereditary disorders

Bleeding or platelet count <20,000/µl

Platelet Transfusions, Apheresis Unit Preferable

Megaloblastic anemia
Drugs, alcohol, estrogens
Viral infections
Paroxysmal nocturnal hemoglobinuria

Treat Underlying Cause Platelet Transfusion if Serious Bleeding

C Increased platelet destruction

Platelet sequestration
Hypersplenism
Hypothermia

Transfuse Platelets if Serious Bleeding

Immune
ITP, acute
ITP, chronic
Alloimmune neonatal thrombocytopenia
HIV+
Post-transfusion purpura*

Consider platelet transfusions for serious hemorrhage; transiently effective

Nonimmune
DIC
TTP
HUS
Drugs
Infection

Treat Underlying Cause of Thrombocytopenia

*Platelet transfusion ineffective.

TRANSFUSION THERAPY: RED BLOOD CELLS

June Clements

RBCs are prepared from a collection of whole blood by removal of plasma. This leaves 250–350 ml RBCs with a hematocrit of 70–75%, containing about 2×10^9 leukocytes. The maximum storage time is 42 days at 1°–6° C.

Transfuse RBCs to increase oxygen-carrying capacity or to replace acute blood loss. One unit should increase the hemoglobin in an adult 1 g/dl or increase the hematocrit by 3%. For immunocompromised patients, irradiated RBCs can prevent transfusion-associated graft-versus-host disease. Directed-donor components from first-degree relatives should also be irradiated regardless of the recipient's immune status (see p 228).

The removal of leukocytes by passage through special filters inhibits HLA alloimmunization for patients who will need future platelet support or transplantation. Leukocyte filters can reduce transfused white cells by 99–99.9%. Leukocyte filters also prevent febrile reactions and possibly transfusion-transmitted cytomegalovirus (CMV) infection.

A. Acute hemorrhage from trauma or GI bleeding may require transfusion of RBCs along with crystalloid solutions.

B. Anemia is not in itself a reason to transfuse RBCs. In patients with chronic anemia, hemoglobins of 6–7 g/dl may be well tolerated. If the patient has clinical signs and symptoms not amenable to specific therapy, transfuse RBCs. Patients with chronic renal failure may respond to erythropoietin therapy. In patients with asymptomatic anemia, investigate and treat the cause. In patients with hemolytic anemia, investigate the cause and treat accordingly. In hereditary hemolytic conditions such as hereditary spherocytosis, splenectomy may be advantageous.

C. Premature infants with compromised pulmonary function may need a hematocrit >40% for adequate oxygen-carrying capacity. Also, in transfusing these infants, consider using either CMV-negative blood components or leukocyte filters.

D. For elective surgery, autologous transfusions (the patient's own blood) are increasingly popular, largely because of increased public awareness of transfusion-associated diseases. Several units of autologous blood can be drawn in the weeks before surgery. Donor restrictions are not as stringent as for homologous blood donations. If the surgery is delayed, give the patient's older units back and draw new ones for surgery ("leap-frogging"). Operative blood salvage techniques involve collection of blood lost during surgery (if the surgical field is sterile) and its return to the patient during or after the procedure.

References

Anderson KC, Weinstein HJ. Transfusion-associated graft versus host disease. N Engl J Med 1990; 323:315.

Eslev AJ. Erythropoietin. N Engl J Med 1991; 324:1339.

Grindon AJ, Tomasulo PS, Bergin JJ, et al. The hospital transfusion committee. JAMA 1985; 253:540.

Legler TJ, Fischer I, Dittmann J, et al. Frequency and causes of refractoriness in multiple transfused patients. Ann Hematol 1997; 74:185.

National Heart, Lung and Blood Institute Expert Panel on the use of Autologous Blood. Transfusion alert: use of autologous blood. Transfusion 1995; 35:703.

RED BLOOD CELL TRANSFUSION Considered

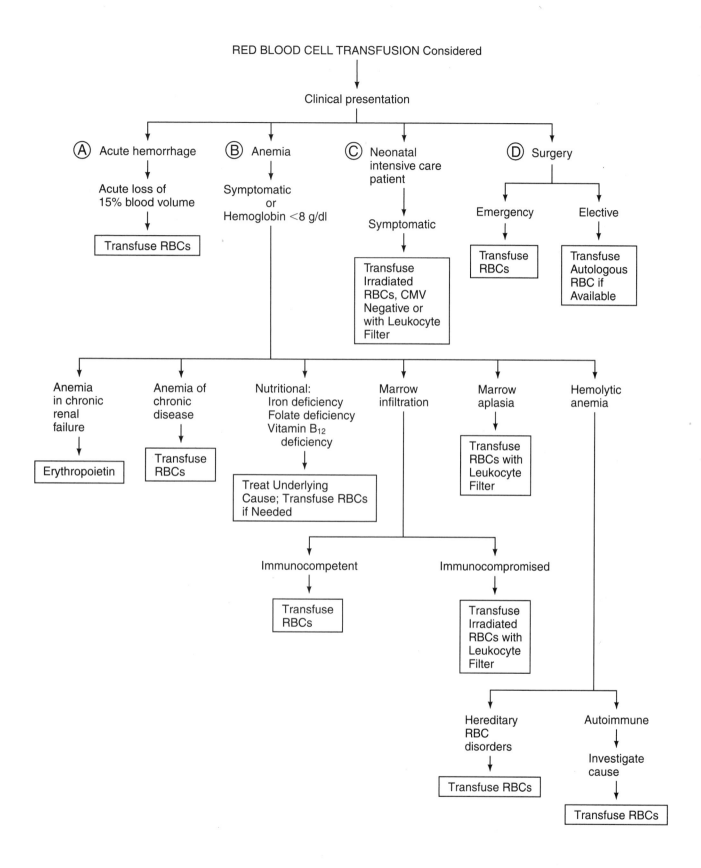

TRANSFUSION THERAPY: GRANULOCYTES

June Clements

Granulocytes are collected by leukapheresis and stored at room temperature. Each concentrate should contain at least 10^{10} granulocytes for a minimal dose of 1.4×10^8/kg for a 70-kg person, which approximates 10% of the daily neutrophil production in a noninfected person. Donors premedicated with corticosteroids provide more neutrophils. Perform transfusion of granulocytes as soon as possible after collection, at least within the first 24 hours.

A. One indication for granulocyte transfusion is an absolute neutrophil count <500/µl in an infected patient. If the count is >1000/µl, granulocyte transfusions are not useful except for abnormal neutrophil function (e.g., chronic granulomatous disease).

B. In neutropenic patients, local or systemic infection justifies granulocyte transfusions, particularly in gram-negative sepsis. However, granulocytes are not useful for fungal infections and may cause complications in persons taking amphotericin B. Prophylactic granulocyte transfusions are not appropriate in uninfected neutropenic patients because adverse effects are likely to exceed the benefits. For example, alloimmunization may compromise future effectiveness of granulocytes, platelets, and bone marrow transplantation. Patients with transient neutropenia and normal bone marrow production are not candidates for granulocyte transfusions. Give appropriate antibiotics to such patients. Patients who are persistently neutropenic with decreased bone marrow production may respond to therapeutic granulocyte transfusions. This is particularly effective in neonatal sepsis with neutropenia and decreased bone marrow reserve.

C. Transfuse granulocytes with caution. A concentrate of granulocytes contains 15–50 ml RBCs and therefore *should be ABO compatible* with the recipient. If not ABO compatible, the RBCs should be removed from the concentrate. Possible adverse reactions include fever, transient hypotension, pulmonary infiltrates, graft-versus-host disease, and various infections (e.g., cytomegalovirus, hepatitis, HIV). In adults, give a trial of antibiotics first if the patient is stable. If there is no improvement, give granulocytes. An adult dosage is one unit of concentrate every 24 hours.

D. If neutrophil dysfunction is suspected, neutrophil function studies may be helpful to characterize any deficiency. Give antibiotics if bacterial infection is present. If there is no improvement, transfuse granulocytes.

References

Dutcher JP. The potential benefit of granulocyte transfusion therapy. Cancer Invest 1989; 7:457.

Huestis DW. The neutrophil in transfusion medicine. Transfusion 1994; 34:630.

Huestis DW, Bove JR, Case J. Practical blood transfusion. 4th ed. Boston: Little, Brown, 1988:337.

Menitove JE, Abrams RA. Granulocyte transfusions in neutropenic patients. Crit Rev Oncol Hematol 1987; 7:89.

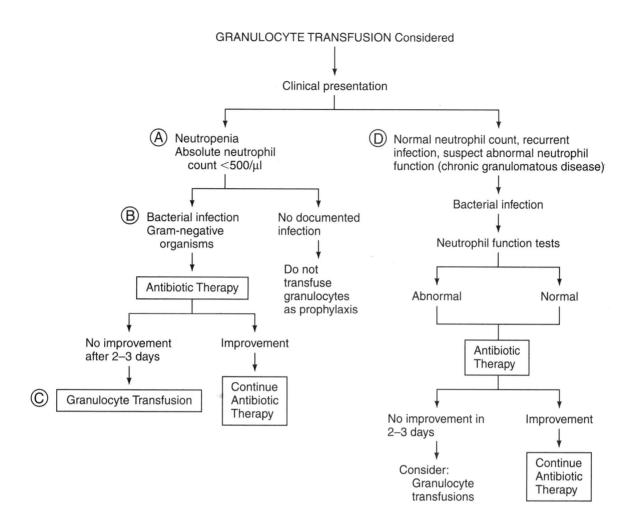

GRANULOCYTE TRANSFUSION Considered

↓

Clinical presentation

(A) Neutropenia
Absolute neutrophil
count <500/µl

(B) Bacterial infection
Gram-negative
organisms

No documented
infection

↓

Antibiotic Therapy

Do not
transfuse
granulocytes
as prophylaxis

No improvement
after 2–3 days

Improvement

(C) Granulocyte Transfusion

Continue
Antibiotic
Therapy

(D) Normal neutrophil count, recurrent
infection, suspect abnormal neutrophil
function (chronic granulomatous disease)

↓

Bacterial infection

↓

Neutrophil function tests

Abnormal   Normal

Antibiotic
Therapy

No improvement in
2–3 days

Improvement

Consider:
Granulocyte
transfusions

Continue
Antibiotic
Therapy

TRANSFUSION REACTIONS AND COMPLICATIONS

June Clements

Transfusion can cause numerous adverse effects. Besides an immediate reaction to various blood components, there also are infectious complications. These include viral hepatitis (90% due to hepatitis C), cytomegalovirus, malaria, syphilis, and HIV. Current screening methods minimize the transmission of such infections. If any adverse reactions occur, stop the transfusion and notify the responsible physician and the blood bank. Recheck the identification of blood and patient at once. Draw a new blood sample and send it with the remaining blood component to the blood bank. The laboratory examines the patient's pre- and post-transfusion serum for evidence of hemolysis, checks the blood types, and does a direct antiglobulin test on the post-transfusion sample.

A. Fever during transfusion may indicate a febrile non-hemolytic reaction, bacterial contamination, noncardiogenic pulmonary edema, or a hemolytic reaction, or may be coincidental. A febrile nonhemolytic reaction is a rise in temperature of 1° C or more. Most occur in previously transfused patients or multiparous women and probably are caused by leukocyte antibodies in the recipient. Febrile reactions can be treated by antipyretics and prevented by leukocyte filters. Bacterial contamination causes sudden high fever, chills, and shock, requiring emergency therapy. Fever and chills may also signify a hemolytic transfusion reaction, usually caused by ABO discrepancies. These reactions may be fatal. A hemolytic transfusion reaction can be due to either intravascular (most often ABO incompatibility) or extravascular (e.g., Rh and other antibodies) RBC destruction. In any case, stop the transfusion and start supportive care immediately.

B. Allergic reactions usually involve itching, hives, and erythema, without fever, caused by reaction to plasma proteins. Stop the transfusion. If the reaction is mild, give an antihistamine. If the hives resolve, the transfusion may be continued. Anaphylactic reactions occasionally occur in IgA-deficient persons.

C. Elderly patients of small body size and those with underlying cardiopulmonary disease sometimes develop congestive heart failure because of volume overload. Symptomatic treatment usually is enough, but occasionally phlebotomy is necessary. Give subsequent transfusions slowly and consider concomitant diuresis.

D. Delayed hemolytic transfusion reaction generally is due to an anamnestic antibody response to certain transfused red cell antigens. This usually does not require clinical support, but the cause of decreasing hemoglobin needs to be identified. Post-transfusion purpura, caused by an antiplatelet antibody response, is rare. Give supportive care and control any bleeding.

References

Brubaker DB. Clinical significance of white cell antibodies in febrile nonhemolytic transfusion reactions. Transfusion 1990; 30:733.

Sazama K. Reports of 355 transfusion-associated deaths: 1976 through 1985. Transfusion 1990; 30:583.

Seeger W, Schneider V, Kreusler B, et al. Reproduction of transfusion-related acute lung injury in an ex vivo lung model. Blood 1990; 76:1438.

Vengelen-Tyler V, ed. Technical manual. 12th ed. Bethesda, MD: American Association of Blood Banks, 1996.

Patient has TRANSFUSION REACTION

↓

Clinical presentation

```
        ┌──────────────────────────────┬────────────────────┬──────────────────┐
   Ⓐ Fever                        Ⓑ Urticaria         Ⓒ Overload      Ⓓ Delayed
                                                                         anemia
```

Ⓐ Fever

High fever Shock Shaking chills	Fever Chills	Fever Chills Back pain Shock Dyspnea Bleeding	Acute respiratory distress Chills Fever

High fever / Shock / Shaking chills
↓
Stop transfusion
↓
No laboratory evidence of acute hemolysis
↓
Consider: Bacterial contamination
↓
Send Donor Blood for Culture Antibiotics Supportive Care

Fever / Chills
↓
Stop transfusion
↓
No laboratory evidence of acute hemolysis
↓
Febrile reaction to donor leukocyte antigens
↓
Prevention: Antipyretic Consider: Leukocyte Filter Washed RBCs

Fever / Chills / Back pain / Shock / Dyspnea / Bleeding
↓
Stop transfusion
↓
Laboratory evidence of acute hemolysis
↓
Hemolytic transfusion reaction to red cell antigens
↓
Maintain: Renal Blood Flow Maintain: Blood Pressure and Blood Volume Consult: Nephrologist

Acute respiratory distress / Chills / Fever
↓
Stop transfusion
↓
No laboratory evidence of acute hemolysis
↓
Reaction to donor leukocyte antigens or Donor plasma antibodies reacting to recipient leukocyte antigens
↓
Supportive Care Prevention: Leukocyte Filters Washed RBCs

Ⓑ Urticaria

Urticaria / Pruritus
↓
Stop transfusion
↓
No laboratory evidence of acute hemolysis
↓
Allergic transfusion reaction to plasma proteins
↓
Prevention: Antihistamines Washed RBCs

Sudden-onset respiratory distress / Shock / Urticaria
↓
Stop transfusion
↓
No laboratory evidence of acute hemolysis
↓
IgA-deficient recipient with anaphylactic reaction to donor plasma IgA
↓
Prevention: Use Components from IgA-Deficient Donors Autologous Blood

Ⓒ Overload

Dyspnea / Cyanosis in a patient with compromised cardiovascular system
↓
Stop transfusion
↓
Volume overload
↓
Supportive Care Diuretic Consider: Phlebotomy O₂

Ⓓ Delayed anemia

Jaundice, unresolved anemia hours to days post-transfusion
↓
Anamnestic response to RBC antigens
↓
Usually no specific treatment needed

HODGKIN'S DISEASE

Carol S. Portlock

Hodgkin's disease typically presents with progressive, non-tender, rubbery lymphadenopathy in supraclavicular, cervical, axillary, or occasionally inguinal regions. Most commonly, patients are 15–35 years of age. Mediastinal adenopathy may be detected incidentally or may lead to symptoms of cough and/or shortness of breath.

A. The diagnosis usually is made on lymph node biopsy; extranodal sites may be confirmatory. The pathology should be reviewed by an expert hematopathologist to rule out benign causes or non-Hodgkin's lymphoma.

B. The following baseline studies are performed in all patients to assess clinical stages: (1) CBC, platelet count; (2) ESR; (3) liver enzymes; (4) serum alkaline phosphatase; (5) renal function tests; (6) chest radiograph (Figure 1); (7) CT of chest, abdomen, and pelvis; (8) lymphography, if abdominal and pelvic CT is equivocal or negative (Figure 2); and (9) bone marrow biopsy.

C. Consider staging laparotomy rarely, only in those patients without favorable features and who are not candidates for combined modality treatment.

D. Radiation therapy may be used without staging laparotomy in designated favorable clinical presentations. If not clearly favorable, staging laparotomy is required when primary irradiation is used. Radiation therapy usually includes mantle and paraaortic fields with doses of 3500–4400 cGy.

E. Because systemic chemotherapy is indicated in all patients with large mediastinal masses and in those with stages IB, IIB, IIIA, IIIB, IVA, and IVB, no staging laparotomy is performed. Treatment is based on clinical staging only. Moreover, in those patients with clinical stage IA and IIA Hodgkin's disease and unfavorable characteristics, combined chemotherapy/radiotherapy is usually used.

F. Combination chemotherapy is indicated in all clinically staged patients as well as those who have been pathologically staged and found to have advanced disease. The standard combination chemotherapy for advanced Hodgkin's disease or as chemotherapy in a combined modality regimen is ABVD (Adriamycin, bleomycin, vinblastine, and dacarbazine).

G. Radiation therapy is given after combination chemotherapy in all stage I and II patients. All patients with large mediastinal masses (>0.3 × the transverse chest diameter) should receive combined modality therapy.

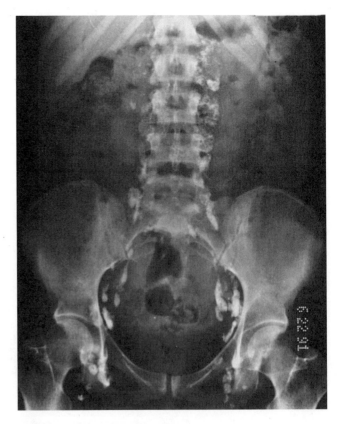

Figure 1 Mediastinal mass >0.3 × the chest diameter.

Figure 2 Abnormal lymphogram in a patient with Hodgkin's disease.

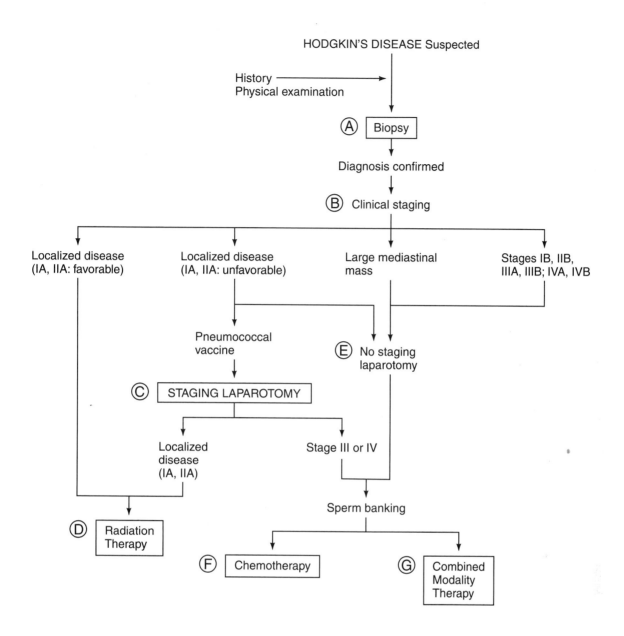

HODGKIN'S DISEASE Suspected

History
Physical examination

(A) Biopsy

Diagnosis confirmed

(B) Clinical staging

Localized disease
(IA, IIA: favorable)

Localized disease
(IA, IIA: unfavorable)

Large mediastinal
mass

Stages IB, IIB,
IIIA, IIIB; IVA, IVB

Pneumococcal
vaccine

(E) No staging
laparotomy

(C) STAGING LAPAROTOMY

Localized
disease
(IA, IIA)

Stage III or IV

Sperm banking

(D) Radiation
Therapy

(F) Chemotherapy

(G) Combined
Modality
Therapy

References

Banks PM. The pathology of Hodgkin's disease. Semin Oncol 1990; 17:683.

Canellos GP. Current strategies for early Hodgkin's disease. Ann Oncol 1996; 7(Suppl 4):91.

Canellos GP, Anderson JR, Propert KJ, et al. Chemotherapy of advanced Hodgkin's disease with MOPP, ABVD, or MOPP alternating with ABVD. N Engl J Med 1992; 327:1478.

Duggan D, Petroni G, Johnson K, et al. MOPP/ABV versus ABVD for advanced Hodgkin's disease—a preliminary report of CALGB 8952 (with SWOG, ECOG, NCIC). Proc Am Soc Clin Oncol 1997; 16:12a.

Leibenhaut MH, Hoppe FT, Efron B. Prognostic indicators of laparotomy findings in clinical stage I, II supradiaphragmatic Hodgkin's disease. J Clin Oncol 1989; 7:81.

Lester TA, Crowther D: Staging for Hodgkin's disease. Semin Oncol 1990; 17:696.

Mauch PM. Management of early stage Hodgkin's disease: the role of radiation therapy and/or chemotherapy. Ann Oncol 1996; 7(Suppl 4):79.

CHRONIC MYELOGENOUS LEUKEMIA

Robert M. Rifkin

Chronic myelogenous leukemia (CML) accounts for about 20% of all leukemias with a death rate of 1.5/100,000 persons per year. The total annual incidence in the United States is approximately 4000 cases per year. The median age of onset is 60 years, but CML may occur at any age. CML results from the malignant transformation of a single cell, yet the causative factors remain unknown. Exposure to ionizing radiation can increase the incidence, but no chemical leukemogens have been identified. Manifestations of CML result from the unrestrained proliferation of granulocytes. Classically, the disease pursues a triphasic course. The chronic phase, which usually lasts 3–5 years, features mild constitutional symptoms that vanish with therapy. The cytogenetic hallmark of CML is the Philadelphia (Ph) chromosome. This product of an unequal reciprocal translocation, t(9;22)(q34:q11), is found in 95% of all CML patients. During the formation of the Ph chromosome, the bulk of the abl-proto-oncogene situated on the long arm of chromosome 9 is detached and translocated onto the fractured genetic locus on 22q–. Transposition of the abl-oncogene to the breakpoint cluster region (bcr) of chromosome 22 creates a chimeric bcr-abl gene. The protein product of the chimeric gene is a 210 kB fusion protein, a tyrosine kinase, and is believed to be a transforming growth factor. CML next evolves into an accelerated phase that becomes resistant to drug therapy. The final or acute phase (blast crisis) resembles acute myeloid leukemia. It exhibits a complex karyotype and pursues a course identical to acute myeloid leukemia. However, this blast crisis is extremely refractory to treatment.

A. Most patients with CML present in the chronic phase with lethargy, symptoms of anemia, or splenomegaly. Sweating and moderate weight loss are common, but fevers are rare in this phase. The most common physical finding is splenomegaly (85% of patients). The size of the spleen is thought to correlate with disease duration. As patients see physicians more often for routine health maintenance, splenomegaly is decreasing in incidence. Hepatomegaly may be noted in up to 50% of patients. Febrile neutrophilia and a dermatosis (Sweet's syndrome) with painful maculonodular violaceous lesions can occur. As the disease transforms, fever, night sweats, weight loss, and bone pain often occur and predominate. Rarely, patients may present in de novo blast crisis.

B. At presentation, the leukocyte count is usually 35,000–300,000/µl but may be >500,000/µl. Thrombocytosis is observed in about one third of cases. Anemia usually is a feature of untreated CML. The observed leukocytosis displays the full spectrum of maturing myeloid cells. Basophilia and eosinophilia are common. Nucleated RBCs often are present and help define the leukoerythroblastic reaction characteristic of CML.

C. Increased levels of uric acid occur in untreated CML but seldom cause problems. Elevated levels of vitamin B_{12} and vitamin B_{12}-binding capacity are common. About 15% of patients have signs or symptoms referable to hyperleukocytosis as a result of vascular flow impedance when the WBC is >300,000/µl. The leukocyte alkaline phosphate (LAP) score usually is decreased in CML. In the past, the LAP was considered a useful diagnostic test because it usually was elevated in other myeloproliferative disorders and infection. However, this test has largely been replaced by the polymerase chain assay for bcr-abl.

D. Bone marrow is hypercellular because of granulocytic hyperplasia with an M/E ratio often >25:1. Mitotic figures are observed easily, and megakaryocyte numbers often are increased with dysplasia. The most commonly observed cell in the bone marrow is the myelocyte. Sea-blue histiocytes resembling Gaucher cells also are present. Marrow fibrosis may be evident and is a poor prognostic feature. In the accelerated phase, ≥20% blasts plus promyelocytes are observed, and in the acute phase, ≥30% blasts plus promyelocytes are observed in the blood or bone marrow. The karyotype of the marrow may serve as a valuable guide to disease progression because a more complex karyotype (more than just the Ph chromosome) is observed as the disease progresses. The bone marrow also may be analyzed for the presence of bcr-abl, and this can be a valuable tool for monitoring the response to therapy and searching for minimal residual disease.

E. Once the diagnosis of CML is established, the triphasic course of the illness must be thoroughly discussed with the patient and an overall therapeutic strategy formulated. The initial objectives of therapy are to alleviate symptoms and to prevent complications. This can be accomplished with hydroxyurea and/or α-interferon. Allopurinol should be given before the institution of therapy to treat hyperuricemia and continued until the WBC count normalizes. Recently the combination of cytarabine arabinoside and hydroxyurea has been found to be extremely effective. Therapy with Busulfan is now reserved for the elderly. The possibility of bone marrow transplantation (BMT) is also evaluated during the initial phases of therapy.

F. In patients ≤60 years of age with a histocompatible sibling, allogeneic stem cell transplantation within 12 months of diagnosis is the preferred treatment. If a sibling donor is unavailable, begin therapy with hydroxyurea to control leukocytosis and symptoms. α-Interferon alone or in combination with cytarabine is then used in an attempt to induce a hematologic remission (normalization of peripheral blood counts) and a cytogenetic response (suppression of the Ph chromosome). This generally requires 6–12 months of therapy. If a cytogenetic remission is achieved, continue interferon therapy. If no remission is observed, consider either an autologous

CHRONIC MYELOGENOUS LEUKEMIA Suspected

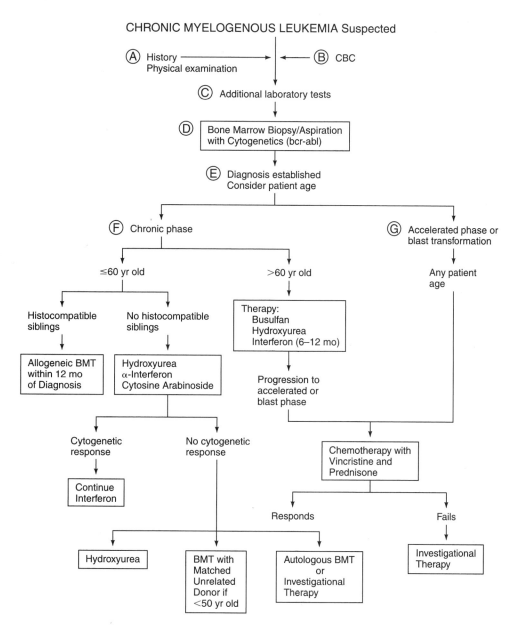

stem cell transplant or a matched-unrelated donor stem cell transplant.

G. Management of the patient with blast crisis must be individualized. If a lymphoblastic transformation is identified (positive tdT), vincristine and prednisone therapy have a 60% initial response rate. If a myeloid transformation (negative tdT) is identified, it usually does not respond to this treatment, and results with conventional leukemia treatment regimens have been dismal. Investigational therapy on a research protocol is strongly suggested in this setting.

References

Giulhot F, Dreyfus B, Brizard A, et al. Cytogenetic remission in chronic myelogenous leukemia using interferon alpha-2a and hydroxyurea with or without low-dose cytosine arabinoside. Leuk Lymphoma 1991; 4:49.

Hehlmann R, Heimpel H, Hasford J, et al. Randomized comparison of busulfan and hydroxyurea in chronic myelogenous leukemia: prolongation of survival by hydroxyurea. Blood 1993; 82:398.

Jandl JH. Chronic myeloproliferative syndromes. In: Jandl JH, ed. Blood—textbook of hematology. 2nd ed. Boston: Little, Brown, 1996:903.

Kantarjian HM, Deisseroth A, Kurzrock R, et al. Chronic myelogenous leukemia: a concise update. Blood 1993; 82:691.

Lichtman MA. Chronic myelogenous leukemia and related disorders. In: Beutler E, Lichtman MA, Coller B, Kipps TJ. William's hematology. 5th ed. New York: McGraw-Hill, 1995:298.

McGlave P, Bartoch G, Anasetti C, et al. Unrelated donor marrow transplantation therapy for chronic myelogenous leukemia. Blood 1993; 81:543.

ABNORMAL SERUM PROTEIN ELECTROPHORESIS

Antonio C. Buzaid
Donna Weber

Monoclonal gammopathy is the presence of a monoclonal protein (M protein) in the serum or urine. It consists of one of the immunoglobulins, a heavy chain, and/or a light chain. Biclonal gammopathy is noted in about 2% of cases. Monoclonal gammopathy may be seen in a variety of diseases, both benign and malignant.

A. The focus of the initial work-up is to recognize, quantitate, and characterize the abnormal protein present in serum and urine using serum protein electrophoresis (SPEP), immunoelectrophoresis (IEP), and urine protein electrophoresis (UPEP), and to determine whether there is evidence of a coexisting disorder that requires treatment. The bone survey and marrow examination are especially helpful in excluding multiple myeloma.

B. Patients with elevated IgG, A, D, or E may have a solitary plasmacytoma of bone, multiple myeloma, amyloidosis, or a monoclonal gammopathy of unknown significance (MGUS). Patients with monoclonal IgM may have MGUS, Waldenström's macroglobulinemia, amyloid, or cryoglobulinemia. The listed screening examinations guide the diagnosis. Statistically, most patients with a monoclonal gammopathy have MGUS. Of the 873 cases of monoclonal gammopathy evaluated at the Mayo Clinic up to 1988, 64% had MGUS and 16% had multiple myeloma. Less common diagnoses were amyloidosis (8%), non-Hodgkin's lymphoma (6%), chronic lymphocytic leukemia (2%), solitary or extramedullary plasmacytoma (2%), and Waldenström's macroglobulinemia (2%).

C. Solitary plasmacytoma of bone occasionally presents with a monoclonal gammopathy (50%) although half the patients show no M component in either serum or urine. The diagnosis is based on histologic evidence of a tumor consisting of plasma cells, identical to those seen in multiple myeloma, and confined to a single bone site. Levels of uninvolved immunoglobulins usually are preserved. In addition to standard studies for myeloma, MRI of the thoracic and lumbo-sacral spine is useful to confirm the absence of additional lytic lesions to exclude the diagnosis of multiple myeloma. Radiotherapy of 45 Gy is the treatment of choice. Although >50% of the patients will be alive at 10 years, the disease-free survival is only 20–30% because most patients develop multiple myeloma. Patients most likely to have prolonged disease-free survival include those with a low serum M protein (<2 g/dl) in whom the M protein completely disappears after radiotherapy. Accordingly, periodic follow-up with SPEP, IEP, and UPEP is indicated in all patients with an abnormality before treatment.

D. Extramedullary plasmacytoma is a plasma cell tumor that arises outside the bone marrow, most often in the upper respiratory tract, including the nasal cavity and sinuses, nasopharynx, and larynx. Patients generally do not have a detectable M component in either serum or urine, so detection of a monoclonal protein usually indicates multiple myeloma. The diagnosis is based on the finding of a plasma cell tumor in an extramedullary site, the absence of multiple myeloma in the bone marrow, and no lytic lesions in the bone survey. Radiotherapy is curative in >50% of patients.

E. Because of more frequent screening of blood chemistries and counts, about 20% of patients with multiple myeloma are now recognized by chance without significant symptoms or signs of disease (asymptomatic multiple myeloma). Asymptomatic disease generally is characterized by the absence of lytic bone lesions, anemia (hemoglobin >10.5 g/dl), hypercalcemia, renal failure attributable to myeloma, and symptoms of disease. The serum M protein is <4.5 g/dl. A subset of these patients may have long-term stability of disease and recently several studies attempting to determine reliable prognostic features have been published. At our center, risk factors include IgA type, M protein >3.0 g/dl, and Bence Jones protein >50 mg/dl. Patients with none of these features may be followed by observation as are patients with MGUS because they remain stable for many years (low risk to progression), whereas patients with two or more features have a median time to progression of 18 months (high risk). To avoid complications of disease, early chemotherapy may be an option for high-risk patients. Patients with one risk feature (intermediate risk) can be separated into low- or high-risk patients by MRI of the spine. An abnormal MRI suggests the patient may be at high risk for early disease progression.

F. The presence of multiple lytic lesions with >10% plasma cells in the bone marrow, any serum M component, and/or light chains in the urine indicates multiple myeloma. Chemotherapy with melphalan-based regimens results in a median survival of 3 years. The most common complications of this disease are bone pain from fractures, hypercalcemia, infection, and renal failure. Significant albuminuria with little or no light chain in the urine suggests a diagnosis of amyloid.

G. MGUS indicates the presence of an M component in patients without multiple myeloma, solitary plasmacytoma of bone, extramedullary plasmacytoma, amyloidosis, macroglobulinemia, or other lymphoproliferative disorders. MGUS is characterized by an M component <2.5 dl, generally preserved uninvolved immunoglobulins, normal CBC, absence of hypercalcemia, and no lytic lesions on bone survey. More important, over a long period the M-component usually remains stable and no additional abnormalities must develop. The incidence of MGUS increases with age, reaching approximately 10% in patients >80 years old. In a large series of 241

Patient with MONOCLONAL GAMMOPATHY

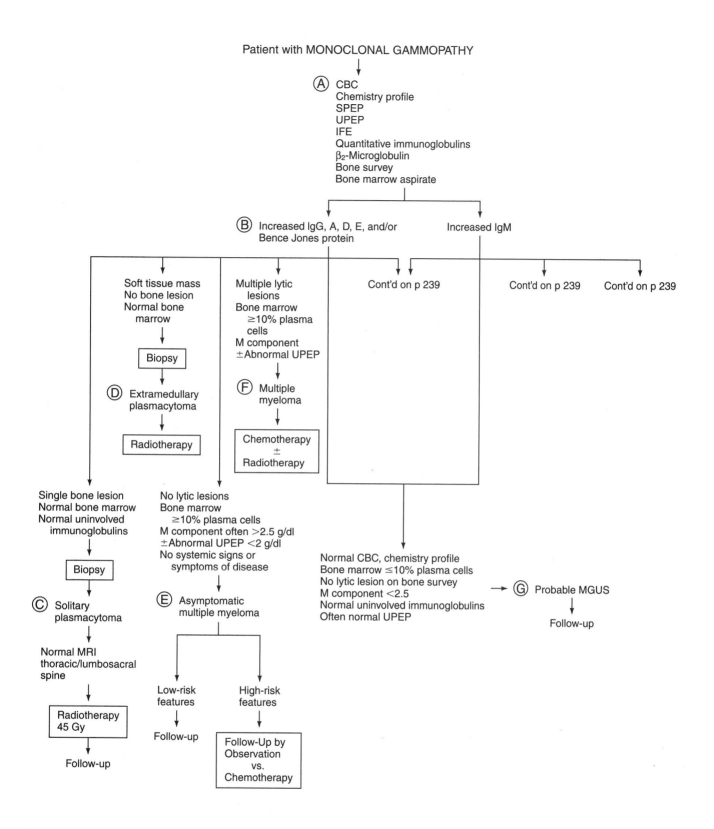

Cont'd on p 239

Cont'd on p 239

Cont'd on p 239

patients with MGUS, the concentration of the M-component was 0.3–3.2 g/dl (median 1.7 g/dl). IEP revealed IgG in 73%, IgA in 11%, and IgM in 14%, and biclonal gammopathy in 2% of patients. About 6% of patients had a urinary Bence Jones protein. The number of plasma cells in the bone marrow was 1–10% (median 3%). Multiple myeloma, amyloidosis, macroglobulinemia, or other lymphoproliferative processes developed in 26% of the patients, with an actuarial rate of 16% at 10 years, 33% at 20 years, and 40% at 25 years. Most patients with progressive disease developed multiple myeloma (68%) 2–29 years from the diagnosis of MGUS (median 10 years), indicating that such patients must be followed indefinitely.

H. The presenting manifestations of primary amyloidosis include weakness, weight loss, ankle edema, dyspnea, paresthesias, light-headedness, syncope, peripheral neuropathy, carpal tunnel syndrome, congestive heart failure, nephrosis, periorbital purpura, arthralgia, orthostatic hypotension, macroglossia, and diarrhea with malabsorption syndrome. Although rectal biopsy has been the classic method of establishing the diagnosis of amyloidosis, a recent study has shown that abdominal fat aspiration at an experienced center, using a 19-gauge needle, can yield positive results in >70% of patients. Prolonged therapy with melphalan and prednisone may be of some benefit in primary amyloidosis, and early reports suggest myeloablative therapy with stem cell support may be of benefit.

I. Patients with an elevated IgM (often <2% g/dl) and peripheral adenopathy often have an underlying B-cell neoplasm. In a series of 430 patients with IgM MGUS diagnosed at the Mayo Clinic between 1956 and 1978, 17% developed lymphoma. The median duration from presentation with MGUS until the diagnosis of the lymphoma was 4 years (range 0.4–22 years). This lymphoma probably can be classified as Waldenström's macroglobulinemia because most patients respond to similar therapy, but the definition of Waldenström's macroglobulinemia remains controversial.

J. Waldenström's macroglobulinemia is a rare disease (one-seventh as common as myeloma) and is the result of an uncontrolled proliferation of lymphocytes and plasma cells in which a large monoclonal IgM is produced. The presenting signs and symptoms include weakness, fatigue, bleeding (especially oozing from the oronasal area), blurred vision, dyspnea, weight loss, paresthesias, retinal lesions ("sausage" or "boxcar" formation), hepatosplenomegaly, and lymphadenopathy. IgM levels often are >3 g/dl. Initial treatment for symptomatic patients traditionally has been with alkylating agents such as chlorambucil. Remission can be achieved in about 50–60% of previously untreated patients. More recently treatment with nucleoside analogs (cladribine and fludarabine) induced responses in 70–80% of previously untreated patients.

References

Alexanian R, Dimopoulos M. The treatment of multiple myeloma. N Engl J Med 1994; 330:484.

Dimopoulos M, Alexanian R. Waldenström's macroglobulinemia. Blood 1994; 83:1452.

Knowling MA, Harwood AR, Bergsagel DE. Comparison of extramedullary plasmacytomas with solitary and multiple plasma cell tumors of bone. J Clin Oncol 1983; 1:255.

Kyle RA. Monoclonal gammopathy of undetermined significance and solitary plasmacytoma. Hematol Oncol Clin North Am 1997; 11:71.

Kyle RA, Greipp PR, O'Fallon WM. Primary systemic amyloidosis: multivariate analysis for prognostic factors in 168 cases. Blood 1986; 68:220.

Weber DM, Dimopoulos MA, Moulopoulos LA, et al. Prognostic features of asymptomatic multiple myeloma. Br J Haematol 1997; 97:810.

Patient with MONOCLONAL GAMMOPATHY
(Cont'd from p 237)

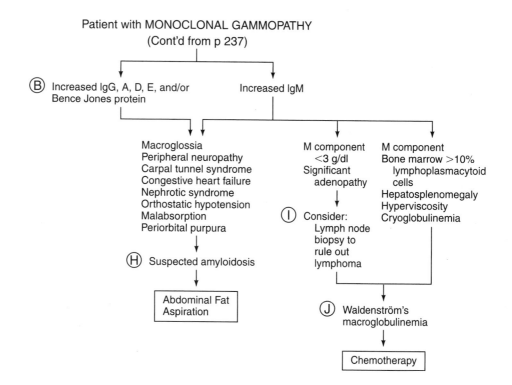

Ⓑ Increased IgG, A, D, E, and/or
Bence Jones protein

Increased IgM

Macroglossia
Peripheral neuropathy
Carpal tunnel syndrome
Congestive heart failure
Nephrotic syndrome
Orthostatic hypotension
Malabsorption
Periorbital purpura

Ⓗ Suspected amyloidosis

Abdominal Fat
Aspiration

M component
<3 g/dl
Significant
adenopathy

Ⓘ Consider:
Lymph node
biopsy to
rule out
lymphoma

M component
Bone marrow >10%
    lymphoplasmacytoid
    cells
Hepatosplenomegaly
Hyperviscosity
Cryoglobulinemia

Ⓙ Waldenström's
macroglobulinemia

Chemotherapy

LYMPHADENOPATHY

Guillermo Gonzalez-Osete
Manuel Modiano

More than 500 lymph nodes in the human body may become enlarged in response to numerous stimuli: (1) infection (bacterial, viral, parasitic, spirochetal, chlamydial, mycobacterial, or fungal), (2) drug reactions (phenytoin, serum sickness), (3) malignancy (head and neck, GI, breast, rectal, lymphoma), and (4) miscellaneous conditions (sarcoidosis, systemic lupus erythematosus).

A. New-onset lymphadenopathy <7 days' duration is unlikely to be malignant.

B. Recurrent or long-term (>7–14 days) lymphadenopathy (unilateral or bilateral) requires a full work-up. Most experienced clinicians see the patient again in 2–4 weeks to determine whether the node is increasing before embarking on a full work-up. The associated symptoms of fever, weight loss, or night sweats suggest malignancy (lymphoma B symptoms) or infection. Regional symptoms such as chest tightness, dysphagia, shortness of breath, and/or facial swelling suggest mediastinal disease and require a CT scan of the chest. Complaints of fullness in the abdomen, early satiety, and pain radiating to the shoulders or back necessitate abdominal CT to rule out pancreatic, renal, or other intraperitoneal lesions. Unilateral leg swelling (after deep vein thrombosis is ruled out) may require pelvic CT to rule out regional lymphadenopathy causing extrinsic compression.

C. Serologic studies and blood cultures help differentiate among infections, collagen vascular disease, and malignancy. Among the most common infectious causes are infectious mononucleosis, toxoplasmosis, syphilis, Epstein-Barr virus, HIV, and cytomegalovirus. If the history is suspicious and the patient is or was living in an endemic area, these causes must be ruled out.

D. Lymph node enlargement in the head and neck area requires a careful ENT evaluation, including biopsy of suspicious lesions; if ENT findings are normal, the patient may need to undergo a triple endoscopy procedure with evaluation of nasal, bronchial, and esophageal passages. Consider fine needle biopsy of the lymph node only if endoscopic findings are normal.

E. The supraclavicular area often is affected by breast cancer, lymphomas (Hodgkin's and non-Hodgkin's), and metastases from the lung and GI tract (esophagus, stomach, pancreas). Supraclavicular nodes are easily biopsied and are highly diagnostic.

F. Enlarged axillary lymph nodes often are a sign of breast or lung cancer. They also are often affected by lymphoma and may be biopsied to obtain a diagnosis if the primary source cannot be found.

G. When inguinal nodes are enlarged, physical examination should focus on the anorectal region, perineum, vulva, penis, and scrotum. Perform sigmoidoscopy to rule out rectal or anal carcinoma, evaluate the genitourinary system by urinalysis. Pelvic CT may provide useful information. If CT findings are normal, proceed with biopsy. Tumor markers CEA, PSA, and OC125 also may provide guidance toward a diagnosis.

H. For a patient with generalized lymphadenopathy but no other signs or symptoms and no other organ involvement, consider biopsy of the most accessible region (not necessarily the largest). The diagnostic yield is better with supraclavicular, axillary, or inguinal nodes (in descending order). A key feature of these biopsies is the need for adequate amounts of tissue with the specimen sectioned to allow for light microscopy, fresh frozen tissue for markers, and a portion in glutaraldehyde for electron microscopy. Patients with nondiagnostic biopsies require close follow-up, especially those with atypical hyperplasia, because many may develop lymphoproliferative disorders. Also, consider angioimmunoblastic lymphadenopathy in patients with "hyperplasia." This can be done by an experienced immunopathologist.

References

Copeland EM, McBride C. Axillary metastases from unknown primary sites. Ann Surg 1973; 178:25.

Faller DV. Diseases of lymph nodes and spleen. In: Bennett JC, Plum F. Cecil textbook of medicine. Philadelphia: WB Saunders, 1996:968.

Moore RD, Weisberger AS, Bowerfind ES. An evaluation of lymphadenopathy in systemic disease. Arch Intern Med 1957; 99:751.

Saltzsein S. The fate of patients with nondiagnostic lymph node biopsies. CA Cancer J Clin 1966; 16:115.

Schroeder K, Franssila KO. Atypical hyperplasia of lymph nodes: a follow-up study. Cancer 1979; 44:1155.

Sinclair S, Beckman E, Eliman L. Biopsy of enlarged superficial lymph nodes. JAMA 1974; 228:602.

Zuelzer W, Kaplan J. The child with lymphadenopathy. Semin Hematol 1975; 12:323.

Patient with LYMPHADENOPATHY

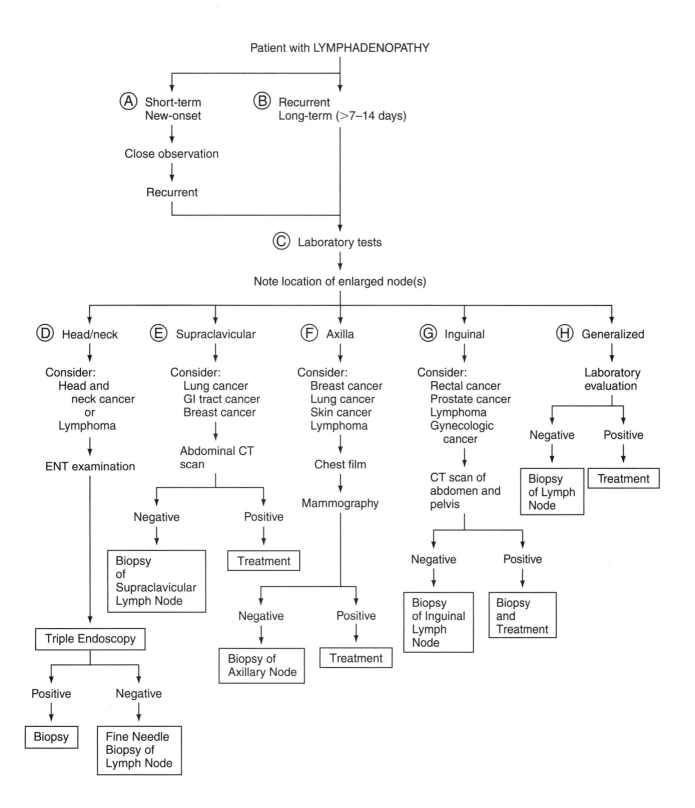

(A) Short-term
New-onset

↓

Close observation

↓

Recurrent

(B) Recurrent
Long-term (>7–14 days)

(C) Laboratory tests

↓

Note location of enlarged node(s)

(D) Head/neck

↓

Consider:
Head and
neck cancer
or
Lymphoma

↓

ENT examination

↓

Triple Endoscopy

Positive → Biopsy

Negative → Fine Needle
Biopsy of
Lymph Node

(E) Supraclavicular

↓

Consider:
Lung cancer
GI tract cancer
Breast cancer

↓

Abdominal CT
scan

Negative → Biopsy
of
Supraclavicular
Lymph Node

Positive → Treatment

(F) Axilla

↓

Consider:
Breast cancer
Lung cancer
Skin cancer
Lymphoma

↓

Chest film

↓

Mammography

Negative → Biopsy of
Axillary Node

Positive → Treatment

(G) Inguinal

↓

Consider:
Rectal cancer
Prostate cancer
Lymphoma
Gynecologic
cancer

↓

CT scan of
abdomen and
pelvis

Negative → Biopsy
of Inguinal
Lymph
Node

Positive → Biopsy
and
Treatment

(H) Generalized

↓

Laboratory
evaluation

Negative → Biopsy
of Lymph
Node

Positive → Treatment

CARCINOMA OF UNKNOWN PRIMARY SITE

Antonio C. Buzaid
Marie C. Abbruzzese
James L. Abbruzzese

Unknown primary carcinoma (UPC) is the presence of documented metastatic cancer in the absence of an identifiable primary tumor site. It constitutes 0.5–7% of referrals to cancer centers. The minimal evaluation necessary to identify an occult primary includes complete history and physical examination, careful pathologic review, basic laboratory studies (including liver function tests, urinalysis, and stool sample for occult blood), chest radiography, CT of the abdomen and pelvis, and mammography in women. Additional studies are recommended only to pursue detected abnormalities. The goal of the evaluation is to identify either the primary site or clinical situations in which potentially curative or effective therapy is available.

A. In the history, focus on symptoms that could lead to the primary site (e.g., abdominal cramps, persistent cough, previous tobacco use) and include family history of cancer. The physical examination should include a careful breast, pelvic, testicular, rectal/prostate, and skin evaluation. Examine lymph node bearing areas for adenopathy.

B. The pathologic examination is the single most important step in determining the primary site or identifying a unique histologic subset amenable to therapy. Provide adequate tissue samples to experienced pathologists who have access to electron microscopy and the most modern techniques in histochemical and immunohistochemical staining. Careful consultation between clinician and pathologist is needed to determine when histochemical and immunohistochemical staining will contribute to the evaluation. These methods are not recommended in every case but are extremely useful in patients diagnosed with undifferentiated or poorly differentiated carcinoma after H & E staining. If pathologic evaluation identifies a specific histologic diagnosis, patients should undergo histology-specific therapy.

C. If the pathologist does not suggest a specific histology (i.e., lymphoma, melanoma, sarcoma) and diagnoses the specimen as adenocarcinoma, carcinoma, squamous cell carcinoma, or neuroendocrine carcinoma, a radiographic evaluation is needed to identify either a primary site or other special clinical presentations that may be amenable to treatment. The baseline work-up including CBC, SMA-20, chest radiography, abdominal and pelvic CT scan, and mammography (in women) effectively achieves this goal. Use of serum tumor markers, such as β-HCG, α-fetoprotein, or prostate-specific antigen, although commonly ordered, remains controversial. When pathological evaluation has been adequate, the tumor markers are rarely helpful.

D. The most common epithelial primary sites identified by a combination of pathology and radiology are lung and pancreas. Most of the primaries identified in this way, with the exception of breast and ovarian cancers, are not very responsive to therapy. Careful screening for these two potential diagnoses is mandatory. Disease specific therapy is indicated.

(Continued on page 244)

Patient with CARCINOMA OF UNKNOWN PRIMARY SITE

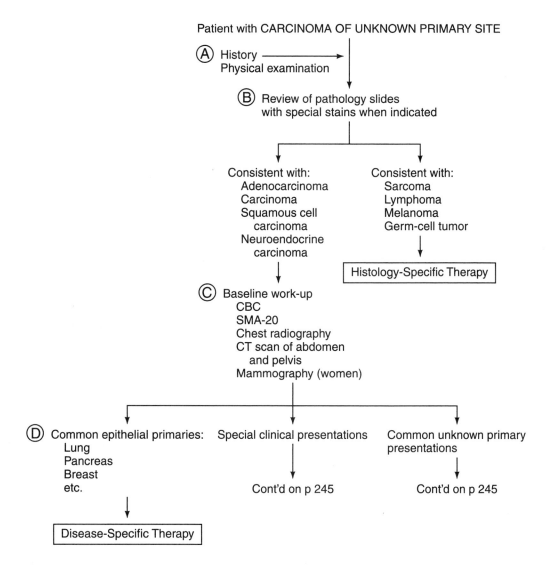

(A) History ——————→
    Physical examination

(B) Review of pathology slides
    with special stains when indicated

Consistent with:
  Adenocarcinoma
  Carcinoma
  Squamous cell
    carcinoma
  Neuroendocrine
    carcinoma

Consistent with:
  Sarcoma
  Lymphoma
  Melanoma
  Germ-cell tumor

Histology-Specific Therapy

(C) Baseline work-up
    CBC
    SMA-20
    Chest radiography
    CT scan of abdomen
      and pelvis
    Mammography (women)

(D) Common epithelial primaries:
    Lung
    Pancreas
    Breast
    etc.

Special clinical presentations

Cont'd on p 245

Common unknown primary
presentations

Cont'd on p 245

Disease-Specific Therapy

E. A special clinical subset includes males <50 years old with rapidly growing, poorly differentiated carcinomas involving predominantly midline structures (mediastinum, retroperitoneum) with or without bilateral pulmonary nodules. Historically, this presentation has been termed the *extragonadal germ cell syndrome*. Adequate pathologic review identifies the patients with germ-cell histologies, who should be treated aggressively with chemotherapy regimens used for testicular cancer. Patients with poorly differentiated carcinomas without any evidence of germ-cell features on cytology are much less responsive to therapy but should be given a trial of platinum-based chemotherapy.

F. Even in the absence of detectable ovarian disease, treat women with peritoneal carcinomatosis according to the guidelines established for therapy of advanced (stage 3) ovarian carcinoma. Cytoreductive surgery followed by cisplatin-based combination chemotherapy produces long-term survival in approximately 10–20% of these patients.

G. The most common cause of adenocarcinoma or poorly differentiated carcinoma confined to the axillary nodes is occult breast cancer. Biopsy material should be analyzed for estrogen and progesterone receptors. The treatment of choice is induction chemotherapy followed by radiation therapy to the ipsilateral breast and lymph nodes and depending on receptor status, adjuvant hormonal therapy. Axillary node dissection is controversial but has been used in some circumstances. Overall *survival* with chemotherapy and radiation therapy appears to be similar to that for stage 2 breast cancer.

H. Inguinal node metastasis of unknown origin is rare. Careful inspection of the skin, endoscopic evaluation of the anal canal and rectum, and gynecologic examination are of major importance. Patients in whom the primary tumor cannot be identified should undergo lymph node dissection of the affected area. Local radiation therapy is often administered after surgery. A 50% long-term survival after surgery was observed in one series of 22 patients.

I. Squamous cell carcinoma is found in >70% of patients whose involved nodes are high in the neck or midneck. The most common occult primary sites include the nasopharynx, tonsil, base of the tongue, and hypopharynx. It often is emphasized that a biopsy of the high or midcervical nodes should not be performed until a search for the primary site has been completed because of increased incidence of wound necrosis and increased risk of local recurrence and even distant metastasis. However, other investigators have not observed such deleterious effects. An alternative is to perform a fine needle aspiration, which often has a high diagnostic yield. If the diagnosis is squamous cell carcinoma, the patient should undergo MRI of the neck and a thorough ENT evaluation. This consists of direct laryngoscopy with random biopsies from the tonsil, nasopharynx, and base of the tongue identified. Patients should undergo neck dissection followed by radiotherapy. Patients with extensive adenopathy often are treated with platinum-based chemotherapy, but the exact role of chemotherapy and the best sequencing of the modalities in these patients is unclear. The 5-year survival rate is 30–50%, depending on the extent of disease at diagnosis.

J. Most patients do not fit into one of the subsets described here. Their diagnostic work-up should be curtailed at this point unless a specific abnormality from the basic evaluation points to further investigation. An extensive "blind" work-up is not cost-effective, yields little in the way of further treatable primaries or subsets, and only delays treatment for a group of patients whose median survival is only 11 months. Consider palliative chemotherapy, with either investigational or standard agents, in patients with good performance status.

References

Abbruzzese JL, Abbruzzese MC, Hess KR, et al. Unknown primary carcinoma: natural history and prognostic factors in 657 consecutive patients. J Clin Oncol 1994; 12:1272.

Abbruzzese JL, Abbruzzese MC, Lenzi R, et al. Analysis of a diagnostic strategy for patients with suspected tumors of unknown origin. J Clin Oncol 1995; 13:2094.

Abbruzzese JL, Raber MN. Unknown primary carcinoma. In: Abeloff MD, Armitage JO, Lichter AS, Niederhuber JE, eds. Clinical oncology. New York: Churchill Livingstone, 1995:1833.

Lenzi R, Hess KR, Abbruzzese MC, et al. Poorly differentiated carcinoma and poorly differentiated adenocarcinoma of unknown origin: favorable subsets of patients with unknown primary carcinoma? J Clin Oncol 1997; 15:2056.

Patient with CARCINOMA OF UNKNOWN PRIMARY SITE

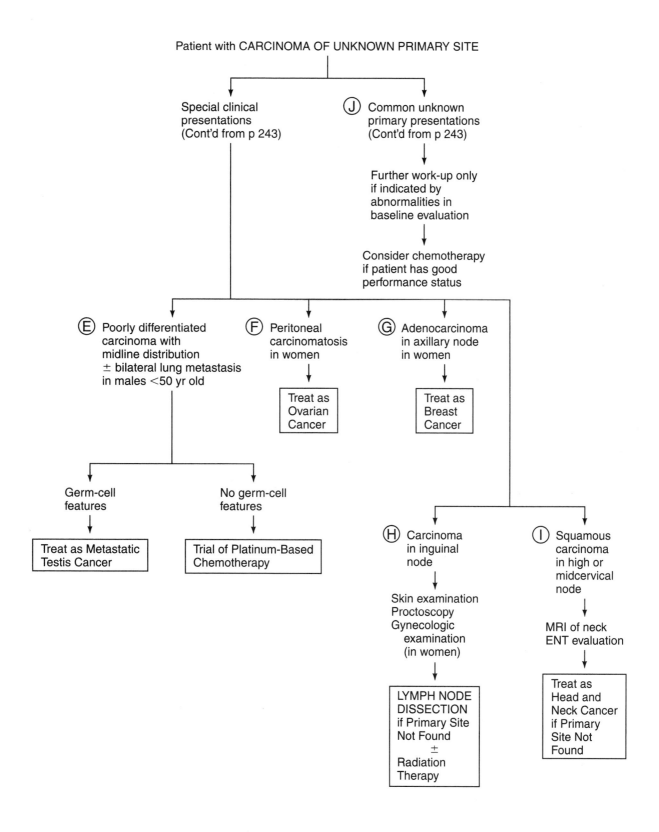

Special clinical
presentations
(Cont'd from p 243)

Ⓙ Common unknown
primary presentations
(Cont'd from p 243)

Further work-up only
if indicated by
abnormalities in
baseline evaluation

Consider chemotherapy
if patient has good
performance status

Ⓔ Poorly differentiated
carcinoma with
midline distribution
± bilateral lung metastasis
in males <50 yr old

Ⓕ Peritoneal
carcinomatosis
in women

Treat as
Ovarian
Cancer

Ⓖ Adenocarcinoma
in axillary node
in women

Treat as
Breast
Cancer

Germ-cell
features

Treat as Metastatic
Testis Cancer

No germ-cell
features

Trial of Platinum-Based
Chemotherapy

Ⓗ Carcinoma
in inguinal
node

Skin examination
Proctoscopy
Gynecologic
examination
(in women)

LYMPH NODE
DISSECTION
if Primary Site
Not Found
±
Radiation
Therapy

Ⓘ Squamous
carcinoma
in high or
midcervical
node

MRI of neck
ENT evaluation

Treat as
Head and
Neck Cancer
if Primary
Site Not
Found

NEUTROPENIA AND FEVER

Antonio C. Buzaid
Issam Raad

Infection during episodes of chemotherapy-induced neutropenia is the most common cause of treatment-related mortality in cancer patients. Most infections originate in the alimentary tract, sinuses, lungs, and skin. The risk of infection in a neutropenic patient primarily is dictated by the severity and duration of neutropenia. The lower the absolute granulocyte nadir and the more prolonged the neutropenia, the greater the risk of serious infection. Fever is common in cancer patients and may have many causes, including infection, the tumor itself, inflammation, transfusion of blood products, and chemotherapeutic and antimicrobial drugs. In neutropenic patients, however, fever (a single temperature ≥38.3° C orally or ≥38° C over at least 1 hour) usually is secondary to infection, especially if they have <500 granulocytes/μl.

A. In addition to a search for localizing symptoms, the medical history should identify any special circumstance or immunologic defect that may predispose the patient to certain opportunistic infections. For example, patients with Hodgkin's disease are at increased risk for herpes zoster and cryptococcal meningitis; those who have undergone bone marrow transplantation are at risk for severe interstitial pneumonia, especially with cytomegalovirus (CMV) or respiratory syncytial virus (RSV); and those on high-dose steroids are at increased risk for pneumocystis pneumonia and fungal infections. Steroid use may further mask the signs and symptoms of infection and cloud the seriousness of the clinical picture. For instance, delirium may be the only manifestation of a serious infection in a patient receiving high-dose steroids.

B. A thorough physical examination must include careful auscultation of the lungs and meticulous evaluation of the oral cavity, genitalia, and perianal region. Evaluate the entire integument, especially sites of vascular access and previous invasive procedures, as potential portals for infection. The characteristic signs and symptoms of infections often are absent in neutropenic patients because they are unable to mount an adequate inflammatory response. For instance, rales may be the only manifestation of pneumonia in a neutropenic patient.

C. Perform the initial medical evaluation rapidly. In addition to routine blood tests, culture blood from two separate sites, culture urine, and order a chest film. Perform other tests such as stool culture, lumbar puncture, abdominal radiography, and bronchoscopy only if clinically indicated. For instance, in patients with diarrhea, culture for bacteria, ova, and parasite, and do a toxic screen for *Clostridium difficile.* Even with a comprehensive evaluation, a specific pathogen is initially identified in only 30–50% of patients. With profound neutropenia (<100 cell/μl), bacteremias can be documented in about 15–20% of febrile episodes.

D. Antimicrobial therapy is directed against the pathogens responsible for most primary infections. Aerobic gram-negative bacilli, especially *Klebsiella, Escherichia coli,* and *Pseudomonas aeruginosa,* account for 30–40% of all culture-confirmed infections. The incidence of gram-positive cocci (e.g., *Staphylococcus aureus,* coagulase-negative staphylococci, streptococci, pneumococci, *Corynebacterium* spp.) has risen significantly, and they now represent 60–70% of isolates in many hospitals. Monotherapy with carbapenems (imipenem or meropenem), cefepime, or occasionally, ceftazidime is acceptable for uncomplicated episodes of fever in neutropenic patients, particularly in those with fever of unknown origin. Aminoglycosides may be given in combination with an antipseudomonal penicillin in all patients with fever and neutropenia. However, aminoglycosides may only need to be added to a third- or fourth-generation cephalosporin or carbapenems in patients who have complicated fever with neutropenia (sepsis syndrome with mental status changes or hypoxemia) or patients with pneumonia or documented *P. aeruginosa* infection. Because of the emergence of vancomycin-resistant gram-positives such as *E. faecium,* add vancomycin only in one of four situations: (1) Obvious catheter-related infection with catheter site inflammation; (2) patients receiving quinolone prophylaxis; (3) severe mucositis; or (4) patients known to have been colonized with methicillin-resistant *S. aureus* or penicillin-resistant *S. pneumoniae.*

E. If the patient becomes rapidly afebrile, no organism is identified, all sites of infection resolve, and the absolute neutrophil count (ANC) is ≥500/μl, discontinue the antibiotic regimen after 5–7 days.

F. If a patient remains neutropenic but has been afebrile for >5 days and is low risk (ANC 100–500/μl, no mucositis and stable vital signs), discontinue antibiotics. If fever spikes again, perform immediate panculture and restart broad-spectrum antibiotics. Neutropenic patients at high risk (ANC <100/μl, mucositis or unstable vital signs) should be continued on antibiotics until ANC is ≥500/μl and the patient is clinically well.

G. Patients who remain neutropenic and febrile at day 4 but are clinically well may continue the same initial regimen for a few more days. However, if there is clinical deterioration, modify the antibiotic regimen depending on the clinical picture. For instance, for patients with severe mucositis or catheter site inflammation who have a high likelihood of a gram-positive infection, vancomycin may be added if not previously included. For patients with pneumonia or sepsis syndrome, add aminoglycoside, IV quinolone (e.g., ciprofloxacin), or trimethoprim-sulfamethoxazole (if not previously included) to cover some of the resistant gram-negatives

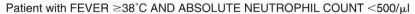

Patient with FEVER ≥38˚C AND ABSOLUTE NEUTROPHIL COUNT <500/μl

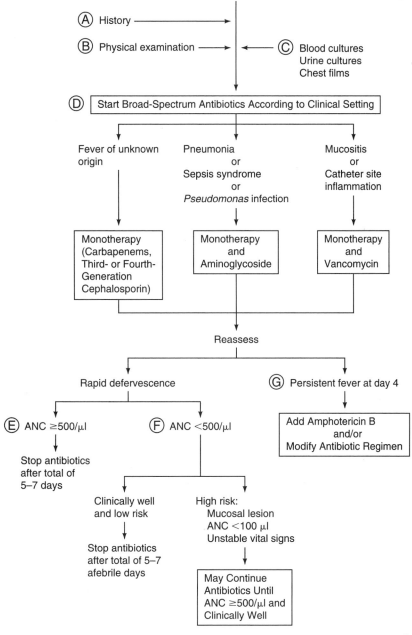

such as *P. aeruginosa* or *Stenotrophomonas malto-philia,* respectively. Add amphotericin B if the patient is febrile through day 5 and resolution of neutropenia is not imminent. Add fluconazole instead of Amphotericin B if *Candida* infection is a possibility and the patient was not receiving fluconazole prophylaxis before the onset of fever. During antibiotic treatment, perform a daily thorough examination including the skin, oral cavity, genitalia, perianal area, and sites of venous access. Take seriously any medical complaint, and pursue the cause without delay. For instance, mild discomfort in the maxillary region often is the first sign of a grave fungal infection, usually caused by *Aspergillus* or *Mucor;* tenderness in the perianal area may indicate a superimposed anaerobic infection; and right-sided abdominal pain may be the first clue to the diagnosis of typhlitis.

References

Bodey GP. Evolution of antibiotic therapy for infection in neutropenic patients: studies at M.D. Anderson Hospital. Rev Infect Dis 1989; 11:1582S.

Hughes WT, Armstrong D, Bodey GP, et al. Guidelines for the use of antimicrobial agents in neutropenic patients with unexplained fever. J Infect Dis 1990; 161:381.

Hughes WT, Armstrong D, Bodey GP, et al. 1997 Guidelines for the use of antimicrobial agents in neutropenic patients with unexplained fever. Clin Infect Dis 1997; 25:551.

Pizzo PA. Management of fever in patients with cancer and treatment-induced neutropenia. N Engl J Med 1993; 328:1323.

PATHOLOGIC FRACTURES

Irwin E. Harris

A. Plain radiography provides most of the information about the underlying lesion and directs future decision making. Technetium-labeled methylenediphosphonate bone scanning is a sensitive indicator of multiple skeletal involvement, except in myeloma, in which little reactive bone is formed. The skeleton is the third most common site of metastasis from adenocarcinoma; skeletal metastases are present in 70% of patients. Diffuse loss of mineral homogeneity throughout the skeleton suggests osteoporosis, osteomalacia, or marrow replacement by leukemia, lymphoma, or myeloma.

B. Of carcinomatous metastases, 90% are solitary, especially those of neuroblastoma and hypernephroma. A solitary bone lesion in a patient >40 years of age is most likely metastasis, whereas it may be a primary bone tumor in a patient <40 years of age.

C. The primary tumor is found in only one third of patients with skeletal metastases; most of those diagnosed have breast or prostate primaries. Undetected primaries are most likely lung or kidney. The recommended diagnostic strategy is history, physical examination, routine laboratory studies, chest radiography, mammography (in women), urinalysis, and ultrasound, CT, or MRI of the kidneys. Additional tests detect primaries in only a few patients.

D. In most cases, tissue diagnosis does not alter the therapy, but it may if the lesion is a primary bone tumor or if the metastatic lesion can justifiably be resected, as in hypernephroma, thyroid carcinoma, or plasmacytoma. Resection of a solitary hypernephroma metastasis may result in a 30% 5-year survival rate.

E. Patients with metastatic disease have a 2-year average life expectancy; 6 months for lung. Internal fixation can be supplemented with methylmethacrylate for immediate stability, and prosthetic replacement can be used even in the young. Treat impending fractures with prophylactic fixation when the lesion is painful, when the lesion is >2.5 cm in diameter, or when the cortex is destroyed >50% across the diameter of the bone on a uniplanar radiograph. Treat shafts of the femur, humerus, tibia, and subtrochanteric femur with intramedullary nail. Intertrochanteric and supracondylar fractures of the femur are treated with nail attached to an intramedullary stem or side plate. Treat the distal tibia and distal humerus with flexible rods and bone cement. Use cemented prosthetic replacement for fractures of the femoral neck, acetabulum, femoral condyler, and distal proximal tibia. Radiotherapy follows fracture stabilization.

F. External beam radiotherapy is used to treat other areas that do not require stabilization and fractures or lesions involving the spine, ribs, or nonarticular pelvis. Systemic treatments for metastatic bone disease include chemotherapy, endocrine therapy, radioisotopes, and bisphosphonates. Tamoxifen is used in postmenopausal women who have estrogen-positive breast tumors, sometimes followed by aromatase inhibitors. Men with metastatic prostate cancer are often treated with bilateral orchiectomy and androgen blockade with leuprolide LHRH-A, flutamide, goserelin acetate, or cyproterone acetate. Site-directed radiotherapy using samarium-153, strontium-89, and rhenium-186 has effectively relieved pain in prostate more than breast lesions. Bisphosphonates, like pamidronate or clodronate, treat hypercalcemia, inhibit osteolysis, relieve pain in 50% of patients, and show radiographic healing in 25% of breast cancer patients.

(Continued on page 250)

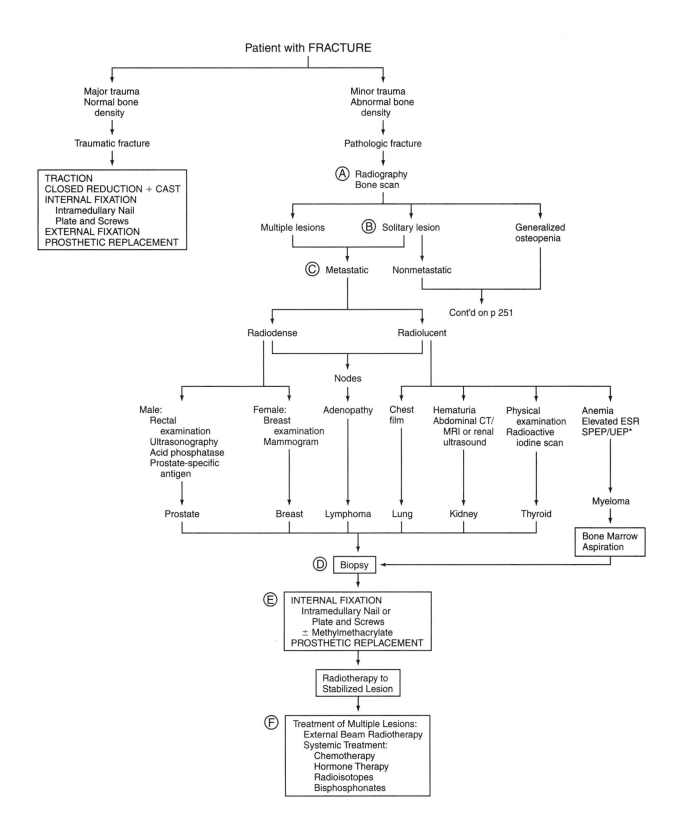

Patient with FRACTURE

Major trauma
Normal bone
density

Traumatic fracture

TRACTION
CLOSED REDUCTION + CAST
INTERNAL FIXATION
  Intramedullary Nail
  Plate and Screws
EXTERNAL FIXATION
PROSTHETIC REPLACEMENT

Minor trauma
Abnormal bone
density

Pathologic fracture

Ⓐ Radiography
   Bone scan

Multiple lesions   Ⓑ Solitary lesion   Generalized
                                                       osteopenia

Ⓒ Metastatic   Nonmetastatic

                      Cont'd on p 251

Radiodense   Radiolucent

                Nodes

Male: Female: Adenopathy   Chest   Hematuria   Physical   Anemia
 Rectal   Breast   film   Abdominal CT/ examination   Elevated ESR
 examination   examination   MRI or renal   Radioactive   SPEP/UEP*
 Ultrasonography   Mammogram   ultrasound   iodine scan
 Acid phosphatase
 Prostate-specific
 antigen

                                                                                         Myeloma

Prostate   Breast   Lymphoma   Lung   Kidney   Thyroid

                                                                          Bone Marrow
                                                                          Aspiration

Ⓓ Biopsy

Ⓔ INTERNAL FIXATION
   Intramedullary Nail or
   Plate and Screws
   ± Methylmethacrylate
   PROSTHETIC REPLACEMENT

   Radiotherapy to
   Stabilized Lesion

Ⓕ Treatment of Multiple Lesions:
   External Beam Radiotherapy
   Systemic Treatment:
     Chemotherapy
     Hormone Therapy
     Radioisotopes
     Bisphosphonates

*SPEP/UEP = Serum protein electrophoresis/Urine electrophoresis

G. The differential diagnosis of a fractured solitary bone lesion is listed. Localized osteopenia from failure to use a limb can occur with pain, reflex sympathetic dystrophy, previous cast immobilization, and paralytic conditions. Fractures often are seen in previously irradiated bone and in Paget's disease. The latter is distinguished from prostatic carcinoma by enlargement of the involved bone and coarsened, rather than destroyed, trabeculation.

H. Benign primary bone tumors often have intact cortex, distinct margins, and solid homogeneous periosteal reactions. Malignant tumors show destruction of cortex, indistinct margins, and lamellated or sunburst periosteal reactions.

I. Cast treatment without biopsy is justified for a benign bone tumor having a diagnostic radiographic appearance and self-healing behavior (e.g., unicameral bone cyst, metaphyseal fibrous cortical defect, eosinophilic granuloma, enchondroma, fibrous dysplasia). Biopsy is indicated when the diagnosis is uncertain or when the lesions are unlikely to heal without resection or curettement and grafting (e.g., aneurysmal bone cysts, giant cell tumor, chondromyxoid fibroma, osteoblastoma, chondroblastoma). A cast may be used for healing of the cortex before definitive treatment. Steroid instillation is effective in obliterating unicameral bone cysts if cast immobilization of a fracture is unsuccessful.

J. Before biopsy, order MRI to determine the extent of marrow and soft tissue involvement in primary malignant tumors of bone, although cortical destruction is better seen on CT. A fracture through a primary bone sarcoma most often necessitates amputation. However, if the cortical fracture is small and displacement is minimal, the patient may still be a candidate for resection and limb salvage, especially if preoperative adjuvant chemotherapy is administered. Treat chondrosarcomas by surgery alone.

K. Both metastatic and metabolic disease may involve the spine, proximal femurs, and ribs. Osteoporosis characteristically results in fractures of the distal radius and femoral neck. Osteomalacia more commonly affects the subtrochanteric femur and successive ribs at the same distance from the spine; 30% of patients with hip fracture have osteomalacia. Osteomalacia, marked by excess of unmineralized osteoid, can be of vitamin D deficiency, poor absorption of calcium or vitamin D enterically, vitamin D–resistant form, or renal osteodystrophy. Osteoporosis can result from immobilization and disuse or from endocrinopathy (hyperthyroidism, hypercortisolism, or hyperparathyroidism), or it may be idiopathic (the type 1 postmenopausal variety is a loss of trabecular more than cortical bone; the type 2 senile variety is an equal loss of both).

References

Albright JA, Gillespie TE, Butard TR. Treatment of bone metastases. Semin Oncol 1980; 17:418.

Berman AT, Hermantin FU, Horowitz SM. Metastatic disease of the hip: evaluation and treatment. J Am Acad Orthop Surg 1997; 5:79.

Harrington KD. Orthopaedic management of extremity and pelvic lesions. Clin Orthop 1995; 312:136.

Houston SJ, Rubens RD. The systemic treatment of bone metastases. Clin Orthop 1995; 312:95.

Mankin HJ. Rickets, osteomalacia, and renal osteodystrophy. An update. Orthop Clin North Am 1990; 21:81.

Simon MA, Bartucci EJ. The search for the primary tumor in patients with skeletal metastases of unknown origin. Cancer 1986; 58:1088.

Yazawa Y, Frassica FJ, Chao EY, et al. Metastatic bone disease; a study of the surgical treatment of 166 pathologic humeral and femoral fractures. Clin Orthop 1990; 251:213.

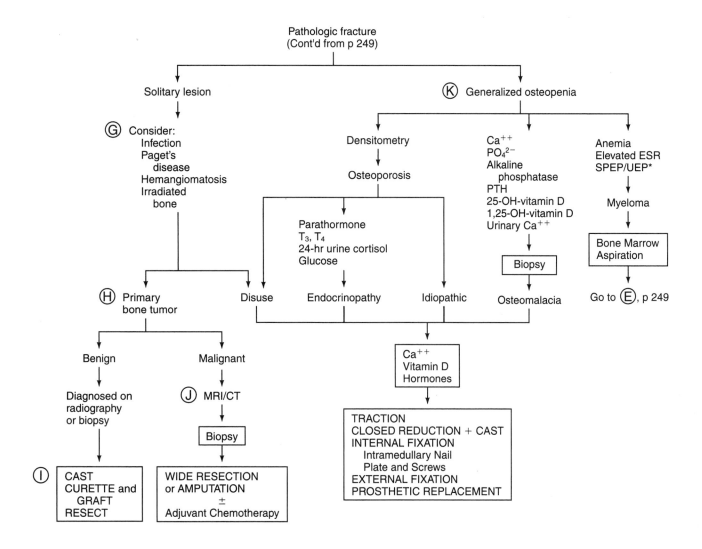

Pathologic fracture
(Cont'd from p 249)

Solitary lesion

(G) Consider:
Infection
Paget's
disease
Hemangiomatosis
Irradiated
bone

(H) Primary
bone tumor

Benign

Diagnosed on
radiography
or biopsy

(I) CAST
CURETTE and
GRAFT
RESECT

Malignant

(J) MRI/CT

Biopsy

WIDE RESECTION
or AMPUTATION
±
Adjuvant Chemotherapy

(K) Generalized osteopenia

Densitometry

Osteoporosis

Parathormone
T_3, T_4
24-hr urine cortisol
Glucose

Disuse   Endocrinopathy   Idiopathic

Ca^{++}
PO_4^{2-}
Alkaline
   phosphatase
PTH
25-OH-vitamin D
1,25-OH-vitamin D
Urinary Ca^{++}

Biopsy

Osteomalacia

Ca^{++}
Vitamin D
Hormones

TRACTION
CLOSED REDUCTION + CAST
INTERNAL FIXATION
   Intramedullary Nail
   Plate and Screws
EXTERNAL FIXATION
PROSTHETIC REPLACEMENT

Anemia
Elevated ESR
SPEP/UEP*

Myeloma

Bone Marrow
Aspiration

Go to (E), p 249

*SPEP/UEP = Serum protein electrophoresis/Urine electrophoresis

CLINICAL CONSIDERATIONS FOR BONE MARROW OR STEM CELL TRANSPLANTATION

Philip A. Lowry

Despite the explosion of agents and techniques for treating patients with cancer, the rate of "cure" remains disappointing. A major limitation of radiation and chemotherapy has been toxicity to the bone marrow, forcing dose limits despite the apparent dose response of at least some tumors. Classic allogeneic bone marrow transplantation (BMT) seeks both to provide a mechanism for dose-escalated treatment and to effect actual replacement of a diseased marrow with cells from a healthy donor. Allogeneic BMT may be useful in treating subsets of patients with hematologic malignancies or with nonmalignant but life-threatening blood and marrow disorders, particularly severe thalassemia, immunodeficiency disorders, and aplastic anemia. Barriers to allogeneic BMT include limited donor availability and technical complications, including graft-versus-host disease (GVHD). With better tissue typing capabilities, alternative transplants from unrelated donors and cord blood can be successfully accomplished. For nonmalignant disorders, simple replacement of marrow function is sufficient. The success of these homologous transplant approaches in treating malignant disease traces not only to the more aggressive therapy delivered before transplant but, probably more important, to immune mechanisms manifested as a "graft-versus-tumor" effect.

With autologous BMT, in which the patient serves as his or her own donor, donor availability and GVHD are not barriers, but the loss of graft-versus-tumor effects and the potential for reinfusion of malignant cells significantly increases post-transplant relapse rates. Autologous BMT is not a transplant so much as it is a means to "rescue" patients from the otherwise potentially fatal effects of higher dosages of chemoradiotherapy. Thus it cannot be used to treat nonmalignant marrow and blood disorders, but it may improve outcomes in selected patients with acute leukemia, Hodgkin's and non-Hodgkin's lymphoma, myeloma, and perhaps chemotherapy-responsive solid tumors such as breast cancer, testicular cancer, and neuroblastoma. Cells mobilized from the peripheral blood may be a superior product for hematopoietic stem cell rescue, particularly in autologous BMT.

A. Early identification of potential transplant candidates is essential. Candidates will benefit most if therapy can be instituted during a more complete remission and before infectious or other complications that increase the risk of transplant occur. When transfusing potential transplant candidates, avoid exposure to cytomegalovirus (CMV) if the patient is CMV negative, and avoid related donors to minimize the potential for patient sensitization and later graft rejection. Do not give transfusions for aplastic anemia; they may decrease transplant success. A long lead time may be required to complete donor and patient evaluation.

B. Transplant candidates must have a disease that has been demonstrated to benefit from the proposed transplant approach or must be enrolled in an appropriately reviewed clinical trial. Review disease stage and response to previous chemotherapy or radiation for their implications for transplant outcome.

C. Transplant candidates must meet minimal criteria for organ function, especially of lung, heart, and kidney, to ensure tolerance of the procedure. They must have no complicating medical illnesses such as HIV infection that might preclude transplant and must be able to give appropriate informed consent.

D. Psychosocial evaluations of both patient and prospective donor and dental and fertility evaluations of the patient should precede commitment to the transplant process.

E. Particularly for patients who will be autologous stem cell donors, cytogenetic marrow evaluation should establish that there is an acceptable potential for harvest of appropriate cells for transplant.

F. The transplant approach should be chosen in consultation with an experienced stem cell transplant center, based on disease type and patient status.

G. For autologous BMT candidates, an appropriate transplant product must be secured, usually via mobilization with chemotherapy and growth factors, followed by appropriately timed apheresis of peripheral stem cells. Cells are preserved and reinfused after additional treatment with high dosages of chemotherapy with or without irradiation. Investigational techniques of stem cell graft manipulation or immune modulation may be applied at the time of transplant.

H. Consider homologous transplant particularly for patients <55 years old with chronic myeloid leukemia, acute leukemia, and nonmalignant blood and marrow disorders. The search for an appropriate donor begins with siblings, focusing particularly on HLA-A, B, and DR matching. Additional consideration is given to the donor's ABO compatibility, degree of potential sensitization (previous pregnancies or blood transfusions), and CMV status (particularly if the patient is CMV negative). The donor should have no complicating medical conditions and be willing and able to undergo stem cell harvest.

I. If a fully matched donor cannot be identified, consider using a partially or phenotypically matched related

Patient Considered for BONE MARROW/STEM CELL TRANSPLANT

(A) Early identification of potential transplant candidate
Appropriate timing of transplant
Appropriate transfusion strategy
Initiation of patient and prospective donor evaluation

(B) Disease and stage review

Potential candidate → Evaluation of patient and donor

Not a transplant candidate → Explore nontransplant options

(C) Organ function
Multigated angiography
Pulmonary functions
D_{LCO}
Renal function
Hepatic function
HIV screen

(D) Psychosocial evaluation

(E) Marrow evaluation with cytogenetics

(F) Contact stem cell transplant center
Choose appropriate transplant type

(G) Autologous transplant candidate
→ Mobilization
→ Stem Cell Collection
→ High-Dose Chemotherapy
→ Stem Cell Reinfusion

(H) Homologous transplant candidate
HLA, ABO, Rh typing, CMV titier of patient and siblings

Appropriate match → ALLOGENEIC TRANSPLANT

No match

(I) Consider:
Other related transplant
Matched unrelated
Autologous transplant
Alternative nontransplant therapies

(J) Long-term follow-up post-transplant
Transfusion support
GVHD prophylaxis (homologous transplant)
Infectious disease treatment and prophylaxis
Inoculations

donor. Simultaneously, initiate a search of unrelated donor and cord blood registries, and evaluate potential matches fully. Searches for and discussion of possible use of such alternative sources should be coordinated through a center experienced in those types of transplants.

J. Follow-up after transplantation focuses initially on hematologic support with transfusion and close observation and care for potential infections. Prophylaxis against GVHD continues for most patients receiving homologous transplants. Patients receive prophylaxis against *Pneumocystis* after transplant. Inoculations against pneumococcus, tetanus, and *Haemophilus* are typically administered on the 1-year anniversary of transplant. For selected diseases, specific consolidative or maintenance strategies may be indicated, such as

post-transplant irradiation of sites of bulk or resistant disease, or long-term suppressive therapy, such as tamoxifen for breast cancer patients or interferon for patients with myeloma. With appropriate care, most patients who do not experience major complications with the first 3 months return to healthy, productive lives.

References

Armitage JO. Bone marrow transplantation. N Engl J Med 1994; 330:827.

Armitage JO, Antman KH. High-dose cancer therapy. 2nd ed. Baltimore: Williams & Wilkins, 1995.

Forman SJ, Blume KG, Thomas ED. Bone marrow transplantation. Boston: Blackwell, 1994.

SECONDARY MALIGNANCIES IN PATIENTS PREVIOUSLY TREATED FOR CANCER

Philip A. Lowry

The increasingly successful treatment of cancer with chemotherapy and radiation has produced an unfortunate byproduct: secondary malignancies that develop as a consequence of the treatment itself. Genetic damage induced by irradiation or by certain classes of chemotherapeutic agents, particularly alkylators (e.g., cyclophosphamide and mechclorethamine) and epipodophyllotoxins (e.g., etoposide), sets into motion a new sequence of cellular degeneration and transformation producing acute leukemia, non-Hodgkin's lymphoma, and virtually the entire spectrum of solid malignancies complicating the late course of cancer treatment. Certain patients, particularly those with Hodgkin's and non-Hodgkin's lymphoma, acute leukemia, retinoblastoma, Wilms' tumor, soft tissue sarcoma, and testicular malignancies, seem to be at particular risk. Although the statistical risk of therapy-induced secondary malignancies in patients with breast cancer is much lower, the number of patients with this disease combined with the threefold increased risk for the development of new, treatment-independent contralateral cancer in breast cancer survivors makes this an important group to monitor for second malignancy.

Secondary malignancies demonstrate important temporal, genetic, and histologic patterns. Epipodophyllotoxin-induced acute leukemias typically develop within 2 years of treatment, demonstrate rearrangements of chromosome 11, and have an M4 or M5 subtype by FAB classification. Alkylator- and radiation-induced acute leukemias peak later (5–9 years after treatment), are often preceded by a period of myelodysplasia, often show abnormalities of chromosomes 5 or 7, and typically show an M1 or M2 subtype. Solid malignancies are especially seen as a consequence of previous irradiation and are delayed ≥10 years in appearance. Bladder cancers may be a particular consequence of previous cyclophosphamide treatment. Non-Hodgkin's lymphomas seen after allogeneic stem cell transplantation may relate to Epstein-Barr virus infection, particularly when treatment has required heavy T-cell immunosuppression.

A. The initial choice of therapy for patients with cancer should take into account the risk of secondary malignancy, such as the choice of ABVD over MOPP in the young patient with Hodgkin's disease.

B. Incorporate appropriate surveillance into the follow-up strategy of patients successfully treated for cancer, particularly because the principles of increased treatability for disease detected earlier may still apply in selected cases of secondary cancer. Follow-up studies should begin with regular evaluation by the physician but also include mammography, particularly for women with previous breast cancer or chest irradiation at a young age, periodic oral-pharyngeal and thyroid examination for patients with neck irradiation, periodic CBCs in patients treated with irradiation or with alkylator or epipodophyllotoxin chemotherapy, periodic urinalysis in patients previously exposed to cytoxan, and thorough skin and lymph node evaluation of all patients.

C. In the patient with new signs or symptoms, evaluation starts with a thorough history and physical examination. Pay particular attention to patient-identified problem areas and potential problems suggested by the previous cancer or treatment regimen. Even subtle findings should prompt an extended evaluation. Suspect lesions should be rigorously pursued and biopsied.

D. Any suspicious skin lesions should be appropriately biopsied.

E. Lymphadenopathy may represent a primary lymphoid malignancy or metastasis from a carcinoma. Surgical biopsy often is required for definitive evaluation because needle aspiration may be inconclusive. Pathologic findings should be closely compared with the patient's original malignancy to distinguish new from recurrent disease.

F. Any organ abnormality suggested by physical or radiologic evaluation should be pursued with appropriate staging work-up and ultimate pathologic evaluation. Appropriate CT scans or other radiologic evaluation combined with the physical examination will both define the extent of disease and suggest the most accessible site for biopsy.

G. Persistent and unexplained cytopenias, elevation of the mean cell volume, or structural hematologic abnormalities suggest a secondary hematologic process. Evaluation should include a thorough review of the peripheral smear, exclusion of vitamin deficiencies (particularly B_{12} deficiency in patients previously treated for gastric cancer with resection), and usually marrow evaluation including marrow for cytogenetics.

H. Previous cytoxan treatment may induce a carcinoma of the bladder. Hematuria may be the initial or sole presenting symptom and should be aggressively pursued with evaluation of urine cytology or cystoscopy.

I. Once a diagnosis has been established, patients should be appropriately and completely staged and discussions regarding prognosis and treatment options initiated with appropriate surgical, medical oncology, and hematologic consultation.

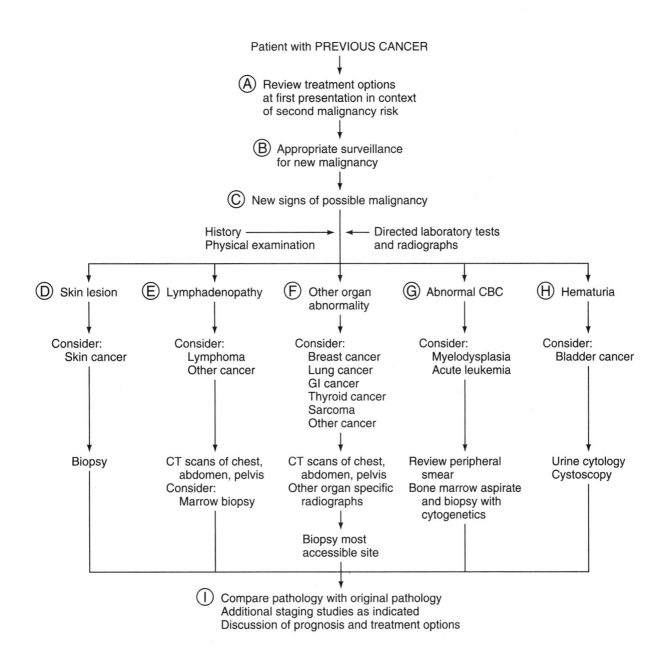

Patient with PREVIOUS CANCER

Ⓐ Review treatment options
at first presentation in context
of second malignancy risk

Ⓑ Appropriate surveillance
for new malignancy

Ⓒ New signs of possible malignancy

History ⟶ ⟵ Directed laboratory tests
Physical examination and radiographs

Ⓓ Skin lesion   Ⓔ Lymphadenopathy   Ⓕ Other organ abnormality   Ⓖ Abnormal CBC   Ⓗ Hematuria

Consider:
Skin cancer

Consider:
Lymphoma
Other cancer

Consider:
Breast cancer
Lung cancer
GI cancer
Thyroid cancer
Sarcoma
Other cancer

Consider:
Myelodysplasia
Acute leukemia

Consider:
Bladder cancer

Biopsy

CT scans of chest,
abdomen, pelvis
Consider:
Marrow biopsy

CT scans of chest,
abdomen, pelvis
Other organ specific
radiographs

Review peripheral
smear
Bone marrow aspirate
and biopsy with
cytogenetics

Urine cytology
Cystoscopy

Biopsy most
accessible site

Ⓘ Compare pathology with original pathology
Additional staging studies as indicated
Discussion of prognosis and treatment options

References

Greene MH, Wilson J. Second cancer following lymphatic and hematopoietic cancers in Connecticut, 1935–1982. Natl Cancer Inst Monograph 1985; 68:191.

Swinnen LJ. Treatment of organ transplant-related lymphoma. Hematol Oncol Clin North Am 1997; 11:963.

Van Leeuwen FE. Second cancers. In: DeVita VT, Hellman S, Rosenberg SA, eds. Cancer: principles and practice of oncology. 5th ed. Philadelphia: Lippincott-Raven, 1997.

Witherspoon, RP, Fisher LD, Schoch G, et al. Secondary cancers after bone marrow transplantation for leukemia or aplastic anemia. N Engl J Med 1989; 321:784.

SUPERIOR VENA CAVAL SYNDROME

Frederick R. Ahmann

A. Obstruction of the superior vena cava (SVC) occurs when this thin-walled vessel is invaded, compressed, or thrombosed. Blockage of the blood flow often leads to development of the easily recognized superior vena caval syndrome (SVCS) with venous distension, facial edema, headache, tachypnea, cyanosis, and plethora. SVCS is commonly characterized as an acute or sub-acute oncologic emergency. Reassessments of published reports, however, suggest that establishing a diagnosis is essential and can be accomplished safely even if biopsies of tissue exposed to elevated venous pressures, and a brief delay in the initiation of therapy, are necessary.

B. In a patient with the above-noted signs and symptoms, confirmation that the SVC is obstructed usually is not required because most patients have a mass visible on imaging studies. However, should confirmation be needed, this can be safely accomplished with either contrast or a nuclear venography. Nuclear venography is preferable because of a lower injection volume of contrast, but both are associated with low complication rates.

C. Since the 1950s, bronchogenic carcinomas have been the leading cause of SVCS. Hence, for many years histologic confirmation of the diagnosis was thought to be unnecessary because palliative therapy was the only treatment possible. Recent advances in the treatment of small cell lung cancer and lymphoproliferative disorders, plus the low incidence of benign causes for which radiotherapy is not palliative and is potentially dangerous, mandate accurate pretherapy assessment. There is little evidence to suggest that diagnostic procedures (including bronchoscopy, lymph node biopsies, mediastinoscopy, and thoracotomies) carry an excessive risk. Therefore, the evaluation of these patients should be similar to that of any patient with a lung mass.

D. Standard palliative therapy for SVCS has been radiotherapy. Some debate persists about the optimal dose, schedule, and fields of treatment, but in general, about 50–70% of treated patients are reported to achieve symptomatic improvement within 2 weeks of initiation of radiotherapy. However, radiotherapy is no longer the sole or even the initial therapy for many patients. In a recent review, 40% of all cases of SVCS were caused by small cell lung cancer; most of the remaining cases were secondary to lymphomas. Thus, up to 50% of all causes of SVCS are malignancies for which combination chemotherapy is needed to accomplish the therapeutic objectives of improved quality of life and prolonged survival. SVCS can cause distressing signs and symptoms that should be palliated in a timely fashion. However, because many such patients may have small cell lung cancer or lymphoma together with a definite incidence of benign etiologies, an accurate histologic diagnosis should be pursued in all patients with SVCS unless there are extenuating circumstances. Only with a definite histologic diagnosis can a rational therapeutic choice be made for both relieving SVCS and maximizing survival potential.

References

Ahmann FR. A reassessment of the clinical implications of the superior vena caval syndrome. J Clin Oncol 1984; 2:961.

Baker GL, Barnes HJ. Superior vena cava syndrome: etiology, diagnosis and treatment. Am J Crit Care 1992; 1:54.

Bigsby R, Greengrass R, Unruh H. Diagnostic algorithm for acute superior vena caval obstruction. J Cardiovasc Surg 1993; 34:347.

Dombernowsky P, Hansen HH. Combination chemotherapy in the management of superior vena caval obstruction in small cell anaplastic carcinoma of the lung. Acta Med Scand 1978; 204:5123.

Perez CA, Presant CA, Van Amburg AL. Management of superior vena cava syndrome. Semin Oncol 1978; 5:123.

SUPERIOR VENA CAVAL SYNDROME Suspected

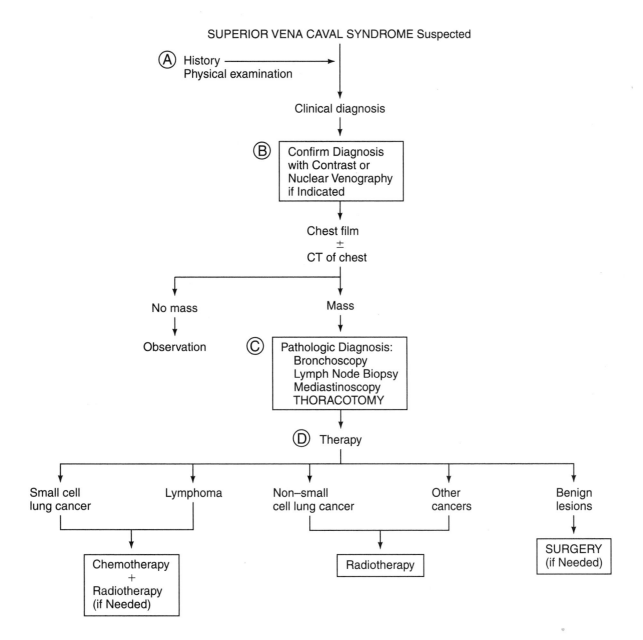

Ⓐ History ——————→
Physical examination

Clinical diagnosis

Ⓑ Confirm Diagnosis
with Contrast or
Nuclear Venography
if Indicated

Chest film
±
CT of chest

No mass

Observation

Mass

Ⓒ Pathologic Diagnosis:
Bronchoscopy
Lymph Node Biopsy
Mediastinoscopy
THORACOTOMY

Ⓓ Therapy

Small cell
lung cancer

Lymphoma

Non–small
cell lung cancer

Other
cancers

Benign
lesions

Chemotherapy
+
Radiotherapy
(if Needed)

Radiotherapy

SURGERY
(if Needed)

SPINAL CORD COMPRESSION

Guillermo Gonzalez-Osete
Manuel Modiano

Approximately 5% of systemic cancers involve the spinal cord. Spinal cord compression is a medical emergency in which a delay in treatment often causes irreversible loss of neurologic function.

A. Tumors that most commonly affect the spinal cord are of lung, breast, prostate, and lymphoma; less common are myeloma, melanoma, and genitourinary tract tumors. An important presenting sign is back pain, either of recent onset or old pain that has returned or increased. Pain is present in 97% of all cord compressions, followed in frequency by weakness (76%) and paresthesias (57%) along a bilateral or unilateral dermatomal distribution. There is associated bowel and bladder dysfunction in 51% of patients with more advanced disease. A few patients have no history of cancer and pain as the initial presentation.

B. Even when the physical examination does not reveal signs of spinal cord compression, obtain plain radiographs of the painful region to rule out neoplastic involvement. If the plain films are negative, consider non-neoplastic causes (rheumatoid arthritis, aortic aneurysm, spondylosis, herniated disc, spinal tuberculosis, osteoarthritis, osteomyelitis). Proceed with a detailed work-up if there is pain with tenderness to percussion over the affected vertebral body, bilateral muscle weakness in the extremities, sensory changes, loss of deep tendon reflexes, or bowel or bladder incontinence.

C. If plain films reveal a lesion in a painful area, follow with MRI or myelography, which have comparable sensitivity and specificity. Myelography is an invasive procedure that requires technical skill and the use of contrast. MRI is not invasive and helps in detecting intramedullary lesions, but patients may have difficulty lying still on the hard table or may have claustrophobia. Also, MRI is not always available. If these studies show a lesion, there is a 90% probability of cord compression.

D. If MRI is negative and clinical findings suggest cord involvement, proceed with myelography. Myelography helps determine the upper and lower extent of the lesion and ascertains whether there is more than one lesion. If a complete block is found on lumbar myelography, cisternal myelography or MRI is required to identify the upper end of the block. If both studies are negative, there is no cord compression.

E. The choice of treatment depends on the type of tumor, the level of the block, the rapidity of onset and duration of symptoms, previous treatment, and the clinical experience available. This medical emergency is treated vigorously with radiation or surgery in addition to steroids. Our current recommendation is to give 10 mg IV dexamethasone immediately, follow with 4 mg every 6 hours daily for at least 72 hours, and then rapidly taper as tolerated. Begin radiotherapy immediately after the diagnosis is established. The earlier a lesion is detected and treated, the better the functional outcome. Response rates are 30–80%. The total dose of radiation is 3000–4000 rad, delivered over 2–4 weeks.

F. Consider surgery (laminectomy, stabilization) when there is (1) no histologic diagnosis and cord compression is the presenting sign of cancer, (2) history of radiation therapy to the affected area, (3) neurologic progression of disease despite steroids and radiotherapy, (4) instability requiring fixation, or (5) a high cervical lesion. After surgery, give radiotherapy to avoid recurrences. Initial response to combined surgery and radiation is 20–100%, depending on tumor type and timing of treatment. The best prognostic index for eventual recovery of function is pretreatment status: 60% of patients who are ambulatory at diagnosis remain so postoperatively, whereas only 7% of those who are paraplegic at diagnosis are ambulatory after treatment.

G. When plain films are negative and physical examination is not definitive, adjust pain medications and observe. If pain persists or worsens or if the history is highly suspicious, perform MRI and proceed accordingly.

References

Gilbert RW, Kim J-H, Posner JB. Epidural spinal cord compression from metastatic tumor: diagnosis and treatment. Ann Neurol 1978; 3:40.

Maranzano E, et al. Radiation therapy in metastatic spinal cord compression. Cancer 1991; 67:1333.

Rodichok L, et al. Early diagnosis of spinal epidural metastases. Am J Med 1981; 70:1181.

Wasserstrom W, Glass PJ, Posner JB. Diagnosis and treatment of leptomeningeal metastases from solid tumors: experience with 90 patients. Cancer 1982; 49:759.

Willson JKV, Masaryk T. Neurologic emergencies in the cancer patient. Semin Oncol 1989; 16:490.

Young RF, Post EM, King GA. Treatment of spinal epidural metastases. J Neurosurg 1980; 53:741.

SPINAL CORD COMPRESSION Suspected

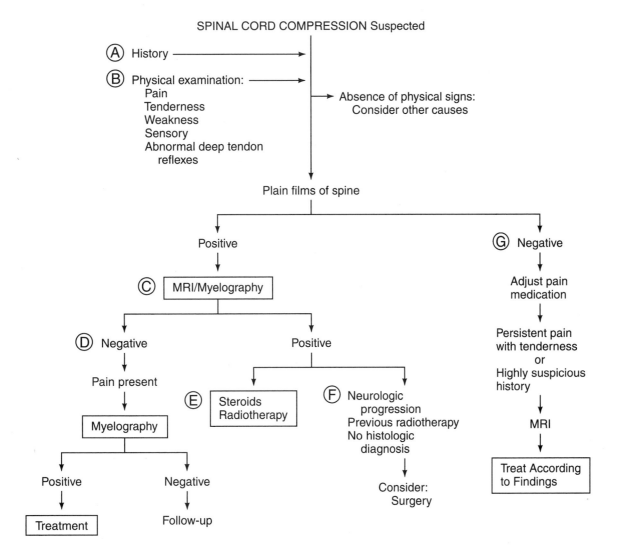

INFECTIOUS DISEASE

FOREIGN TRAVEL: IMMUNIZATIONS AND INFECTIONS

Rodney D. Adam

A. Ascertain the patient's travel plans to determine the risk of exposure to various infections and the appropriate precautions. This includes countries of travel, whether city or rural, and purpose and duration of trip. Determine which illnesses are endemic or epidemic in the region to be visited and whether chloroquine-resistant *Plasmodium falciparum* is present. Malaria is not found in most cities outside equatorial Africa, but the water supply may be contaminated in urban or rural areas. In general, exposure to endemic infections is greater during longer trips and visits to more rural areas.

B. Common means of acquiring infections include endogenous food and water and mosquitos; exposure to these sources should be limited as much as possible. HIV infection, endemic in many parts of the world, is spread sexually and by blood transfusion and reused needles. Other STDs, including gonorrhea and chancroid, also are common in many areas. Sexual abstinence, condom use, and avoidance of contaminated needles or transfusion of untested blood limit exposure to these agents.

C. Hepatitis A vaccine is highly effective for 6–12 months. The vaccine should be given 1 month before travel; however, most people develop antibodies within 2 weeks, so vaccination 2 weeks before travel may be sufficient. For shorter lead times, gamma globulin may be administered alone or along with the vaccine. The oral and new injectable typhoid vaccines are better tolerated than the old two-dose injectable phenol-inactivated vaccines and are preferred. The oral vaccine has a longer duration of immunity (5 years vs. 2 years), but consists of live attenuated organisms, generating theoretical concerns regarding use in immunocompromised people. Cholera vaccine has poor efficacy and high toxicity, and cholera is uncommon in most areas. Canine rabies is common in many areas, and human diploid vaccine for postexposure prophylaxis is not readily available. In highly endemic areas where exposure is possible, consider pre-exposure immunization. Hepatitis B is common in many areas; consider vaccination for travelers with potential occupational (e.g., medical workers) or sexual exposure.

D. Malaria is common in most tropical and subtropical regions. Most cases are caused by *P. falciparum* and *P. vivax*. Chloroquine is effective preventive therapy for *P. vivax* (except in New Guinea/Irian Jaya, where mefloquine should be used) and chloroquine-sensitive *P. falciparum*. Mefloquine is the recommended preventive agent in 1998 for chloroquine-resistant *P. falciparum* (except in northern Thailand, where doxycycline should be used). Doxycycline is a reasonable alternative to mefloquine. Recommendations are continually changing, so consult current CDC recommendations.

E. Febrile illnesses in returning travelers may be the result of routine viral infections. However, malaria is a common, treatable, and often fatal infection and is thus a primary consideration.

F. If the malaria smear is positive but does not definitively identify the species, the patient should be presumed to have *P. falciparum* infection, which should be assumed to be drug resistant if the person received preventive therapy. Patients with definite or probable *P. falciparum* malaria should be hospitalized for treatment. The recommended treatment changes often; consult current recommendations (e.g., CDC).

G. The infections in the decision tree are only a partial list and are geographically variable. For example, scrub typhus (rickettsial) is common in Malaysia, and several viral causes of hemorrhagic fever (e.g., Lassa fever) are found in equatorial Africa. If a hemorrhagic fever is suspected on the basis of thrombocytopenia, leukopenia, or coagulopathy, contact the CDC for proper isolation precautions.

H. Diarrhea occurring during travel or within a few days of return is most commonly caused by pathogenic *Escherichia coli* but may be caused by *Shigella, Salmonella, Campylobacter,* or other agents. Bloody diarrhea suggests shigellosis or amebiasis and stool WBCs are found with *Shigella,* invasive *E. coli, Campylobacter,* and some *Salmonella* infections. In the absence of specific findings, empiric therapy with trimethoprim-sulfamethoxazole or a quinolone is appropriate. Further diagnostic steps or changes in therapy depend on initial findings and response to therapy.

I. Diarrhea with malabsorption but no blood or WBCs suggests giardiasis, cryptosporidiosis, isosporiasis, strongyloidiasis, or tropical sprue. *Entamoeba histolytica* causes a colitis (as do *Shigella, Campylobacter,* and sometimes *Salmonella*) characterized by rectal pain and bloody stools but an absence of WBCs. Initial studies include stools for ova and parasites (O&P), WBCs, and culture.

J. This partial list includes infections that are uncommon in short-term travelers but may be seen in long-term travelers or immigrants from endemic areas.

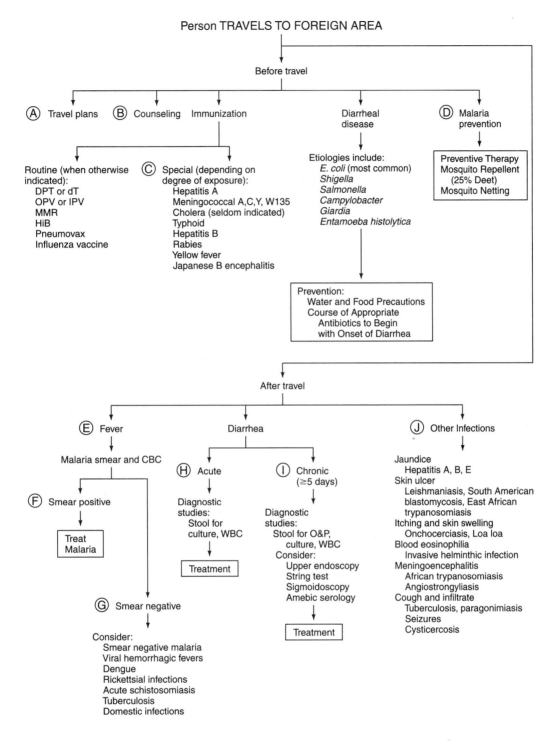

Person TRAVELS TO FOREIGN AREA

Before travel

(A) Travel plans (B) Counseling Immunization

Diarrheal disease

(D) Malaria prevention

Routine (when otherwise indicated):
DPT or dT
OPV or IPV
MMR
HiB
Pneumovax
Influenza vaccine

(C) Special (depending on degree of exposure):
Hepatitis A
Meningococcal A,C,Y, W135
Cholera (seldom indicated)
Typhoid
Hepatitis B
Rabies
Yellow fever
Japanese B encephalitis

Etiologies include:
E. coli (most common)
Shigella
Salmonella
Campylobacter
Giardia
Entamoeba histolytica

Preventive Therapy
Mosquito Repellent (25% Deet)
Mosquito Netting

Prevention:
Water and Food Precautions
Course of Appropriate Antibiotics to Begin with Onset of Diarrhea

After travel

(E) Fever

Diarrhea

(J) Other Infections

Malaria smear and CBC

(F) Smear positive

(H) Acute

(I) Chronic (≥5 days)

Treat Malaria

Diagnostic studies:
Stool for culture, WBC

Treatment

Diagnostic studies:
Stool for O&P, culture, WBC
Consider:
Upper endoscopy
String test
Sigmoidoscopy
Amebic serology

Treatment

(G) Smear negative

Consider:
Smear negative malaria
Viral hemorrhagic fevers
Dengue
Rickettsial infections
Acute schistosomiasis
Tuberculosis
Domestic infections

Jaundice
Hepatitis A, B, E
Skin ulcer
Leishmaniasis, South American blastomycosis, East African trypanosomiasis
Itching and skin swelling
Onchocerciasis, Loa loa
Blood eosinophilia
Invasive helminthic infection
Meningoencephalitis
African trypanosomiasis
Angiostrongyliasis
Cough and infiltrate
Tuberculosis, paragonimiasis
Seizures
Cysticercosis

References

Barnett ED, Chen R. Children and international travel: immunizations. Pediatr Infect Dis J 1995; 14:982.

Centers for Disease Control and Prevention. Health Information for International Travel 1996–97. Atlanta: Centers for Disease Control and Prevention, 1997 (new edition every 1 or 2 years).

Committee on Infectious Diseases. 1997 Red Book: report of the Committee on Infectious Diseases. Elk Grove Village, IL: American Academy of Pediatrics, 1997 (new edition every 3 years).

Gardner P, Eickhoff T, Poland GA, et al. Adult immunizations. Ann Intern Med 1996; 124:35.

Salam I, Katelaris P, Leigh-Smith S, Farthing MJ. Randomised trial of single-dose ciprofloxacin for travellers' diarrhoea. Lancet 1994; 344:1537.

Wyler DJ. Malaria chemoprophylaxis for the traveler. N Engl J Med 1993; 329:31.

ACUTE AND SUBACUTE MENINGITIS

Richard M. Mandel

A. Papilledema and/or focal neurologic deficits in a patient with meningeal symptoms suggests the possibility of a cerebral abscess. In this setting, lumbar puncture may disturb intracranial pressures and precipitate herniation.

B. Common underlying conditions in patients with brain abscess and other parameningeal foci include endocarditis, lung abscess, sinusitis, middle ear infection, and antecedent head trauma or neurosurgery. Therefore, obtain blood cultures and design empiric therapy according to likely pathogens (see E–I).

C. If the CNS imaging procedure reveals a mass lesion, a neurologic and/or neurosurgical evaluation may be indicated. In patients with focal neurologic findings, altered sensorium, and temporal horn cerebritis, consider herpes simplex encephalitis and institute empiric therapy pending diagnostic confirmation. Brain biopsy may be indicated, depending on the clinical circumstances.

D. In patients with signs and symptoms of acute meningitis, initiation of emergent antibiotic therapy within 30 minutes is critical in treating the potentially lethal progression of this disease. Waiting for CT scan or CSF Gram stain may waste valuable therapeutic time. Start patients on empiric antibiotics on the basis of minimal data; further revision of the antimicrobial regimen may be undertaken after evaluation of the complete history, physical examination, and CSF analysis.

E. In normal immunocompetent hosts the most likely organisms include *Streptococcus pneumoniae, Neisseria meningitidis,* and (less likely) *Haemophilus influenzae.* Elderly patients may present in a more subtle fashion, encountering the usual organisms and others such as *Staphylococcus aureus, Listeria monocytogenes,* and gram-negative bacilli.

F. Common etiologic agents in compromised hosts include (1) in diabetic and oncology patients, *S. pneumoniae, S. aureus,* gram-negative bacilli, *Cryptococcus neoformans;* (2) in alcoholic patients, *S. pneumoniae;* (3) in steroid-treated and AIDS patients, *C. neoformans, Mycobacterium tuberculosis;* and (4) in AIDS patients, acute HIV meningitis.

G. Patients with closed head trauma encounter *S. pneumoniae* as well as gram-negative bacilli.

H. After open head trauma or neurosurgery, be concerned about *Staphylococcus* spp. and gram-negative bacilli. In procedures that traverse sinuses, upper respiratory flora are common.

I. Intraventricular shunt devices are associated with organisms such as *Staphylococcus epidermidis, Propionibacterium acnes,* diphtheroids, and gram-negative bacilli.

(Continued on page 264)

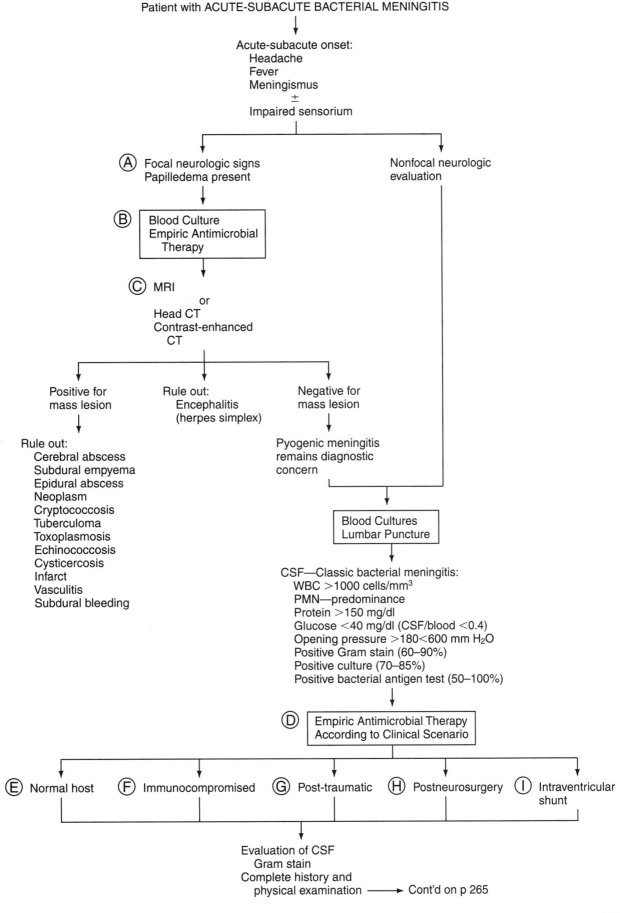

Patient with ACUTE-SUBACUTE BACTERIAL MENINGITIS

Acute-subacute onset:
    Headache
    Fever
    Meningismus
    ±
    Impaired sensorium

(A) Focal neurologic signs
    Papilledema present

Nonfocal neurologic evaluation

(B) Blood Culture
    Empiric Antimicrobial Therapy

(C) MRI
    or
    Head CT
    Contrast-enhanced CT

Positive for mass lesion

Rule out: Encephalitis (herpes simplex)

Negative for mass lesion

Rule out:
    Cerebral abscess
    Subdural empyema
    Epidural abscess
    Neoplasm
    Cryptococcosis
    Tuberculoma
    Toxoplasmosis
    Echinococcosis
    Cysticercosis
    Infarct
    Vasculitis
    Subdural bleeding

Pyogenic meningitis remains diagnostic concern

Blood Cultures
Lumbar Puncture

CSF—Classic bacterial meningitis:
    WBC >1000 cells/mm³
    PMN—predominance
    Protein >150 mg/dl
    Glucose <40 mg/dl (CSF/blood <0.4)
    Opening pressure >180<600 mm H_2O
    Positive Gram stain (60–90%)
    Positive culture (70–85%)
    Positive bacterial antigen test (50–100%)

(D) Empiric Antimicrobial Therapy
    According to Clinical Scenario

(E) Normal host   (F) Immunocompromised   (G) Post-traumatic   (H) Postneurosurgery   (I) Intraventricular shunt

Evaluation of CSF
    Gram stain
    Complete history and
        physical examination ——→ Cont'd on p 265

J. At this juncture, re-evaluate empiric therapy and start appropriate antimicrobial therapy based on Gram stain evaluation. Centrifuged CSF is positive in 60–90% of cases of culture-positive meningitis. Positive cultures further guide therapy.

K. If no bacteria are seen on Gram stain, the differential diagnosis expands. Cryptococcal meningitis can be ruled out by India ink preparation, cryptococcal antigen determination, and fungal culture.

L. In the absence of cryptococcal disease and if the CSF demonstrates a normal sugar level and absent or minimal cells, investigate a parameningeal focus.

M. Polymorphonuclear leukocytes in the CSF may indicate partially treated bacterial disease or viral meningitis.

N. If the CSF demonstrates leukocytes with a mononuclear cell response, the glucose can be used to discriminate between viral meningitis and partially treated bacterial, fungal, or tuberculous meningitis. If partially treated bacterial meningitis is a diagnostic consideration, continue antimicrobial therapy.

O. Treatment for tuberculous meningitis is indicated if there is strong ancillary evidence for this infection. Note that an appropriate CSF-AFB smear and culture result from the spun sediment of 10 ml of CSF. The AFB cultures may take 6 weeks to turn positive; therefore, consider empiric therapy when clinical suspicion is high. Note that many of these presentations may not be classic and it is important to call in consultants to help with the subtle nuances of this extensive differential diagnosis.

References

Kaufman BA. Meningitis in the neurosurgical patient. Infect Dis Clin North Am 1990; 4:677.

Tunkel A, Scheld WM. Acute meningitis. In: Mandell GL, et al, eds. Principles and practice of infectious diseases. 4th ed. New York: Churchill Livingstone, 1995:831.

Wispelwey B, Tunkel AR, Scheld WM. Bacterial meningitis in adults. Infect Dis Clin North Am 1990; 4:645.

Patient with ACUTE-SUBACUTE BACTERIAL MENINGITIS
(Cont'd from p 263)

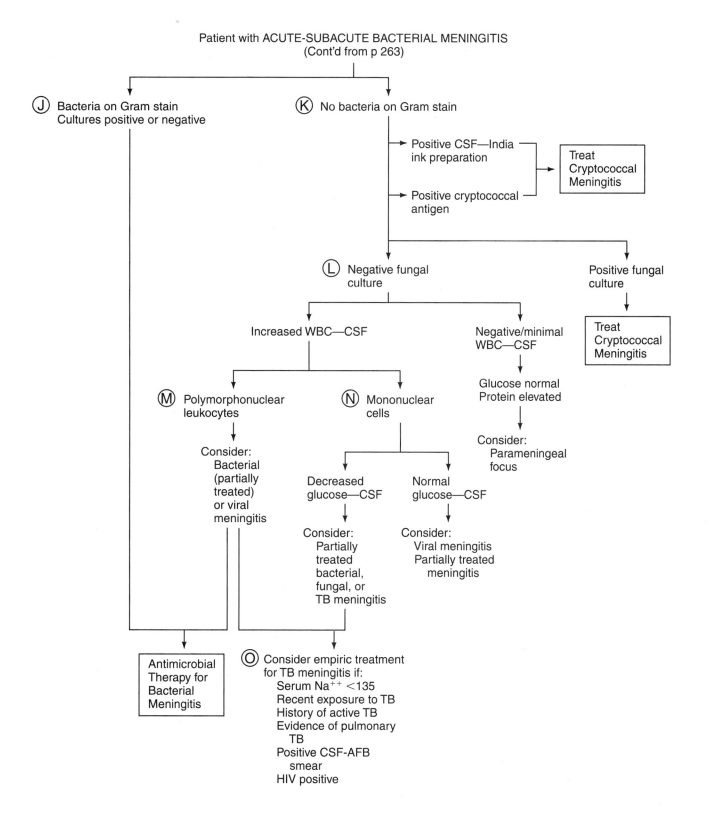

Ⓙ Bacteria on Gram stain
Cultures positive or negative

Ⓚ No bacteria on Gram stain

Positive CSF—India ink preparation

Positive cryptococcal antigen

Treat Cryptococcal Meningitis

Ⓛ Negative fungal culture

Positive fungal culture

Treat Cryptococcal Meningitis

Increased WBC—CSF

Negative/minimal WBC—CSF

Glucose normal
Protein elevated

Consider:
Parameningeal focus

Ⓜ Polymorphonuclear leukocytes

Ⓝ Mononuclear cells

Consider:
Bacterial (partially treated) or viral meningitis

Decreased glucose—CSF

Normal glucose—CSF

Consider:
Partially treated bacterial, fungal, or TB meningitis

Consider:
Viral meningitis
Partially treated meningitis

Antimicrobial Therapy for Bacterial Meningitis

Ⓞ Consider empiric treatment for TB meningitis if:
Serum Na^{++} <135
Recent exposure to TB
History of active TB
Evidence of pulmonary TB
Positive CSF-AFB smear
HIV positive

CHRONIC MENINGITIS

Jeffrey L. Silber
Mark J. DiNubile

A. In patients with chronic meningitis there is the insidious onset of headache, often accompanied by fever, nausea, vomiting, lethargy, and confusion. By convention, symptoms and CSF abnormalities must be present for at least 4 weeks. Differentiate chronic or persistent meningitis from the syndrome of recurrent meningitis.

B. Order CT or MRI of the brain in all patients with suspected chronic meningitis. The scan may identify a mass lesion, hydrocephalus, and/or contrast enhancement of the basilar meninges. If not contraindicated, perform a lumbar puncture. The CSF profile characteristically shows elevated protein and lymphocytic pleocytosis. The formula is never in itself diagnostic, but certain findings may suggest particular causes (e.g., hypoglycorrhachia is common in carcinomatous, tuberculous, and fungal meningitis).

C. In most cases the history is nonspecific. Travel, outdoor activity, sexual habits, or other exposures occasionally help focus the evaluation. Abrupt neurologic deterioration in a previously stable patient suggests an anatomic abnormality, such as hydrocephalus. Previous antimicrobial therapy may obscure bacterial infections such as endocarditis.

D. The physical examination sometimes reveals signs of associated systemic illness. Eye examination may reveal choroid tubercles, uveitis, sarcoid granulomas, or papilledema. Focality in the neurologic examination may help localize lesion. Cranial nerve abnormalities suggest a basilar meningitis. If accessible lesions outside the CNS are found, these are amendable to biopsy and culture.

E. Tuberculosis (TB), sarcoid, or tumor may be found by chest radiography. Cytologic, microbiologic, or histopathologic examination of tissue, sputum, or fluid obtained from other body sites may confirm a diagnosis of a mycobacterial, fungal, or malignant process. Skin tests have minimal use and should be limited to a PPD and anergy panel. Serologic tests for certain infections and connective tissue diseases can be helpful in the appropriate clinical context. Any patient with a positive serum serology specific for *Treponema pallidum* (e.g., FTA, MHA-TP, HATTS) may have neurosyphilis, even if the serum RPR and CSF VDRL are negative. Obtain blood cultures to exclude bacterial endocarditis. Additional studies, such as mammography and endoscopy, may be indicated in selected cases.

F. Stains and cultures of CSF for bacteria, mycobacteria, and fungi are mandatory and often must be repeated. Large volumes (>10 ml) should be processed to maximize detection of fungi, mycobacteria, and tumor cells. Fungi can sometimes be demonstrated in ventricular CSF, even when lumbar fluid is negative. Additional CSF studies may be diagnostic, such as serologic tests for syphilis, Lyme disease, and certain fungi; cytology for malignancies; and India ink and antigen detection for cryptococcal organisms. The role of polymerase chain reaction (PCR) in identifying etiologic organisms continues to grow, as illustrated by Whipple's disease.

G. If all attempts at diagnosis prove futile, consider a directed biopsy of brain and meninges. The yield of blind meningeal biopsy is low, and this invasive procedure is usually reserved for undiagnosed patients who have a focal lesion or an unrelenting decline in neurologic function.

H. If empiric therapy is undertaken, certain principles guide the strategy of therapeutic trials: (1) diagnostic efforts must continue during therapy; (2) therapeutic response is difficult to interpret because recovery is always protracted, even with the use of appropriate drugs; (3) trials should be made sequentially, not concurrently; (4) amphotericin B should be used last; and (5) corticosteroids should be used cautiously because they confound interpretation of a therapeutic trial and potentially worsen any untreated infection. A trial of antituberculous therapy is indicated in most undiagnosed cases. Despite all diagnostic and therapeutic efforts, sometimes no cause can be determined. Some cases can be categorized retrospectively as "chronic benign lymphocytic meningitis," a self-limited illness in which spontaneous clinical remission usually ensues within 6 months. Other patients have persistent neurologic symptoms and CSF abnormalities. Malignancy and collagen vascular disease are common in this group. Certain patients with "idiopathic" chronic meningitis have a poor prognosis; the etiology often remains undefined, despite postmortem examination.

References

Anderson NE, Willoughby EW, Synek BJ. Leptomeningeal and brain biopsy in chronic meningitis. Aust N Z J Med 1995; 25:703.

Gripshover B, Ellner JJ. Chronic meningitis. In: Mandell GL, Bennett JE, Dolin R, eds. Principles and practice of infectious diseases. 4th ed. New York: Churchill Livingstone, 1995:865.

Peacock JE Jr. Persistent neutrophilic meningitis. Infect Dis Clin North Am 1990; 4:747.

Verdon R, Chevret S, Laissy JP, Wolff M. Tuberculous meningitis in adults: review of 48 cases. Clin Infect Dis 1996; 22:982.

Patient with HEADACHE ± FEVER ± CHANGE IN MENTAL STATUS

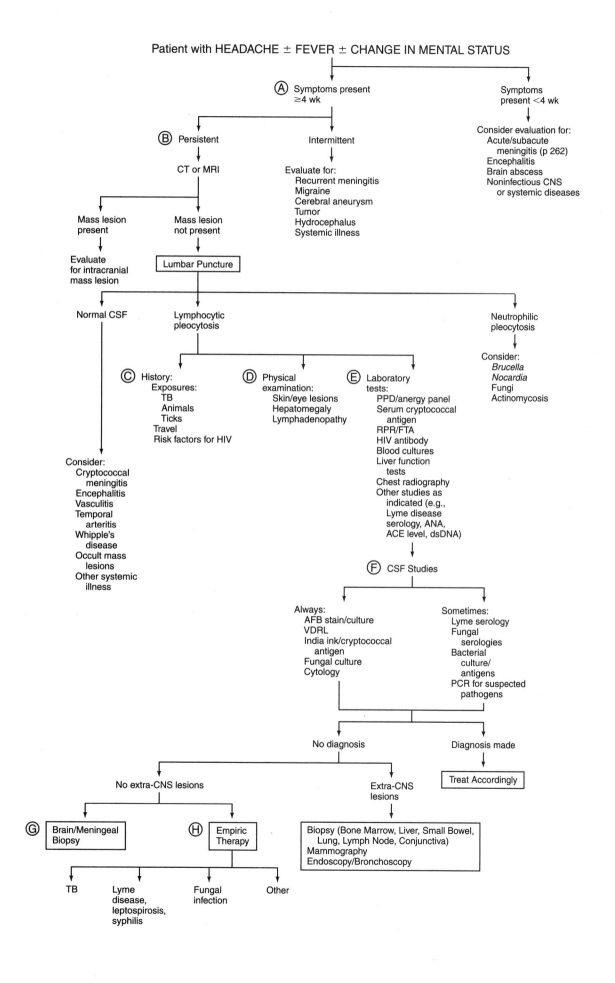

(A) Symptoms present ≥4 wk

Symptoms present <4 wk

Consider evaluation for:
  Acute/subacute
    meningitis (p 262)
  Encephalitis
  Brain abscess
  Noninfectious CNS
    or systemic diseases

(B) Persistent

Intermittent

CT or MRI

Evaluate for:
  Recurrent meningitis
  Migraine
  Cerebral aneurysm
  Tumor
  Hydrocephalus
  Systemic illness

Mass lesion present

Mass lesion not present

Evaluate for intracranial mass lesion

Lumbar Puncture

Normal CSF

Lymphocytic pleocytosis

Neutrophilic pleocytosis

Consider:
  Brucella
  Nocardia
  Fungi
  Actinomycosis

(C) History:
  Exposures:
    TB
    Animals
    Ticks
    Travel
    Risk factors for HIV

(D) Physical examination:
  Skin/eye lesions
  Hepatomegaly
  Lymphadenopathy

(E) Laboratory tests:
  PPD/anergy panel
  Serum cryptococcal antigen
  RPR/FTA
  HIV antibody
  Blood cultures
  Liver function tests
  Chest radiography
  Other studies as indicated (e.g., Lyme disease serology, ANA, ACE level, dsDNA)

Consider:
  Cryptococcal meningitis
  Encephalitis
  Vasculitis
  Temporal arteritis
  Whipple's disease
  Occult mass lesions
  Other systemic illness

(F) CSF Studies

Always:
  AFB stain/culture
  VDRL
  India ink/cryptococcal antigen
  Fungal culture
  Cytology

Sometimes:
  Lyme serology
  Fungal serologies
  Bacterial culture/antigens
  PCR for suspected pathogens

No diagnosis

Diagnosis made

Treat Accordingly

No extra-CNS lesions

Extra-CNS lesions

(G) Brain/Meningeal Biopsy

(H) Empiric Therapy

Biopsy (Bone Marrow, Liver, Small Bowel, Lung, Lymph Node, Conjunctiva)
Mammography
Endoscopy/Bronchoscopy

TB

Lyme disease, leptospirosis, syphilis

Fungal infection

Other

ASEPTIC MENINGITIS

Deborah L. Goldsmith
Richard M. Mandel

A. The history and physical examination are the most useful tools to determine the likely causes of aseptic meningitis. Consider host factors such as immunosuppression, medical history, sexual history and other HIV risk factors, age, medication use, and immunizations. Note epidemiologic factors such as recent travel, ill contacts, exposure to insects or animals, and time of year. Examine the patient for rashes, sinusitis, otitis, herpetic lesions, or evidence of sexually transmitted diseases.

B. MRI in particular can help identify the parietal hemorrhage associated with herpes simplex virus encephalitis, one of the few treatable encephalitides.

C. Order a lumbar puncture (LP) when meningitis is considered. If there is evidence of increased intracranial pressure or focal neurologic signs, obtain a CT or MRI scan before LP to rule out a mass lesion. Measure an opening pressure. At a minimum, obtain cell count and differential, glucose, protein, Gram stain, and bacterial culture. If Gram stain findings are negative, the CSF contains <500 WBCs with a monocyte or lymphocyte predominance, and protein and glucose levels are normal, it is reasonable to observe the patient when he or she is not receiving therapy, especially during summer and fall, when most viral meningitis is contracted. If these criteria are not met or there is doubt, institute empiric antibacterial therapy. If the patient is immunocompromised, is elderly, or has recently been taking antibiotics, treat with antibiotics for 48–72 hours while awaiting cultures. Consider counterimmunoelectrophoresis for bacterial antigens (*Streptococcus pneumoniae, Neisseria meningitidis,* and *Haemophilus influenzae*) if available. Polymerase chain reaction (PCR) is a rapid, sensitive way to detect enteroviruses; this test likely will soon be used commercially for diagnosis of aseptic meningitis.

D. There are numerous noninfectious causes of meningitis. NSAIDs are most often implicated; patients with systemic lupus erythematosus (SLE) are at particular risk.

The antibiotic trimethoprim and the sulfonamides also have been associated with aseptic meningitis; unfortunately, the recent use of antibiotics may lead to negative CSF cultures because of partially treated bacterial meningitis, giving a similar clinical and laboratory picture. There have been rare reports of penicillin-, ciprofloxacin-, and isoniazid-associated aseptic meningitis. Intravenous immunoglobulin, azathioprine, and muromonab CD-3 also have been implicated. Drugs injected intrathecally can cause direct chemical irritation of the meninges. Mollaret's (benign endothelioleukocytic) aseptic meningitis usually is mild and self-limited but can recur. Malignancy, collagen vascular disease (SLE, Sjögren's disease), heavy metal poisoning, and subarachnoid hemorrhage may have associated aseptic meningitis. Miscellaneous causes include Behçet's syndrome, Kawasaki disease, multiple sclerosis, postvaccination (measles, mumps), and sarcoidosis.

E. Evaluate patients in endemic areas with serologic tests for Lyme disease, coccidioidomycosis, and histoplasmosis. For those with known malignancy or compatible history, have CSF spun down for cytologic study. Recent freshwater swimmers are at risk for amebic infection.

References

Connolly KJ, Hammer SM. The acute aseptic meningitis syndrome. Infect Dis Clin North Am 1990; 4:599.

Elmore JG, Horwitz RI, Quagliarello VJ. Acute meningitis with a negative Gram's stain: clinical and management outcomes in 171 episodes. Am J Med 1996; 100:78.

Lipton JD, Schafermeyer RW. Central nervous system infections—the usual and unusual. Emerg Med Clin North Am 1995; 13:41.

Marinac JS. Drug and chemical-induced aseptic meningitis: a review of the literature. Ann Pharmacother 1992; 26:813.

Yerly S, Gervaix A, Simonet V, et al. Rapid and sensitive detection of enterovirus in specimens from patients with aseptic meningitis. J Clin Microbiol 1996; 34:199.

Patient with SIGNS/SYMPTOMS OF MENINGITIS (FEVER, HEADACHE, STIFF NECK, PHOTOPHOBIA)

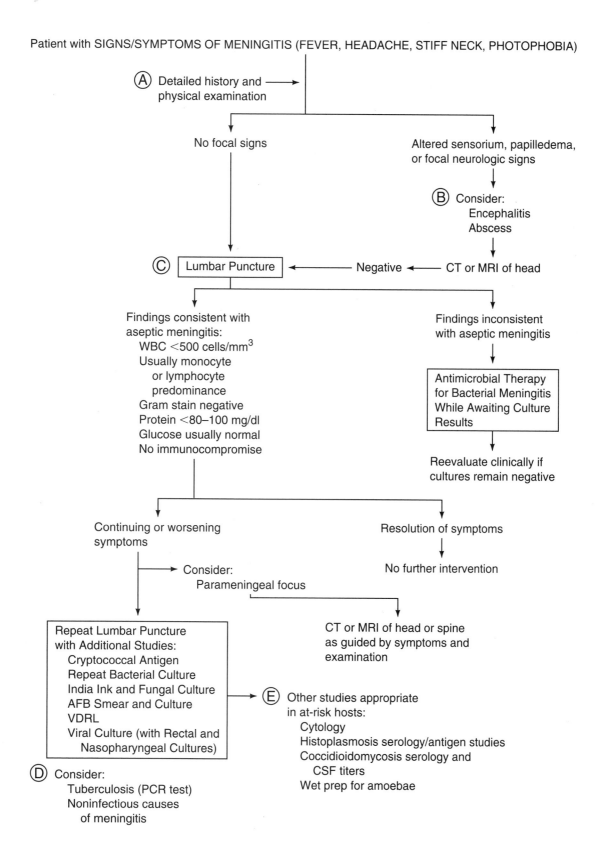

Ⓐ Detailed history and physical examination

No focal signs

Altered sensorium, papilledema, or focal neurologic signs

Ⓑ Consider:
Encephalitis
Abscess

Ⓒ Lumbar Puncture ← Negative ← CT or MRI of head

Findings consistent with aseptic meningitis:
WBC <500 cells/mm³
Usually monocyte or lymphocyte predominance
Gram stain negative
Protein <80–100 mg/dl
Glucose usually normal
No immunocompromise

Findings inconsistent with aseptic meningitis

Antimicrobial Therapy for Bacterial Meningitis While Awaiting Culture Results

Reevaluate clinically if cultures remain negative

Continuing or worsening symptoms

Consider:
Parameningeal focus

Resolution of symptoms

No further intervention

Repeat Lumbar Puncture with Additional Studies:
Cryptococcal Antigen
Repeat Bacterial Culture
India Ink and Fungal Culture
AFB Smear and Culture
VDRL
Viral Culture (with Rectal and Nasopharyngeal Cultures)

CT or MRI of head or spine as guided by symptoms and examination

Ⓔ Other studies appropriate in at-risk hosts:
Cytology
Histoplasmosis serology/antigen studies
Coccidioidomycosis serology and CSF titers
Wet prep for amoebae

Ⓓ Consider:
Tuberculosis (PCR test)
Noninfectious causes of meningitis

SEXUALLY TRANSMITTED DISEASES

Dianna L. Rynkiewicz

Symptoms of STDs include genital lesions, discharges, and GU complaints. High-risk characteristics include age <25 years, low socioeconomic status, female gender, unmarried status, illicit drug use, and STD history.

A. Elicit sexual history, nature of the primary lesion (vesicle, papule), duration of lesion, history of recurrence, and associated symptoms (pruritus, fevers, malaise). Examine skin, throat, lymph nodes, lower abdomen, external and internal genitalia, rectum and perirectal area, and other sites as indicated.

B. Screen sexually active adolescent males for urethritis. Urinary leukocyte esterase is 46–100% sensitive and 83–93% specific for urethritis in males. Follow up a positive leukocyte esterase test with a urethral Gram stain. A presumptive diagnosis of nongonococcal urethritis (NGU) is made with urethral Gram stain showing >4 leukocytes per oil immersion field.

C. Because >70% of women infected with chlamydia may be asymptomatic, the CDC recommends screening for cervicitis in high-risk females: all sexually active women <20 years old; 20–24 years old with new or >1 sexual partner within the past 3 months or irregular barrier contraceptive use; and >24 years old with both of the above criteria.

D. Presumptive diagnosis of chlamydial cervicitis is made with cervical Gram stain showing >10 leukocytes per oil immersion field. Cervical Gram stain is not very sensitive for the diagnosis of *Neisseria gonorrhoeae* (NG). Cervical culture is highly sensitive and is the recommended diagnostic assay. Diagnostic tests for chlamydia include direct fluorescent antibody (DFA), enzyme-linked immunosorbent assay (ELISA), DNA hybridization, and nucleic acid amplification. Cervical culture for chlamydia is about 70% sensitive and highly dependent on adequate specimen, transport, and storage; its yield increases if pooled with urethral culture. Nonculture methods for identifying NG are available and are more rapid but compromise sensitivity or specificity and do not allow for susceptibility testing. Confirm all nonculture methods for identifying chlamydia and NG in low-prevalence populations with culture or a second nonculture test.

E. The clinical examination is insensitive in identifying the cause of ulcers and discharges. Confirmatory laboratory testing is imperative.

F. Human papillomavirus (HPV) types 16, 18, 31, 33, and 35 have been strongly associated with the development of cervical dysplasia and cancer.

G. Up to 10% of genital ulcers have more than one cause; therefore pursue a complete evaluation on all ulcers of unknown cause.

H. A positive darkfield examination (DFE) is diagnostic for syphilis. Three consecutive DFEs are required before a lesion can be considered negative. Debris and antiseptics may cause a false-negative result. Order nontreponemal syphilis serology initially for all ulcers; 1- and 3-month follow-up serology is optional. HIV-infected patients are more likely to have false-negative serologic results, especially if the CD4 cell count is <200.

I. A complement fixation titer of >256 strongly suggests lymphogranuloma venereum.

J. Enriched selective medium improves the isolation rate of *Haemophilus ducreyi*. Gram stain may show characteristic "school of fish" gram-negative coccobacilli.

K. Up to 30% of syphilitic chancres may be tender; frank pain is common with superinfection.

L. Granuloma inguinale is rare in the United States (<40 cases/year).

M. Treatment is based on local susceptibility patterns, patient allergies, and pregnancy status. It includes partner notification/screening and empiric treatment, education on STD prevention and risk reduction, and HIV test counseling. Perform a screening nontreponemal syphilis test on all persons diagnosed with an STD.

N. Noninvasive methods for screening males for chlamydia are ELISA and urine polymerase chain reaction (PCR; 94% sensitivity, 99–100% specificity). Nonculture methods for identifying NG are more rapid but compromise sensitivity or specificity and do not allow for susceptibility testing. All nonculture methods for identifying chlamydia and NG in low-prevalence populations should be confirmed with culture or a second nonculture test.

O. Less common causes of NGU are *Ureaplasma urealyticum, Mycoplasma hominis, Trichomonas,* and rarely herpes simplex virus.

P. Chlamydial infection is present in 20–50% of cases of gonococcal infection; therefore empiric cotreatment is recommended.

Q. Anaerobic bacteria and trichomonads give off an amine odor when drops of 10% KOH are added to infected vaginal secretions.

(Continued on page 272)

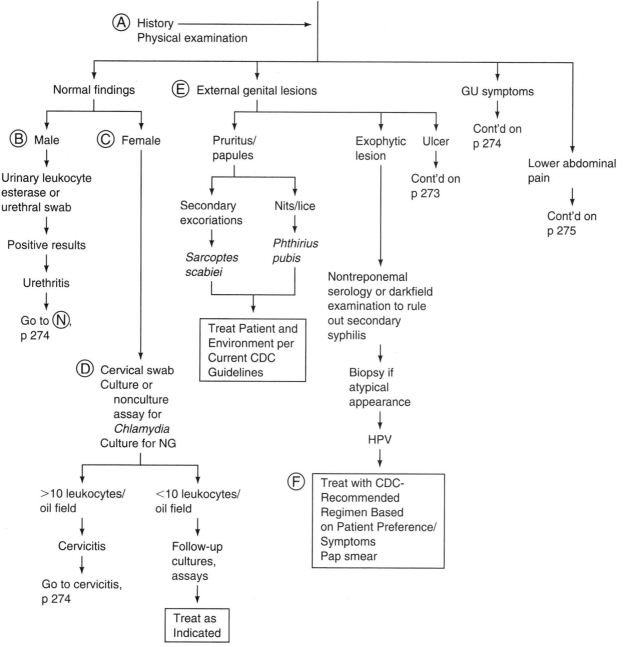

Patient with Suspected SEXUALLY TRANSMITTED DISEASE
(Patient with symptoms, asymptomatic high-risk patient
in STD or primary-care clinic, or partner of STD-infected patient)

(A) History
Physical examination

Normal findings

(E) External genital lesions

GU symptoms

(B) Male   (C) Female

Pruritus/
papules

Exophytic
lesion

Ulcer

Cont'd on
p 274

Urinary leukocyte
esterase or
urethral swab

Secondary
excoriations

Nits/lice

Cont'd on
p 273

Lower abdominal
pain

Positive results

Sarcoptes
scabiei

Phthirius
pubis

Nontreponemal
serology or darkfield
examination to rule
out secondary
syphilis

Cont'd on
p 275

Urethritis

Go to (N),
p 274

Treat Patient and
Environment per
Current CDC
Guidelines

Biopsy if
atypical
appearance

(D) Cervical swab
Culture or
nonculture
assay for
Chlamydia
Culture for NG

HPV

>10 leukocytes/
oil field

<10 leukocytes/
oil field

(F) Treat with CDC-
Recommended
Regimen Based
on Patient Preference/
Symptoms
Pap smear

Cervicitis

Follow-up
cultures,
assays

Go to cervicitis,
p 274

Treat as
Indicated

271

R. Clue cells are epithelial cells coated with large numbers of bacteria.

S. Treat the partner of a patient with candidiasis or bacterial vaginosis only if the patient has frequent recurrences with the same partner.

T. Silent pelvic inflammatory disease (PID), a sequela of chlamydia infection, underlies most cases of tubal infertility and ectopic pregnancy.

References

Black CM. Current methods of laboratory diagnosis of *Chlamydia trachomatis* infections. Clin Microbiol Rev 1997; 10:160.

Centers for Disease Control and Prevention. 1993 Sexually transmitted diseases treatment guidelines. MMWR 1993; 42(RR-14):1.

Mandell GL, Douglas RG, Bennett JE, eds. Principles and practice of infectious diseases. 4th ed. New York: McGraw-Hill, 1995.

Morse SA, Moreland AA, Holmes KK, eds. Atlas of sexually transmitted diseases and AIDS. 2nd ed. London: Mosby-Wolfe, 1996.

Quinn TC, Zenilman J, Rompalo A. Sexually transmitted diseases: advances in diagnosis and treatment. Adv Intern Med 1994; 39:149.

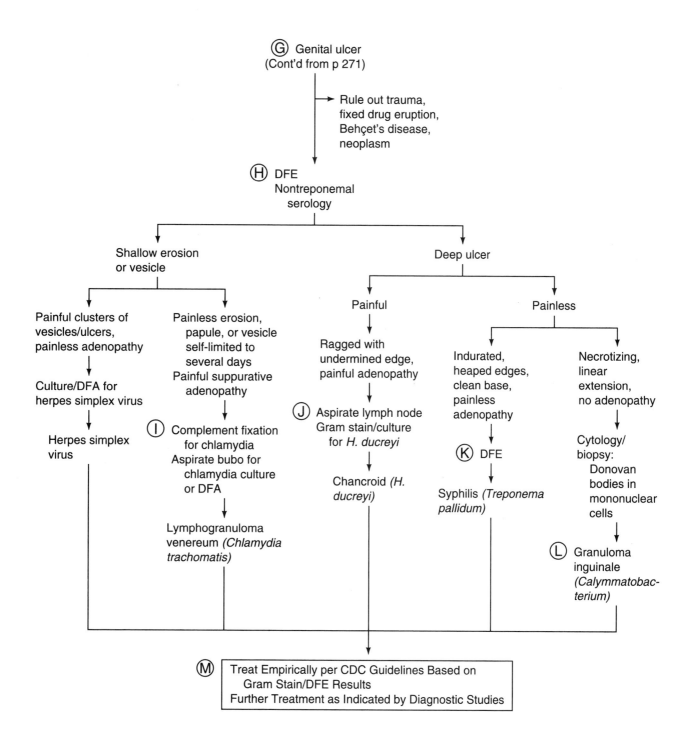

G Genital ulcer
(Cont'd from p 271)

→ Rule out trauma,
fixed drug eruption,
Behçet's disease,
neoplasm

H DFE
Nontreponemal
serology

Shallow erosion or vesicle

Painful clusters of vesicles/ulcers, painless adenopathy

Culture/DFA for herpes simplex virus

Herpes simplex virus

Painless erosion, papule, or vesicle self-limited to several days
Painful suppurative adenopathy

I Complement fixation for chlamydia
Aspirate bubo for chlamydia culture or DFA

Lymphogranuloma venereum *(Chlamydia trachomatis)*

Deep ulcer

Painful

Ragged with undermined edge, painful adenopathy

J Aspirate lymph node Gram stain/culture for *H. ducreyi*

Chancroid *(H. ducreyi)*

Painless

Indurated, heaped edges, clean base, painless adenopathy

K DFE

Syphilis *(Treponema pallidum)*

Necrotizing, linear extension, no adenopathy

Cytology/ biopsy:
Donovan bodies in mononuclear cells

L Granuloma inguinale *(Calymmatobacterium)*

M Treat Empirically per CDC Guidelines Based on
Gram Stain/DFE Results
Further Treatment as Indicated by Diagnostic Studies

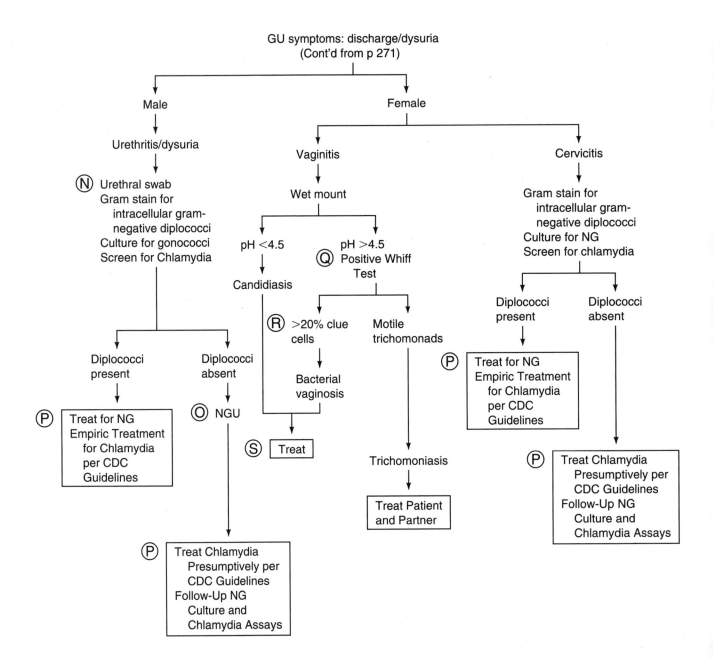

GU symptoms: discharge/dysuria
(Cont'd from p 271)

Male

Urethritis/dysuria

Ⓝ Urethral swab
Gram stain for
intracellular gram-
negative diplococci
Culture for gonococci
Screen for Chlamydia

Diplococci present

Ⓟ Treat for NG
Empiric Treatment
for Chlamydia
per CDC
Guidelines

Diplococci absent

Ⓞ NGU

Ⓟ Treat Chlamydia
Presumptively per
CDC Guidelines
Follow-Up NG
Culture and
Chlamydia Assays

Female

Vaginitis

Wet mount

pH <4.5

Candidiasis

pH >4.5
Ⓠ Positive Whiff
Test

Ⓡ >20% clue cells

Bacterial vaginosis

Ⓢ Treat

Motile trichomonads

Trichomoniasis

Treat Patient
and Partner

Cervicitis

Gram stain for
intracellular gram-
negative diplococci
Culture for NG
Screen for chlamydia

Diplococci present

Ⓟ Treat for NG
Empiric Treatment
for Chlamydia
per CDC
Guidelines

Diplococci absent

Ⓟ Treat Chlamydia
Presumptively per
CDC Guidelines
Follow-Up NG
Culture and
Chlamydia Assays

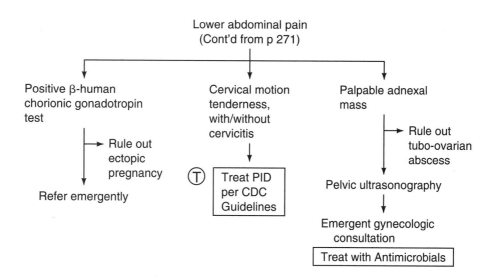

Lower abdominal pain
(Cont'd from p 271)

Positive β-human
chorionic gonadotropin
test

→ Rule out
ectopic
pregnancy

Refer emergently

Cervical motion
tenderness,
with/without
cervicitis

(T) Treat PID
per CDC
Guidelines

Palpable adnexal
mass

→ Rule out
tubo-ovarian
abscess

Pelvic ultrasonography

Emergent gynecologic
consultation

Treat with Antimicrobials

APPROACH TO THE NEWLY DIAGNOSED HIV-POSITIVE PATIENT

J. Kevin Carmichael

HIV infection is most commonly diagnosed by detection of serum antibodies. The most commonly used test is the enzyme-linked immunosorbent assay (ELISA), which has both a sensitivity and specificity >98%. The predictive power of a positive ELISA varies with the prevalence of HIV in the population tested. A positive test in a person with a history of high-risk behaviors is probably a true positive, and a positive test in a person without such a history is likely a false positive. Consequently a person should not be definitively diagnosed as HIV-infected until a confirmatory test such as a Western blot or an HIV immunofluorescence assay is also positive.

A. Counseling the HIV-infected person is a continuous process beginning with pretest counseling and lasting throughout the infection. There are certain "imperatives" as follows: (1) the distinction between HIV infection and AIDS, (2) the natural history of HIV infection and available intervention/treatment measures, (3) methods of transmission and the prevention of transmission, and (4) referral to community resources. The burden of counseling rests with the physician, but many other resources often are available and should be used to complement physician counseling.

B. Obtain a general history. Pay special attention to any history of and treatment of STDs, mycobacterial infections, and AIDS-defining illnesses. Also obtain an immunization review (Table 1).

C. Order baseline laboratory testing. Specific complaints may require additional testing for evaluation.

D. An HIV-focused review of systems is critical in HIV management. Review of systems should include fatigue, weight loss, anorexia, anxiety, depression, fever, chills, night sweats, adenopathy, skin rash or bruising, headache, sinus or ear pain, visual changes, oral sores, odynophagia, dysphagia, shortness of breath, dyspnea on exertion, cough, abdominal pain, diarrhea, genital-rectal sores or pain, arthritis, muscle weakness, forgetfulness, and discoordination.

E. The CD4 lymphocyte number correlates well with immune function and is used to gauge the risk for opportunistic infections and the need for opportunistic infection prophylaxis (see H). In addition, all patients with a CD4 <500 on two occasions separated by >1 month should be offered antiretroviral therapy. Plasma HIV-1 RNA levels correlate strongly with the risk of progression to AIDS and death. Treatment-induced changes in these levels may be used to measure and monitor the efficacy of antiretroviral therapy. Patients with HIV-1 RNA >5000–10,000 copies/ml should also be offered antiretroviral therapy regardless of CD4 count. Patients who are symptom free and have a CD4 >500 and lower HIV-1 RNA levels should be monitored every 3–6 months; some experts recommend antiretroviral therapy for any person with detectable virus who is wiling to commit to a long-term regimen.

(Continued on page 278)

TABLE 1 Immunization of HIV-Infected Adults

Streptococcus pneumoniae: Recommended for all patients.
Influenza: Recommended for all patients annually before influenza season.
Hepatitis B: Recommended for all susceptible patients (anti-HBc negative).
Patients with a CD4 <200 may not mount a protective humoral response to immunization, and vaccination should be considered optional. There have been reports of transient increases in HIV replication after immunization of patients not receiving antiretroviral therapy. The clinical significance of these transient elevations is unclear and immunization is still recommended because the benefits appear to outweigh the risks.

NEWLY DIAGNOSED HIV-POSITIVE PATIENT

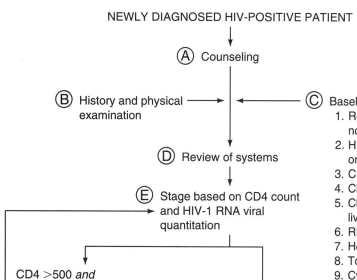

Ⓐ Counseling

Ⓑ History and physical ⟶ ⟵ Ⓒ Baseline laboratory testing:
examination
　　1. Repeat HIV-1 antibody testing if documentation
　　　 not available
　　2. HIV-1 RNA quantitation by either PCR, bDNA,
Ⓓ Review of systems　　　 or NASBA methodology
　　3. CD4 enumeration
　　4. CBC with platelets
Ⓔ Stage based on CD4 count　　5. Chemistry panel including albumin to assess
　 and HIV-1 RNA viral　　　 liver and kidney function and nutritional status
　 quantitation　　6. RPR
　　7. Hepatitis B serology
　　8. Toxoplasmosis IgG
　　9. Cytomegalovirus IgG
CD4 >500 and　　10. Chest radiograph
HIV-1 RNA <5000–10,000　　11. Tuberculin skin test unless there is a reliable
　　　 history of a previous positive test or of treatment
　　　 for tuberculosis
Repeat CD4　　12. Cervical Pap smear in women
and HIV-1 RNA
viral quantitation
q3–6mo　　　　　　Cont'd on p 279

277

TABLE 2 Antiretroviral Agents

Nucleoside reverse transcriptase inhibitors

Didanosine (ddI)	Videx	200 mg bid*
Lamivudine (3TC)	Epivir	150 mg bid
Stavudine (d4T)	Zerit	40 mg bid*
Zalcitabine (ddC)	Hivid	0.75 mg tid
Zidovudine (AZT, ZDV)	Retrovir	200 mg tid or 300 mg bid

Non-nucleoside reverse transcriptase inhibitors

Nevirapine	Viramune	200 mg bid
Delaviradine	Rescriptor	400 mg tid
Protease inhibitors		
Indinavir	Crixivan	800 mg q8h
Nelfinavir	Viracept	750 mg tid
Ritonavir	Norvir	600 mg bid
Saquinavir	Invirase	600 mg tid
	Fortovase	1200 mg tid

*Reduce dose if patient is <60 kg.

TABLE 3 Opportunistic Infection Prophylaxis

Organism	Indication	Preferred Prophylactic Agent
Mycobacterium tuberculosis	Tuberculin skin test >5 mm Active tuberculosis excluded	Isoniazid × 12 mo
Pneumocystis carinii	CD4 <200, unexplained fever >100° F for >2 wk, or oral candidiasis	Trimethoprim-sulfamethoxazole
Toxoplasma gondii	IgG antibody to toxoplasma and CD4 <100	Trimethoprim-sulfamethoxazole
Mycobacterium avium complex	CD4 <50	Clarithromycin or azithromycin
Varicella virus	Significant exposure to chicken pox or zoster with no history of either	Varicella-zoster immune globulin within 96 hr of exposure

F. The goal of antiretroviral therapy is to maximally inhibit viral replication and minimize the development of resistant strains of HIV. There are currently three classes of antiretroviral medications: nucleoside reverse transcriptase inhibitors, non-nucleoside reverse transcriptase inhibitors, and protease inhibitors. Nucleoside reverse transcriptase inhibitors compete with nucleoside triphosphates and, when incorporated, cause premature termination of viral-DNA chain synthesis. Non-nucleoside reverse transcriptase inhibitors are noncompetitive inhibitors of reverse transcriptase and bind directly to reverse transcriptase, changing conformation and inactivating the catalytic site. Protease inhibitors inhibit HIV protease, which is responsible for cleaving viral precursor proteins into the final viral elements.

The rapid rate of viral replication allows for the rapid acquisition of antiretroviral resistance in the face of suboptimal therapy. Combination therapy has emerged as the standard of care, but the optimal number of agents to be used is not yet known. The current recommendation is to use three-drug therapy. Recommended combinations include two nucleoside analogs such as zidovudine/didanosine, zidovudine/zalcitabine, zidovudine/lamivudine, or stavudine/lamivudine, and plus either a protease inhibitor or a non-nucleoside reverse transcriptase inhibitor (Table 2).

G. Plasma HIV-1 RNA quantification allows for the monitoring of the magnitude and the duration of antiretroviral activity. HIV-1 RNA levels should be measured 4 weeks after initiating or changing therapy. The assay has a biologic variability of about 0.3 log and an intra-assay variability of about 0.2 log and consequently the minimum reduction in HIV-1 RNA levels needed to demonstrate antiretroviral activity is 0.5 log. The goal of antiretroviral therapy is a decline in HIV-1 RNA of >0.5 log and a decline to <5000. Although the greatest treatment-induced changes in HIV-1 RNA occur in the first 4 weeks, it may take up to 6 months to see the maximal effects. Stable patients receiving antiretroviral therapy should have HIV-1 RNA and CD4 count measured every 3 months. CD4 changes are now thought to be of less use in guiding antiretroviral therapy than HIV-1 RNA levels, but they are still necessary to determine the need for prophylaxis and as a secondary measure of antiretroviral efficacy.

H. Despite the improving efficacy of antiretroviral therapy, appropriate prophylaxis against opportunistic infection remains a clinical imperative in the care of persons with HIV infection. Prophylaxis against *Mycobacterium tuberculosis*, *Pneumocystis carinii*, *Toxoplasma gondii*, *Mycobacterium avium* complex, Varicella virus, and immunization against *Streptococcus pneumoniae* are strongly recommended as standard of care (Table 3).

References

Carpenter CJ, Fischl MR, Hammer SM, et al. Antiretroviral therapy for HIV infection in 1997. JAMA 1997; 377:1962.

Guidelines for the use of antiretroviral agents in HIV-infected adults and adolescents. November 5, 1997.

Kaplan JE, Masur H, Holmes KK, et al. USPHS/IDSA guidelines for the prevention of opportunistic infections in persons infected with human immunodeficiency virus. Clin Infect Dis 1997; 25(suppl 3):S299.

NEWLY DIAGNOSED HIV-POSITIVE PATIENT
(Cont'd from p 277)

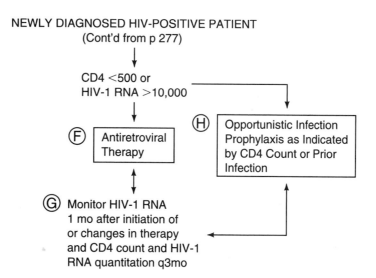

THE ACUTELY ILL HIV-POSITIVE PATIENT

Deborah L. Goldsmith
Richard M. Mandel

A. A meticulous history can point out specific risks such as ill contacts, recent diet, travel, sexual activity, and medication compliance. A careful review of systems often directs the work-up. Physical examination should be thorough, including skin, lymph nodes, eyes, mouth, face/sinuses, heart, lungs, abdomen, genitalia, and nervous system.

B. Although fever is common in HIV-positive patients, a cause can be found in >80% with careful work-up. Admit patients who appear toxic or are neutropenic for thorough evaluation and empiric antibiotic therapy. If there are no localizing signs or symptoms, consider the AIDS-defining illnesses of occult *Pneumocystis carinii* pneumonia (PCP), *Mycobacterium avium*-complex bacteremia, toxoplasmosis, lymphoma, cryptococcal meningitis, cytomegalovirus (CMV), or tuberculosis. Catheter infections, sinusitis, dental abscess, and pelvic inflammatory disease also can cause fever with few other symptoms. Always consider drug fever.

C. Acute visual changes require immediate evaluation by funduscopy. In patients with <100 CD4 cells, referral to an ophthalmologist is imperative if no cause is found by direct funduscopy.

D. Retinal hemorrhage or exuberant yellow exudate is suspicious for CMV retinitis; empiric therapy and immediate ophthalmologic referral are warranted. Other infectious causes of retinitis include *P. carinii* (especially if the patient has been taking inhaled pentamidine for PCP prophylaxis), *Toxoplasma gondii,* and syphilis. Cotton-wool spots are common in the HIV-positive patient and merely need close follow-up; they are not sight threatening.

E. The HIV-positive patient may be acutely ill from sudden profuse diarrhea or from severe dehydration and inanition from chronic diarrhea. Patients who are orthostatic or unable to maintain euvolemia at home should be admitted to the hospital.

F. Initial evaluation of acute diarrhea includes routine culture for enteric pathogens *(Salmonella, Shigella, Campylobacter jejuni)* and evaluation of stool for fecal leukocytes, *Clostridium difficile* toxin if the patient has had recent antibiotic therapy, with or without examination for ova and parasites. Obtain blood cultures in the febrile patient. Consider empiric antibiotic therapy if the patient appears toxic. If the diarrhea is chronic, evaluation of stool for ova and parasites, *Cryptosporidium* and *Microsporidium* assays, acid-fast bacilli smear and cultures, and blood cultures for *Mycobacterium* are warranted.

G. If stool studies are negative and diarrhea persists, consider lower GI tract endoscopy with biopsies for CMV, mycobacteria, fungi, and parasites and electron microscopy for *Microsporidium.* Upper GI endoscopy for routine histopathology and biopsy for CMV and *Giardia* may be more appropriate for the patient with watery diarrhea, no cramps, blood, or fecal leukocytes. Remember noninfectious causes of diarrhea such as pancreatic insufficiency and lactose intolerance. If no sources are found, treat with antimotility agents.

H. HIV-positive patients are prone to rash and other dermatologic complications. Infections such as herpes simplex virus (HSV) and varicella-zoster virus (VZV) can present with perioral, oral, perirectal, or genital lesions. Nonmucosal skin may also be affected, especially with VZV. Brown or purple papules are seen in Kaposi's sarcoma (KS) and bacillary angiomatosis *(Bartonella henselae).* Treat psoriasis, ichthyosis, tinea, and seborrheic dermatitis as in the non-HIV patient. Scabies often causes an exuberant keratotic reaction (Norwegian scabies) that may require multiple treatments. Drug eruptions are common. Maintain a very low threshold for dermatology referral and biopsy.

I. Odynophagia and dysphagia are common in HIV-positive patients. A thorough oral examination to assess for abscesses, ulcers, vesicles, or thrush is necessary. If thrush is seen, empiric treatment for esophageal candidiasis is reasonable. If there is no response, perform upper GI endoscopy for direct visualization and biopsies for CMV, HSV, and fungal cultures. KS, giant aphthous ulcers, other malignancies, or gastroesophageal reflux disease may be diagnosed.

References

Friedburg DN. Cytomegalovirus retinitis: diagnosis and status of systemic therapy. J Acquir Immune Defic Syndr Hum Retrovirol 1997; 14(Suppl 1):S1.

Lew E, Dieterich D, Poles M, Scholes J. Gastrointestinal emergencies in the patient with AIDS. Crit Care Clin 1995; 11:531.

Sande MA, Volberding PA. The medical management of AIDS. 5th ed. Philadelphia: WB Saunders, 1997.

Sepkowitz KA, Telzak EE, Carrow M, Armstrong D. Fever among outpatients with advanced human immunodeficiency virus infection. Arch Intern Med 1993; 153:1909.

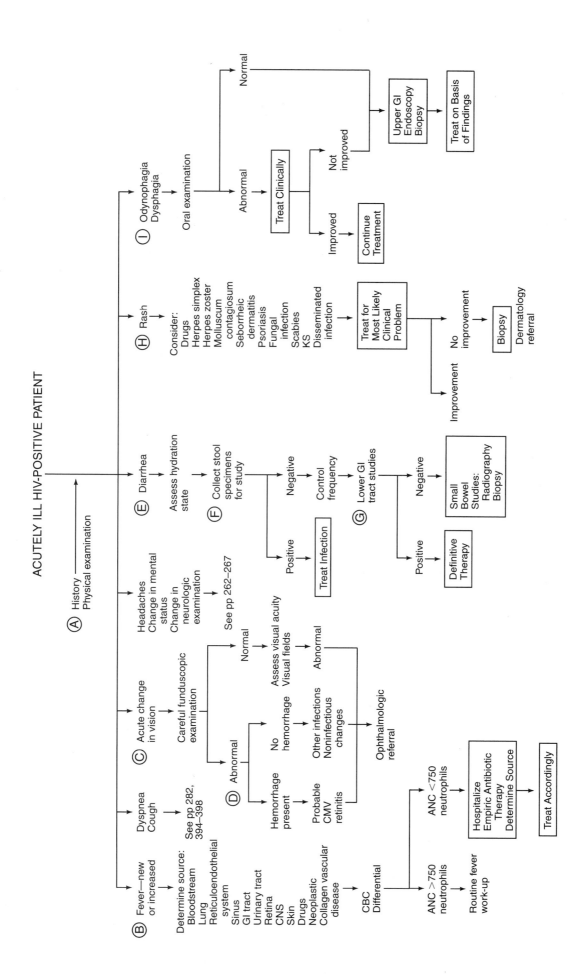

ACUTELY ILL HIV-POSITIVE PATIENT

Ⓐ History — Physical examination

Ⓑ Fever—new or increased

Determine source:
Bloodstream
Lung
Reticuloendothelial system
Sinus
GI tract
Urinary tract
Retina
CNS
Skin
Drugs
Neoplastic
Collagen vascular disease

CBC Differential

ANC >750 neutrophils → Routine fever work-up

ANC <750 neutrophils → Hospitalize Empiric Antibiotic Therapy Determine Source → Treat Accordingly

Dyspnea Cough → See pp 282, 394–398

Ⓒ Acute change in vision → Careful funduscopic examination

Normal → Assess visual acuity Visual fields

Ⓓ Abnormal

Hemorrhage present → Probable CMV retinitis

No hemorrhage → Other infections Noninfectious changes

Abnormal → Ophthalmologic referral

Headaches Change in mental status Change in neurologic examination → See pp 262–267

Ⓔ Diarrhea → Assess hydration state

Ⓕ Collect stool specimens for study

Positive → Treat Infection

Negative → Control frequency

Ⓖ Lower GI tract studies

Positive → Definitive Therapy

Negative → Small Bowel Studies: Radiography Biopsy

Ⓗ Rash

Consider:
Drugs
Herpes simplex
Herpes zoster
Molluscum contagiosum
Seborrheic dermatitis
Psoriasis
Fungal infection
Scabies
KS
Disseminated infection

→ Treat for Most Likely Clinical Problem

Improvement

No improvement → Biopsy Dermatology referral

Ⓘ Odynophagia Dysphagia → Oral examination

Normal → Upper GI Endoscopy Biopsy → Treat on Basis of Findings

Abnormal → Treat Clinically

Improved → Continue Treatment

Not improved → Upper GI Endoscopy Biopsy → Treat on Basis of Findings

PULMONARY INFILTRATES IN HIV-INFECTED PATIENTS

Karam C. Mounzer
Ian Woolley
Mark J. DiNubile

A. Pulmonary disease is the most common reason for presentation and the major cause of death in HIV-infected patients. Staging of such patients with regard to their HIV status is essential because most opportunistic infections are less likely to occur in patients with CD4+ lymphocyte count $\geq 200/mm^3$. These infections become increasingly frequent as the CD4+ count drops below 200 and/or when patients develop wasting, persistent fever, oral thrush, or other opportunistic infections. Despite prophylaxis, *Pneumocystis carinii* pneumonia (PCP) remains the most common opportunistic infection in these patients; failures are uncommon but still occur in compliant patients taking daily trimethoprim-sulfamethoxazole as a prophylaxis.

Fever is commonly but not invariably present in HIV-infected patients with respiratory complaints. However, it is a nonspecific finding because patients with advanced HIV disease are often febrile in the absence of localized signs and symptoms.

Pulmonary, extrapulmonary, and disseminated tuberculosis is increasingly recognized in HIV-infected persons, especially in those who acquire their infection through drug use or sex with drug users. The pulmonary manifestations are often atypical, and infiltrates may not involve the upper lobes. When pulmonary tuberculosis is suspected (as it should be whenever patients with any stage of HIV infection present from a high-risk environment with a subacute or chronic illness in association with cough and localized pulmonary infiltrates), the patient should be placed in respiratory isolation until the diagnosis is effectively excluded. Atypical myobacteria are much less likely than *M. tuberculosis* to present with a predominantly respiratory illness.

B. Although not diagnostic, a chest x-ray (CXR) is a useful guide to the work-up of respiratory symptoms. A CXR with diffuse infiltrates is highly suggestive of PCP in a patient with advanced HIV infection and a subacute illness. However, as many as 20% of patients with clinical PCP have normal CXRs. Focal infiltrates are unusual with PCP, except when involving the upper lobe(s) in patients taking aerosolized pentamidine for PCP prophylaxis. Prominent pleural effusions and intrathoracic adenopathy are seldom encountered in PCP and suggest a different (or coexistent) diagnosis.

Pneumococcal pneumonia, a common complication of HIV infection at any stage, presents acutely as lobar or segmental consolidation. Other causes of localized or diffuse infiltrates in HIV-infected patients include *Haemophilus influenzae*, *Legionella* sp., *Rhodococcus equi*, *Nocardia asteroides*, endemic and opportunistic fungi, *Toxoplasma gondii*, some viruses, and tumors. Episodic bronchospasm and/or recurrent fleeting infiltrates in a patient from an endemic area raises the suspicion of migratory larvae of *Strongyloides stercoralis*; unfortunately the presence or absence of eosinophilia has little diagnostic use.

C. The degree of oxygen desaturation can be both a helpful diagnostic tool in patients without pulmonary infiltrates and an important prognostic factor in patients with PCP. If the patient's Po_2 when breathing room air is within normal limits for his or her age, measure O_2 saturation after treadmill exercise (or the equivalent). A drop in O_2 saturation $\geq 5\%$ is considered abnormal. Evaluate patients with O_2 desaturation, even with a normal CXR, and treat empirically for PCP. An (A-a) gradient ≥ 35 and/or a $Po_2 < 70$ mm Hg on room air are indications for adjunctive corticosteroids (along with specific anti-PCP therapy) in patients in whom the diagnosis of PCP is secure. Cytomegalovirus (CMV) often is found in the lungs of patients with PCP but only rarely affects the clinical outcome.

D. Most patients with PCP have a dry cough and cannot produce a deep sputum specimen. In these cases, sputum can best be induced with 3% to 5% saline administered via a nebulizer for 10–20 minutes. The recovered sample is stained with Papanicolaou (Pap) or similar reagents to look for alveolar macrophages (as markers of the adequacy of the specimen) and with Gomori methenamine silver (GMS) for *P. carinii* cysts. The diagnostic sensitivity of this approach varies from 50–80%, largely depending on technical expertise. Indirect immunofluorescence and polymerase chain reaction tests for *P. carinii* are more sensitive techniques but less readily available. PCP sometimes can be identified in respiratory tract specimens from asymptomatic persons with AIDS or may cause disease concurrently with other opportunistic pathogens.

(Continued on page 284)

HIV-INFECTED PATIENT WITH RESPIRATORY COMPLAINTS
(COUGH, DYSPNEA, FEVER, AND/OR CHEST PAIN)

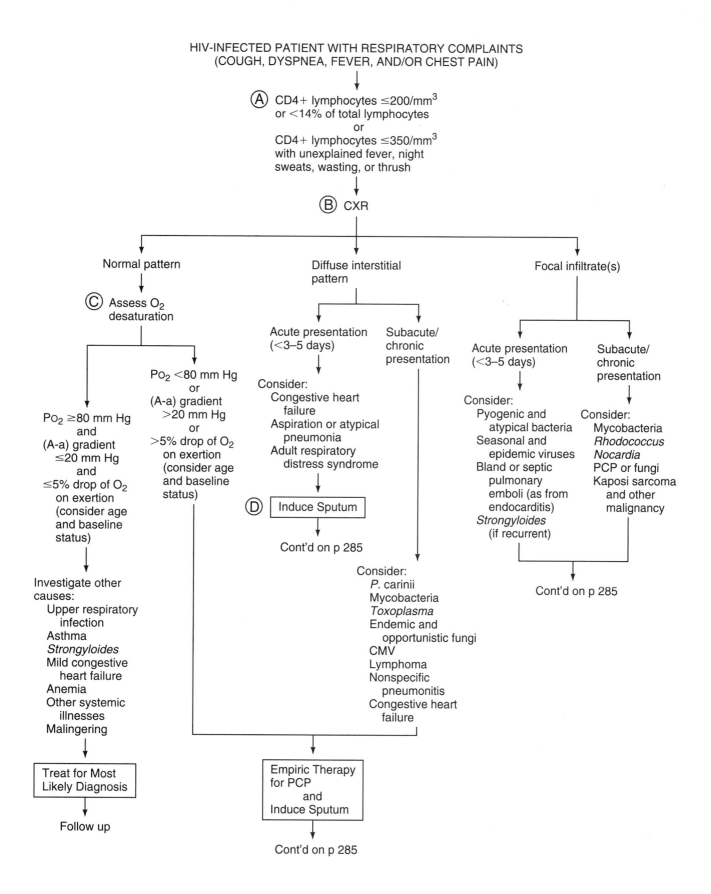

A CD4+ lymphocytes ≤200/mm³
or <14% of total lymphocytes
or
CD4+ lymphocytes ≤350/mm³
with unexplained fever, night
sweats, wasting, or thrush

B CXR

Normal pattern

C Assess O₂ desaturation

Po_2 <80 mm Hg
or
(A-a) gradient
>20 mm Hg
or
>5% drop of O₂
on exertion
(consider age
and baseline
status)

Po_2 ≥80 mm Hg
and
(A-a) gradient
≤20 mm Hg
and
≤5% drop of O₂
on exertion
(consider age
and baseline
status)

Investigate other
causes:
  Upper respiratory
    infection
  Asthma
  Strongyloides
  Mild congestive
    heart failure
  Anemia
  Other systemic
    illnesses
  Malingering

Treat for Most
Likely Diagnosis

Follow up

Diffuse interstitial pattern

Acute presentation
(<3–5 days)

Consider:
  Congestive heart
    failure
  Aspiration or atypical
    pneumonia
  Adult respiratory
    distress syndrome

D Induce Sputum

Cont'd on p 285

Subacute/
chronic
presentation

Consider:
  P. carinii
  Mycobacteria
  Toxoplasma
  Endemic and
    opportunistic fungi
  CMV
  Lymphoma
  Nonspecific
    pneumonitis
  Congestive heart
    failure

Empiric Therapy
for PCP
and
Induce Sputum

Cont'd on p 285

Focal infiltrate(s)

Acute presentation
(<3–5 days)

Consider:
  Pyogenic and
    atypical bacteria
  Seasonal and
    epidemic viruses
  Bland or septic
    pulmonary
    emboli (as from
    endocarditis)
  Strongyloides
    (if recurrent)

Subacute/
chronic
presentation

Consider:
  Mycobacteria
  Rhodococcus
  Nocardia
  PCP or fungi
  Kaposi sarcoma
    and other
    malignancy

Cont'd on p 285

E. The diagnostic evaluation and empiric choice of therapy depend on the most likely etiologic pathogens suggested by the patient's clinical presentation, epidemiology, and HIV risk factors. The stage of the patient's HIV disease accurately predicts the risk for many opportunistic infections (e.g., adult patients with PCP almost always have CD4+ counts near or below 200/mm^3, while CD4+ counts in patients with disseminated *Mycobacterium avium* complex or CMV infections are typically <100/mm^3). Diagnostic testing in mildly symptomatic patients may be limited to induced sputum and other simple noninvasive tests, followed by a therapeutic trial aimed at the most likely diagnosis; however, in moderately to severely ill patients, more aggressive evaluation with early bronchoscopy versus percutaneous, thoracoscopic or open lung biopsy is prudent if induced sputum findings are nondiagnostic. Under most circumstances, specimens should be sent for Gram, standard AFB with or without modified AFB, Pap, and GMS stains (along with corresponding cultures). Direct fluorescent antibody (DFA) staining of lung tissue or secretions for *Legionella* species can provide a quick and accurate diagnosis. Blood cultures are helpful when pyogenic (or certain fungal) pneumonias or endocarditis is suspected. Testing for fungal antigens in blood and urine of patients with suspected cryptococcosis and histoplasmosis is more sensitive than sputum stains and cultures for these organisms. Urinary antigen testing for *Legionella pneumophila* type I can detect almost 70% of cases caused by *Legionella* species. Bone marrow or liver biopsy often is a helpful diagnostic tool in selected patients with systemic mycobacterial and fungal infections as well as with non-Hodgkin's lymphoma.

F. A careful history (including the epidemiologic context) and physical examination can help direct appropriate empiric therapy. A detailed social, travel, and exposure history is mandatory. Any induration at the site of purified protein derivative (PPD) skin testing in HIV-infected patients should be interpreted as potential evidence of exposure to *Mycobacterium tuberculosis*. An acute onset of fever with pleuritic chest pain suggests pyogenic pneumonias (e.g., pneumococcal pneumonia) or right-sided endocarditis or pyophlebitis with septic pulmonary emboli (e.g., tricuspid valve endocarditis caused by *Staphylococcus aureus*). The latter infection is common in injecting drug users with hemoptysis and/or multifocal nodular pulmonary infiltrates. Pneumonia from resistant organisms (e.g., *Pseudomonas aeruginosa*) occasionally develops in patients taking antibiotics for prophylaxis (e.g., trimethoprim-sulfamethoxazole to prevent PCP).

Patients with the insidious onset of dyspnea and diffuse infiltrates deserve empiric treatment for PCP while awaiting confirmation with induced sputum or bronchoalveolar lavage (BAL). Unexplained hypoxemia in a patient with advanced disease, even with a normal CXR, also should be treated as PCP while attempts are made to establish a diagnosis. A subacute to chronic evolution of systemic symptoms in patients with associated respiratory complaints who are not responding to traditional antibiotic therapy (especially if they have been taking PCP prophylaxis regularly) suggests mycobacterial or fungal infection, lymphoma, Kaposi sarcoma, or uncontrolled HIV disease.

G. If the patient deteriorates, remains hypoxemic after 3–5 days of empiric therapy, or responds suboptimally to therapy, an invasive procedure is needed to secure the diagnosis and exclude another coexistent process. The specific choice of procedure is decided case by case and could be a bronchoscopy with BAL and transbronchial biopsy (TBB) or an open lung biopsy. Tissue should be sent to both the pathology and microbiology laboratories.

References

Baughman RP, Dohn MN, Frame PT. The continuing utility of bronchoalveolar lavage to diagnose opportunistic infection in AIDS patients. Am J Med 1994; 97:515.

Boswell SL, van Gorder M. A 38-year-old man with AIDS and cavitary pulmonary lesions. N Engl J Med 1997; 337:619.

Brenner M, Ognibene FP, Lack EE, et al. Prognostic factors and life expectancy of patients with acquired immunodeficiency syndrome and *Pneumocystis carinii* pneumonia. Am Rev Respir Dis 1987; 136:1199.

Burack JH, Hahn JA, Saint-Maurice D, et al. Microbiology of community-acquired bacterial pneumonia in persons with and at risk for human immunodeficiency virus type I infection. Arch Intern Med 1994; 154:2589.

Hirschtick RE, Glassroth J, Jordan MC, et al. Bacterial pneumonia in persons infected with HIV. N Engl J Med 1995; 333:845.

Tu JV, Biem HV, Detsky AS. Bronchoscopy versus empirical therapy in HIV-infected patients with presumptive *Pneumocystis carinii* pneumonia. Am Rev Respir Dis 1993; 148:370.

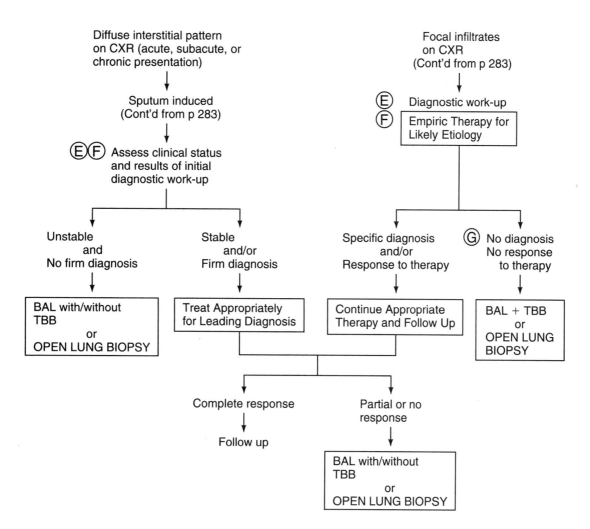

Diffuse interstitial pattern
on CXR (acute, subacute, or
chronic presentation)

Sputum induced
(Cont'd from p 283)

Ⓔ Ⓕ Assess clinical status
and results of initial
diagnostic work-up

Unstable
and
No firm diagnosis

Stable
and/or
Firm diagnosis

BAL with/without
TBB
or
OPEN LUNG BIOPSY

Treat Appropriately
for Leading Diagnosis

Complete response

Follow up

Partial or no
response

BAL with/without
TBB
or
OPEN LUNG BIOPSY

Focal infiltrates
on CXR
(Cont'd from p 283)

Ⓔ Diagnostic work-up
Ⓕ Empiric Therapy for
Likely Etiology

Specific diagnosis
and/or
Response to therapy

Ⓖ No diagnosis
No response
to therapy

Continue Appropriate
Therapy and Follow Up

BAL + TBB
or
OPEN LUNG
BIOPSY

CENTRAL NERVOUS SYSTEM INFECTION IN THE HIV-INFECTED PATIENT

Deborah L. Goldsmith

A. In history taking, focus on evidence of opportunistic infection, systemic illness, sexually transmitted disease, or metabolic insults. Staging of HIV by history and by CD4 cell count helps determine for which infections or neoplasms the patient is at risk. A detailed physical examination elucidates opportunistic infections or focal neurologic signs. Pay special attention to the patient's mental status, which may show subtle changes. Patients with focal signs must have an MRI or CT scan before lumbar puncture to rule out a dangerous mass effect from a lesion.

B. The appearance and number of lesions present help focus the differential diagnosis. Multiple, ring-enhancing lesions, especially in the basal ganglia or cortex, are most consistent with toxoplasmosis. Nonenhancing or weakly enhancing single lesions, especially in the periventricular white matter, are more consistent with primary CNS lymphoma.

C. Begin empiric therapy for toxoplasmosis in the patient with consistent radiographic evidence. Positive serum toxoplasmosis IgG is supporting evidence but is unnecessary. Negative serologic results make this diagnosis unlikely.

D. If a single lesion is apparent on CT scan, obtain MRI, which is more sensitive, to look for multiple lesions. If they are found, consider empiric toxoplasmosis treatment. If the lesion is truly solitary, primary CNS lymphoma is the most likely diagnosis. Also consider pyogenic abscess, cryptococcoma, and tuberculoma.

E. Another entity presenting with multiple lesions is progressive multifocal leukoencephalopathy. This condition tends to have nonenhancing, characteristic subcortical lesions that appear white on T2 MRI and black on T1 MRI.

F. Obtain opening pressure, cell count and differential, protein, glucose, VDRL test, cryptococcal antigen test, and bacterial and fungal cultures. It is advisable to hold a tube of CSF for additional studies suggested by new information or clinical progression. Consider acid-fast bacilli (AFB) smear and culture and cytology.

G. Treat an HIV-infected patient with positive CSF VDRL test with appropriate high-dose CNS-active antibiotics per the current CDC guidelines. A patient with negative CSF findings but positive serum VDRL test and abnormal findings on lumbar puncture should be treated for neurosyphilis if there is no other clear explanation for the CSF findings.

H. The India ink test is not sensitive; cryptococcal antigen and culture must be used. CSF findings are often unimpressive, although low glucose and high protein levels can be seen. A WBC count in CSF $<20/mm^3$ is a poor prognostic sign.

I. Polymerase chain reaction tests for tuberculosis and cytomegalovirus are available. Consider cytologic studies for lymphoma. Other fungal infections such as coccidioidomycosis or histoplasmosis are possible and can be checked by culture and appropriate serologic studies.

References

Aronow HA, Brew BJ, Price RW. The management of the neurological complications of HIV infection and AIDS. AIDS 1988; 2(Suppl 1):S151.

Petty RKH. Recent advances in the neurology of HIV infection. Postgrad Med J 1994; 70:393.

Simpson D, Tagliati M. Neurologic manifestations of HIV infection. Ann Intern Med 1994; 121:769.

Whiteman ML, Post MJ, Berger JR, et al. Progressive multifocal leukoencephalopathy in 47 HIV-seropositive patients: neuroimaging with clinical and pathological correlation. Radiology 1993; 187:233.

HIV-POSITIVE PATIENT WITH SUSPECTED CNS INFECTION

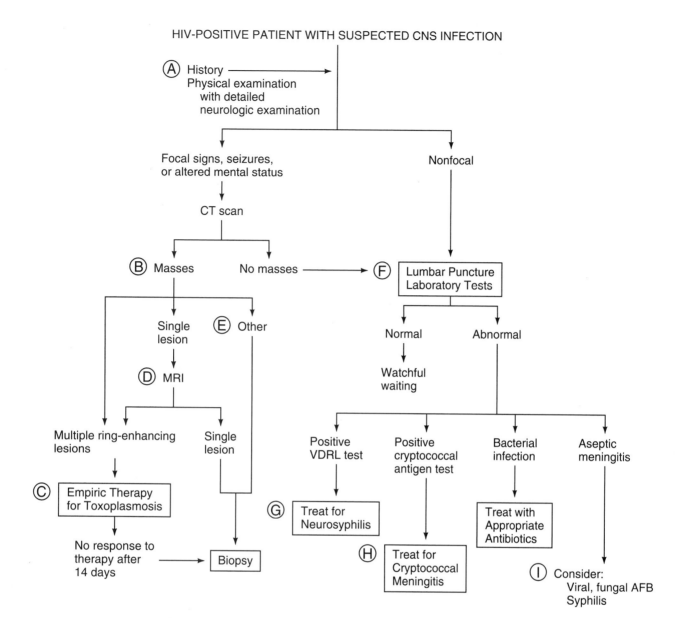

SEPSIS

Richard M. Mandel

A. No standardized definitions embrace the concepts of sepsis and septic shock. *Sepsis* may be defined as the clinical evidence of infection with fever or hypothermia, tachypnea, tachycardia, and leukocytosis or impaired leukocyte response. The *sepsis syndrome* is a more severe manifestation encompassing sepsis with evidence of inadequate organ perfusion, such as the inability to maintain adequate oxygenation, oliguria, elevated serum lactate, and altered mentation. *Septic shock* is the sepsis syndrome with hypotension. Manifestation of the sepsis syndrome with or without shock can be attributed to host-derived inflammatory cytokines that are part of the host defense system but in the end may prove injurious to the patient. Although gram-negative aerobic bacilli are the most common cause of the syndrome, any number of pathogenic organisms, including gram-positive bacteria, fungi, and parasites may produce the same physiologic response. Blood cultures may be positive in 33–50% of septic patients.

B. The basic approach to managing a patient with presumed sepsis involves three steps. First, attempt to restore the patient to physiologic normalcy. Intravascular volume should be repleted to maintain adequate BP. In less severe cases, this is done by administering crystalloid fluids. With severe hypotension it may be necessary to add pressor agents to IV fluids to maintain adequate BP and renal function. To optimize pressor efficacy the patient should have a pH >7.3 and adequate preload and calcium and glucose levels. Adrenocortical insufficiency must be recognized and treated. Administer supplemental oxygen; in severe cases intubation and mechanical ventilation may be required. Pulmonary end-expiratory pressure may be needed to maintain adequate arterial oxygenation. Finally, correct metabolic abnormalities. Many clinicians administer sodium bicarbonate if serum pH falls to ≤7.2, but others believe this may be harmful. Monitor hyperglycemia, hypoglycemia, electrolyte disorders, and coagulopathy and correct when indicated.

C. Once basic support has been achieved, seek the cause of the infection. A thorough history and physical examination elucidate the cause in most patients. Direct special attention to prior surgery, trauma, burn injuries, transplantation, and neutropenia/chemotherapy. The most common causes of sepsis include urinary tract infection, pneumonia, and IV line infection. Occasionally a GI catastrophe such as perforation, ischemic colitis, or intra-abdominal abscess is the cause. Based on history and physical findings, obtain appropriate radiographs, including an initial chest film. Standard laboratory tests include CBC, ABG, measurement of serum electrolytes, BUN and creatinine, and urinalysis.

D. Draw blood cultures in all cases, at least two different sets from different venipuncture sites to ensure that a contaminating organism is not mistaken for a pathogen and to increase the likelihood of detecting true bacteremia. Although some clinicians advise waiting 20 minutes between each set, it is appropriate in the septic patient to obtain them one after another. Obtain other cultures based on the history and on physical and radiographic findings. If there is evidence of pneumonia, attempt a Gram stain and culture of sputum. If the urinalysis demonstrates pyuria and/or bacteriuria, obtain a culture and if possible a Gram stain of urine.

E. Once basic support has been provided, the source of infection assessed, and appropriate cultures obtained, begin empiric antibiotic therapy. Ideally, in the critically ill patient the time between initial contact and initiation of antibiotic therapy should not be >30 minutes. The choice of antimicrobial agent depends on the source of infection, the most likely organism involved, and local/regional antibiotic resistance patterns. Host factors such as neutropenia, recent chemotherapy, HIV/AIDS, breaches in anatomic host defenses, or renal or liver disease may influence the initial choice of antimicrobial therapy. In all cases therapy may have to be modified subsequently based on the patient's response to treatment and the results of cultures. To date, high-dose corticosteroids have not proved beneficial and are not recommended for treatment of sepsis or septic shock. In general, abscesses should be drained. When feasible and clinically indicated, remove prosthetic materials.

References

Bone RC. Sepsis, the sepsis syndrome, multi-organ failure: a plea for comparable definitions. Ann Intern Med 1991; 114:332.

Parker MM. Current management of septic shock. Infect Med 1989; March/April:47.

The Veterans Administration Systemic Sepsis Cooperative Study Group. Effect of high-dose glucocorticoid therapy on mortality in patients with clinical signs of systemic sepsis. N Engl J Med 1987; 317:659.

Wenzel RP, et al. Current understanding of sepsis. Clin Infect Dis 1996; 2:407.

Young L. Sepsis syndrome. In: Mandell G, Bennet J, Dolin R, eds. Principles and practice of infectious diseases. New York: Churchill Livingstone, 1995:690.

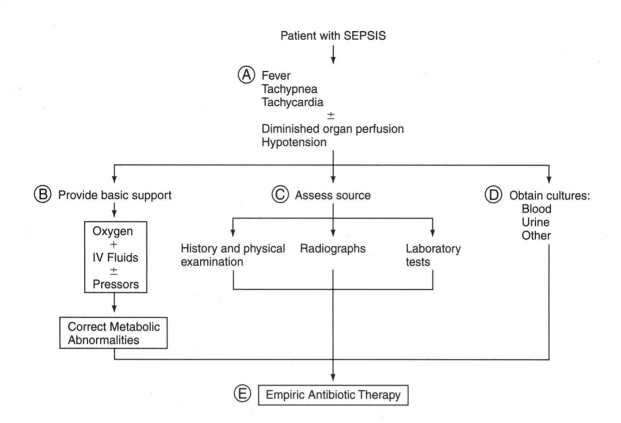

Patient with SEPSIS

(A) Fever
Tachypnea
Tachycardia
±
Diminished organ perfusion
Hypotension

(B) Provide basic support

Oxygen
+
IV Fluids
±
Pressors

Correct Metabolic
Abnormalities

(C) Assess source

History and physical   Radiographs   Laboratory
examination   tests

(D) Obtain cultures:
Blood
Urine
Other

(E) Empiric Antibiotic Therapy

TOXIC SHOCK SYNDROME

Richard M. Mandel

Toxic shock syndrome (TSS) is the name given to the myriad of clinical findings caused by infection with an exotoxin-producing species of *Staphylococcus aureus,* first described in 1978 in children. Afflicted adults had similar clinical features of high fever, erythroderma, and hypotension along with variable organ system dysfunction, including nausea, vomiting, diarrhea, mental confusion, renal failure, hepatic failure, and thrombocytopenia. In 1980 it was noted that this syndrome occurred with increasing frequency in young menstruating females, particularly those who used super-absorbent tampons. Surgical and nonsurgical wounds, post-partum infection, augmentation mammoplasty, arthroscopy, abscesses, osteomyelitis, pneumonia, sinusitis, and influenza have been reported to cause nonmenstrual TSS. Contraceptive sponge and diaphragm use has also been impli-cated in a few cases of TSS. Nonmenstrual TSS is often nosocomial. Renal and CNS complications are common.

A. It is essential to determine the presence or absence of hypotension, with implications not only for treatment, but for early exclusion of some of the exanthems of various other diseases that may masquerade as the erythroderma of TSS (Table 1). Measles is most promi-nent in children and young adults but can occur in any age group. Prodromal symptoms of measles include high fever, malaise, irritability, conjunctivitis, photopho-bia, hacking cough, nasal discharge, and (variably) Koplik's spots are followed in 3–4 days by a red maculopapular rash. Within 3 days the rash spreads from the face to the trunk and extremities; it may coalesce in areas, giving the appearance of erythro-derma. The rash typically persists for 6 days and disap-pears in the order in which it appeared. Measles can be differentiated from TSS by the absence of hypotension. Rocky Mountain spotted fever (RMSF), an acute febrile illness caused by infection with *Rickettsia rickettsiae,* is transmitted by tick bite and is characterized by the abrupt onset of fever, headache, chills, and a pink macular rash on the extremities. This progresses over 2–3 weeks to a deep red maculopapular rash on the trunk and extremities. Again, the history and the rare presence of hypovolemic hypotension differentiate RMSF from TSS. Leptospirosis is an acute febrile illness caused by infection with the spirochete *Leptospira,* usually via contact with infected animal urine or tissue. Farmers, trappers, and abattoir workers are at increased risk. The onset is sudden with fever and chills, headache, myalgia, pharyngeal and conjunctival injection, and a macular/maculopapular/urticarial rash on the trunk. Hypotension is absent.

B. If hypotension is present with a fever >38.9° C, consider an infectious process leading to sepsis (see p 288). Perform a thorough work-up with blood cultures, chest film, urinalysis, and lumbar puncture if there are signs of CNS involvement. The presence of classical erythro-derma narrows the possible diagnoses to TSS and "toxic streptococcus" syndrome. The erythroderma may be delayed, localized, or evanescent; therefore continue to suspect TSS.

C. A different entity, redescribed in the mid-1980s and associated with many of the signs and symptoms of TSS, is the "toxic streptococcus" syndrome. Caused by an exotoxin-producing species of group A β-hemolytic streptococcus *(S. pyogenes)* isolated from a normally sterile site, it too is characterized by fever, hypotension, rash, and multiple organ failure. This syndrome, how-ever, often is secondary to an obvious source of infec-tion; search for cellulitis, fasciitis/myositis, gangrene, or a pulmonary source leading to the systemic illness.

D. The CDC definition of TSS is given in Table 1. Fever, hypotension, and rash consisting of a diffuse erythro-derma, often described as sunburn, are major charac-teristics, along with multiple organ involvement: GI, muscular, renal, liver, blood, CNS, and mucous mem-brane abnormalities. In most cases of TSS, desquama-tion of rash-afflicted areas occurs about 1 week after the onset. In the absence of desquamation, all three major criteria plus more than five organ systems involved must be present to comply with the CDC definition. If desqua-mation is present, all three major criteria plus more than three organ systems involved are sufficient for diagnosis.

E. The diagnosis is made on the basis of clinical findings and associated tampon use. An obvious infectious source is present only in a minority of patients, although a thorough search for such a source should be made. Blood cultures are rarely positive. Treatment hinges on early diagnosis, vigorous fluid replacement, pressor and ventilatory support if needed, tampon removal, vaginal douche, drainage of abscesses, and antibiotic therapy

TABLE 1   CDC Criteria for Diagnosis of TSS

Temperature >38.9° C
Systolic BP <90 mm Hg
Rash with subsequent desquamation, especially on palms and soles
Involvement of ≥3 of the following organ systems:
  GI: vomiting, profuse diarrhea
  Muscular: severe myalgias or more than fivefold increase in creatine kinase
  Mucous membranes (vagina, conjunctivae, or pharynx): frank hyperemia
  Renal insufficiency: BUN or creatinine at least twice upper limit of normal, with pyuria in absence of urinary tract infection
  Liver: hepatitis, bilirubin, SGOT, SGPT at least twice upper limit of normal
  Blood: thrombocytopenia <100,000/mm^3
  CNS: disorientation without focal neurological signs
Negative results of serologic tests for Rocky Mountain spotted fever, leptospirosis, and measles

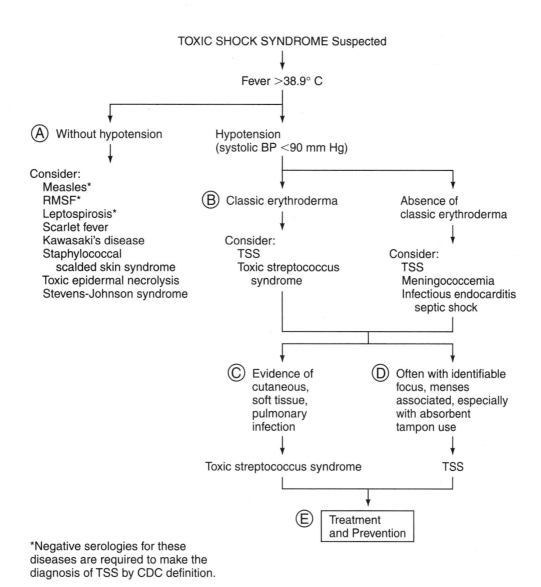

TOXIC SHOCK SYNDROME Suspected

Fever >38.9° C

Ⓐ Without hypotension

Consider:
　Measles*
　RMSF*
　Leptospirosis*
　Scarlet fever
　Kawasaki's disease
　Staphylococcal
　　scalded skin syndrome
　Toxic epidermal necrolysis
　Stevens-Johnson syndrome

Hypotension
(systolic BP <90 mm Hg)

Ⓑ Classic erythroderma

Consider:
　TSS
　Toxic streptococcus
　　syndrome

Absence of
classic erythroderma

Consider:
　TSS
　Meningococcemia
　Infectious endocarditis
　　septic shock

Ⓒ Evidence of
　cutaneous,
　soft tissue,
　pulmonary
　infection

Ⓓ Often with identifiable
　focus, menses
　associated, especially
　with absorbent
　tampon use

Toxic streptococcus syndrome

TSS

Ⓔ Treatment
　and Prevention

*Negative serologies for these
diseases are required to make the
diagnosis of TSS by CDC definition.

with a penicillinase-resistant penicillin. Prevention interventions should center on education about the use of catamenial products.

References

Barter T, Dascal A, Carrol K, Curley FJ. Toxic strep syndrome—a manifestation of group A streptococcal infection. Arch Intern Med 1988; 148:1421.

Broome CV. Epidemiology of TSS in the US: overview. Rev Infect Dis 1989; 11(suppl 1):S14.

Centers for Disease Control and Prevention. Summary of notifiable diseases—1995. MMWR 1996; 44:53.

Chesney PJ. Clinical aspects and spectrum of illness of TSS: overview. Rev Infect Dis 1989; 11(suppl 1):S1.

Waldvogel F. *Staphylococcus aureus*—including toxic shock syndrome. In: Mandell G, Bennett JE, Dolin R, eds. Principles and practice of infectious diseases. 4th ed. New York: Churchill Livingstone, 1995:1766.

STAPHYLOCOCCUS AUREUS BACTEREMIA

Jeffrey L. Silber
Mark J. DiNubile

Staphylococcus aureus is one of the most common causes of both community-acquired and nosocomial bacteremia. In most cases, *S. aureus* bacteremia is a consequence of a local infection that enters the bloodstream after an insult to normally protective skin structures. Serious complications and poor outcome are common despite the availability of potent antistaphylococcal antibiotics.

Once in the bloodstream, *S. aureus* has the propensity to infect both normal and damaged organs, including heart valves, viscera, bones, and joints, in addition to shunts and orthopedic hardware. Patients with *S. aureus* bacteremia who have no overt evidence of endocarditis or metastatic infection may still harbor occult infection of vital structures. It was previously recommended that all patients with *S. aureus* bacteremia be treated for at least 4 weeks. Although the diagnosis of endocarditis can never be totally excluded, the clinical settings in which patients are at low risk of endocarditis can be defined (Table 1). The challenge is to identify patients unlikely to have endocarditis or other hidden foci of infection after *S. aureus* bacteremia and who are therefore candidates for shorter courses (usually 10–14 days) of antibiotic therapy.

A. The approach to patients with *S. aureus* bacteremia should emphasize the primary site of infection. The absence of a demonstrable initial focus of infection suggests endocarditis. If the bacteremia was clearly related to a removable focus (e.g., an intravascular line), the patient is relatively less likely to have or develop endocarditis.

B. When blood cultures remain persistently positive for >48 hours or, in presumed line-related bacteremia, 24 hours after the line has been removed, the patient usually should be treated as though endovascular infection were present.

C. Injecting drug users with *S. aureus* bacteremia almost always have endovascular infection. A patient with a prosthetic device (especially if intravascular) generally should be treated as if that prosthesis has been seeded. Bacteremic patients with a visceral abscess, pneumonia, osteomyelitis, or septic arthritis are assumed to have endocarditis (unless there is evidence of direct inoculation). Although it often is unclear whether these infected foci are the source or the result of the ongoing bacteremia, a long course of therapy is indicated in either case.

D. Echocardiography is occasionally helpful but not routinely indicated. The presence of a vegetation usually mandates 4 weeks of treatment. Although transesophageal echocardiography is more sensitive than transthoracic, neither study is required in most cases.

E. Patients considered for short-course therapy should show no evidence of active infection on repeated evaluations, including a careful examination at the end of 10–14 days of treatment. Patients with a removable primary focus of infection, short-lived bacteremia, no prosthetic devices, and a "negative" echocardiogram (if done) who have responded promptly to antibiotic therapy and show no evidence of ongoing infection may be treated with appropriate antistaphylococcal antibiotics for 2 weeks. Most other patients require longer courses of therapy. In some, surgical intervention (e.g., incision and drainage, valve replacement) may also be indicated. On completion of therapy, all patients (especially those receiving short-course therapy) need close clinical follow-up for several weeks. Re-treat those who relapse with longer courses of antibiotics and evaluated for endovascular or other foci of infection.

TABLE 1   Risk of Deep Infection after *S. aureus* Bacteremia

High	Low
Community acquired	Hospital acquired
No apparent primary focus	Identifiable primary focus
Injecting drug use	Removable focus
Metastatic foci	No identified metastatic foci
Abnormal heart valves*	Normal heart valves
Intravascular or other prosthetic device	No intravascular or other prosthetic device
Slow clinical response	Rapid clinical response
Persistent bacteremia	Short-lived bacteremia

*Previous bacterial endocarditis, most congenital cardiac malformations, hypertrophic cardiomyopathy, rheumatic and other acquired valvular dysfunction, and mitral valve prolapse with regurgitation, as per American Heart Association indications for endocarditis prophylaxis before surgical, dental, and endoscopic procedures (Dajani AS, Taubert KA, Wilson W, et al. JAMA 1997; 277:1794).

References

Bayer AS, Lam K, Gintzon L, et al. *Staphylococcus aureus* bacteremia: clinical, serologic, and echocardiographic findings in patients with and without endocarditis. Arch Intern Med 1987; 147:457.

Dajani AS, Taubert KA, Wilson W, et al. Prevention of bacterial endocarditis. Recommendations by the American Heart Association. JAMA 1997; 277:1794.

Malanoski GJ, Samore MH, Pefanis A, Karchmer AW. *Staphylococcus aureus* catheter–associated bacteremia: minimal effective therapy and unusual infectious complications associated with arterial sheath catheters. Arch Intern Med 1995; 155:1161.

Mylotte JM, McDermott C, Spooner JA. Prospective study of 114 consecutive episodes of *Staphylococcus aureus* bacteremia. Rev Infect Dis 1987; 9:891.

Sheagren JN. *Staphylococcus aureus:* the persistent pathogen. N Engl J Med 1984; 310:1368, 1437.

Patient with *S. aureus* BACTEREMIA

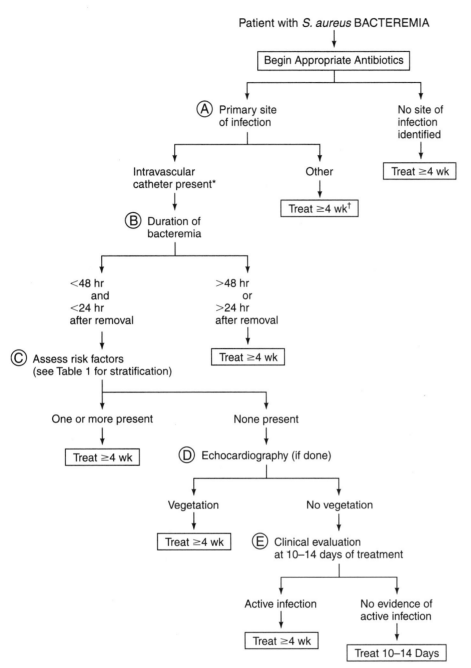

*Intravascular catheters should be removed promptly in most patients with *S. aureus* bacteremia.

†Patients with a skin or soft tissue source of infection may be candidates for short-course therapy. For these selected patients, management should proceed as for intravascular catheter–derived infection.

HEPATITIS EXPOSURE

Stephen J. Gluckman
Mark J. DiNubile

Hepatitis is inflammation of the liver that can result from infections or other causes. Some infections are contagious, and a subset of these are potentially preventable after a significant exposure. It is impossible to advise a patient after exposure to hepatitis without ascertaining the relevant historical information. Three particularly important questions must be addressed: (1) *Type of hepatitis* (e.g., A, B, C, Epstein-Barr virus, cytomegalovirus, alcohol, or drug)— each type has its own specific risks for transmission and strategies for prevention. (2) *Any history of hepatitis*—if a person has already had the type of viral hepatitis to which he or she has been exposed, there is no risk of acquiring it again. (3) *Type of exposure*—each type of infectious hepatitis has particular modes of transmission. Not only does a person have to be "exposed," but the contact must be sufficient for transmission of infection to occur.

A. If a person exposed to hepatitis A has already had the infection or the vaccine >3–4 weeks before the exposure, only reassurance is required.

B. If the exposed person is not known to have had hepatitis A, the type of exposure becomes important. Hepatitis A is spread via the fecal-oral route. Persons at increased risk for the disease are close personal, household, or day-care contacts. In addition, this virus has been responsible for epidemics related to contaminated food or water. If the exposure has not occurred in one of these settings, no intervention is necessary. If the exposure has been of one of these types and has occurred within the previous 2 weeks, immune globulin (IG), 0.02 ml/kg, is indicated. The efficacy of inactivated hepatitis A vaccine administered within a few days of exposure is being investigated, given recent successful experiments in marmosets.

C. If a person exposed to hepatitis B has already had the infection there is no further risk.

D. If the exposed person is not known to have had hepatitis B, the type of exposure becomes critical. If the exposure was via a contaminated blood transfusion, interventions are unlikely to be effective. If the situation involves a newborn of a mother with hepatitis B, the child should receive 0.5 ml of hepatitis B immune globulin (HBIG) within 12 hours of birth, and active immunization should be started.

E. If the exposure was via a contaminated needlestick or permucosal exposure to infectious blood within the past week or through sexual contact in the previous 2 weeks, and if the patient has never received hepatitis B vaccine, prophylaxis is indicated. The proper approach is to obtain a tube of blood to test for hepatitis B core antibody (HBcAb) and administer a dose of HBIG (0.06 ml/kg). If the antibody test is positive, the patient has already had hepatitis B and no further prophylaxis is indicated. If negative, active immunization against hepatitis B usually should be initiated within 1 week of exposure. If the patient has already received hepatitis B vaccine, ascertain the response to the vaccine. In a known responder, the level of hepatitis B surface antibody (HBsAb) should be determined. If the levels are adequate (≥10 sample ratio units [SRU]), no further prophylaxis is needed. If the levels are <10 SRU, a booster dose of vaccine is indicated. A known nonresponder should usually receive HBIG (0.06 ml/kg) on two occasions 1 month apart. When patients do not know their response status to the vaccine, check the level of HBsAb: If ≥10 SRU, nothing further is required; if <10 SRU, give HBIG (0.06 ml/kg) and a single booster dose of the vaccine.

F. If a person exposed to hepatitis C has already had it, there is no further risk.

G. There are no proven interventions after exposure to hepatitis C. Hepatitis C is a major cause of posttransfusion hepatitis, but any intervention after transfusion is unlikely to be effective. The virus also appears to be contagious via sticks from contaminated needles and permucosal contact with blood. Infection as a consequence of sexual relations occurs much less often.

H. When a person has had exposure to hepatitis but the contact cannot be determined, evaluation and treatment should proceed based on the type of exposure and the general epidemiologic context. Coincident exposure to HIV should always be considered when there is blood exposure.

References

Clemens R, Safary A, Hepburn A, et al. Clinical experience with an inactivated hepatitis A vaccine. J Infect Dis 1995; 171(suppl 1):S44.

Prevention of hepatitis A through active or passive immunization: recommendations of the Advisory Committee on Immunization Practices (ACIP). MMWR 1997; 45:1.

Protection against viral hepatitis: recommendations of the Advisory Committee on Immunization Practices (ACIP). MMWR 1990; 39:1.

Recommendations for follow-up of health-care workers after occupational exposure to hepatitis C virus. MMWR 1997; 46:603.

Update: recommendations to prevent hepatitis B virus transmission—United States. MMWR 1995; 44:574.

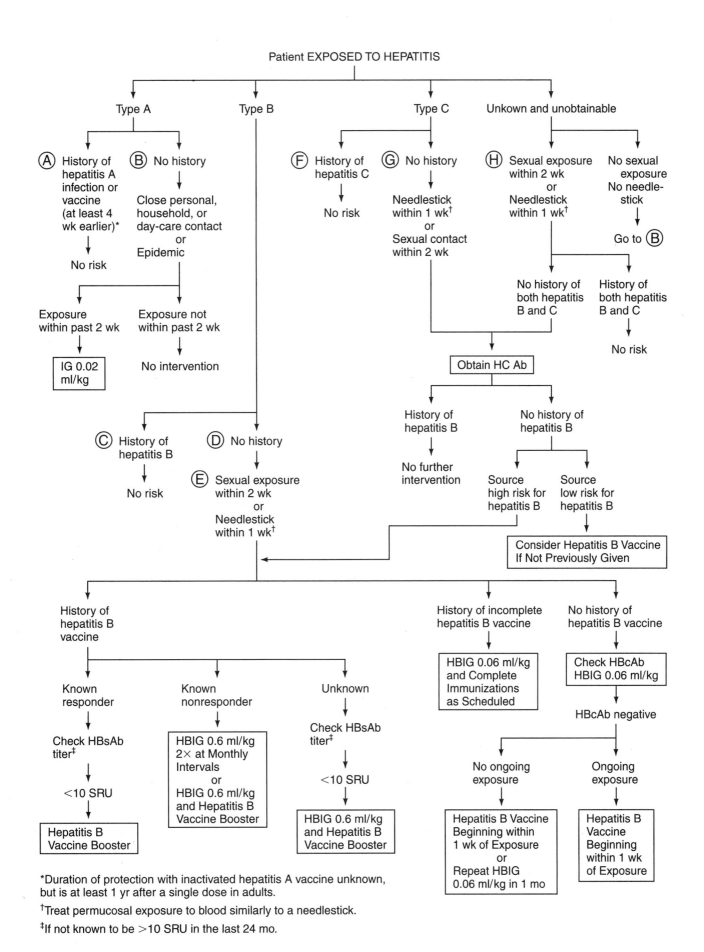

Patient EXPOSED TO HEPATITIS

Type A Type B Type C Unkown and unobtainable

(A) History of hepatitis A infection or vaccine (at least 4 wk earlier)*

(B) No history

No risk

Close personal, household, or day-care contact or Epidemic

Exposure within past 2 wk

Exposure not within past 2 wk

IG 0.02 ml/kg

No intervention

(F) History of hepatitis C

No risk

(G) No history

Needlestick within 1 wk† or Sexual contact within 2 wk

(H) Sexual exposure within 2 wk or Needlestick within 1 wk†

No sexual exposure No needle-stick

Go to (B)

No history of both hepatitis B and C

History of both hepatitis B and C

No risk

Obtain HC Ab

History of hepatitis B

No history of hepatitis B

No further intervention

Source high risk for hepatitis B

Source low risk for hepatitis B

Consider Hepatitis B Vaccine If Not Previously Given

(C) History of hepatitis B

No risk

(D) No history

(E) Sexual exposure within 2 wk or Needlestick within 1 wk†

History of hepatitis B vaccine

History of incomplete hepatitis B vaccine

No history of hepatitis B vaccine

HBIG 0.06 ml/kg and Complete Immunizations as Scheduled

Check HBcAb HBIG 0.06 ml/kg

HBcAb negative

Known responder

Known nonresponder

Unknown

Check HBsAb titer‡

HBIG 0.6 ml/kg 2× at Monthly Intervals or HBIG 0.6 ml/kg and Hepatitis B Vaccine Booster

Check HBsAb titer‡

<10 SRU

<10 SRU

Hepatitis B Vaccine Booster

HBIG 0.6 ml/kg and Hepatitis B Vaccine Booster

No ongoing exposure

Ongoing exposure

Hepatitis B Vaccine Beginning within 1 wk of Exposure or Repeat HBIG 0.06 ml/kg in 1 mo

Hepatitis B Vaccine Beginning within 1 wk of Exposure

*Duration of protection with inactivated hepatitis A vaccine unknown, but is at least 1 yr after a single dose in adults.

†Treat permucosal exposure to blood similarly to a needlestick.

‡If not known to be >10 SRU in the last 24 mo.

295

FEVER OF UNKNOWN ORIGIN

Seth D. Weissman
Richard M. Mandel

A working definition of fever of unknown origin (FUO) is (1) duration of at least 2–3 weeks, (2) temperature >38.3° C on several occasions, and (3) unknown cause after routine work-up. These criteria tend to eliminate protracted viral illness or other self-limited etiologies from being classified as FUO. In addition to the classic FUO discussed here, there have been further subclassifications of nosocomial FUO (hospitalized patients who were apparently uninfected and afebrile on admission), neutropenic FUO (in patients with absolute granulocyte count <500/mm^3), and HIV-associated FUO.

Instruct patients to check their temperature at least twice daily. Sustained fever is seen with typhoid fever or miliary tuberculosis (TB). Intermittent fever most often is seen with abscesses and other pyogenic infections. In the absence of other symptoms (chills, sweats, and tachycardia) or abnormal results on initial work-up, consider diagnoses such as exaggerated circadian temperature rhythm and factitious fever. Although the pattern of fever generally is not helpful in determining the cause of FUO, it may aid in diagnosing cases of tertian or quartan malaria, cyclic neutropenia, or Hodgkin's disease (with the Pel-Ebstein fever characterized by 5–10 days of fever alternating with 5–10 days of afebrility). Fever lasting >6 months suggests granulomatous disease or adult Still's disease.

A. Most associated symptoms are nonspecific (e.g., malaise, sweats, weight loss, myalgias). Obtain a thorough history of travel (especially to regions where malaria, tuberculosis, or certain mycoses are endemic), animal exposure (zoonotic infections), insect bites (rickettsial infections), previous surgery, and occupational exposures (berylliosis).

B. Physical examination must be painstakingly thorough and often repeated. Pay particular attention to skin, eyes, teeth, sinuses, lymph nodes, heart, abdomen, pelvis, rectum, and extremities.

C. Resist the urge to "shotgun" the work-up. Reasonable routine testing includes CBC with differential, hepatic and muscle enzymes, multiple (up to three sets over 24 hours) blood cultures, and urine for analysis and culture (including three morning specimens for AFB analysis). Stool examination for ova and parasites may be indicated. The choice of serologic tests is guided by the history and physical examination. Consider VDRL and HIV antibody tests in patients with appropriate risk factors. Other serologies may include a streptozyme panel, antibody titers to mycoses, agents responsible for many zoonotic infections, amebiasis, as well as to cytomegalovirus (CMV), Epstein-Barr virus, and the hepatitis viruses. Do not order these tests for every patient. If there is a low pretest probability of the specific disease, expect more false than true positives. Serum should be frozen and saved for potential use in comparing acute and con-valescent titers. In the absence of clinical suspicion of disease, ANA, rheumatoid factor, and serum protein electrophoresis are seldom diagnostic. ESR is nonspecific. Although ESR >100 mm/hr suggests vasculitis, it can also be seen with neoplasm, TB, or pyogenic infection. Skin testing may reveal a positive purified protein derivative (PPD), exposure to fungal pathogens, or anergy, which suggests sarcoidosis, miliary TB, Whipple's disease, Hodgkin's disease, or another malignancy. Chest films are routine. Examination of CSF in the absence of specific CNS signs or symptoms usually is not indicated initially.

D. Infection is the most common cause of FUO in adults. However, as the duration of FUO increases, the probability of an infectious etiology decreases. Two important systemic infections to consider are TB and infectious endocarditis (IE). When TB presents as FUO, extrapulmonary involvement predominates. Patients with miliary TB may have a negative PPD and a normal chest film. Bone marrow and liver biopsies may be necessary for diagnosis. IE is rare in the absence of a murmur, and only 5% are truly culture negative. Four to six negative blood cultures (obtained at least 5–10 days after the patient stops taking antibiotics) should eliminate this possibility. Peripheral stigmata of IE may suggest the diagnosis. Transthoracic echocardiography is helpful if vegetations are seen, transesophageal echocardiography has sensitivity approaching 95%.

E. Intra-abdominal abscesses are the most common type of localized infection to cause FUO. Use abdominal and pelvic CT and ultrasonography to investigate this possibility; consider sites of previous surgeries as potential foci of the occult infection. Osteomyelitis is commonly encountered as FUO. Radionuclide bone scan reveals abnormalities earlier than plain radiographs. Also consider odontogenic abscess and infections of the biliary tree, urinary tract, sinuses, and prostate.

F. Innumerable other infectious agents may cause FUO. Except for CMV or HIV, viruses rarely cause FUO. The search for other infectious agents must be tailored to the patient, but spirochetes (e.g., *Borrelia*) and fungal and parasitic diseases need to be considered in certain cases.

G. Neoplasm is the second most common cause of FUO in adults; lymphoma is the most common neoplasm. Fever also occurs with leukemia, myelodysplasia, and solid tumors, including renal cell carcinoma, hepatoma, adenocarcinoma of the colon, carcinomatosis, and atrial myxoma.

H. Among the collagen vascular or autoimmune etiologies are systemic lupus erythematosus (fever as the only presenting symptom in <5%), Still's disease, vasculitis,

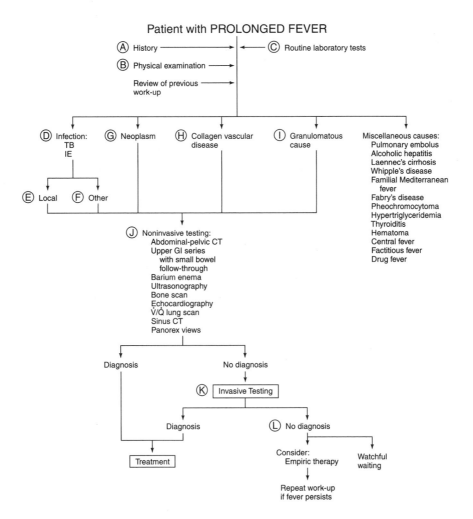

Patient with PROLONGED FEVER

and drug hypersensitivity reactions. Strongly consider temporal arteritis in elderly patients, even in the absence of classical physical findings. Patients often have an ESR of >100 mm/hr. Erythema multiforme, rheumatic fever, and polymyalgia rheumatica occasionally present with fever as the chief complaint.

I. In one study of patients with FUO lasting >1 year, granulomatous causes were more common than neoplastic or autoimmune ones. Entities include granulomatous hepatitis of unknown etiology, sarcoidosis, and Crohn's disease. When granulomas are found on liver biopsy, rule out other infectious and noninfectious causes before diagnosing granulomatous hepatitis of unknown etiology.

J. The noninvasive work-up should be thorough but tempered by one's best judgment of clinical probabilities.

K. If the work-up to this point is still unrevealing, proceed with biopsies of bone marrow and liver. Culture for bacteria, mycobacteria, viruses, and fungi, and send samples for histologic study. Other biopsy sites may include skin, lymph nodes, muscle, temporal artery, or any organ or bodily fluid found to be suspicious on work-up. Temporal artery biopsy can be considered early in older patients with elevated ESR and fever, even in the absence of other symptoms. Reserve laparotomy

for patients with fever and abdominal pain whose etiology remains unknown after noninvasive study.

L. The cause may remain unknown in 5–15% of patients even after thorough evaluation. These patients tend to have a low mortality rate and good prognosis, and fever often resolves spontaneously. Therapeutic trials tend to obscure the picture and there probably is no role for empiric antibiotics in FUO. Trials of antipyretics, NSAIDs, and even corticosteroids (if a noninfectious etiology is certain) may bring symptomatic improvement. The work-up may need to be repeated in several weeks to months if fever persists.

References

Gelfand JA, Wolff SM. Fever of unknown origin. In: Mandel GL, Bennett JE, Dolin R, eds. Principles and practice of infectious diseases. 4th ed. New York: Churchill Livingstone, 1995:536.

Hirschmann JV. Fever of unknown origin in adults. Clin Infect Dis 1997; 24:291.

Larson EB, Featherstone HJ, Petersdorf RG. Fever of undetermined origin: diagnosis and follow-up of 105 cases, 1970–80. Medicine 1982; 61:269.

Swartz MN, Simon HB. Fever of undetermined origin. Sci Am Med 1996; 7:6.

NEPHROLOGY

CHRONIC RENAL FAILURE

Anwar Al-Haidary
Joy L. Logan

A. Renal ultrasonography is a sensitive, noninvasive test that defines kidney size and rules out chronic obstruction. Small kidneys (<10 cm long) indicate chronic renal failure, but normal to large kidneys may be present in chronic renal failure as a result of diabetes, amyloidosis, or light-chain disease. Polycystic kidney disease also causes chronic renal failure and renomegaly, but the renal cysts are clearly discernible by ultrasonography after the age of 18 years. Cysts also may be found by ultrasound examination of the liver, pancreas, and ovaries of patients with polycystic kidney disease.

B. Pertinent historical data in chronic renal failure include symptoms or signs of extrarenal manifestations of connective tissue diseases or vasculitides (e.g., skin rashes, joint pains, neurologic complaints). Respiratory symptoms prompt consideration of antineutrophil cytoplasmic antibody (ANCA)–associated diseases or Goodpasture's syndrome. A history of high-risk behaviors heightens consideration of chronic glomerulopathies resulting from hepatitis B, hepatitis C, or HIV. These diagnoses are supported by serologic studies (antinuclear antibody, C3/C4, ANCA, anti–glomerular basement membrane antibodies, cryoglobulins, HIV, hepatitis B surface antigen, and hepatitis C antibody). Other historical factors pertinent to the differential diagnosis of chronic renal failure include a family history of renal disease, long-standing hypertension, or recurrent urinary tract infection (UTI). A drug history is also important because analgesics, some antibiotics, amphotericin B, cyclosporin A, and other agents may lead to chronic renal injury.

C. A lack of historical clues in a patient with small kidneys suggests a subclinical glomerulopathy as the cause of chronic renal failure, whether primary or secondary. Also consider chronic interstitial nephritis resulting from disorders of calcium or urate metabolism, as well as occult small vessel occlusion from cholesterol emboli. A long-standing history of hypertension suggests nephrosclerosis, whereas hypertension in a patient with peripheral or coronary vascular disease suggests ischemic nephropathy.

D. Identification of light chains by urine protein electrophoresis suggests myeloma, amyloidosis, or light-chain disease. The urinary protein in amyloidosis usually is in the nephrotic range, and the diagnosis is confirmed by peritoneal fat pad aspiration or rectal biopsy. Light-chain disease and myeloma can be confirmed by bone marrow examination and skeletal radiographs. Diabetic nephropathy usually presents with proteinuria and hypertension, and the diagnosis is strongly supported by the finding of associated diabetic retinopathy.

E. After the initial evaluation of renal function and the exclusion of reversible factors (fluid overload/contraction, hypertension, UTI, obstruction), evaluate the patient periodically for signs or symptoms of uremia or fluid imbalance. Regularly assess renal function by determining creatinine clearance and/or serum creatinine, BUN, electrolytes, calcium, phosphate, albumin, full blood counts, ferritin, PTH, and bone radiographs.

F. Stable patients with slow deterioration of renal function and minor uremic symptoms (pruritus, anemia, volume and/or electrolyte abnormalities responsive to conservative treatment, renal osteodystrophy) may be managed conservatively with appropriate pharmacologic and dietary therapy. Erythropoietin may be administered to correct the anemia.

G. Unanticipated deterioration in renal function prompts additional searches for reversible factors. Appearance of major uremic symptoms (e.g., nonresponsive volume overload, pericarditis, progressive neuropathy, anorexia with malnutrition) in a patient without reversible factors requires consideration of renal replacement therapy via dialysis or transplantation. Dialysis also is considered appropriate in patients with a creatinine clearance <10 ml/min independent of uremic symptoms.

References

Baldwin DS. Chronic glomerulonephritis: nonimmunologic mechanisms of progressive glomerular damage. Kidney Int 1982; 21:109.

Eschbach JW, Adamson JW. Recombinant human erythropoietin: implications for nephrology. Am J Kidney Dis 1988; 11:203.

Hostetter TH, Olson JL, Rennke HG, et al. Hyperfiltration in remnant nephrons: a potentially adverse response to renal ablation. Am J Physiol 1981; 241:F85.

Krowlewski AS, Canessa M, Warren JH, et al. Predisposition to hypertension and susceptibility to renal disease in insulin-dependent diabetes mellitus. N Engl J Med 1988; 318:140.

Meyer TW, Anderson SA, Rennke HG, Brenner BM. Reversing glomerular hypertension stabilizes established glomerular injury. Kidney Int 1987; 31:752.

Morris PJ. Renal transplantation: indications, outcome, complications, and results. In: Schrier RW, Gottschalk CW, eds. Diseases of the kidney. 4th ed. Boston: Little, Brown, 1988:3229.

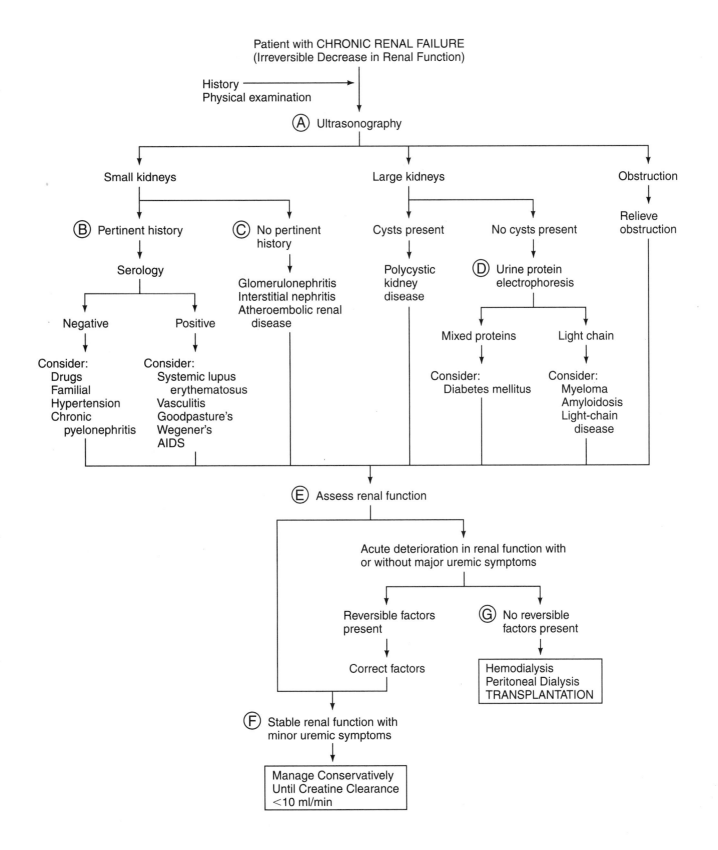

Patient with CHRONIC RENAL FAILURE
(Irreversible Decrease in Renal Function)

History
Physical examination

Ⓐ Ultrasonography

Small kidneys

Large kidneys

Obstruction

Relieve obstruction

Ⓑ Pertinent history

Ⓒ No pertinent history

Cysts present

No cysts present

Serology

Glomerulonephritis
Interstitial nephritis
Atheroembolic renal disease

Polycystic kidney disease

Ⓓ Urine protein electrophoresis

Negative

Positive

Mixed proteins

Light chain

Consider:
  Drugs
  Familial
  Hypertension
  Chronic
    pyelonephritis

Consider:
  Systemic lupus
    erythematosus
  Vasculitis
  Goodpasture's
  Wegener's
  AIDS

Consider:
  Diabetes mellitus

Consider:
  Myeloma
  Amyloidosis
  Light-chain
    disease

Ⓔ Assess renal function

Acute deterioration in renal function with or without major uremic symptoms

Reversible factors present

Ⓖ No reversible factors present

Correct factors

Hemodialysis
Peritoneal Dialysis
TRANSPLANTATION

Ⓕ Stable renal function with minor uremic symptoms

Manage Conservatively
Until Creatine Clearance
<10 ml/min

ACUTE RENAL FAILURE

Anwar Al-Haidary
David B. Van Wyck

Acute renal failure (ARF) in hospitalized patients often involves multiple potential etiologies. The challenge is therefore to identify and correct dominant reversible factors and to prevent the complications anticipated after sudden loss of renal function. The history and physical examination should aim to identify or exclude evidence of systemic inflammatory disease, infection, volume and hemodynamic disturbances, medications, and allergies. Renal ultrasonography should be undertaken if historical or physical evidence suggests malignancy, urinary stone disease, solitary kidney (including transplanted), neurogenic bladder, or bladder outlet obstruction. Careful examination of a fresh urine specimen is essential.

A. In the patient with ARF, muddy brown casts and epithelial cell casts suggest acute tubular necrosis (ATN), WBC casts acute interstitial nephritis (AIN), and RBC casts rapidly progressive glomerulonephritis (RPGN). Obtain a random urine sample for analysis of sodium (U_{Na}, P_{Na}) and creatinine (U_{cr}, P_{cr}) concentration, and calculation of fractional excretion of sodium (Fe_{Na}):

$$Fe_{Na}(\%) = \frac{U_{Na} \times P_{cr}}{U_{cr} \times P_{Na}} \times 100$$

B. ATN results from ischemic or toxic damage to renal tubular epithelium. Ischemia usually can be identified by inspection of the patient and recent blood pressure recordings. The most common causes of nephrotoxic ATN include drugs (especially aminoglycosides, amphotericin B, cisplatin), radiocontrast material, heavy metals (mercury, lead), hemoglobin, myoglobin (see A), and multiple myeloma (with light-chain deposition). Because the BUN and P_{cr} rise proportionately in ATN, a normal ratio of 10–20:1 often is seen. U_{Na} >20 mEq/L or Fe_{Na} >1.0% supports the diagnosis of ATN, but lower values for either test may be seen, particularly early in the course of ischemic ATN.

C. Although myoglobin is not directly nephrotoxic, luminal obstruction of the renal tubules with myoglobin casts and intense myoglobin-mediated intrarenal vasoconstriction often combine to produce ARF after breakdown of muscle tissue (rhabdomyolysis). The diagnosis of rhabdomyolysis is suggested by high serum concentrations of other intracellular constituents, including potassium, phosphate, and urate, and is confirmed by elevated plasma creatine kinase levels, a positive urine dipstick test for heme without urinary RBCs by microscopy, and a positive test for myoglobinuria. The relatively rapid rise of P_{cr} and low BUN/P_{cr} ratio that characterize rhabdomyolysis-related ARF probably reflect the generous muscle mass, and higher creatinine production rates, of physically active individuals, who are most prone to this mode of injury. The risk of ARF after rhab-

domyolysis is increased by hypotension or dehydration; vigorous efforts to maintain brisk urinary output are accordingly indicated. Common causes of rhabdomyolysis include trauma, drug overdose (alcohol and cocaine), and heat stroke. Although decreased protein intake, drugs (including sulfamethoxazole and cimetidine), and acidosis can also lower the BUN/P_{cr} ratio, these laboratory abnormalities usually are not associated with ARF.

D. Inflammation of the tubulointerstitial region of the kidney may be associated with acute or chronic renal failure. If the etiology is bacterial, as in pyelonephritis, treatment requires appropriate antibiotics. The most common noninfectious cause of interstitial nephritis is a drug-induced allergic reaction. Methicillin, penicillin, cephalothin, NSAIDs, and cimetidine are strongly associated with AIN. Other penicillins and cephalosporins, as well as the sulfonamides, thiazides, and furosemides, are also likely offenders. In most patients, partial to full recovery is expected after withdrawal of the responsible agent. Because the role of steroid therapy in AIN is uncertain, give prednisone (60 mg/day with rapid taper) only to patients with severe disease (P_{cr} >2.5–3.0 mg/dl).

E. Consider RPGN when rapid deterioration in renal function is accompanied by RBC casts and proteinuria. Serologic examination is the key to differential diagnosis. In particular, low plasma complement levels often are found in immune complex–mediated diseases, including postinfectious glomerulonephritis, membranoproliferative glomerulonephritis, cryoglobulinemia, and (in the presence of antinuclear antibodies) systemic lupus erythematosus; a positive test for antineutrophil cytoplasmic antibody strongly suggests either Wegener's granulomatosis or a necrotizing systemic vasculitis. Definitive diagnosis is established by renal biopsy, in which RPGN is histologically defined as crescent formation involving >50% of glomeruli.

F. In prerenal disease, enhanced tubular reabsorption of solutes and water predominates over the rather modest fall in glomerular filtration rate. Because urea and creatinine are both filtered, but urea is avidly reabsorbed and creatinine is not, an elevated BUN/P_{cr} ratio results. U_{Na} <10 mEq/L or Fe_{Na} <1% provides further evidence that intrinsic renal function is intact and that prerenal causes for azotemia, including volume depletion, hypotension, congestive heart failure, cirrhosis, NSAID administration, and severe bilateral renal artery stenosis, should be sought. In hepatorenal syndrome, ARF in association with cirrhosis and ascites is characterized by low U_{Na} (often <10 mEq/L) and Fe_{Na} (<1%). The interpretation of BUN/P_{cr} ratios may be rendered unreliable by disorders of protein metabolism. For example, hepatic cirrhosis and protein malnutrition are associated

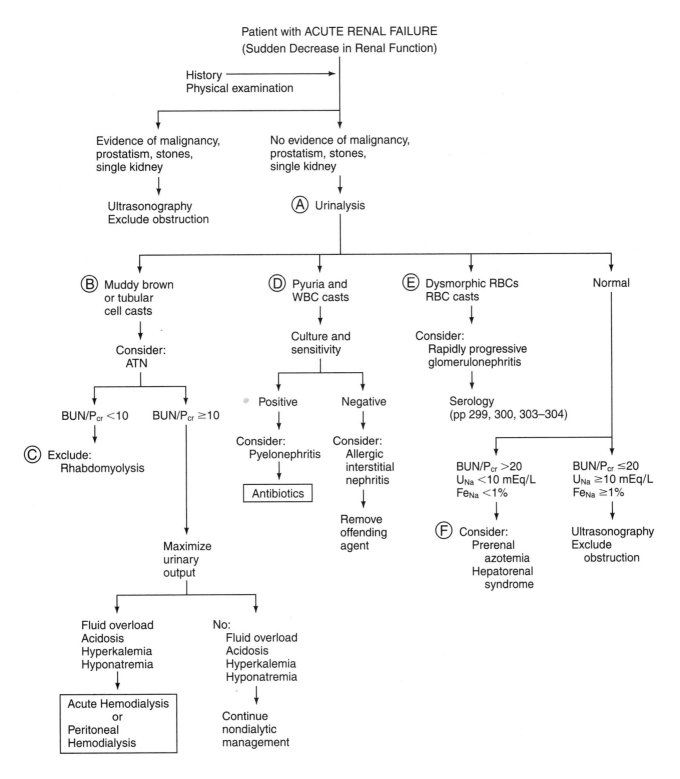

Patient with ACUTE RENAL FAILURE
(Sudden Decrease in Renal Function)

History
Physical examination

Evidence of malignancy, prostatism, stones, single kidney

No evidence of malignancy, prostatism, stones, single kidney

Ultrasonography
Exclude obstruction

(A) Urinalysis

(B) Muddy brown or tubular cell casts

(D) Pyuria and WBC casts

(E) Dysmorphic RBCs RBC casts

Normal

Consider: ATN

Culture and sensitivity

Consider: Rapidly progressive glomerulonephritis

$BUN/P_{cr} < 10$ $BUN/P_{cr} \geq 10$

Positive   Negative

Serology (pp 299, 300, 303–304)

(C) Exclude: Rhabdomyolysis

Consider: Pyelonephritis

Consider: Allergic interstitial nephritis

$BUN/P_{cr} > 20$
$U_{Na} < 10$ mEq/L
$Fe_{Na} < 1\%$

$BUN/P_{cr} \leq 20$
$U_{Na} \geq 10$ mEq/L
$Fe_{Na} \geq 1\%$

Antibiotics

Remove offending agent

(F) Consider: Prerenal azotemia Hepatorenal syndrome

Ultrasonography Exclude obstruction

Maximize urinary output

Fluid overload Acidosis Hyperkalemia Hyponatremia

No: Fluid overload Acidosis Hyperkalemia Hyponatremia

Acute Hemodialysis or Peritoneal Hemodialysis

Continue nondialytic management

with low BUN levels, whereas GI bleeding, hypercatabolism, high protein intake (often from parenteral nutrition), and corticosteroid administration are all associated with elevated BUN levels.

References

Ebert TH. Hematuria. In: Greene HL, ed. Clinical medicine. 2nd ed. St. Louis: Mosby, 1996:584.

Espinal CH, Gregory AW. Differential diagnosis of acute renal failure. Clin Nephrol 1980; 13:73.

Falk RJ, Hogan S, Carey TS, Jennette C. Clinical course of anti-neutrophil cytoplasmic antibody-associated glomerulonephritis and systemic vasculitis. Ann Intern Med 1990; 113:656.

Galpin JE, Shinaberger JH, Stanley TM, et al. Acute interstitial nephritis due to methicillin. Am J Med 1978; 65:756.

Thadhani R, Pascual M, Bonventre JV. Acute renal failure. N Engl J Med 1996; 334:1448.

PROTEINURIA

Anwar Al-Haidary
David B. Van Wyck

A. Proteinuria is the presence of >150 mg/day of protein in the urine. Perform protein electrophoresis of a 24-hour urine specimen in any patient with proteinuria identified by dipstick urine examination because quantification and characterization of the protein excreted are essential to differential diagnosis and treatment.

B. The presence of nephrotic range proteinuria (>3.5 g/day) implies glomerular disease or glomerulonephritis (GN). Characteristically, the main component of glomerular proteinuria is albumin, and there is no monoclonal protein component. Diabetes is one of the most common causes of nephrotic syndrome in adults. It can be readily excluded by history, physical examination (with particular attention to retinal changes), and normal fasting blood glucose. Rarely, diabetic retinopathy can be excluded only by fluorescein angiography.

C. In the absence of diabetes, the most common causes of nephrotic syndrome in adults include focal sclerosing GN, membranous GN, and amyloidosis, which can be distinguished only by tissue examination (renal biopsy). Serologic investigation may be rewarding, nevertheless. Systemic lupus erythematosus (SLE) is characterized by elevated ANA. Complement components C3 and C4 may be low in SLE, postinfectious GN, cryoglobulinemia, and membranoproliferative GN. Positive antinuclear neutrophil cytoplasmic antibody (ANCA), formerly thought to be specific for Wegener's granulomatosis, is known to be associated also with the GN of systemic vasculitis. Hepatitis B virus or HIV antigenemia are well described causes of nephrotic syndrome, and the presence of either renders further diagnostic studies unnecessary. A number of drugs, including gold, penicillamine, phenytoin, captopril, and NSAIDs, have been shown to cause nephrotic syndrome; withdrawal of the offending agents generally prompts resolution of proteinuria.

D. Renal biopsy remains the best means of establishing the definitive diagnosis of most causes of nephrotic syndrome. Treatment is aimed at the underlying condition, control of excessive protein losses, and managing the expected complications of nephrotic syndrome (edema, ascites, and increased risk of infections and deep venous thrombosis). A low-protein diet, angiotensin III converting enzyme (ACE) inhibitors, and calcium channel blockers have proved effective in decreasing proteinuria in patients with nephrotic syndrome from a wide range of causes.

E. Although patients showing proteinuria of <3.5 g/day may have the same disorders of glomerular function seen in nephrotic syndrome, low-grade proteinuria also is commonly seen in patients with primarily extrarenal disorders such as congestive cardiac failure or uncontrolled hypertension. Similarly, significant proteinuria that arises during a febrile illness or after heavy exercise does not suggest a pathologic condition. Orthostatic proteinuria is a benign condition that usually remits spontaneously and is characterized by significant proteinuria only when the patient is active and in the upright position. Like transient and benign persistent forms, orthostatic proteinuria has a typically benign course.

F. The presence of monoclonal protein in the urine and in plasma suggests plasma cell dyscrasia. Further examination by immunoelectrophoresis, bone marrow aspiration, and skeletal radiography is needed to exclude multiple myeloma. In the absence of evidence for myeloma, consider secondary amyloidosis, light-chain disease, and B-cell lymphoproliferative disorders. Definitive diagnosis of amyloidosis may require tissue biopsy. Management consists of treating the underlying disorder.

References

Ahmed Z, Lee J. Asymptomatic urinary abnormalities: hematuria and proteinuria. Med Clin North Am 1997; 81:641.

Clive DM. Proteinuria. In: Greene HL, ed. Clinical medicine. 2nd ed. St. Louis: Mosby, 1996:591.

Rose BD. Pathophysiology of renal disease. 2nd ed. New York: McGraw-Hill, 1987.

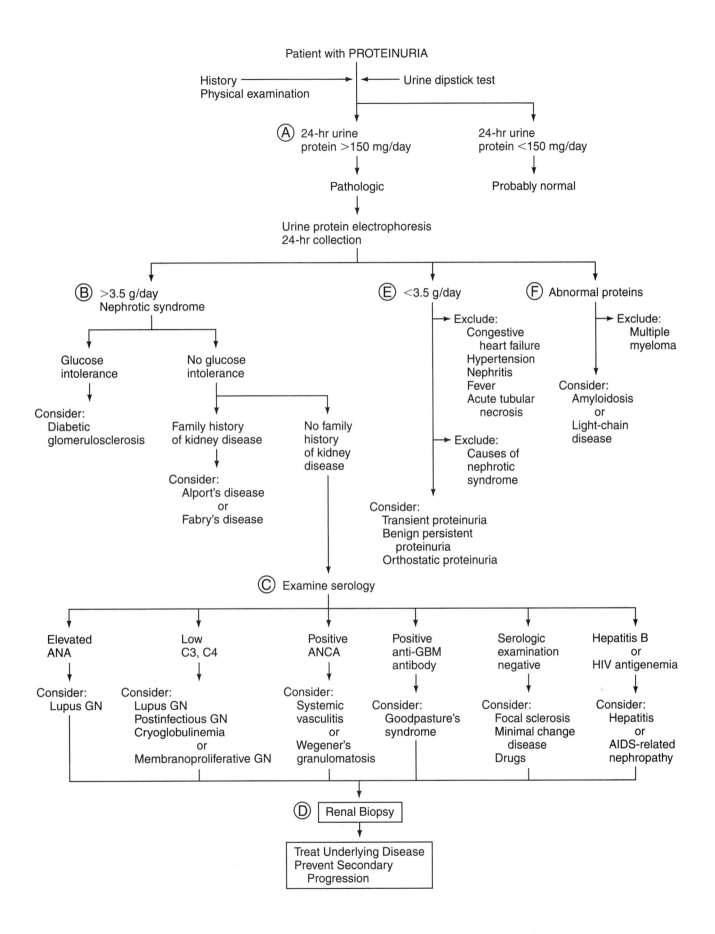

Patient with PROTEINURIA

History
Physical examination → ← Urine dipstick test

(A) 24-hr urine protein >150 mg/day

24-hr urine protein <150 mg/day

Pathologic

Probably normal

Urine protein electrophoresis
24-hr collection

(B) >3.5 g/day
Nephrotic syndrome

Glucose intolerance

No glucose intolerance

Consider:
Diabetic glomerulosclerosis

Family history of kidney disease

No family history of kidney disease

Consider:
Alport's disease
or
Fabry's disease

(E) <3.5 g/day

Exclude:
Congestive heart failure
Hypertension
Nephritis
Fever
Acute tubular necrosis

Exclude:
Causes of nephrotic syndrome

Consider:
Transient proteinuria
Benign persistent proteinuria
Orthostatic proteinuria

(F) Abnormal proteins

Exclude:
Multiple myeloma

Consider:
Amyloidosis
or
Light-chain disease

(C) Examine serology

Elevated ANA

Low C3, C4

Positive ANCA

Positive anti-GBM antibody

Serologic examination negative

Hepatitis B or HIV antigenemia

Consider:
Lupus GN

Consider:
Lupus GN
Postinfectious GN
Cryoglobulinemia
or
Membranoproliferative GN

Consider:
Systemic vasculitis
or
Wegener's granulomatosis

Consider:
Goodpasture's syndrome

Consider:
Focal sclerosis
Minimal change disease
Drugs

Consider:
Hepatitis
or
AIDS-related nephropathy

(D) Renal Biopsy

Treat Underlying Disease
Prevent Secondary Progression

HEMATURIA

Anwar Al-Haidary
David B. Van Wyck

A. Because the presence or absence of cellular urinary casts is pivotal to the evaluation of patients with hematuria, several freshly voided urine sediments should be closely examined. The presence of RBC casts virtually establishes the diagnosis of glomerulonephritis (GN) or vasculitis. Dysmorphic changes in urinary RBCs, best observed under interference phase-contrast microscopy, likewise suggest glomerular origin.

B. Perform serologic tests (antinuclear antibody for systemic lupus erythematosus [SLE], cryoglobulins for essential mixed cryoglobulinemia, antineutrophil cytoplasmic antibody for Wegener's and vasculitis, and anti–glomerular basement membrane antibodies for Goodpasture's syndrome) as soon as glomerular disease is detected. Also, examine the plasma C3 and C4 components of complement because low levels are a hallmark of GN associated with SLE, infections, cryoglobulinemia, and membranoproliferative GN.

C. If the serologic examination is unrewarding and the patient has normal renal function, normal blood pressure, and proteinuria <300 mg/day, consider the diagnosis of IgA nephropathy (Berger's disease). This relatively common presentation of GN has a typically benign course. Hypertension, renal insufficiency, or high-grade proteinuria, regardless of the pathologic diagnosis, suggests a less favorable prognosis and, in the opinion of many nephrologists, requires tissue evaluation.

D. Normal-shaped RBCs and the absence of cellular casts, acellular casts, or significant proteinuria (>300 mg/day) suggest extraglomerular bleeding. The common causes of extraglomerular hematuria in adults include prostatic disease, kidney and urinary stones, malignancy, and trauma. In children, urinary stones and trauma are main causes of nonglomerular hematuria.

E. Pyuria, >4 WBCs per high-power field (hpf), is commonly associated with bacteriuria. Pyuria without evidence of infection suggests the diagnosis of interstitial nephritis. Acute interstitial nephritis is characterized by fever, skin rash, eosinophilia, and eosinophiluria, most commonly in association with antibiotic administration. Chronic interstitial nephritis is found in association with a wide variety of drugs, heavy metal intoxication, metabolic abnormalities, and therapeutic radiation.

References

Ahmed Z, Lee J. Asymptomatic urinary abnormalities: hematuria and proteinuria. Med Clin North Am 1997; 81:641.

Ebert TH. Hematuria. In: Greene HL, ed. Clinical medicine. 2nd ed. St. Louis: Mosby, 1996:584.

Falk RJ, Hogan S, Carey TS, Jennette C. Clinical course of antineutrophil cytoplasmic antibody–associated glomerulonephritis and systemic vasculitis. Ann Intern Med 1990; 113:656.

Rodicio JL. Idiopathic IgA nephropathy. Kidney Int 1984; 25:717.

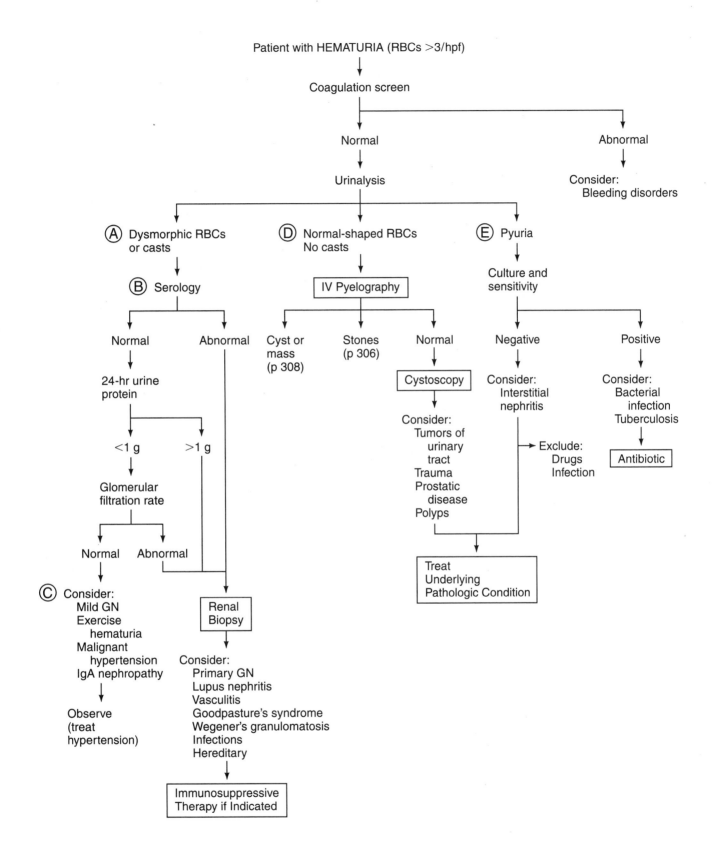

Patient with HEMATURIA (RBCs >3/hpf)

Coagulation screen

Normal

Abnormal

Consider:
Bleeding disorders

Urinalysis

Ⓐ Dysmorphic RBCs
or casts

Ⓓ Normal-shaped RBCs
No casts

Ⓔ Pyuria

Ⓑ Serology

IV Pyelography

Culture and
sensitivity

Normal

Abnormal

Cyst or
mass
(p 308)

Stones
(p 306)

Normal

Negative

Positive

24-hr urine
protein

Cystoscopy

Consider:
Interstitial
nephritis

Consider:
Bacterial
infection
Tuberculosis

<1 g

>1 g

Consider:
Tumors of
urinary
tract
Trauma
Prostatic
disease
Polyps

Exclude:
Drugs
Infection

Antibiotic

Glomerular
filtration rate

Normal

Abnormal

Treat
Underlying
Pathologic Condition

Ⓒ Consider:
Mild GN
Exercise
hematuria
Malignant
hypertension
IgA nephropathy

Renal
Biopsy

Observe
(treat
hypertension)

Consider:
Primary GN
Lupus nephritis
Vasculitis
Goodpasture's syndrome
Wegener's granulomatosis
Infections
Hereditary

Immunosuppressive
Therapy if Indicated

KIDNEY STONES

James L. McGuire
David B. Van Wyck

Kidney stones are commonly manifested by sharp colicky pain radiating to the groin, testicle, or tip of the urethra, often accompanied by gross hematuria. Common clinical presentations also include nephrocalcinosis, renal damage, and staghorn calculi. Although urinary stone disease is common, approximately 40% of patients have only a single episode of stone passage. Therefore intensive investigation and treatment is directed toward patients with special risk factors, including family history of stone disease, history of major stone complication, solitary kidney, age at onset <20 years, and associated predisposing conditions such as renal tubular acidosis, urinary infection with urea-splitting organisms, and malabsorption syndromes. Chemical analysis is useful in distinguishing the four main stone types. Struvite or infection stones account for 20% of all stones and are found in urine infected with urea-splitting organisms. Urate stones account for 5% and commonly arise in the setting of hyperuricemia and gout. Cystine stones comprise 3% of the total and result from a renal tubular defect promoting urinary cystine loss. Clinical setting and chemical analysis render the diagnosis of these disorders readily apparent. The pathogenesis and treatment of calcium- and uric acid–containing stones are detailed in the decision tree.

A. A detailed history is useful in identifying high calcium intake, usually from dairy products; high salt intake, which promotes calcium excretion; fluid intake inadequate to match losses; malabsorption syndromes, which are associated with calcium oxalate stones; previous urinary tract infections or procedures; or use of medications such as vitamin D or calcium-containing antacids.

B. A 24-hour urine collection for calcium, urate, creatinine, and pH may be the single most important test in patients with calcium kidney stones. The demonstration of hypercalciuria is pivotal. In the absence of major reversible causes of hypercalciuria, consider the diagnosis of idiopathic hypercalciuria from hyperabsorption of calcium. A low urinary volume (<1 L/day) may aggravate the degree of urinary supersaturation in patients with

stones. High urate excretion predisposes patients to stone formation, whether pure urate or mixed. Most patients with calcium oxalate nephrolithiasis show urine pH values >6.5. In approximately 50% of patients, no obvious abnormality is apparent on routine urine collection. In some of these remaining patients, urinary levels of the stone inhibitor citrate may be low. Hypocitraturia most commonly is associated with distal renal tubular acidosis and may be profound. Consider other disorders associated with acidification defects, including chronic renal failure, diarrhea, and hypokalemia.

C. Treatment strategies for patients with calcium-containing stones should begin with generous fluid intake (>2 L/day) and, in the presence of hypercalciuria, dietary restriction of calcium and sodium. Thiazide (e.g., hydrochlorothiazide, 25–50 mg/day) lowers both calcium and oxalate excretion. Cellulose sodium phosphate (Calcibind) has been suggested for idiopathic calcium hyperabsorption, but its cost and the high level of GI intolerance has limited its use. Give allopurinol (300 mg/day, adjusted downward for renal insufficiency) for hyperuricosuria.

References

Coe FI, Parks JH. Pathophysiology of kidney stones and strategies for treatment. Hosp Pract 1988; 23:185.

Kupin WL. A practical approach to nephrolithiasis. Hosp Pract (Off Ed) 1995; 30:57.

McGuire JL, Lee YSL. Kidney stones. In: Greene HL, ed. Clinical medicine. St. Louis: Mosby, 1996:603.

Pak CYC, Fuller C. Idiopathic hypocitrauric calcium-oxalate nephrolithiasis successfully treated with potassium citrate. Ann Intern Med 1986; 104:33.

Preminger GM, Pak CYC. The practical evaluation and selective medical management of nephrolithiasis. Semin Urol 1985; 3:170.

Saklayen MG. Medical management of nephrolithiasis. Med Clin North Am 1997; 81:785.

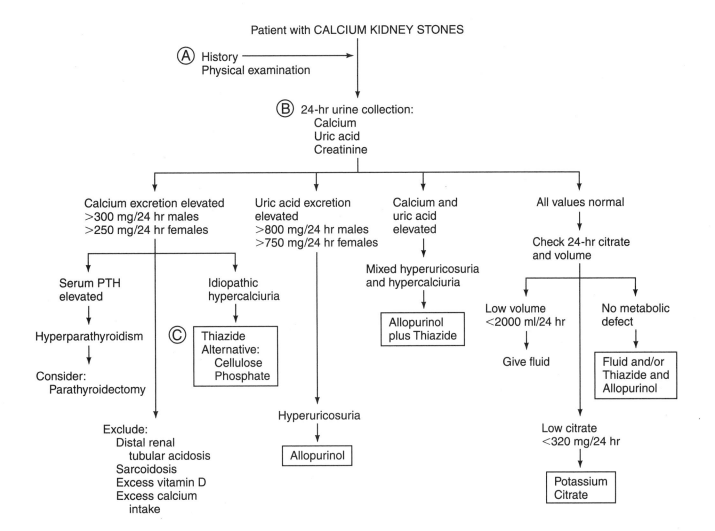

Patient with CALCIUM KIDNEY STONES

Ⓐ History
Physical examination

Ⓑ 24-hr urine collection:
Calcium
Uric acid
Creatinine

Calcium excretion elevated
>300 mg/24 hr males
>250 mg/24 hr females

Uric acid excretion
elevated
>800 mg/24 hr males
>750 mg/24 hr females

Calcium and
uric acid
elevated

All values normal

Serum PTH
elevated

Idiopathic
hypercalciuria

Hyperparathyroidism

Ⓒ Thiazide
Alternative:
Cellulose
Phosphate

Consider:
Parathyroidectomy

Exclude:
Distal renal
tubular acidosis
Sarcoidosis
Excess vitamin D
Excess calcium
intake

Hyperuricosuria

Allopurinol

Mixed hyperuricosuria
and hypercalciuria

Allopurinol
plus Thiazide

Check 24-hr citrate
and volume

Low volume
<2000 ml/24 hr

No metabolic
defect

Give fluid

Fluid and/or
Thiazide and
Allopurinol

Low citrate
<320 mg/24 hr

Potassium
Citrate

RENAL CYSTS AND MASSES

David B. Van Wyck

A. Flank pain, palpable abdominal mass, or hematuria often heralds a renal mass or cystic disease. Begin evaluation of patients with these findings with a CT scan or ultrasonography (US). In general, superior sensitivity renders CT sufficient for the definitive diagnosis of most lesions and necessary when US evidence is equivocal. When CT is inconclusive, arteriography or needle aspiration may be required.

B. Simple renal cysts are the most common renal masses, occurring in 50% of patients >50 years of age. Although usually asymptomatic and discovered incidentally on a plain film of the abdomen, intravenous pyelography (IVP), or renal US, simple cysts occasionally cause flank or abdominal pain. There may be a single cyst or multiple cysts involving both kidneys. Distinguishing simple cysts from two more serious conditions, polycystic kidney disease (PKD) and solid masses, such as renal cell carcinoma or a renal abscess, is the most important task in the differential diagnosis and is aided by criteria established for the use of US and CT. The criteria favoring a simple cyst on US are (1) sharp margins with smooth walls, (2) no echoes (anechoic) within the cyst, and (3) a strong posterior wall echo, indicating good transmission through the water-filled cyst. When all three criteria are fulfilled, the likelihood of a malignancy is extremely small and no further evaluation is required. When there is incomplete renal visualization, evidence of calcifications or septa, or multiple cysts that may obscure a potential carcinoma, CT is required. A simple cyst is considered to be present on CT if (1) the cyst is sharply demarcated from the surrounding parenchyma and has smooth, thin walls; (2) the fluid within the cyst is homogeneous (like water) with a density of 0–20 Hounsfield units; and (3) there is no enhancement of the cyst fluid after administration of radiocontrast media. The need for cyst puncture is virtually eliminated by the use of US and CT and should be considered only if the initial, noninvasive procedures cannot confirm a benign cyst.

C. Single or multiple cysts may arise in the course of chronic renal failure. Although acquired cystic disease occasionally is found in patients before dialysis, its incidence may be >50% among patients who have undergone dialysis for >3 years. The relatively high incidence of neoplasia associated with acquired cystic disease has prompted recommendations to regularly monitor end-stage renal disease (ESRD) patients sonographically. The diagnostic approach to simple cysts should also be used in patients with acquired renal cystic disease.

D. Adult PKD is responsible for 10–12% of cases of ESRD. Inherited as an autosomal-dominant disorder and progressing uniformly to chronic renal failure, adult PKD occurs in approximately 1 of every 1250 live births. Penetrance is complete if the patient lives to 80 years of age. Symptoms of flank pain, abdominal discomfort, and hematuria often do not become apparent until the age of 40–50 years, when they may be associated with hypertension and renal insufficiency. Diagnosis by US is straightforward in advanced disease but may be less reliable in the early stages: A negative US cannot with complete certainty rule out PKD in patients <40 years old. However, CT can detect smaller cysts, lowering the age at which a negative study virtually excludes disease to about 20–25 years.

E. Medullary cystic disease, unlike the previously mentioned disorders, is rare. Occurring in children, it progresses inevitably to ESRD by the age of 20–40 years. Because the course of disease is slow and largely asymptomatic, patients often have evidence of advanced renal disease. The diagnosis of medullary cystic disease often is made by inference from the clinical presentation and the common feature of a positive family history. Multiple small and occasional large cysts at the corticomedullary junction are distinctive features on US.

F. Because patients with medullary sponge kidney often are asymptomatic, the diagnosis may never be made unless urinary tract infection or passage of a stone prompt IVP. With the exception of stone formation, medullary sponge kidney is a benign disorder with an excellent long-term prognosis, and no specific therapy is needed. Recurrent stone formers may benefit from a thiazide diuretic for hypercalciuria, allopurinol for hyperuricosuria, or potassium citrate for hypocitraturia (p 306).

G. Renal cell carcinoma may arise as a mass lesion, cystic degeneration of a mass, or malignant conversion of a cyst. Symptoms often are absent or not specific to the kidney, so most tumors are discovered during evaluation of hematuria; the full triad of flank pain, palpable mass, and hematuria is seen in <10% of patients. Associated findings include fever, either anemia or erythrocytosis, hepatic dysfunction, and hypercalcemia. CT is pivotal in the diagnosis and staging of renal cell carcinoma and has largely replaced arteriography as the definitive diagnostic study. Lesions <2 cm may be detected before distortion of the renal outline by abnormal heterogeneous enhancement after injection of contrast.

References

Black RM. Rose and Black's manual of clinical problems in nephrology. Boston: Little, Brown, 1995.

Gardner KD. Cystic kidneys. Kidney Int 1988; 33:610.

Grantham JJ. Polycystic kidney disease: an old problem in a new context. N Engl J Med 1988; 319:944.

Warshauer DM, McCarthy SM, Street L, et al. Detection of renal masses: sensitivities and specificities of excretory urography/linear tomography, US and CT. Radiology 1988; 169:363.

Patient with RENAL MASS OR CYSTIC DISEASE

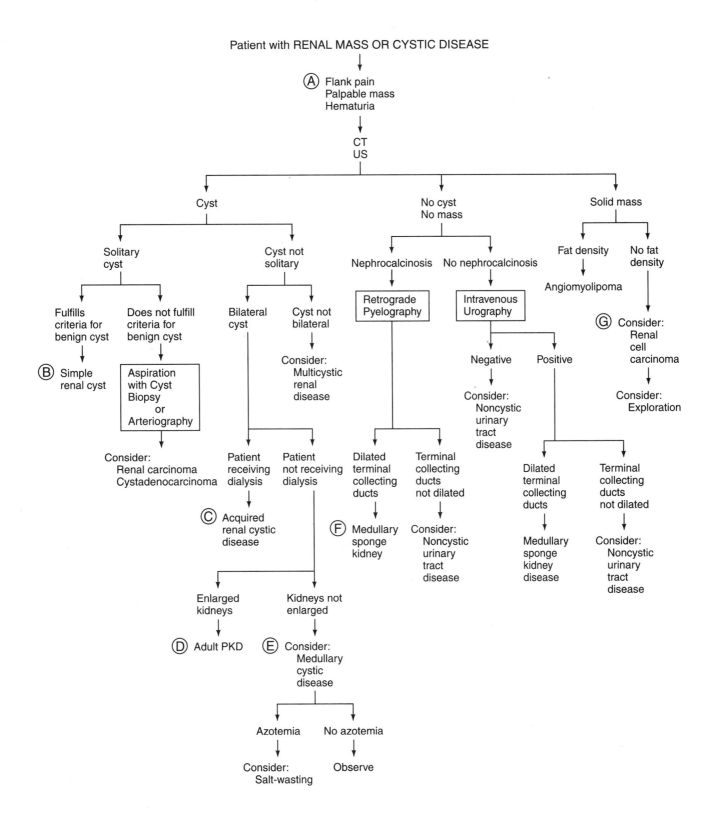

METABOLIC ACIDOSIS

Hillary Don

A. Metabolic acidosis is a decrease in measured blood bicarbonate accompanied by the appearance of a base deficit. It does not include the small, immediate, mandatory physiologic response to *acute respiratory alkalosis* (change $HCO_3^- = 0.2 \times$ change $Paco_2$), which is not associated with a base deficit. At normal $Paco_2$, the CO_2 combining power measured with plasma electrolytes should be 1.0–1.5 mEq greater than the HCO_3^- calculated with the blood gas determination: Greater differences suggest discrepant sampling times or excess heparin or processing time for the blood gas sample. When serum HCO_3^- is low but blood pH is >7.43, the metabolic acidosis is likely to be in partial compensation for a respiratory alkalosis (change in $HCO_3^- = 0.5 \times$ change $Paco_2$). On the other hand, when serum HCO_3^- is low and pH is <7.39, assume metabolic acidosis to be the primary disorder and expect a secondary respiratory alkalosis (change $Paco_2 = 1.1 \times$ change HCO_3^-). When pH is between these two values, mixed defects are present and the primary lesion must be distinguished by the clinical setting.

B. The physiologic anion gap (AG) ($AG = Na^+ - [Cl^- + HCO_3^-]$) is 12 mEq/L. An increase in circulating organic acid anions such as lactate or acetoacetate produces a rise in AG that matches the fall in serum HCO_3^- milliequivalent for milliequivalent. If the fall in HCO_3^- exceeds the increase in AG, a mixed AG and non-AG acidosis is present; this may arise when there are renal and extrarenal disorders or, more commonly, during early or resolving phases of ketoacidosis when the ketoacid clearance rate exceeds the rate at which depleted HCO_3^- buffers are regenerated. Metabolic acidoses showing an elevated AG are limited to (1) a short list of drug and poison ingestions, including methanol, salicylates, ethylene glycol, paraldehyde, paracetamol, and butanone and, (2) in the absence of suspicious ingestions, the diabetic and alcoholic ketoacidoses or lactic acidosis.

C. The use of $NaHCO_3$ to correct metabolic acidosis is controversial because it may transiently increase $Paco_2$, increase cerebral acidosis, decrease serum K^+, increase Na^+, shift the oxyhemoglobin curve to the left, and contribute to a postrecovery overshoot metabolic alkalosis. However, in certain instances the correction of acidemia may improve cardiac function and potentiate the action of vasoactive drugs. Some authors therefore advise cautious administration of $NaHCO_3$ (base deficit $\times 0.1 \times$ kg body weight) when pH is <7.2 and volume replacement with saline has failed. The pH should not be corrected above 7.25 with $NaHCO_3$.

D. Predisposing factors for lactic acidosis are tissue hypoxia (shock, hypotension, congestive heart failure, hypoxemia), systemic disorders (sepsis, liver failure, leukemia, convulsions, strychnine poisoning, abnormal gut flora), drugs or toxins (butanone, paracetamol, ritodrine), and inborn errors of metabolism (glucose-6 phosphatase deficiency). D-Lactate is not detected by the usual enzymatic methods for lactate and requires special analysis. Treat the underlying cause, but a pH <7.2 may need to be partially corrected with $NaHCO_3$ (see C). Dichloroacetate stimulates pyruvate dehydrogenase and has been used successfully to treat lactic acidosis. Treat D-lactate with a nonabsorbable antibiotic such as vancomycin.

E. Non-AG acidosis (hyperchloremic metabolic acidosis) results from either increased loss of HCO_3^- or insufficient acid excretion and HCO_3^- production by the kidney. Non-AG acidosis can be caused by administration of acid (NH_4Cl, $CaCl_2$, arginine HCl), by loss of HCO_3^- through the GI tract (diarrhea, small bowel fistula, ileostomy), or by loss through the kidney (renal tubular acidosis, mineralocorticoid deficiency states such as Addison's disease, carbonic anhydrase inhibition). Aldosterone deficiency is suspected by the clinical picture (weight loss, increased skin pigmentation, hypotension) or previous administration of steroids. Treatment of the underlying condition whenever possible is the key. Unlike the situation in elevated AG acidoses, $NaHCO_3$ therapy is mandatory in most non-AG acidoses.

References

Black RM. Acid base disturbances. In: Dale DC, Federman DD, eds. Scientific American medicine. New York: Scientific American 1996; 10, II, 1–23.

DuBose TD Jr. Clinical approach to patients with acid-base disorders. Med Clin North Am 1983; 67:799.

Lever E, Jaspan JB. Sodium bicarbonate therapy in severe diabetic ketoacidosis. Am J Med 1983; 75:263.

Stacpoole PW, Harman EM, Curry SH, et al. Treatment of lactic acidosis with dichloroacetate. N Engl J Med 1983; 309:390.

Stolberg L, Rolfe R, Gitlin N, et al. D-Lactic acidosis due to abnormal gut flora. Diagnosis and treatment of two cases. N Engl J Med 1982; 306:1344.

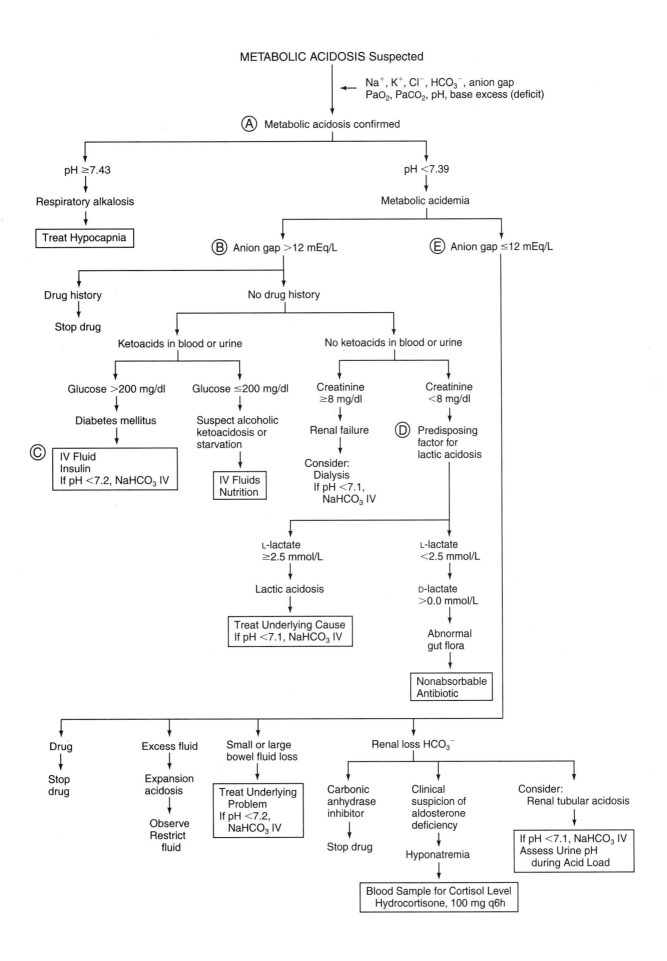

METABOLIC ACIDOSIS Suspected

Na⁺, K⁺, Cl⁻, HCO₃⁻, anion gap
PaO₂, PaCO₂, pH, base excess (deficit)

Ⓐ Metabolic acidosis confirmed

pH ≥7.43

Respiratory alkalosis

Treat Hypocapnia

pH <7.39

Metabolic acidemia

Ⓑ Anion gap >12 mEq/L

Ⓔ Anion gap ≤12 mEq/L

Drug history

Stop drug

No drug history

Ketoacids in blood or urine

No ketoacids in blood or urine

Glucose >200 mg/dl

Diabetes mellitus

Ⓒ IV Fluid
Insulin
If pH <7.2, NaHCO₃ IV

Glucose ≤200 mg/dl

Suspect alcoholic
ketoacidosis or
starvation

IV Fluids
Nutrition

Creatinine
≥8 mg/dl

Renal failure

Consider:
Dialysis
If pH <7.1,
NaHCO₃ IV

Creatinine
<8 mg/dl

Ⓓ Predisposing
factor for
lactic acidosis

ʟ-lactate
≥2.5 mmol/L

Lactic acidosis

Treat Underlying Cause
If pH <7.1, NaHCO₃ IV

ʟ-lactate
<2.5 mmol/L

ᴅ-lactate
>0.0 mmol/L

Abnormal
gut flora

Nonabsorbable
Antibiotic

Drug

Stop
drug

Excess fluid

Expansion
acidosis

Observe
Restrict
fluid

Small or large
bowel fluid loss

Treat Underlying
Problem
If pH <7.2,
NaHCO₃ IV

Renal loss HCO₃⁻

Carbonic
anhydrase
inhibitor

Stop drug

Clinical
suspicion of
aldosterone
deficiency

Hyponatremia

Blood Sample for Cortisol Level
Hydrocortisone, 100 mg q6h

Consider:
Renal tubular acidosis

If pH <7.1, NaHCO₃ IV
Assess Urine pH
during Acid Load

METABOLIC ALKALOSIS

Hillary Don

When alkalemia is severe, metabolic alkalosis produces paresthesias, obtundation, tetany, and convulsions. Cardiac arrhythmias may be precipitated, particularly in the presence of digitalis, and volume depletion is common. The oxygen-hemoglobin dissociation curve is shifted to the left, impeding tissue oxygen uptake.

A. Metabolic alkalosis is confirmed by an increase in measured blood bicarbonate, a reciprocal decrease in Cl^-, and an increase in base excess. It does not include the small, immediate, mandatory physiologic increase in HCO_3^- in response to *acute respiratory acidosis* (change $HCO_3^- = 0.1 \times$ change $Paco_2$). At normal $Paco_2$, the CO_2 combining power measured with plasma electrolytes should be 1.0–1.5 mEq greater than the HCO_3^- calculated with the blood gas determination: Greater differences suggest discrepant sampling times, or excess heparin or processing time for the blood gas sample. Elevated plasma HCO_3^- with a blood pH <7.39 suggests that the metabolic alkalosis is secondary, compensating for a primary chronic respiratory acidosis. Because compensation is slow in onset and slow to resolve, metabolic alkalosis may persist after rapid correction of respiratory acidosis. A pH >7.43 suggests a primary metabolic alkalosis with alkalemia. When pH lies between these two levels, a mixed lesion is present and the primary deficit must be distinguished by information gained from the clinical setting. A modest compensatory respiratory acidosis with reduction in tidal volume and maintained respiratory rate (change in $Paco_2 = 0.7 \times$ change in HCO_3^-) usually accompanies the metabolic alkalemia. However, the $Paco_2$ rarely exceeds 60 mm Hg, and total absence of compensation is not abnormal for moderate degrees of metabolic alkalosis. Hypoxemia may be present, requiring titration of Fio_2 to maintain adequate O_2 saturation. Mechanical ventilation is unnecessary; if it is already in use for some other reason, take care to restrict minute ventilation to prevent a compounding respiratory alkalosis.

B. Metabolic alkalosis may occur from exogenous sources of alkali, including administration of oral citrate (Shohl's) solution, citrated blood, acetate in IV hyperalimentation, excessive $NaHCO_3$ during treatment of metabolic acidosis, and absorbable antacids. Cation exchange resins (Kayexalate) and possibly neutral phosphate (Neutra-Phos) potentiate absorption of otherwise nonabsorbable antacids. Alkalosis caused by administered alkali, loss of acid from the stomach, or diuretics (thiazides, ethacrynic acid, furosemide) usually is associated with hypovolemia, which prevents renal bicarbonate excretion. Selective dehydration (water loss) causes a rise in HCO_3^- concentration, a condition called contraction alkalosis. Treatment with IV normal saline, coupled with cautious KCl replacement, restores effective renal perfusion, permits renal excretion of bicarbonate, and thereby corrects alkalemia (saline responsive).

C. High urine Cl^-, in the absence of diuretics, provides evidence that volume depletion is not present and that alkalosis therefore will not be corrected by saline infusion (so-called saline unresponsive). A high urine Cl^- therefore turns attention to the possibility of hypermineralocorticolism (primary or secondary to corticosteroid ingestion). Renal failure plus alkali administration, and severe K^+ deficiency, also may be suspected. If renal function is intact, an aldosterone antagonist (aldactone) may be effective. Rarely, correction of severe alkalemia requires intravenous HCl (0.2 mol/L). Other forms of titratable H^+ are available but may precipitate hepatic coma (NH_4Cl) and may increase intracellular alkalosis (NH_4Cl, arginine HCl). Alternatively, hemodialysis and peritoneal dialysis readily correct metabolic alkalosis and may be the safest and most expeditious treatment when hypervolemia is present, particularly in the presence of renal failure.

References

Black RM. Acid base disturbances. In: Dale DC, Federman DD, eds. Scientific American medicine. New York: Scientific American, 1996; 10, II, 1–23.

Cogan MG, Liu F, Berger BE, et al. Metabolic alkalosis. Med Clin North Am 1983; 67:903.

Javaheri S, Shore NS, Rose B, Kazemi H. Compensatory hypoventilation in metabolic alkalosis. Chest 1982; 81:296.

Madias NE, Levey AS. Metabolic alkalosis due to absorption of "nonabsorbable" antacids. Am J Med 1983; 74:155.

Rothe KF. Hydrochloric acid for metabolic alkalosis. Lancet 1983; 1:1332.

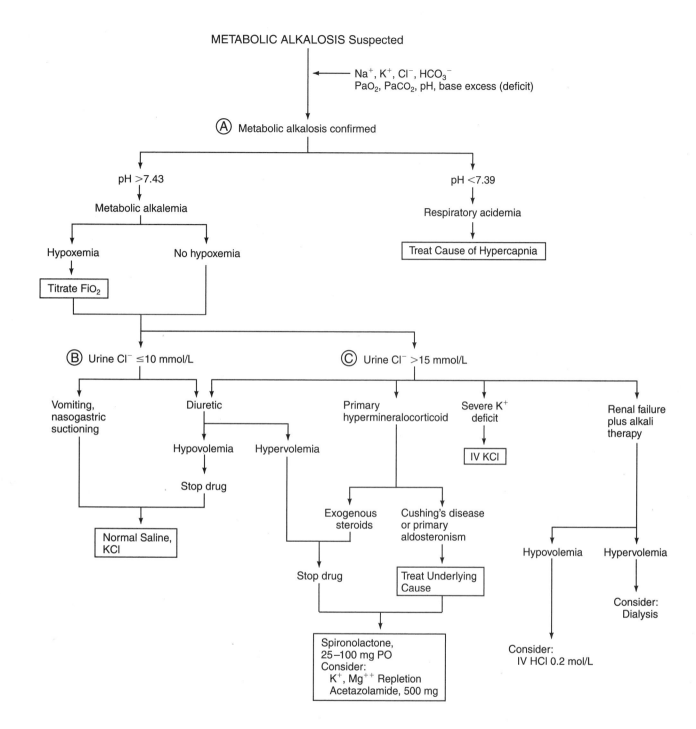

METABOLIC ALKALOSIS Suspected

Na⁺, K⁺, Cl⁻, HCO₃⁻
PaO₂, PaCO₂, pH, base excess (deficit)

Ⓐ Metabolic alkalosis confirmed

pH >7.43

Metabolic alkalemia

Hypoxemia

Titrate FiO₂

No hypoxemia

pH <7.39

Respiratory acidemia

Treat Cause of Hypercapnia

Ⓑ Urine Cl⁻ ≤10 mmol/L

Vomiting, nasogastric suctioning

Diuretic

Hypovolemia

Stop drug

Hypervolemia

Normal Saline, KCl

Ⓒ Urine Cl⁻ >15 mmol/L

Primary hypermineralocorticoid

Severe K⁺ deficit

IV KCl

Renal failure plus alkali therapy

Exogenous steroids

Cushing's disease or primary aldosteronism

Stop drug

Treat Underlying Cause

Spironolactone, 25–100 mg PO
Consider:
  K⁺, Mg⁺⁺ Repletion
  Acetazolamide, 500 mg

Hypovolemia

Hypervolemia

Consider: Dialysis

Consider: IV HCl 0.2 mol/L

HYPONATREMIA

Anwar Al-Haidary

A. Sodium concentrations may be spuriously low when excess lipid or protein displaces sodium and water from plasma (so-called pseudohyponatremia). Simple inspection of plasma samples reveals the lactescence of hyperlipidemia and increased viscosity of hyperproteinemic states. Plasma osmolality remains normal.

B. When both plasma sodium and plasma osmolality are low, true hypotonic hyponatremia exists. The important diagnostic task is to determine whether the apparent free water excess is absolute or relative; despite hyponatremia, total body sodium may be low (hypovolemia), normal (euvolemic), or high (hypervolemia).

C. In hypovolemic states the renal imperative to maintain effective circulating blood volume overrides its role in regulating plasma osmolality. Despite decreased plasma osmolality, hypovolemic hyponatremia is characterized by nonosmotic secretion of antidiuretic hormone (ADH) secretion and avid salt and water retention. Direct management at correcting the underlying disorder and re-establishing normal effective circulating volume.

D. Euvolemic hyponatremia is caused by persistent nonosmotic secretion of ADH in the absence of evidence of either volume depletion or salt retention. Total body sodium is normal and the U_{Na} reflects daily intake of sodium. Water restriction with treatment of the underlying disorder is the cornerstone of treatment. If hyponatremia is accompanied by seizures or mental status changes, initial therapy should include infusion of 3% saline, with diuretics if volume overload is threatened, sufficient to raise the plasma sodium 0.75–1.0 mEq/L/hr until the plasma sodium rises above 120 mEq/L, followed by water restriction. The syndrome, which has been termed *reset osmostat,* generally is not severe and does not require specific therapy.

E. Hypo-osmolar states associated with excess total body sodium and extracellular fluid expansion are easily recognized by evidence of pulmonary or peripheral edema. When renal function is intact, the pathophysiology resembles that in hypovolemic hyponatremia: Decreased effective circulating volume brought on by heart failure, liver disease, or nephrotic syndrome causes avid retention of both salt and water; if the resultant total body increase in water is greater than that of salt, hyponatremia develops. Low U_{Na} excretion is the key finding. When acute or chronic renal failure is present, salt and water excretion are both limited and the low plasma sodium concentration reflects greater intake of water than of salt. Treatment entails water restriction, diuretics, and therapy for the underlying condition. Severe hyponatremia with mental status changes, hypervolemia, and renal failure may require emergency dialysis.

F. Hyponatremia associated with hypertonic states reflects the presence of impermeant nonsodium solutes circulating in high concentrations in plasma. These substances draw fluid from the intracellular into the extracellular space to maintain osmotic equilibrium across cell membranes, thereby diluting plasma sodium: For example, it is calculated that for every 100 mg/dl in blood sugar, the S_{Na} decreases by 1.6 mEq/L.

References

Anderson RJ. Hospital associated hyponatremia. Kidney Int 1986; 29:1237.

Arieff AI. Hyponatremia, convulsions, respiratory arrest, and permanent brain damage after elective surgery in healthy women. N Engl J Med 1986; 314:1529.

Buckalew VM Jr. Hyponatremia: pathogenesis and management. Hosp Pract 1986; 21:49.

Cluitmans FHM. Management of severe hyponatremia: rapid or slow correction? Am J Med 1990; 88:161.

Lohr JW. Osmotic demyelination syndrome: association with hypokalemia. Am J Med 1994; 96:408.

Schrier RW. Renal and electrolyte disorders. 5th ed. Philadelphia: Lippincott-Raven, 1997.

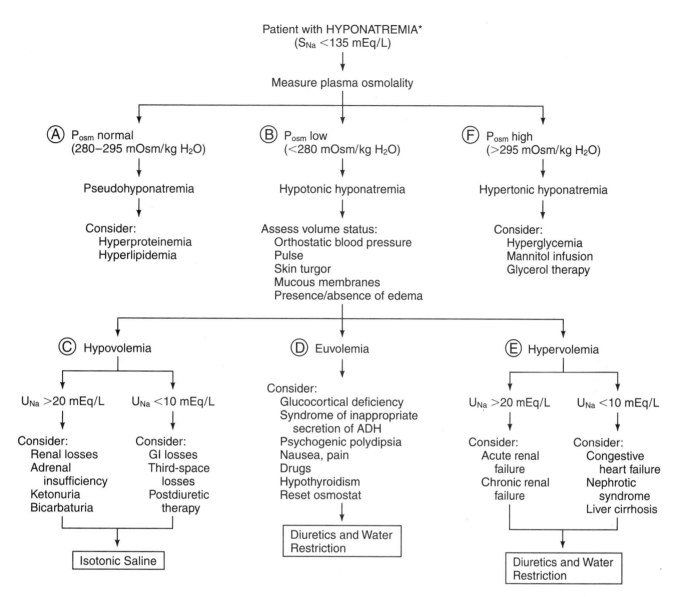

Patient with HYPONATREMIA*
(S_{Na} <135 mEq/L)

Measure plasma osmolality

(A) P_{osm} normal
(280–295 mOsm/kg H_2O)

Pseudohyponatremia

Consider:
  Hyperproteinemia
  Hyperlipidemia

(B) P_{osm} low
(<280 mOsm/kg H_2O)

Hypotonic hyponatremia

Assess volume status:
  Orthostatic blood pressure
  Pulse
  Skin turgor
  Mucous membranes
  Presence/absence of edema

(F) P_{osm} high
(>295 mOsm/kg H_2O)

Hypertonic hyponatremia

Consider:
  Hyperglycemia
  Mannitol infusion
  Glycerol therapy

(C) Hypovolemia

U_{Na} >20 mEq/L

Consider:
  Renal losses
  Adrenal
    insufficiency
  Ketonuria
  Bicarbaturia

U_{Na} <10 mEq/L

Consider:
  GI losses
  Third-space
    losses
  Postdiuretic
    therapy

Isotonic Saline

(D) Euvolemia

Consider:
  Glucocortical deficiency
  Syndrome of inappropriate
    secretion of ADH
  Psychogenic polydipsia
  Nausea, pain
  Drugs
  Hypothyroidism
  Reset osmostat

Diuretics and Water
Restriction

(E) Hypervolemia

U_{Na} >20 mEq/L

Consider:
  Acute renal
    failure
  Chronic renal
    failure

U_{Na} <10 mEq/L

Consider:
  Congestive
    heart failure
  Nephrotic
    syndrome
  Liver cirrhosis

Diuretics and Water
Restriction

*Adapted from Humes HD, ed. Pathophysiology of electrolyte disorders.
Churchill Livingstone, 1986:55; with permission.

315

HYPERNATREMIA

Anwar Al-Haidary

Disorders of plasma sodium concentration often reflect either a net gain or loss of body water or an imbalance between the change in body water and the change in total body sodium. Because hypernatremia, regardless of fluid status, is a potent stimulus for thirst, it must be assumed that the patient with hypernatremia has either a diminished thirst reflex (as in organic brain disease) or limited access to water (severe debilitation). The diagnostic approach centers on careful assessment of body fluid status, using both the physical examination and laboratory information. Treatment is guided by the etiology of the disorder. Because compensatory mechanisms to prevent brain shrinkage are slow to reverse, correction of chronic hypernatremia should be timed accordingly to be completed over 1–3 days.

A. In hypovolemic hypernatremia, substantial loss of hypotonic fluids without water replacement has occurred. Water loss therefore exceeds sodium loss, but both water and sodium deficits exist. The hypotonic fluid loss could be of renal origin, as suggested by high U_{Na} (>20 mEq/L) and low U_{osm} (<300 mOsm/L), or extrarenal origin as evidenced by low U_{Na} (<10 mEq/L) and high U_{osm}. Isotonic saline should be administered until volume depletion has been reversed, followed by hypotonic saline infusion until the electrolyte disorder has been corrected. Approximate water deficit can be calculated by the following formula:

Water deficit = $0.5 \times$ Body weight (kg) $\times$ ([P_{Na}/140] $-$ 1),

assuming that total body water in a volume-depleted patient is approximately 50% of body weight.

B. When there is pure water loss and total body sodium remains normal, isovolemic hypernatremia results. Excessive water loss can occur when there is a defect in the production or release of antidiuretic hormone (ADH) (e.g., in central diabetes insipidus [DI]) or in renal response to ADH (nephrogenic DI). The hallmark of this disorder is polyuria with low U_{osm}. On the other hand, normal renal function ensures that when the water loss is due to extrarenal factors such as respiratory or skin losses, the U_{osm} will be elevated. Appropriate management entails gradual rehydration with 5% dextrose in water and treatment of the underlying disorder.

C. When sodium salts are added abruptly and in massive amounts to extracellular fluid (ECF), hypernatremia results. Administration of hypertonic $NaHCO_3$ during cardiac resuscitation, excessive infusion of hypertonic saline, and enteric tube feeding each has been implicated in iatrogenic hypernatremia. The rapid ECF volume expansion and intracellular fluid volume contraction that follows hypertonic sodium infusion may lead to pulmonary edema. Diuretics should therefore be given promptly and the resultant sodium and water losses replaced with equal volumes of dextrose in water. Patients with poor renal function who remain oliguric in response to diuretics require dialysis.

References

Borra SI, Beredo R, Kleinfeld M. Hypernatremia in the aging: causes, manifestations, and outcome. J Natl Med Assoc 1995; 87:220.

Marsden PA, Halperin ML. Pathophysiological approach to patients presenting with hypernatremia. Am J Nephrol 1985; 5:229.

Palevsky PM, Bhagrath R, Greenberg A. Hypernatremia in hospitalized patients. Ann Intern Med 1996; 124:197.

Schrier RW. Renal and electrolyte disorders. 5th ed. Philadelphia: Lippincott-Raven, 1997.

Synder NA, Feigal EW, Arieff AL. Hypernatremia in elderly patients. Ann Intern Med 1987; 107:309.

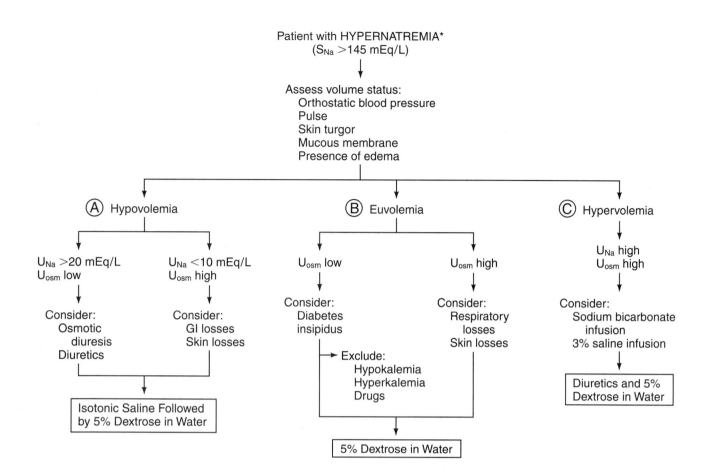

Patient with HYPERNATREMIA*
(S_{Na} >145 mEq/L)

Assess volume status:
Orthostatic blood pressure
Pulse
Skin turgor
Mucous membrane
Presence of edema

Ⓐ Hypovolemia

U_{Na} >20 mEq/L
U_{osm} low

Consider:
Osmotic
diuresis
Diuretics

U_{Na} <10 mEq/L
U_{osm} high

Consider:
GI losses
Skin losses

Isotonic Saline Followed
by 5% Dextrose in Water

Ⓑ Euvolemia

U_{osm} low

Consider:
Diabetes
insipidus

Exclude:
Hypokalemia
Hyperkalemia
Drugs

U_{osm} high

Consider:
Respiratory
losses
Skin losses

5% Dextrose in Water

Ⓒ Hypervolemia

U_{Na} high
U_{osm} high

Consider:
Sodium bicarbonate
infusion
3% saline infusion

Diuretics and 5%
Dextrose in Water

*Adapted from Humes HD, ed. Pathophysiology of electrolyte
disorders. Churchill Livingstone, 1986:68; with permission.

HYPOKALEMIA

Catherine S. Thompson
David M. Clive

Two factors influence the serum potassium (K^+) level. The *total body potassium content,* also called the *external potassium balance,* reflects the balance between K^+ intake and excretion. The *internal potassium balance* refers to the distribution of K^+ in the body. Normally, about 98% of the body's K^+ is intracellular. Potassium fluxes across cell membranes can change the serum K^+ level independent of changes in total body K^+ content. Hypokalemia usually arises through some disorder in the external potassium balance. Of the 70–100 mEq of potassium per day ingested by the average American, virtually all is absorbed and 80% is excreted through the kidneys; the rest is lost in the feces, largely through intestinal secretion. Dietary deficiency of potassium is uncommon in American society. Generally, it is seen only in chronically ill and malnourished people or in alcoholics. Any state characterized by metabolic alkalosis leads to hypokalemia. The shift of K^+ from the extracellular space into the intracellular space during alkalosis not only lowers the plasma K^+ level but also enhances the gradient for K^+ excretion in the distal tubule of the kidney. The major effects of hypokalemia are on electrically excitable cells, particularly skeletal and cardiac muscle cells. Muscle weakness is common in severe hypokalemia, and rhabdomyolysis may actually occur. Marked hypokalemia produces characteristic ECG changes. Cardiac arrhythmias are the most dangerous complication of hypokalemia. Hypokalemia has effects on the kidney itself. In potassium deficiency states, the kidneys lose the ability to concentrate urine, which leads to polyuria (e.g., nephrogenic diabetes insipidus).

A. Ask hypokalemic patients about dietary ingestion of potassium and use of medications, including diuretics or laxatives, that can cause potassium depletion. Symptoms such as vomiting or diarrhea or a family history of hypokalemia also are important features. The physical examination provides clues if the patient has signs of volume depletion (hypotension or tachycardia) or if it detects GI fistulas, a nasogastric drainage tube, or ureterosigmoidostomy. Hypertension may suggest the presence of primary hyperaldosteronism or a related disorder.

B. Initial laboratory assessment of hypokalemic patients includes an electrolyte profile, blood pH, and urine electrolytes, ($U_{Na}/K^+/Cl$). Serum aldosterone and renin level tests occasionally are helpful.

C. Hypokalemia is caused by one of two mechanisms (Table 1). The first is extrarenal (increased extrarenal losses or reduced potassium intake); the second is increased renal losses. The two mechanisms are differentiated on the basis of urine K^+ content: a urine K^+ level >20 mEq/L in the presence of hypokalemia indicates excess renal loss.

D. Extrarenal potassium losses may occur as a result of diarrhea, vomiting, continuous nasogastric suction, or profuse sweating.

E. Hypokalemia is common in patients being treated with diuretics. The K^+ losses are attributable to the increased distal delivery of sodium, which occurs as a result of the renal tubular actions of the diuretic. The metabolic "contraction" alkalosis, which these medications engender, also contributes to K^+ wasting. Disorders characterized by glucocorticoid or mineralocorticoid excess (e.g., Cushing's syndrome, Conn's syndrome, and Bartter's syndrome) also are causes of K^+ loss. In these patients kaliuresis is driven by the mineralocorticoid effects of the hormones on the tubular cells and by the metabolic alkalosis that occurs in these physiologic states.

F. Adequate treatment of hypokalemia caused by true K^+ depletion requires identification of the underlying cause of the disorder and then specific interventions to replete K^+ stores (Table 2). Correct volume depletion in hypokalemic individuals with excessive GI fluid losses; discontinue medications that aggravate hypokalemia, specifically diuretics. In most cases K^+ repletion can be accomplished with oral K^+ supplements. In patients with

TABLE 1   Causes of Hypokalemia

Reduced potassium intake
Renal losses
   Tubular defects (renal tubular acidosis)
   Metabolic alkalosis
   Diuretics
   Mineralocorticoid excess
   Edematous disorders
   Bartter's syndrome
   Magnesium deficiency
   Filtered, nonreabsorbable anions
   Leukemia
Extrarenal losses
   Vomiting, nasogastric suction
   Losses from large intestine
   Biliary drainage
   Profuse sweating

TABLE 2   Treatment of Hypokalemia

Acute
   IV replacement (potassium chloride or potassium phosphate) ≤20 mEq/hr or 200 mEq/day
Chronic
   Increased dietary supply (e.g., citrus fruits)
   Oral solutions (potassium chloride, potassium citrate)
   Oral tablets (avoid enteric-coated preparations)
   Potassium-sparing agents (spironolactone, triamterene)

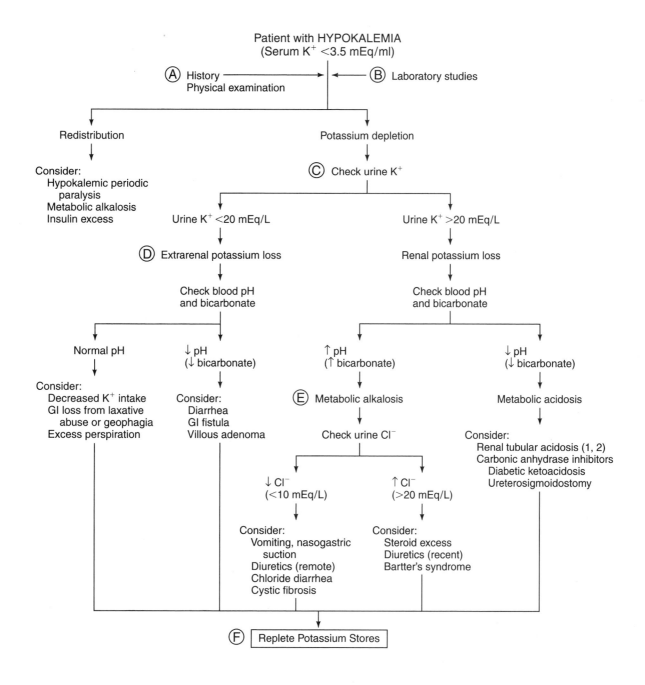

Patient with HYPOKALEMIA
(Serum K^+ <3.5 mEq/ml)

Ⓐ History → ← Ⓑ Laboratory studies
Physical examination

Redistribution

↓

Consider:
Hypokalemic periodic
paralysis
Metabolic alkalosis
Insulin excess

Potassium depletion

↓

Ⓒ Check urine K^+

Urine K^+ <20 mEq/L

Ⓓ Extrarenal potassium loss

↓

Check blood pH
and bicarbonate

Normal pH

↓

Consider:
Decreased K^+ intake
GI loss from laxative
abuse or geophagia
Excess perspiration

↓ pH
(↓ bicarbonate)

↓

Consider:
Diarrhea
GI fistula
Villous adenoma

Urine K^+ >20 mEq/L

Renal potassium loss

↓

Check blood pH
and bicarbonate

↑ pH
(↑ bicarbonate)

↓

Ⓔ Metabolic alkalosis

↓

Check urine Cl^-

↓ Cl^-
(<10 mEq/L)

↓

Consider:
Vomiting, nasogastric
suction
Diuretics (remote)
Chloride diarrhea
Cystic fibrosis

↑ Cl^-
(>20 mEq/L)

↓

Consider:
Steroid excess
Diuretics (recent)
Bartter's syndrome

↓ pH
(↓ bicarbonate)

↓

Metabolic acidosis

↓

Consider:
Renal tubular acidosis (1, 2)
Carbonic anhydrase inhibitors
Diabetic ketoacidosis
Ureterosigmoidostomy

Ⓕ Replete Potassium Stores

severe hypokalemia (K^+ <2.5 mEq/L) or with cardiac arrhythmias referable to hypokalemia, IV repletion is indicated. In these patients, administer K^+ salts no faster than 10–20 mEq/hr; pay close attention to cardiac rhythm and serum K^+ concentration.

References

Brown RS. Extrarenal potassium homeostasis. Kidney Int 1986; 30:116.

DeFronzo R. Hyperkalemia and hyporeninemic hypoaldosteronism. Kidney Int 1980; 17:118.

Gabow PA, Peterson LN. Disorders of potassium metabolism. In: Schrier RW, ed. Renal and electrolyte disorders. 5th ed. Philadelphia: Lippincott-Raven, 1997.

Mandal AK. Hypokalemia and hyperkalemia. Med Clin North Am 1997; 81:611.

Stein JH. Hypokalemia: common and uncommon causes. Hosp Pract 1988; 23:55.

Tannen RL. Potassium disorders. In: Kokko JP, Tannen RL, eds. Fluids and electrolytes. 3rd ed. Philadelphia: WB Saunders, 1996.

HYPERKALEMIA

Catherine S. Thompson
David M. Clive

Hyperkalemia is potentially the most rapidly lethal of all electrolyte disturbances. ECG changes may be seen when the plasma potassium (K^+) concentration rises to ≥ 5.5 mEq/L. With further increases in serum K^+ concentration, cellular irritability and eventually lethal arrhythmias develop.

A. Question hyperkalemic patients closely about dietary intake of potassium, including the use of salt substitutes (KCl). Some drugs, including potassium-sparing diuretics, β-adrenergic blockers, NSAIDs, and angiotensin-converting enzyme inhibitors, can aggravate a hyperkalemic tendency in certain patients. A history of renal disease or recent reduction in urinary output is also important.

B. Laboratory assessment should include serum electrolytes, creatinine, BUN, and acid-base status. Additional tests such as aldosterone and renin levels may provide information about renal tubular disorders that lead to hyperkalemia. "Spurious" hyperkalemia can be excluded by obtaining a plasma K^+ level, which will be normal if the hyperkalemia is the result of cell lysis after the blood specimen is obtained.

C. An elevated plasma K^+ level confirms hyperkalemia. The three chief mechanisms of hyperkalemia are increased excretory load, decreased excretory capacity, and transcellular K^+ movement (Table 1).

D. Eating a potassium-rich diet is unlikely to provoke hyperkalemia. Acutely, the body rapidly mobilizes the K^+ load into cells. Over the course of each day, the kidney is capable of excreting large amounts of excess potassium. However, the combination of renal insufficiency plus a normal or high potassium intake may lead to hyperkalemia, a constant concern in patients with kidney disease. Diets must be modified accordingly.

E. Disorders leading to decreased urinary K^+ excretion include glucocorticoid and mineralocorticoid deficiency, renal tubule secretory defects, and renal failure.

F. Hyperkalemia also arises from perturbations in the internal mechanism of K^+ balance. Metabolic acidosis can provoke hyperkalemia through transcellular shifting of K^+ stores. Tissue necrosis or toxic injury to cells can also cause leakage of K^+ into the extracellular space. K^+ deficiency, with or without hyperglycemia, can lead to impaired cellular K^+ intake.

G. The treatment of hyperkalemia exploits both the internal and external pathways of K^+ disposition (Table 2). Internal mechanisms are the fastest acting (i.e., one can engender shifts of potassium into cells more quickly than one can remove potassium from the body). Thus, rapidly administer insulin and alkalinizing agents (sodium bicarbonate) to patients with life-threatening degrees of hyperkalemia. β-Adrenergic agonists, such as albuterol, which stimulate K^+ uptake by cells, may also be used. Calcium salts also may be administered because these have a membrane-stabilizing effect, although they do not engender K^+ movement in and of themselves. To reduce total body K^+ stores, introduce ion-exchange resins like sodium polystyrene sulfate (e.g., Kayexalate) into the GI tract. These absorb potassium from the gut and release, in exchange, a sodium molecule. For hyperkalemic patients with renal insufficiency, emergent dialysis may be required.

References

Brown RS. Extrarenal potassium homeostasis. Kidney Int 1986; 30:116.

Cox M, Sterns R, Singer I. The defense against hyperkalemia: the roles of insulin and aldosterone. N Engl J Med 1978; 299:525.

DeFronzo R. Hyperkalemia and hyporeninemic hypoaldosteronism. Kidney Int 1980; 17:118.

Gabow PA, Peterson LN. Disorders of potassium metabolism. In: Schrier RW, ed. Renal and electrolyte disorders. 5th ed. Philadelphia: Lippincott-Raven, 1997.

Goldfarb S, et al. Acute hyperkalemia induced by hyperglycemia: hormonal mechanisms. Ann Intern Med 1976; 84:426.

Mandal AK. Hypokalemia and hyperkalemia. Med Clin North Am 1997; 81:611.

Rose BD. Clinical physiology of acid-base and electrolyte disorders. 4th ed. New York: McGraw-Hill, 1994.

Stein JH. Hypokalemia: common and uncommon causes. Hosp Pract 1988; 23:55.

Tannen RL. Potassium disorders. In: Kokko JP, Tannen RL, eds. Fluids and electrolytes. 3rd ed. Philadelphia: WB Saunders, 1996.

Valtin H. Renal function: mechanisms preserving fluid and solute balance in health. 3rd ed. Boston: Little, Brown, 1995.

TABLE 1 Causes of Hyperkalemia

Increased excretory load
  Dietary excess
  Iatrogenic
  Tissue breakdown
Decreased excretory ability
  Acute and chronic renal failure
  Mineralocorticoid insufficiency
  Hyporeninemic hypoaldosteronism
  Potassium-sparing diuretics
  Renal tubular defects (acute interstitial nephritis, transplant kidney)
Transcellular potassium movement
  (Metabolic) acidosis
  Exercise
  Endocrine abnormalities (diabetes mellitus)
  Periodic paralyses
  Drugs (e.g., succinylcholine, digitalis)
  Osmolar load

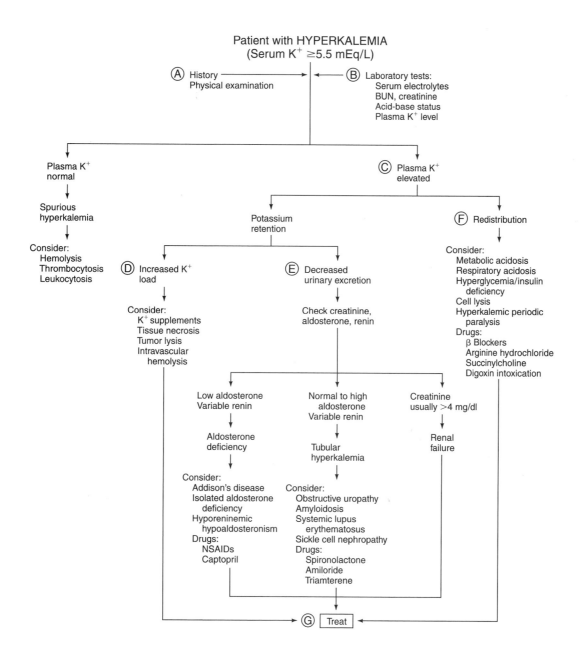

Patient with HYPERKALEMIA
(Serum K⁺ ≥5.5 mEq/L)

Ⓐ History ——— Ⓑ Laboratory tests:
Physical examination ——— Serum electrolytes
BUN, creatinine
Acid-base status
Plasma K⁺ level

Plasma K⁺ normal

Ⓒ Plasma K⁺ elevated

Spurious hyperkalemia

Potassium retention

Ⓕ Redistribution

Consider:
Hemolysis
Thrombocytosis
Leukocytosis

Ⓓ Increased K⁺ load

Ⓔ Decreased urinary excretion

Consider:
Metabolic acidosis
Respiratory acidosis
Hyperglycemia/insulin deficiency
Cell lysis
Hyperkalemic periodic paralysis
Drugs:
β Blockers
Arginine hydrochloride
Succinylcholine
Digoxin intoxication

Consider:
K⁺ supplements
Tissue necrosis
Tumor lysis
Intravascular hemolysis

Check creatinine, aldosterone, renin

Low aldosterone
Variable renin

Normal to high aldosterone
Variable renin

Creatinine usually >4 mg/dl

Aldosterone deficiency

Tubular hyperkalemia

Renal failure

Consider:
Addison's disease
Isolated aldosterone deficiency
Hyporeninemic hypoaldosteronism
Drugs:
NSAIDs
Captopril

Consider:
Obstructive uropathy
Amyloidosis
Systemic lupus erythematosus
Sickle cell nephropathy
Drugs:
Spironolactone
Amiloride
Triamterene

Ⓖ Treat

TABLE 2 Treatment of Hyperkalemia

Drug	Dose	Time of Onset	Duration of Action	Mechanism
Calcium gluconate	1 amp, 10% solution	1–5 min	30–120 min	Membrane stabilization
NaHCO₃	1–2 amp (bolus)	5–10 min	2 hr	Redistribution
Glucose/insulin	50 g dextrose, 10 units regular insulin	Rapid	Variable	Redistribution
β₂-Agonist (albuterol)	Depends on preparation	Rapid	2–3 hr	Redistribution
Sodium polystyrene sulfonate resin (Kayexalate)	15–30 g PO or rectally	10–60 min	As long as continued	Increased excretion
Mineralocorticoid replacement	For specific indications	—	—	Increased excretion
Dialysis	For severe hypokalemia	—	—	—

HYPOMAGNESEMIA

Anwar Al-Haidary
David B. Van Wyck

Hypomagnesemia is common in patients hospitalized with severe disease. Because several factors, including hyperaldosteronism and cisplatin therapy, enhance renal excretion of both magnesium and potassium and because hypomagnesemia may provoke both potassium and calcium depletion, hypomagnesemia should be suspected whenever hypokalemia or hypocalcemia is resitant to supplementation. Increased renal loss of magnesium is the most common pathogenesis of hypomagnesemia, but excessive extrarenal losses or transcellular redistribution are also seen.

A. Redistribution of magnesium from the extracellular space to the bone may be responsible for acute hypomagnesemia after parathyroidectomy (so-called hungry bone syndrome). Similarly, saponification of magnesium has been thought responsible for hypomagnesemia in acute pancreatitis.

B. Hypomagnesemia often complicates management of chronic alcoholism. Although acutely rising alcohol levels may increase renal magnesium excretion, the pathogenesis of hypomagnesemia among most alcoholics is most likely the result of poor dietary intake, coupled with increased stool losses with diarrhea and increased renal losses with hypophosphatemia, if present. Increased intestinal losses are responsible for hypomagnesemia associated with intestinal malabsorption, chronic diarrhea, laxative abuse, short bowel syndrome, inflammatory bowel syndromes, and biliary fistulas.

C. Defective tubular reabsorption of magnesium has been identified in patients developing hypomagnesemia after cisplatin therapy and may contribute to magnesium wasting during recovery from acute tubular necrosis, urinary obstruction, and renal transplant rejection. Because renal tubular reabsorption of magnesium is impaired by natriuresis or calciuresis, magnesium depletion may complicate the course of diuretic therapy (particularly with loop diuretics), high-volume saline infusion, hyperaldosteronism, hypercalcemia, and hyper vitaminosis D.

D. Initiate treatment of chronic hypomagnesemia caused by malabsorption and renal magnesium wasting with oral magnesium replacement (magnesium oxide, 250–500 mg qid). Acute hypomagnesemia, or chronic hypomagnesemia unresponsive to oral supplements, is appropriately managed with a 3-day replacement plan requiring IV therapy as follows: *Day 1:* Dilute 12 ml of a 50% solution of $MgSO_4$ in 1000 ml of a glucose-containing solution, and infuse over 3 hours; follow with 10 ml in each of two 1000-ml solutions, and infuse through the remainder of the first day. *Day 2:* Dilute 10 ml of $MgSO_4$ in the daily IV fluid volume, and infuse over the second day. *Day 3:* Same as day 2.

References

Brautbar N, Gruber HE. Magnesium and bone disease. Nephron 1986; 44:1.

Flink EB. Therapy of magnesium deficiency. Ann NY Acad Sci 1969; 162:901.

Lim P, Jacob E. Magnesium deficiency in patients on long-term diuretic therapy for heart failure. BMJ 1972; 3:620.

Schrier RW. Renal and electrolyte disorders. 5th ed. Philadelphia: Lippincott-Raven, 1997.

Whang R. Magnesium deficiency: pathogenesis, prevalence and clinical implications. Am J Med 1987; 82(suppl 3A):25.

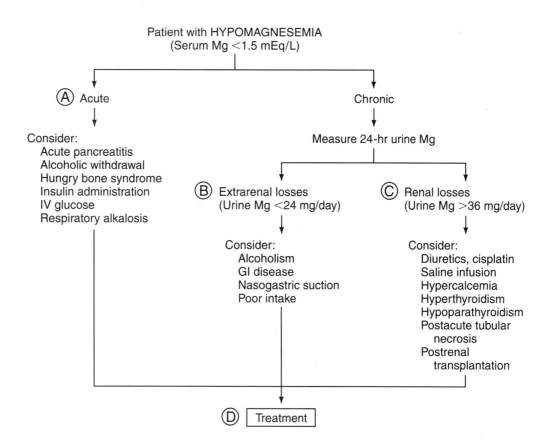

Patient with HYPOMAGNESEMIA
(Serum Mg <1.5 mEq/L)

(A) Acute

Consider:
    Acute pancreatitis
    Alcoholic withdrawal
    Hungry bone syndrome
    Insulin administration
    IV glucose
    Respiratory alkalosis

Chronic

Measure 24-hr urine Mg

(B) Extrarenal losses
(Urine Mg <24 mg/day)

Consider:
    Alcoholism
    GI disease
    Nasogastric suction
    Poor intake

(C) Renal losses
(Urine Mg >36 mg/day)

Consider:
    Diuretics, cisplatin
    Saline infusion
    Hypercalcemia
    Hyperthyroidism
    Hypoparathyroidism
    Postacute tubular
      necrosis
    Postrenal
      transplantation

(D) Treatment

HYPOPHOSPHATEMIA

Mark S. Siskind
Robert F. Klein
Steven T. Harris

Although phosphate is predominantly an intracellular anion, cell function and integrity are determined by both its intracellular and extracellular concentrations. Serum phosphate concentrations >1.5 mg/dl rarely produce symptoms. When phosphate levels fall below this threshold, widespread evidence of cell dysfunction may be seen, manifested by muscle weakness (including heart failure and respiratory insufficiency), rhabdomyolysis, hemolytic anemia, impaired leukocytic chemotaxis and phagocytosis, and diminished platelet aggregation. CNS findings may range from anorexia and malaise to ataxia, delirium ("hypophosphatemic madness"), seizures, and coma.

A. Asymptomatic hypophosphatemia can be treated orally with skim milk (0.9 mg phosphate/ml), Neutra-Phos (3.33 mg/ml), or Phospho-Soda (129 mg/ml) (Table 1). Unfortunately, diarrhea often complicates oral phosphate repletion. Phosphate should be replaced parenterally when hypophosphatemia is symptomatic or complicated or when the patient is asymptomatic but oral therapy has failed or is not a practical option. An appropriate regimen for uncomplicated hypophosphatemia is 2.5 mg phosphorus/kg IV over 6 hours, with a dosage increase to 5 mg phosphorus/kg IV over 6 hours in symptomatic patients. Stop parenteral administration when the serum phosphate level reaches 2.0 mg/dl. Monitoring blood levels should be particularly painstaking during phosphate repletion in patients with renal failure because fatal hyperphosphatemia may occur. Calcium and (if hypomagnesemia also is present) magnesium supplementation may be required during phosphate repletion to prevent hypocalcemic tetany. The calcium must not be added to phosphate-containing solutions, or precipitation of calcium salts will occur. Other potential hazards of parenteral phosphate administration include hypotension, as well as hyperkalemia and hypernatremia, which may result from the particular phosphate preparation used.

B. The cause of hypophosphatemia usually is readily apparent from inspection of the patient and the clinical setting. Hypophosphatemia arises from either total body phosphate depletion or movement of phosphate from the extracellular to the intracellular space. Phosphate depletion may occur after reduced dietary intake (starvation, chronic alcoholism), increased renal losses (renal "leak," hypomagnesemia, hyperparathyroidism), or increased nonrenal losses (secretory diarrhea, vomiting, laxative abuse). Diabetic ketoacidosis is associated with both low intake of dietary phosphate and high urinary losses. Iatrogenic causes are common, however. Phosphate absorption is blocked by phosphate-binding antacids, diuretic therapy enhances renal phosphate excretion, and profound transcellular shifts of phosphate often occur during nutritional refeeding with IV glucose solutions or hyperalimentation. The hypophosphatemia accompanying respiratory alkalosis is caused by a shift of phosphate into the intracellular compartment, is associated with neither phosphate depletion nor symptoms, and requires no phosphate replacement. Because only a small fraction of total body phosphate resides in the extracellular fluid space, the degree of body phosphate deficit cannot be reliably assessed by serum level alone. Therefore, patients at greatest risk for hypophosphatemia require careful monitoring of serum phosphate, especially during inception of nutritional therapy. Hyperalimentation fluids should contain a phosphate concentration of 12–15 mmol/L to provide an adequate amount of phosphate.

TABLE 1 Therapeutic Phosphorus Preparations

Preparation	Phosphate (mmol/ml)	Phosphorus (mg/ml)	Sodium (mEq/ml)	Potassium (mEq/ml)
Oral				
Whole cow's milk	0.029	0.9	0.025	0.035
Neutra-Phos	0.107	3.33	0.095	0.095
Phospho-Soda	4.15	128.65	4.822	0
Acid Na phosphate	1.018	35.54	1.015	0
Neutral Na phosphate	0.673	20.86	1.214	0
Parenteral				
Neutral Na phosphate	0.09	2.8	0.161	0
Neutral Na, K phosphate	0.1	3.1	0.162	0.019
Na phosphate	3.0	93.0	4.0	0
K phosphate	3.003	93.11	0	4.36

From Klein RF, Harris ST. Hypophosphatemia. In: Don H, ed. Decision making in critical care. Philadelphia: BC Decker, 1985:170.

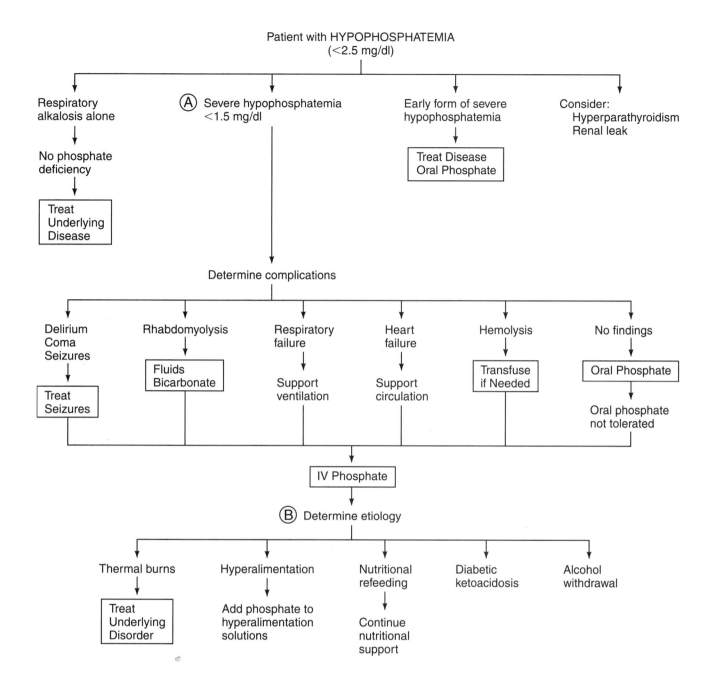

Patient with HYPOPHOSPHATEMIA
(<2.5 mg/dl)

Respiratory alkalosis alone → No phosphate deficiency → Treat Underlying Disease

Ⓐ Severe hypophosphatemia <1.5 mg/dl

Early form of severe hypophosphatemia → Treat Disease Oral Phosphate

Consider: Hyperparathyroidism Renal leak

Determine complications

Delirium Coma Seizures → Treat Seizures

Rhabdomyolysis → Fluids Bicarbonate

Respiratory failure → Support ventilation

Heart failure → Support circulation

Hemolysis → Transfuse if Needed

No findings → Oral Phosphate → Oral phosphate not tolerated

IV Phosphate

Ⓑ Determine etiology

Thermal burns → Treat Underlying Disorder

Hyperalimentation → Add phosphate to hyperalimentation solutions

Nutritional refeeding → Continue nutritional support

Diabetic ketoacidosis

Alcohol withdrawal

References

Fitzgerald FT. Clinical hypophosphatemia. Annu Rev Med 1978; 29:177.

Knochel JP. The pathophysiology and clinical characteristics of severe hypophosphatemia. Arch Intern Med 1977; 137:203.

Knochel JP. Hypophosphatemia and phosphorus depletion. In: Brenner BM, Rector FC, eds. Brenner and Rector's the kidney. 5th ed. Philadelphia: WB Saunders, 1997.

Lentz RD, Brown DM, Kjelistrand CM. Treatment of severe hypophosphatemia. Ann Intern Med 1978; 89:941.

CHOOSING A CHRONIC DIALYSIS MODALITY

Joseph I. Shapiro

Patients with end-stage renal disease (ESRD) may be successfully treated with renal transplantation (p 328), hemodialysis, or peritoneal dialysis.

A. Both peritoneal dialysis and hemodialysis may safely be performed at home in some patients at less expense than in-center therapy. Moreover, although peritoneal dialysis may be performed in-center, it is not economically feasible for extended periods and is not truly a therapeutic option.

B. Next, it must be decided whether hemodialysis or peritoneal dialysis is superior. Both of the basic dialysis modalities have several advantages and disadvantages. Hemodialysis requires adequate vascular access, which is preferably an arteriovenous fistula and less desirably a Gore-Tex graft. Semipermanent venous catheters ("permacaths") may also be used, although they do not function as well or remain patent as long as arteriovenous fistulas. Hemodialysis also requires a relatively stable blood pressure during the therapy. In-center facilities generally are expert in optimizing hemodynamics of patients during hemodialysis and still report a considerable incidence of symptomatic hypotension with dialysis treatments. Candidates for home hemodialysis should have exceptionally stable hemodynamics. Peritoneal dialysis patients must have a suitable peritoneal membrane for dialysis therapy to be effective. Although patients who have had considerable abdominal surgery or a number of peritoneal infections may have an unsuitable peritoneal membrane, it probably is wrong to exclude most of these patients without a therapeutic trial.

C. Peritoneal dialysis may be prescribed as chronic ambulatory peritoneal dialysis that involves very long dwell times spaced throughout the day, or chronic cycling peritoneal dialysis in which the patient has relatively rapid exchanges performed with the aid of a mechanical cycler, usually at night during sleep. The former has the advantage of better middle molecule clearance and less total expense (because no cycler is necessary), with the negative features of more connections and disconnections (which increase the risk of infection) and greater protein losses across the membrane. Depending on the permeability characteristics of the peritoneal membrane and the efficiency of abdominal lymphatic absorption of dialysate, one may be preferable to the other.

D. In deciding between home and in-center hemodialysis and peritoneal dialysis, psychological and social considerations are as important as the medical factors. Home dialysis requires increased motivation of the patient, and often the patient's family, especially for home hemodialysis in which a hemodialysis partner is essential. Home dialysis also requires a suitable dwelling place with adequate space for peritoneal dialysis or hemodialysis supplies and a water supply suitable for hemodialysis. Patient compliance with prescribed therapy and communication with dialysis physicians and staff must be good for home dialysis to be a reasonable alternative. Because of these constraints and other issues, home dialysis appears to be gradually losing popularity in the United States.

E. The choice of one modality does not necessarily exclude a subsequent switch to another. Patients often develop frustration with in-center hemodialysis over time and may desire a home-based alternative, although at the onset of their need for dialytic therapy, involvement with home hemodialysis or peritoneal dialysis seemed overwhelming. Conversely, other patients may develop complications or find difficulties, both medical and social, with home dialysis and subsequently choose to dialyze in center. Therefore a certain empiricism may be justified in choosing dialysis modalities in the knowledge that it is relatively easy to switch to an alternative.

References

de Fijter CW, Oe LP, Nauta JJ, et al. Clinical efficacy and morbidity associated with continuous cyclic compared with continuous ambulatory peritoneal dialysis. Ann Intern Med 1994; 120:264.

Goeree R, Manalich J, Grootendorst P, et al. Cost analysis of dialysis treatments for end-stage renal disease. Clin Invest Med 1995; 18:455.

Hirth RA, Turenne MN, Woods JD, et al. Predictors of type of vascular access in hemodialysis patients. JAMA 1996; 76:1303.

Maher JF. Physiology of the peritoneum: implications for peritoneal dialysis. Med Clin North Am 1990; 74:985.

Mattern WD, McGaghie WC, Rigby RJ, et al. Selection of ESRD treatment: an international study. Am J Kidney Dis 1989; 13:457.

Nolph KD. Peritoneal dialysis update 1994. J Postgrad Med 1994; 40:151.

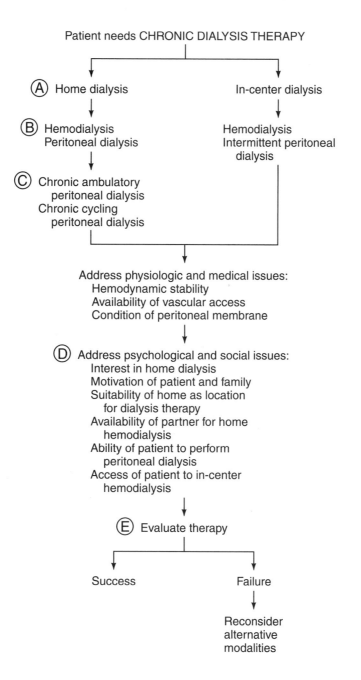

Patient needs CHRONIC DIALYSIS THERAPY

Ⓐ Home dialysis

In-center dialysis

Ⓑ Hemodialysis
Peritoneal dialysis

Hemodialysis
Intermittent peritoneal
dialysis

Ⓒ Chronic ambulatory
peritoneal dialysis
Chronic cycling
peritoneal dialysis

Address physiologic and medical issues:
Hemodynamic stability
Availability of vascular access
Condition of peritoneal membrane

Ⓓ Address psychological and social issues:
Interest in home dialysis
Motivation of patient and family
Suitability of home as location
for dialysis therapy
Availability of partner for home
hemodialysis
Ability of patient to perform
peritoneal dialysis
Access of patient to in-center
hemodialysis

Ⓔ Evaluate therapy

Success

Failure

Reconsider
alternative
modalities

SELECTION OF PATIENTS FOR TRANSPLANTATION

Joseph I. Shapiro

Most transplant nephrologists believe it is the right of every patient with end-stage renal disease (ESRD) to be considered for renal transplantation, a procedure that in the long run is less expensive than chronic hemodialysis therapy. Moreover, although a definite survival advantage of renal transplantation over chronic hemodialysis or peritoneal dialysis has been difficult to demonstrate, most patients enjoy a considerably better quality of life with a renal transplant than with alternative ESRD therapy. A relative shortage of organs still exists, but with improvements in organ harvesting and storage and improved awareness of potential organ donors, it is possible that most patients with ESRD may ultimately receive a renal transplant.

A. To determine whether the patient is interested in a renal transplant, first educate the patient about the risks and benefits of renal transplantation. If a patient is willing to consider renal transplantation, the transplant team must address the risks and benefits for that patient, and first determine the safety of the procedure for him or her.

B. Perform a detailed history and physical examination as well as baseline laboratory values (CBC, prothrombin time, partial thromboplastin time, chemistry panel, HIV antibody, hepatitis B surface antigen, cytomegalovirus [CMV] antibody, urine culture, urinalysis) and other screening tests (chest film, ECG) in all potential kidney transplant recipients. Pay careful attention to the nature of the underlying renal disease and the presence of extrarenal disease that would be relevant to either the transplant procedure itself or the chronic immunosuppression required. Diseases that recur in high incidence in the transplant kidney (e.g., focal glomerulosclerosis, Goodpasture's syndrome, oxalosis) are relative but not absolute contraindications to renal transplantation. Diseases of relevance to the procedure include diabetes mellitus (which increases the likelihood of coronary artery disease or neurogenic bladder) and abnormalities of the urinary tract architecture. Diseases of relevance to the chronic immunosuppression required include HIV infection, an absolute contraindication to renal transplantation; the presence of noncutaneous cancer, a very strong contraindication to a transplant; infection or lack of infection with CMV, which could influence management of the recipient if given a CMV-positive kidney; or a history of psychosocial difficulties, which might suggest potential difficulties for the patient in complying with a transplantation medical regimen.

C. In selected patients, further evaluation of potential problems is indicated before transplantation. Diabetic patients should receive a detailed cardiac evaluation even if there is no history of chest discomfort because of the high incidence of silent myocardial ischemia in these patients. Similarly, vesicoureterography is warranted in diabetic patients because of the high incidence of neurogenic bladder and reflux in this population. A multidisciplinary approach is needed in patients with significant extrarenal diseases. Age itself is not a contraindication to renal transplantation, but the likelihood of significant extrarenal disease that could adversely affect the success and safety of transplantation does increase with age.

D. If transplantation is determined to be safe for the patient, the next step is to decide between a living related and a cadaveric transplant. In general, living related transplants have little survival advantage over cadaveric transplants unless the tissue match is excellent (e.g., a six-antigen or two-haplotype match). Other reasons to favor a living related transplant are high plasma renin activity, making it difficult to obtain a cadaveric transplant, or the patient's failure to thrive with alternative therapy. Because waiting times (and waiting list lengths) vary considerably among centers, the enthusiasm for living related transplants for this latter indication also varies. Potential living related kidney donors should not be considered if they have significant extrarenal disease or a significant possibility of developing renal disease. Hypertension is still considered a contraindication to donating a kidney. In addition, any reluctance of the potential donor to go through the organ donation procedure should dampen the enthusiasm for the transplant considerably. The choice of living nonrelated transplants is controversial at this time because of the considerable ethical issues surrounding this practice.

References

Carpenter CB, Lazarus JM. Dialysis and transplantation in the treatment of renal failure. In: Fauci AS, Braunwald E, Isselbacher KJ, eds. Harrison's principles of internal medicine. 14th ed. New York: McGraw-Hill, 1997:1520.

Holley JL, McCauley C, Doherty B, et al. Patients' views in the choice of renal transplant. Kidney Int 1996; 49:494.

McKay DB. Clinical aspects of renal transplantation. In: Brenner BM, Rector FC, eds. Brenner and Rector's the kidney. 5th ed. Philadelphia: WB Saunders, 1996:2602.

Riehle RA Jr, Steckler R, Naslund EB, et al. Selection criteria for the evaluation of living related renal donors. J Urol 1990; 144:845.

Terasaki PI, Cecka JM, Gjertson DW, Takemoto S. High survival rates of kidney transplants from spousal and living unrelated donors. N Engl J Med 1995; 333:333.

Yoshimura N, Oka T. Medical and surgical complications of renal transplantation: diagnosis and management. Med Clin North Am 1990; 74:1025.

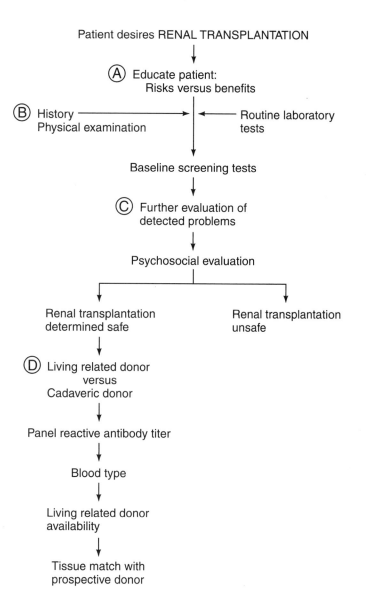

Patient desires RENAL TRANSPLANTATION

(A) Educate patient:
Risks versus benefits

(B) History ——————→ ←—— Routine laboratory
Physical examination   tests

Baseline screening tests

(C) Further evaluation of
detected problems

Psychosocial evaluation

Renal transplantation   Renal transplantation
determined safe   unsafe

(D) Living related donor
versus
Cadaveric donor

Panel reactive antibody titer

Blood type

Living related donor
availability

Tissue match with
prospective donor

FEVER IN A TRANSPLANT PATIENT

Joseph I. Shapiro

A. Fever in a transplant patient offers a considerable differential diagnosis, including virtually all the conventional causes of fever as well as special considerations related to the immunosuppressive agents used to prevent or treat allograft rejection, plus allograft rejection itself. This can be simplified somewhat by examining the clinical situation in which the fever occurred. Fevers may be related to rejection, infection, drug reactions, malignancies, or collagen vascular diseases.

B. Infections must be considered first and, because of the impaired ability of immunosuppressed transplant recipients to combat infection, must be addressed with expediency and aggressiveness. Infections can be categorized as conventional and opportunistic (i.e., related primarily to the immunosuppression used). The likelihood of a given infectious agent causing fever is related to duration of time since the transplant. In the early posttransplant period, the most likely infectious causes of fever are bacterial, most commonly urinary tract infections and wound infections with the usual pathogens. Urinary infections may lead to pyelonephritis with a higher than usual incidence because of the high incidence of reflux into the transplant ureter and kidney as well as the immunosuppressive agents used. Pyelonephritis in a transplant patient typically is associated with renal failure, in contrast to native kidney pyelonephritis in which the contralateral kidney usually maintains renal function at normal. Opportunistic infections in this period are not common, although herpes simplex may occur. When a cytomegalovirus (CMV)-negative recipient receives a CMV-positive kidney, primary CMV infection is likely. Therefore CMV prophylaxis with immunoglobulin may be indicated in this setting. In the intermediate period, opportunistic infections are more likely than conventional bacterial infections. *Pneumocystis* infections were once extremely common during this period, but their incidence has become low with the common use of either trimethoprim-sulfamethoxasole or inhaled pentamidine prophylaxis. CMV reactivations remain a common infectious cause of fever during this time. The likelihood of this infection becoming symptomatic is directly related to the amount of immunosuppression the patient has received. *Nocardia* and fungal infections such as cryptococcosis and aspergillosis also may complicate overimmunosuppression. Conventional infections in this time period. Later, after transplant, infections in general are considerably less common, and opportunistic and conventional infections occur with comparable frequency. *Pneumocystis* infections are unlikely >6 months after transplant whether or not prophylaxis has been used.

C. Acute rejection is another cause of fever in transplant recipients. This may be seen with hyperacute rejection (extremely uncommon) or with acute rejection. Even patients with severe chronic rejection leading to reinstitution of dialysis therapy may develop fever when immunosuppression is tapered off. With cyclosporin A immunosuppression, fever accompanies rejection less often than before this agent became available.

D. Drug reactions may cause fever in transplant recipients, although this is uncommon, possibly because of the immunosuppressive agents (which also are anti-inflammatory) used.

E. Similarly, collagen vascular disorders such as systemic lupus erythematosus or polyarteritis nodosa may cause fever in transplant recipients, but this is less likely because of the immunosuppressive agents used.

F. Malignancies may complicate renal transplant care, especially when excessive amounts of immunosuppression are used. Although skin tumors represent a considerable percentage of these malignancies, lymphoproliferative disorders occur with considerably increased incidence compared with age-matched controls. These are particularly likely to occur in the late post-transplant period and appear to be related to the net amount of immunosuppression received. Polyclonal B-cell lymphomas related to Epstein-Barr virus infection have been described in renal transplant recipients. These infections may show a response to lower dosages of immunosuppression and antiviral therapy initially but are extremely difficult to treat in later stages, especially when they become monoclonal.

References

Basgoz N, Preiksaitis JK. Post-transplant lymphoproliferative disorder. Infect Dis Clin North Am 1995; 9:901.

Fischer SA, Trenholme GM, Levin S. Fever in the solid organ transplant patient. Infect Dis Clin North Am 1996; 10:167.

Kontoyiannis DP, Rubin RH. Infection in the organ transplant recipient: an overview. Infect Dis Clin North Am 1995; 9:811.

Paya CV. Fungal infections in solid-organ transplantation. Clin Infect Dis 1993; 16:677.

Penn I. Depressed immunity and the development of cancer. Cancer Detection Prev 1994; 18:241.

Solez K, Racusen LE, Billingham ME. Solid organ transplant rejection: mechanisms, pathology, and diagnosis. New York: Marcel Dekker, 1996.

Tolkoff-Rubin NE, Rubin RH. Infection in renal transplant recipients. In: Glassock RJ, ed. Current therapy in nephrology and hypertension. 4th ed. St. Louis: Mosby, 1998:368.

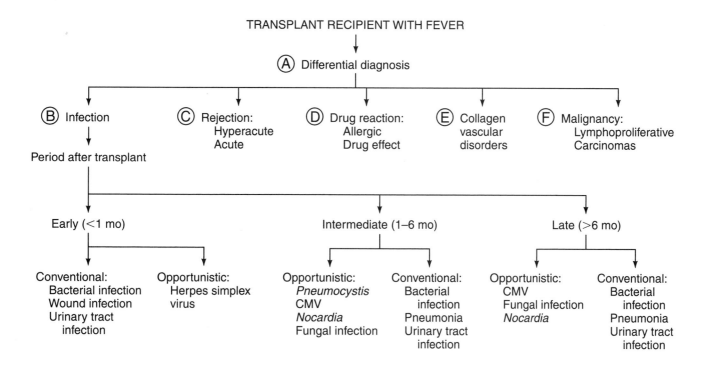

TRANSPLANT RECIPIENT WITH FEVER

Ⓐ Differential diagnosis

Ⓑ Infection

Period after transplant

Ⓒ Rejection:
Hyperacute
Acute

Ⓓ Drug reaction:
Allergic
Drug effect

Ⓔ Collagen
vascular
disorders

Ⓕ Malignancy:
Lymphoproliferative
Carcinomas

Early (<1 mo)

Conventional:
Bacterial infection
Wound infection
Urinary tract
infection

Opportunistic:
Herpes simplex
virus

Intermediate (1–6 mo)

Opportunistic:
Pneumocystis
CMV
Nocardia
Fungal infection

Conventional:
Bacterial
infection
Pneumonia
Urinary tract
infection

Late (>6 mo)

Opportunistic:
CMV
Fungal infection
Nocardia

Conventional:
Bacterial
infection
Pneumonia
Urinary tract
infection

NEUROLOGY

ACUTE HEADACHE

Jeanette K. Wendt

Headache is a common complaint in Western society, but fortunately most patients with acute headache have benign conditions.

A. Patients with sudden onset of headache and no history of head trauma require a full neurologic evaluation to exclude a subarachnoid hemorrhage. Perform a CT scan of the head first. This can be negative in up to 15% of those with subarachnoid hemorrhage. Most neurologists perform a lumbar puncture in all patients with sudden onset of severe headache who have a negative CT scan, regardless of the presence or absence of nuchal rigidity. If subarachnoid hemorrhage is seen on CT, a lumbar puncture is not necessary.

B. Every patient with a recent history of head trauma who has focal neurologic complaints or findings or has altered mental status should undergo a head CT. Those patients with no focal complaints and a normal neurologic examination can be observed and treated symptomatically. However, if their condition deteriorates or if they fail to improve with conservative treatment, perform CT. Skull radiography has limited usefulness in the evaluation of head trauma.

C. Sinusitis is an overdiagnosed cause of headache. The diagnosis of sinus headache should be made only in the context of recent upper respiratory illness, purulent nasal discharge, fever, and localized tenderness over the sinus area. Sinus radiography can confirm the diagnosis but is seldom necessary for the initial evaluation and treatment.

D. The most common category of headache in patients presenting to emergency rooms is the nonmigrainous vascular headache secondary to systemic infection. These patients typically are febrile and have other symptoms of systemic illness. The neurologic examination is normal, and there is no nuchal rigidity.

E. In patients with no history of headache, a new headache may represent a first migraine or tension headache. For the initial migraine headache it is often necessary to perform a complete neurologic evaluation, including CT. The role of hypertension in headache is not clearly understood, and it is probably overdiagnosed as a cause of headache. When diastolic blood pressure is >120 mm Hg, this may be the source of headache. Patients in pain from any cause may have elevated blood pressure. Therefore exclude other causes in patients with headache and high blood pressure.

F. In individuals >50 years of age who have headache, exclude temporal arteritis as a cause. The headache may be uni- or bilateral and the temporal arteries are often thickened and tender. It is important to make an early diagnosis to prevent the visual loss that can occur from thrombosis of the ophthalmic artery. The ESR usually is elevated, but a temporal artery biopsy is diagnostic. Treatment consists of high-dose prednisone.

References

Edmeads J. Emergency management of headache. Headache 1988; 28:675.

Little N. Acute head pain. Emerg Med Clin North Am 1987; 5:687.

Mathew NT. Serotonin 10 (5-HT10) agonists and other agents in acute migraine (review). Neurol Clin 1997; 15:61.

Robbins LD. Management of headache and headache medications. New York: Springer-Verlag, 1994.

Patient with HEADACHE OF RECENT ONSET

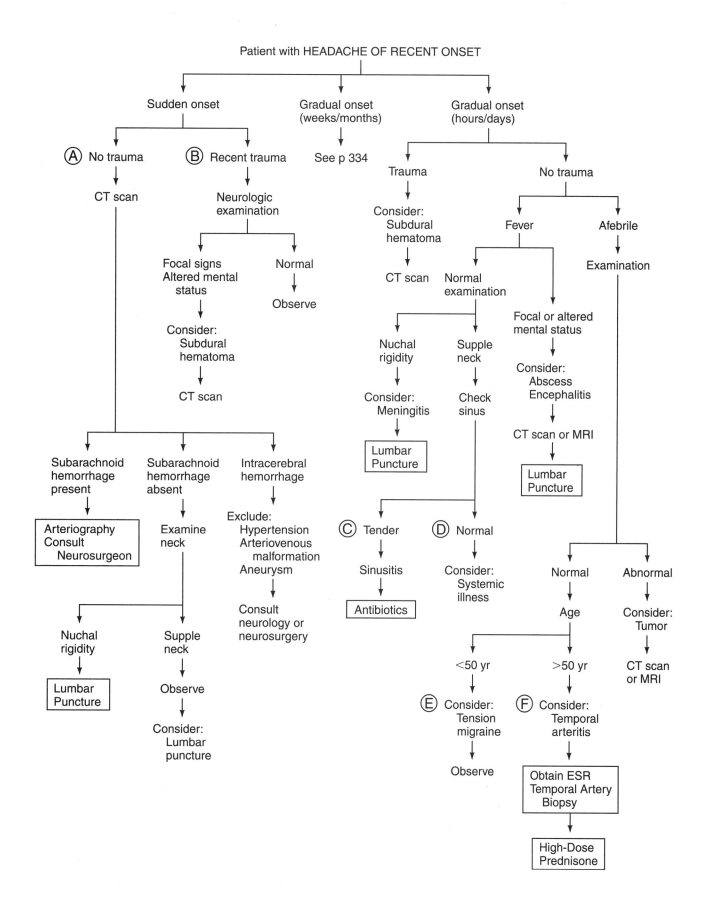

CHRONIC HEADACHE

Jeanette K. Wendt

Most patients with chronic headache have benign conditions. Those with more serious neurologic disorders usually can be diagnosed on the basis of a careful history and examination.

A. A careful history is the most important aspect in the evaluation of headache patients because there are no diagnostic tests for most headache disorders. Important aspects of the history include rapidity of onset, location, age, constancy of the pain, symptoms of systemic illness, and focal neurologic complaints.

B. Migraine headaches are more common in women than in men, with onset before age 50 years. Classic migraine is a headache preceded by a focal neurologic deficit, usually lasting 15–30 minutes. The most common auras are visual, but sensory, motor, speech, or brainstem symptoms may occur. The headache is usually but not always unilateral; is throbbing and accompanied by nausea and/or vomiting, photophobia, and phonophobia; is typically aggravated by physical activity; and lasts hours to a few days.

C. Individuals who have ≤1 migraine per month usually can be treated with abortive and symptomatic medications only. The most effective abortive agents are sumatriptan; ergotamine; isometheptene, usually in combination with dichloralphenazone; high dosages of NSAIDs; or dihydroergotamine. Symptomatic medications include antiemetics, NSAIDs, mild tranquilizers, and narcotic analgesics.

D. Patients with >1 migraine headache per month should be given prophylactic medications, including valproic acid, tricyclic antidepressants, β blockers, and calcium channel blockers. Methysergide usually is reserved for patients who do not respond to or cannot take other prophylactic medications. Each prophylactic agent should be given in adequate doses and for 3–4 weeks before its effectiveness is determined.

E. Cluster headaches are severe, unilateral, usually periorbital, dull, boring pain that is relatively short in duration (usually 45 minutes to 1 hour) but may recur many times during a day and often wakes the patient from sleep. Cluster headaches are more common in men than in women, may be precipitated by alcohol, and must be associated with at least one related symptom such as lacrimation, rhinorrhea, conjunctival injection, nasal congestion, forehead and facial sweating, ptosis, or miosis. The attacks occur in clusters, each cluster lasting an average of 2–3 months. Acute headaches can be treated with ergotamine and high-flow oxygen. Treat cluster headaches prophylactically in all patients because of their severity.

F. Patients with analgesic rebound headaches take daily or almost daily analgesics. These may be the simple analgesics such as acetaminophen or aspirin or those combined with caffeine and minor tranquilizers. Overuse of these medications perpetuates and escalates the headache cycle. Only by discontinuing the offending medications can effective prophylactic treatment be found. Some patients require hospitalization during the withdrawal period for symptomatic treatment of the often severe withdrawal headache and the associated nausea, vomiting, and dehydration. An aggressive prophylactic treatment program is necessary after withdrawal of the analgesics.

G. Patients with ergotamine dependency have daily or almost daily headaches alleviated only by ergotamine. When attempts to discontinue the ergotamine are made, a severe and protracted withdrawal headache occurs. Prophylactic medications usually are ineffective while the excessive ergotamine use continues. These patients usually require hospitalization. An effective treatment of the withdrawal headache consists of IV phenothiazines or metoclopramide and IV dihydroergotamine. Once the patient has been withdrawn from the ergotamine, institute an aggressive prophylactic regimen.

H. Tension headache is common. The typical description is of a bilateral-pressure, dull, bandlike pain associated with neck muscle tightness and often precipitated by emotional stress. There is often associated scalp tenderness but not nausea, vomiting, photophobia, or phonophobia. Carefully search for aggravating or precipitating factors. Relaxation and biofeedback can lessen the severity and frequency of the headaches. Some patients may require prophylactic medications such as tricyclic antidepressants or β blockers.

References

Rapoport AM. Analgesic rebound headache. Headache 1988; 28:662.

Ryan CW. Evaluation of patients with chronic headache (review). Am Fam Physician 1996; 54:1051.

Saper JR. Ergotamine dependency: a review. Headache 1987; 27:435.

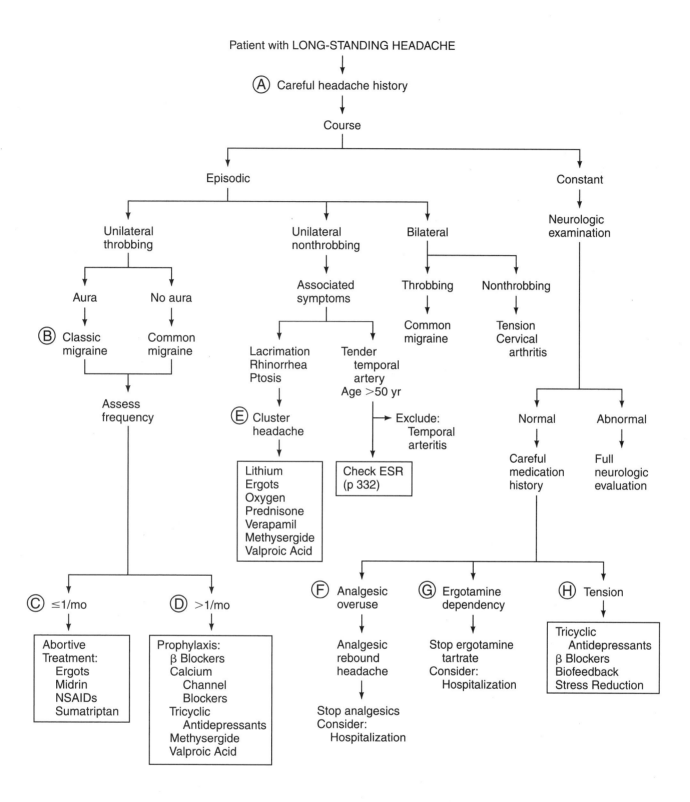

Patient with LONG-STANDING HEADACHE

Ⓐ Careful headache history

Course

Episodic / Constant

Episodic:

Unilateral throbbing
- Aura → Ⓑ Classic migraine
- No aura → Common migraine

Assess frequency
- Ⓒ ≤1/mo → Abortive Treatment: Ergots, Midrin, NSAIDs, Sumatriptan
- Ⓓ >1/mo → Prophylaxis: β Blockers, Calcium Channel Blockers, Tricyclic Antidepressants, Methysergide, Valproic Acid

Unilateral nonthrobbing
Associated symptoms
- Lacrimation, Rhinorrhea, Ptosis → Ⓔ Cluster headache → Lithium, Ergots, Oxygen, Prednisone, Verapamil, Methysergide, Valproic Acid
- Tender temporal artery, Age >50 yr → Exclude: Temporal arteritis → Check ESR (p 332)

Bilateral
- Throbbing → Common migraine
- Nonthrobbing → Tension, Cervical arthritis

Constant:

Neurologic examination
- Normal → Careful medication history
  - Ⓕ Analgesic overuse → Analgesic rebound headache → Stop analgesics Consider: Hospitalization
  - Ⓖ Ergotamine dependency → Stop ergotamine tartrate Consider: Hospitalization
  - Ⓗ Tension → Tricyclic Antidepressants, β Blockers, Biofeedback, Stress Reduction
- Abnormal → Full neurologic evaluation

335

TRANSIENT ISCHEMIC ATTACKS

M. Kanter Carolin

Transient ischemic attacks (TIAs) are brief episodes of focal neurologic deficits caused by interruption of blood flow to the brain that does not last long enough to cause permanent infarction. The deficit must resolve within 24 hours to be classified as a TIA and usually lasts <1 hour. TIAs are an important indicator of cerebrovascular and cardiovascular disease. The risk of cerebral infarction is highest in the first few months after a TIA; thus, early intervention and treatment are crucial. Myocardial infarction (MI) is the most common cause of death in patients with TIA; therefore a thorough cardiac history and evaluation are indicated.

A. Focal neurologic deficits occur in a number of conditions other than vascular ischemic events. Vascular events have an abrupt onset; the maximal effect usually is seen within minutes. Conditions such as subdural hematoma, metabolic abnormalities, demyelinating disorders, brain abscesses, and brain tumors often have a more insidious onset. Occasionally they present with transient deficits, but more commonly persistent abnormalities remain. A focal seizure or migraine may present with transient focal neurologic deficits but usually is accompanied by other symptoms. Involuntary movements, loss of consciousness, incontinence, or confusion suggests a seizure. Visual scintillations or severe headache occur in transient episodes in migraine patients.

B. The pattern of neurologic deficits indicates the vascular territory involved. Carotid artery ischemia causes weakness or sensory loss that may involve the contralateral face, arm, and leg. If the speech center is affected, aphasia may be present. Blindness in one eye (amaurosis fugax) is seen with carotid artery disease (p 338). Vertebrobasilar TIAs usually involve a combination of ataxia, diplopia, dysarthria, complete blindness, dysphagia, and varying patterns of limb weakness.

C. When a TIA is in the vertebrobasilar distribution, evaluation includes imaging of the brain to exclude nonvascular causes (e.g., hemorrhage, arteriovenous malformation, tumor). This can be done with a CT scan; however, MRI gives a more detailed view of the cerebellum and brainstem and is the procedure of choice. Hematologic evaluation includes CBC (differential, platelet count), prothrombin and activated partial thromboplastin times, VDRL (FTA) test, ESR, fasting glucose, electrolytes, liver and kidney function, lipid profile, and urinalysis. Cardiac evaluation includes chest film and ECG. If these are abnormal or if there is clinical evidence of cardiac disease, transthoracic echocardiography and/or a Holter monitor may identify thrombi or arrhythmias. In patients <45 years old, those with left atrial abnormalities, and those with suspected embolic disease, transesophageal echocardiography can identify left atrial thrombi.

D. The same hematologic and risk factor evaluation is performed for carotid artery TIAs. CT of the head rules out nonvascular causes. Noninvasive neurovascular testing is important in these patients. Carotid duplex ultrasonography, including B-mode and Doppler evaluation of the extracranial carotid system, is the procedure of choice for initial evaluation; it assesses the degree of stenosis present and plaque characteristics. Ultrasonography can be used as a screening procedure to determine the need for surgical evaluation; it also is a noninvasive method for follow-up evaluation. If surgery is considered, perform cerebral arteriography. This visualizes the intra- and extracranial vessels, providing an accurate assessment of the degree of extracranial stenosis and amount of intracranial vascular disease.

E. Management includes modification of risk factors such as hypertension, diabetes mellitus, hypercholesterolemia, smoking, and obesity. Treat vertebrobasilar TIAs with aspirin, 325 mg/day. Other antiplatelet options are ticlopidine, 250 mg bid, or clopidogrel, 75 mg/day. If TIAs persist with antiplatelet therapy, consider low-intensity anticoagulation with heparin and then low-dose warfarin (INR 2-3) for 3–6 months.

Management of carotid artery TIAs involves determining the degree of carotid stenosis. If there is an ipsilateral stenosis of ≥70%, carotid endarterectomy along with best medical treatment is more beneficial than medical therapy alone. Best medical treatment is usually aspirin, 325–1300 mg/day; lower dosages cause fewer GI side effects. The two other options for antiplatelet therapy are ticlopidine and clopidogrel. Ticlopidine (250 mg bid) is useful in patients whose symptoms persist with aspirin, those who are aspirin allergic, and those with a history of peptic ulcer. Because of the risk of neutropenia, CBC must be checked every 2 weeks for the first 3 months. Clopidogrel (75 mg/day) is a new antiplatelet agent, chemically related to ticlopidine, that has been shown in a randomized, blinded trial to be effective in reducing the risk for ischemic stroke and is as safe as medium-dose aspirin therapy. Anticoagulant therapy is beneficial when a cardiac source is identified. Consider anticoagulation for patients with a thrombus, prosthetic valve, recent MI, or chronic arrhythmia. Less-well-established indications are crescendo TIAs and persistent TIAs with aspirin therapy. Use low-dose anticoagulation for 3–6 months and then re-evaluate the need for it. Because long-term anticoagulation may increase the risk of hemorrhagic complications, a retrial

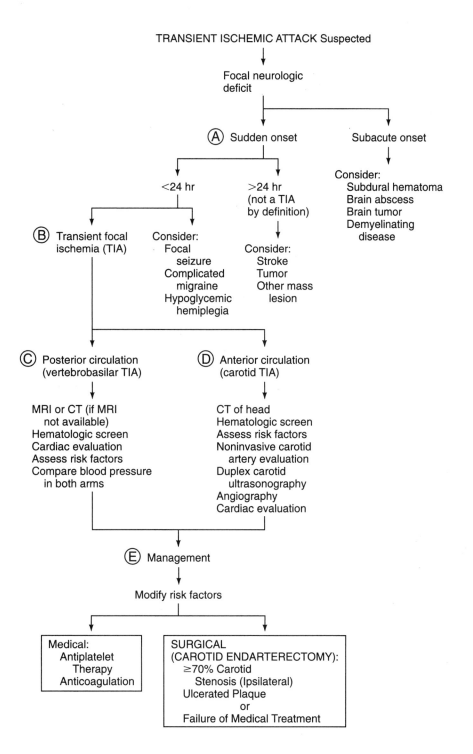

TRANSIENT ISCHEMIC ATTACK Suspected

Focal neurologic deficit

(A) Sudden onset

Subacute onset

Consider:
  Subdural hematoma
  Brain abscess
  Brain tumor
  Demyelinating
    disease

<24 hr

>24 hr
(not a TIA
by definition)

(B) Transient focal
ischemia (TIA)

Consider:
  Focal
    seizure
  Complicated
    migraine
  Hypoglycemic
    hemiplegia

Consider:
  Stroke
  Tumor
  Other mass
    lesion

(C) Posterior circulation
(vertebrobasilar TIA)

(D) Anterior circulation
(carotid TIA)

MRI or CT (if MRI
  not available)
Hematologic screen
Cardiac evaluation
Assess risk factors
Compare blood pressure
  in both arms

CT of head
Hematologic screen
Assess risk factors
Noninvasive carotid
  artery evaluation
Duplex carotid
  ultrasonography
Angiography
Cardiac evaluation

(E) Management

Modify risk factors

Medical:
  Antiplatelet
    Therapy
  Anticoagulation

SURGICAL
(CAROTID ENDARTERECTOMY):
  ≥70% Carotid
    Stenosis (Ipsilateral)
  Ulcerated Plaque
    or
  Failure of Medical Treatment

of antiplatelet therapy often is used. Check CBC every 2 weeks for the first 3 months.

References

Antiplatelet Trialists' Collaboration. Collaborative overview of randomized trials of antiplatelet therapy: 1. Prevention of death, myocardial infarction and stroke by prolonged antiplatelet therapy in various categories of patients. BMJ 1994; 308:81.

CAPRIE Steering Committee. A randomised, blinded trial of clopidogrel versus aspirin in patients at risk of ischaemic events (CAPRIE). Lancet 1996; 348:1329.

Sherman DG, Dyken ML, Gent M, et al. Antithrombotic therapy for cerebrovascular disorders: an update. Chest 1995; 108:444S.

Ticlopidine Aspirin Stroke Study Group. Ticlopidine vs. aspirin for stroke prevention: on-treatment results from the ticlopidine—aspirin stroke study. J Stroke Cerebrovasc Dis 1993; 3:168.

TRANSIENT MONOCULAR VISUAL LOSS

M. Kanter Carolin

Patients with transient monocular visual loss require urgent evaluation. The risk of permanent visual loss from temporal arteritis is approximately 35%, and timely evaluation and treatment can prevent further visual loss. If the temporary visual loss is caused by vascular ischemia, it commonly is called *amaurosis fugax* (AF). An episode of AF is an indicator of increased risk of stroke similar to that of a hemispheric transient ischemic attack (TIA). In the presence of carotid artery disease, AF is a marker of increased risk of cardiac death.

A. Temporal arteritis may cause blindness as a result of thrombosis of the central retinal artery secondary to giant cell arteritis. Presentation usually includes headache, visual loss or changes, and symptoms of fever, anorexia, and weight loss. Leukocytosis, anemia, and elevated ESR are common. The disease process is self-limited over a period of months. Therapy with high-dose steroids can prevent further visual impairment, although restoration of vision is variable. Other disorders that can present with unilateral visual changes and headache include migraine and occipital seizures. These often have a homonymous hemianopsia that has been misinterpreted by the patient as a monocular loss of vision. A positive visual phenomenon such as scintillating scotoma may be seen in migraine or seizure patients.

B. AF typically is described as impairment of vision that begins in the upper field of vision of one eye and progresses to involve the entire visual field of that eye. It usually lasts seconds to minutes. AF occasionally stops with a hemifield loss, ascends, or rarely progresses across the visual field laterally. Repeat episodes of AF tend to follow a stereotyped pattern for each patient.

C. Vascular ocular diseases causing anterior ischemic optic neuropathy, occlusion of the central retinal vein, and malignant arterial hypertension sometimes begin with attacks of AF. Nonvascular causes of AF include hemorrhage, increased intraorbital pressure, and congenital anomalies. Optic neuritis and glaucoma can present with transient visual loss. Papilledema from any cause can present with visual obscurations. These disorders can be identified with the aid of a careful opthalmologic examination showing abnormal ocular findings with a normal retina.

D. Laboratory evaluation of patients with a history of transient monocular visual loss includes CBC differential and platelet count (polycythemia, leukemia, thrombocytosis); Westergren sedimentation rate (evidence of arteritis; giant cell or Takayasu's); fasting glucose (diabetes mellitus); prothrombin and partial thromboplastin times (if prolonged, check antiphospholipid antibodies); and lipid profile (hyperlipidemia).

E. Noninvasive carotid artery studies include duplex (B mode and Doppler) ultrasonography, transcranial Doppler, pneumoplethysmography, transcranial Doppler, pneumoplethysmography, and ophthalmodynamometry. Identification of the percent stenosis and plaque characteristics helps assess the need for further, more invasive, evaluation. Carotid artery stenosis ≥70% indicates surgical intervention (ipsilateral carotid endarterectomy). Surgical intervention was recently shown to be far superior to medical treatment in a multicenter randomized trial. The trial is continuing to assess the risks and benefits of surgical versus medical treatment in patients with ipsilateral carotid stenoses of 30–69% who have had an ischemic event (stroke, TIA, AF). Total occlusion seen by duplex ultrasonography is not as accurate as arteriography; therefore perform arteriography in all patients who show no flow on Doppler ultrasound to evaluate the possibility of a very high-grade stenosis. The treatment is different for patients with total occlusion (best medical therapy) and those with tight stenosis (surgical therapy). The other noninvasive studies mentioned can provide further information about intracranial stenosis in patients in whom arteriography is not performed. CT or MRI scans can reveal clinically silent cerebral infarctions and nonvascular lesions.

F. If the ipsilateral carotid artery is normal, further evaluation to identify a source may include cardiac evaluation. Cardiac emboli may cause unilateral visual loss, although they usually are larger emboli and do not occlude the ophthalmic vessels. Hypoperfusion from low cardiac output occasionally can cause AF, particularly with severe ipsilateral carotid disease.

References

Feinberg AW. Recognition and significance of amaurosis fugax. Heart Dis Stroke 1993; 2:382.

Fox AJ. Carotid endarterectomy trials. Neuroimag Clin North Am 1996; 6:931.

Miller NR. Walsh and Hoyt's clinical neuro-ophthalmology. 4th ed. Baltimore: Williams & Wilkins, 1991:2300.

Streifler JY, Eliaziw M, et al. The risk of stroke in patients with first-ever retinal vs hemispheric transient ischemic attacks and high-grade stenosis. Arch Neurol 1995; 52:246.

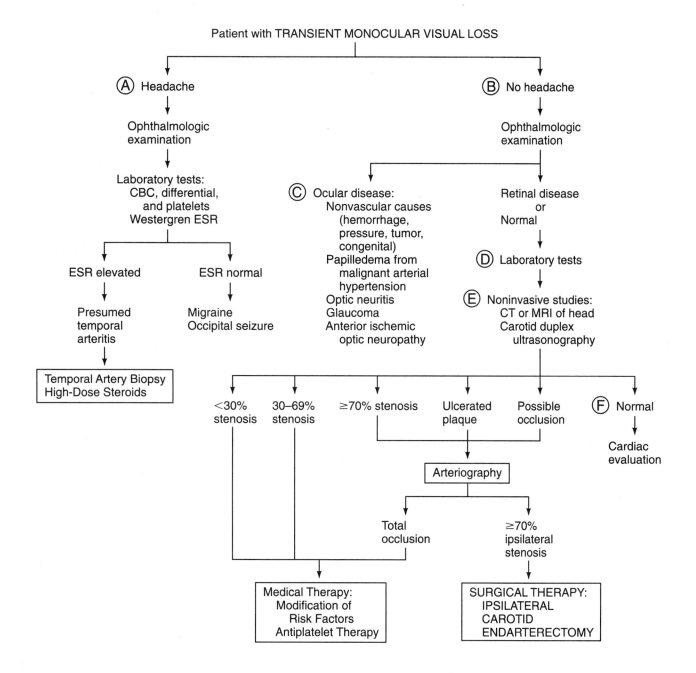

Patient with TRANSIENT MONOCULAR VISUAL LOSS

Ⓐ Headache

Ophthalmologic examination

Laboratory tests:
CBC, differential, and platelets
Westergren ESR

ESR elevated

ESR normal

Presumed temporal arteritis

Migraine
Occipital seizure

Temporal Artery Biopsy
High-Dose Steroids

Ⓑ No headache

Ophthalmologic examination

Ⓒ Ocular disease:
Nonvascular causes (hemorrhage, pressure, tumor, congenital)
Papilledema from malignant arterial hypertension
Optic neuritis
Glaucoma
Anterior ischemic optic neuropathy

Retinal disease
or
Normal

Ⓓ Laboratory tests

Ⓔ Noninvasive studies:
CT or MRI of head
Carotid duplex ultrasonography

<30% stenosis

30–69% stenosis

≥70% stenosis

Ulcerated plaque

Possible occlusion

Ⓕ Normal

Cardiac evaluation

Arteriography

Total occlusion

≥70% ipsilateral stenosis

Medical Therapy:
Modification of Risk Factors
Antiplatelet Therapy

SURGICAL THERAPY:
IPSILATERAL CAROTID ENDARTERECTOMY

COMPLETED STROKE

M. Kanter Carolin

A. Ischemia of a complete vascular region at the onset of symptoms causes a completed stroke. This may occur in the anterior circulation, where most commonly the middle cerebral artery is occluded and causes a hemiparesis and sensory loss contralateral to the lesion. In the posterior circulation, infarctions involving the lower brainstem are most common and cause a constellation of symptoms, including ataxia, dysarthria, diplopia, and facial weakness. It is important to differentiate among other focal neurologic deficits by using the history, physical examination, and neuroimaging (p 336). Seizures with Todd's paralysis or complicated migraine may present with sudden onset of focal neurologic deficits.

B. In completed stroke patients who are candidates for anticoagulation, it is important to evaluate any evidence of cerebral hemorrhage. Patients considered for anticoagulation are those at high risk for embolic strokes (i.e., cardiac source or recurrent strokes). Repeat a CT scan approximately 48 hours after the event. If there is no hemorrhagic transformation and the infarct is small to moderate, acute anticoagulation (heparin) followed by warfarin therapy is indicated. If hemorrhagic transformation has occurred, postpone anticoagulation for 8–10 days. Re-evaluate the patient after the hemorrhage has resolved. This includes repeat CT of the head and reassessment of the medical, neurologic, and social risk factors for anticoagulation.

C. Thrombolytic therapy has been the focus of much recent clinical research in acute stroke. Tissue plasminogen activator (t-PA) was approved by the FDA in 1996 for use in patients with acute ischemic stroke within 3 hours of onset. This acute therapy is effective and of overall benefit in carefully selected patients, but it carries substantial risk. Approximately 1 in 15–20 patients given t-PA suffers serious brain hemorrhage, even if t-PA is given according to strict guidelines (see Adams reference below). This includes early detection and intervention within 3 hours of stroke onset, a normal head CT scan (i.e., no evidence of early edema or necrosis), admission to an acute stroke unit that allows for close neurologic/cardiovascular observation, and arterial blood pressure monitoring. Although there are no other proven effective interventions for acute ischemic stroke, t-PA should be given with caution. Controlled investigations continue with other fibrinolytic agents, and in the future there may be other options available for acute therapy of ischemic stroke.

References

Adams HP Jr, Brott TG, Furlan AJ, et al. Guidelines of thrombolytic therapy for acute stroke: a supplement to the guidelines for the management of patients with acute ischemic stroke. A statement for healthcare professionals from a Special Writing Group of the Stroke Council, American Heart Association. Stroke 1996; 27:1711.

Feinberg W. Primary and secondary stroke prevention. Curr Opin Neurol 1996; 9:46.

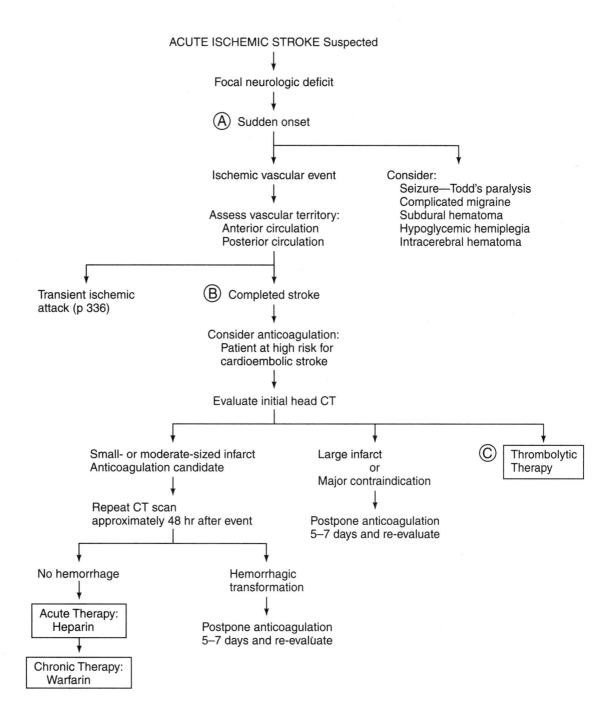

ACUTE ISCHEMIC STROKE Suspected

Focal neurologic deficit

(A) Sudden onset

Ischemic vascular event

Consider:
    Seizure—Todd's paralysis
    Complicated migraine
    Subdural hematoma
    Hypoglycemic hemiplegia
    Intracerebral hematoma

Assess vascular territory:
    Anterior circulation
    Posterior circulation

Transient ischemic attack (p 336)

(B) Completed stroke

Consider anticoagulation:
Patient at high risk for cardioembolic stroke

Evaluate initial head CT

Small- or moderate-sized infarct
Anticoagulation candidate

Large infarct
or
Major contraindication

(C) Thrombolytic Therapy

Repeat CT scan
approximately 48 hr after event

Postpone anticoagulation
5–7 days and re-evaluate

No hemorrhage

Hemorrhagic transformation

Acute Therapy:
Heparin

Postpone anticoagulation
5–7 days and re-evaluate

Chronic Therapy:
Warfarin

PROGRESSING STROKE

M. Kanter Carolin

An ischemic stroke is a focal neurologic deficit that persists >24 hours. If only a portion of the vascular territory is involved (partial stroke), the stroke may worsen after its initial onset. Deterioration may occur over hours to days after the initial event. There are a variety of causes of worsening or progressing stroke, including both cerebral and systemic factors.

A. Patients who show neurologic deterioration after a partial stroke require re-examination, including thorough neurologic, cardiac, and pulmonary evaluations. Clinical or laboratory evidence of infection, renal or hepatic failure, congestive heart failure, arrhythmias, or pulmonary embolism may cause significant worsening of neurologic symptoms. In addition, overzealous lowering of blood pressure can cause early neurologic deterioration in a patient who usually is hypertensive and now has compromised cerebral autoregulation because of ischemia. A repeat head CT scan is important in assessing the size of the infarction, recurrent strokes, edema, and secondary hemorrhage.

B. Cerebral causes of a progressive stroke include progressing thrombosis or recurrent emboli. If there are no contraindications to anticoagulation (systemic or cerebral hemorrhage, uncontrolled hypertension, large infarction) in the presence of progressing thrombosis or recurrent emboli, use IV heparin. Worsening neurologic deficits in patients with partial strokes in the posterior circulation are more often the result of progressing thrombosis. About 30–40% of patients with partial posterior circulation ischemia go on to develop thrombosis. Use acute therapy with heparin anticoagulation to prevent further ischemia. However, a thorough evaluation to exclude other causes of deterioration is important before considering anticoagulation.

C. If there is early CT evidence of hemorrhage or edema, intensive supportive care is needed. If the edema compromises brainstem function or causes alteration of consciousness (i.e., a herniation syndrome), use hyperventilation and osmotic diuresis to control raised intracranial pressure.

D. Acute hydrocephalus or early seizure activity can occur, particularly in association with hemorrhage. Hydrocephalus can be treated and monitored with a ventriculoperitoneal shunt. Clinical deterioration caused by a rapid increase in intracranial pressure because of an intracerebral hemorrhage warrants consideration of surgical evacuation of the hematoma.

References

Biller J, Bruno A. Acute ischemic stroke. In: Johnson RT, Griffin JW, eds. Current therapy in neurologic disease. 5th ed. St. Louis: Mosby, 1997:191.

Slibka A, Levy D. Natural history of progressive ischemic stroke in a population treated with heparin. Stroke 1990; 21:1657.

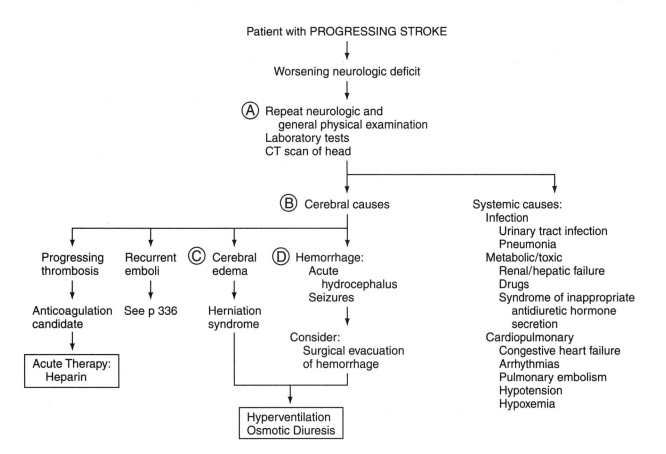

Patient with PROGRESSING STROKE

Worsening neurologic deficit

Ⓐ Repeat neurologic and
    general physical examination
Laboratory tests
CT scan of head

Ⓑ Cerebral causes

Progressing thrombosis	Recurrent emboli	Ⓒ Cerebral edema	Ⓓ Hemorrhage:

Progressing
thrombosis

Recurrent
emboli

Ⓒ Cerebral
edema

Ⓓ Hemorrhage:
   Acute
      hydrocephalus
   Seizures

Anticoagulation
candidate

See p 336

Herniation
syndrome

Consider:
   Surgical evacuation
   of hemorrhage

Acute Therapy:
Heparin

Hyperventilation
Osmotic Diuresis

Systemic causes:
   Infection
      Urinary tract infection
      Pneumonia
   Metabolic/toxic
      Renal/hepatic failure
      Drugs
      Syndrome of inappropriate
        antidiuretic hormone
        secretion
   Cardiopulmonary
      Congestive heart failure
      Arrhythmias
      Pulmonary embolism
      Hypotension
      Hypoxemia

MEMORY LOSS

Geoffrey L. Ahern

The pure amnestic syndrome is a disturbance of memory function with four characteristics: (1) the patient is alert, attentive, and motivated (i.e., not confused or depressed) and cognitive functions other than memory (e.g., language, visuospatial functions) are intact; (2) there is an anterograde amnesia (moving forward in time from the ictal event) in which there is impairment of new learning; (3) there is a retrograde amnesia in which information acquired before the ictus is not accessible—this accessibility is variable, with older memories more easily retrieved than more recently formed ones (Ribot's law); (4) confabulation (the production of implausible answers to questions about unretrievable information) may be present. The foregoing description is useful as a reference point, but keep in mind that memory disturbance can be seen with a number of other neuropsychological abnormalities, particularly disorders of higher-order attention and concentration.

The amnestic syndrome appears to depend on damage to the limbic system, especially the temporal lobe (including the hippocampus and amygdala), dorsomedial nucleus of the thalamus, hypothalamus (particularly the mamillary bodies), and mesial portions of the frontal lobes and basal forebrain. The responsible lesions usually are (although not necessarily) bilateral and may result from a number of different insults.

A. Exogenous substance abuse (intentional or otherwise) may compromise memory functions. If a toxic screen results in a positive test for alcohol, consider a number of entities. First, the patient may be experiencing an alcoholic blackout. Second, alcoholics are subject to trauma; consider the entities discussed under B. Finally, the Wernicke-Korsakoff syndrome usually is encountered in alcoholics who have poor nutrition (thiamine deficiency). Wernicke's encephalopathy (confusion, ataxia, ophthalmoplegia, and nystagmus) may progress to Korsakoff's syndrome in which a chronic amnestic state is present (often accompanied by confabulation, particularly in the early stages). Thiamine replacement may be useful if given early; glucose may precipitate a deficiency state and therefore should not be given until thiamine is administered. In other populations, consider different substances (particularly prescription and over-the-counter medications). The elderly are particularly susceptible to cognitive side effects of common medications. Perhaps the best examples of this are anticho-linergic compounds, which have been shown to interfere with memory processes.

B. Probably the most common cause of amnesia seen in clinical practice is head trauma. The damage done to the temporal lobe and orbitofrontal areas often affects memory processes. Concussion/contusion of the brain is the most likely etiology in these cases, but also keep in mind the possibility of more severe injury, including subdural, epidural, and intracerebral hematomas. Accompanying alterations in attention and concentration are possible and perhaps even likely.

C. The tissues of the CNS are very sensitive to metabolic derangements. This is particularly true for those structures subserving higher-order attention/concentration and memory. Therefore any insult, whether anoxic (e.g., cardiorespiratory arrest, carbon monoxide poisoning), hypoglycemic, or ischemic, may result in an amnestic state, with or without accompanying changes in attention and concentration. Herpes simplex encephalitis demonstrates a preference for attacking the temporal lobes. The resulting hemorrhagic encephalitis may lead to an amnestic state. Also consider mass lesions in the differential diagnosis of the amnestic syndrome. Entities in this group include aneurysms of the anterior communicating artery, pituitary lesions, and colloid cysts of the third ventricle.

D. Psychogenic amnesia does not resemble the organic amnesias. Rather than there being clear anterograde and retrograde amnestic gradients, the patient may forget only selective events from the past, usually of an unpleasant or traumatic nature. Selective biographical information may be lost, including personal identity (which is almost always preserved in organic amnesias). A remarkable indifference to their own deficits may be observed in these patients. Although psychogenic amnesia generally is thought to be a form of hysterical conversion, temporolimbic epilepsy or even frank malingering may produce a similar picture. Psychotherapy, hypnosis, or amobarbital (Amytal) interview may be useful in these cases; if epilepsy is suspected, EEG and appropriate anticonvulsant treatment may be indicated. Finally, memory impairment may be seen after a course of electroconvulsive therapy (ECT).

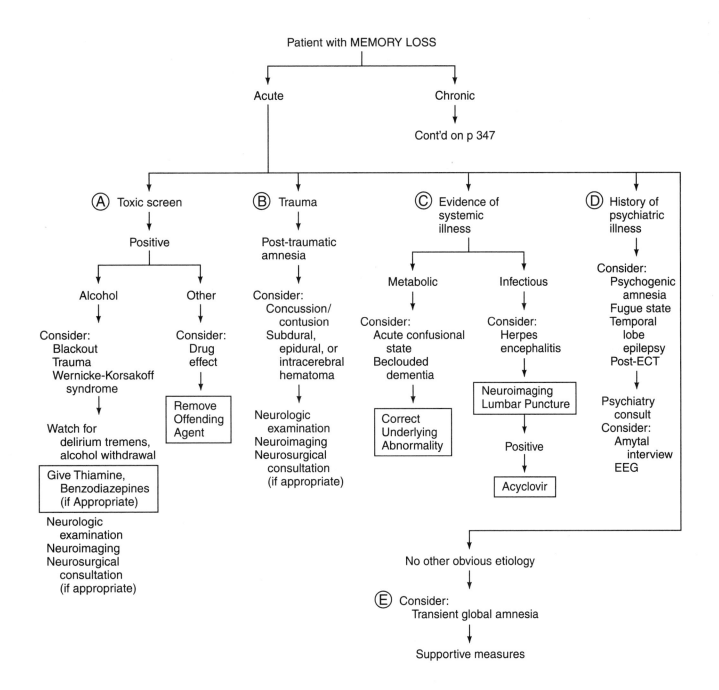

Patient with MEMORY LOSS

Acute

Chronic

Cont'd on p 347

Ⓐ Toxic screen

Positive

Alcohol

Consider:
Blackout
Trauma
Wernicke-Korsakoff
syndrome

Watch for
delirium tremens,
alcohol withdrawal

Give Thiamine,
Benzodiazepines
(if Appropriate)

Neurologic
examination
Neuroimaging
Neurosurgical
consultation
(if appropriate)

Other

Consider:
Drug
effect

Remove
Offending
Agent

Ⓑ Trauma

Post-traumatic
amnesia

Consider:
Concussion/
contusion
Subdural,
epidural, or
intracerebral
hematoma

Neurologic
examination
Neuroimaging
Neurosurgical
consultation
(if appropriate)

**Ⓒ Evidence of
systemic
illness**

Metabolic

Consider:
Acute confusional
state
Beclouded
dementia

Correct
Underlying
Abnormality

Infectious

Consider:
Herpes
encephalitis

Neuroimaging
Lumbar Puncture

Positive

Acyclovir

**Ⓓ History of
psychiatric
illness**

Consider:
Psychogenic
amnesia
Fugue state
Temporal
lobe
epilepsy
Post-ECT

Psychiatry
consult
Consider:
Amytal
interview
EEG

No other obvious etiology

**Ⓔ Consider:
Transient global amnesia**

Supportive measures

E. Transient global amnesia (TGA) usually is seen in middle-aged individuals. It may occur after physical exertion. The onset is abrupt and the patient often appears very confused and anxious, sometimes repeating the same questions over and over. The anterograde component can last several hours; the retrograde component may span hours to years. The total episode may last 12–72 hours and generally does not recur. Vascular insufficiency has been suggested as the usual cause, but migraine, epilepsy, tumors, and diazepam overdose also have been implicated. Should a case of what appears to be classic TGA last >3 days, consider the possibility of an irreversible cerebrovascular event involving the posterior cerebral circulation.

F. Chronic memory loss is most likely to result from a degenerative dementing process. The best known of these entities is senile dementia of the Alzheimer's type (SDAT). Although it is true that the syndrome usually begins with an amnestic disorder, other higher-cortical functions (e.g., language, constructional abilities) are eventually compromised as well. SDAT sometimes is characterized as one of the "cortical" dementias, in contrast to the "frontal-subcortical" dementias that occasionally accompany extrapyramidal disorders such as Parkinson's disease or progressive supranuclear palsy (PSP). The amnestic problem seen in the frontal-subcortical dementias often is less of a true amnesia, per se, than "forgetting to remember"; in other words, the memory traces are there, but the patient has great difficulty retrieving them. Depression can look much the same as a frontal-subcortical dementia and should be considered in the differential diagnosis. It is important not to miss the diagnosis of depression because it is one of the few causes of memory loss that can be treated (as opposed to the degenerative dementias discussed above). Multi-infarct dementia may show elements characteristic of either the cortical or frontal-subcortical dementias, depending on the areas involved. Stepwise progression, a pseudobulbar syndrome, and focal neurologic deficits sometimes are found. Finally, the same entities that can cause an acute confusional state may go on to produce a chronic confusional state if they are not alleviated. Here too, it is important not to miss the diagnosis because some amelioration of the impaired cognitive status may be possible if the condition is treated.

References

Ahern GL, Daffner KR, Duffy JD, Mesulam MM. Selected topics in behavioral neurology. In: Hyman SE, Jenike MA, eds. Manual of clinical problems in psychiatry. Boston: Little, Brown, 1990:111.

Bauer RM, Tobias B, Valenstein E. Amnesic disorders. In: Heilman KM, Valenstein E, eds. Clinical neuropsychology. 3rd ed. New York: Oxford, 1993:523.

Kapur N. Memory disorders in clinical practice. Washington, DC: Psychology Press, 1994.

Signoret JL. Memory and amnesias. In: Mesulam MM, ed. Principles of behavioral neurology. Philadelphia: FA Davis, 1985:169.

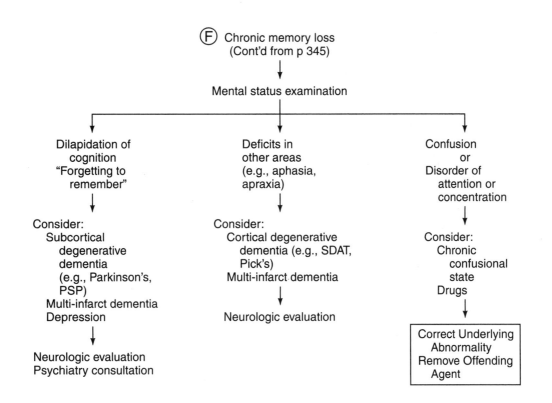

F Chronic memory loss
(Cont'd from p 345)

↓

Mental status examination

Dilapidation of cognition "Forgetting to remember"

↓

Consider:
  Subcortical degenerative dementia (e.g., Parkinson's, PSP)
  Multi-infarct dementia
  Depression

↓

Neurologic evaluation
Psychiatry consultation

Deficits in other areas (e.g., aphasia, apraxia)

↓

Consider:
  Cortical degenerative dementia (e.g., SDAT, Pick's)
  Multi-infarct dementia

↓

Neurologic evaluation

Confusion or Disorder of attention or concentration

↓

Consider:
  Chronic confusional state
  Drugs

↓

Correct Underlying Abnormality
Remove Offending Agent

DIZZINESS

William A. Sibley

Complaints of dizziness from a patient may mean near-syncope, including hyperventilation/anxiety attacks (p 544); a peripheral vestibular disorder (e.g., vestibular neuronitis, labyrinthitis, Meniere's disease, internal auditory artery thrombosis, nonspecific vascular disturbances in the inner ear, or benign paroxysmal positional vertigo); a central vestibular disturbance (brainstem disorders: multiple sclerosis, lateral medullary infarction; temporal lobe disturbance: e.g., vertigo as the aura of a complex partial seizure); or ataxia (p 360).

A. The sensation of dizziness from near-syncope or hyperventilation/anxiety commonly is called *giddiness.*

B. When there is a false sense of motion, the sensation is called *vertigo,* and this symptom usually implies dysfunction of the vestibular system. The most common type of vertigo is rotary. When vertigo is severe, it often is associated with nausea and vomiting.

C. In Meniere's disease, there is distension of the membranous labyrinth in one or both ears that fluctuates in severity. During a period of increased pressure in the labyrinth, patients typically have a feeling of fullness in the affected ear, an increase in the chronic tinnitus and deafness in that ear, and acute vertigo. The severity of each attack varies greatly; at the onset of very severe vertigo, some patients lose consciousness briefly. The duration typically is hours to a few days. With repeated attacks, deafness increases. In most patients with Meniere's disease, deafness precedes the episodic vertigo, but in some, episodes of vertigo precede the deafness. Acoustic neuromas and other posterior fossa tumors seldom produce episodic vertigo of this kind.

D. Acute labyrinthitis, from either bacterial or viral infection, is much less common, and there is hearing loss associated with the vertigo.

E. Benign paroxysmal positional vertigo is a fairly common disorder thought to be caused by a loose or dislodged otolith in one ear. Vertigo occurs only in certain positions of the head (e.g., looking up, lying on the right side) and usually starts after a brief latent interval (a few seconds) after the head assumes the offending position. Changing position usually relieves symptoms rapidly. Most cases begin suddenly, without apparent cause; others follow head trauma. In older persons the syndrome may be caused by vascular insults in the inner ear. Symptoms commonly subside in a few months but may recur.

F. Vestibular neuronitis is an acute illness lasting 6–8 weeks. There usually is rapid onset of rotary vertigo, which is almost always worse on the first day of the illness. There is no hearing loss. After the first day the severity of vertigo rapidly subsides, and in the later weeks of the illness it occurs only with rapid head movement. Vestibular neuronitis is a syndrome rather than a disease and probably has a variety of causes.

G. Multiple sclerosis may produce an attack of vertigo lasting several days (seldom longer) that is caused by a new plaque in the floor of the fourth ventricle. In addition to nystagmus, patients usually have other typical symptoms or signs of the illness: double vision, extraocular muscle palsies, Babinski sign. In older individuals a lateral medullary infarct (Wallenberg's syndrome) often is heralded by vertigo; examination also shows Horner's syndrome, unilateral palatal weakness, and ipsilateral loss of pain in the face and opposite side of the body.

H. To distinguish when a complaint of dizziness is really caused by ataxia, always question whether it is present only when walking. When the sensation also is present while sitting, recumbent, or standing, it cannot be explained as ataxia.

References

Baloh RW, Honrubia V. Clinical neurophysiology of the vestibular systems. 2nd ed. Philadelphia: FA Davis, 1990.

Froehling DA, Silverstein MD, Mohr DN, Beatty CW. Does this dizzy patient have a serious form of vertigo? JAMA 1994; 271:585.

Sloane PD, Dallara J, Roach C, et al. Management of dizziness in primary care. J Am Board Fam Pract 1994; 7:1.

Weinstein BE, Devons CA. The dizzy patient: stepwise workup of a common complaint. Geriatrics 1995; 50:42.

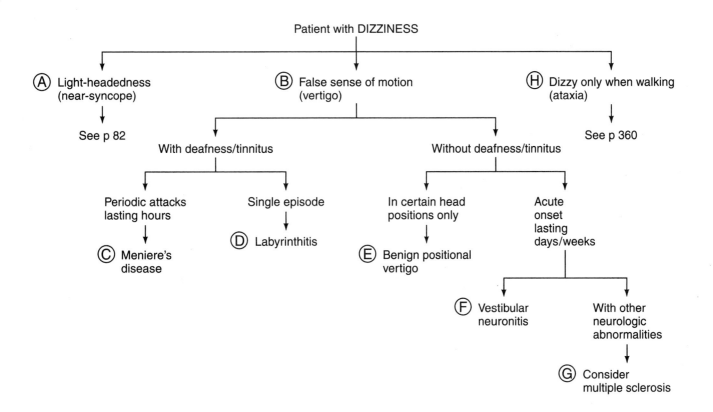

Patient with DIZZINESS

(A) Light-headedness (near-syncope) → See p 82

(B) False sense of motion (vertigo)

   With deafness/tinnitus
- Periodic attacks lasting hours → (C) Meniere's disease
- Single episode → (D) Labyrinthitis

   Without deafness/tinnitus
- In certain head positions only → (E) Benign positional vertigo
- Acute onset lasting days/weeks
  - (F) Vestibular neuronitis
  - With other neurologic abnormalities → (G) Consider multiple sclerosis

(H) Dizzy only when walking (ataxia) → See p 360

SEIZURES

K.J. Oommen

A seizure is the subjective or objective behavioral manifestation of an abnormal, often excessive, neural discharge within the CNS. The focus of origin and nature of this discharge determine its phenomenology and clinical presentation. The advent of closed circuit television monitoring and simultaneous EEG led to the classification of seizures by the International League Against Epilepsy (ILAE) in 1981 and of Epilepsies and Epileptic Syndromes in 1985.

A. After an initial seizure, take a careful history. If there is evidence of previous undiagnosed episodes of seizures, consider this a recurrent seizure disorder or epilepsy. Search for precipitating factors such as sleep deprivation and use of alcohol or stimulant drugs, including over-the-counter preparations. Look for underlying diseases that by themselves or because of their treatment would cause seizures. Thus, a patient with a history of diabetes may develop hyperglycemia resulting in seizures or may have hypoglycemia as a result of overdose of insulin or hypoglycemic agents. Treatment for hypertension with diuretics may cause hyponatremia, and patients with hypoparathyroidism may develop hypocalcemia, tetani, and seizures. Direct treatment toward the underlying cause of the problem. A history of recurrent abdominal pain and seizures should raise the suspicion of acute intermittent porphyria. In addition to neurologic evaluation, perform EEG, MRI, and a complete metabolic screen.

B. With seizures of focal onset, first ask whether awareness is preserved or impaired during the seizure. When awareness of the surroundings or consciousness is impaired, it is a complex partial seizure; if not, it is a simple partial seizure. Simple partial sensory seizures consist of paresthesias, special sensory symptoms (smell or taste), affective symptoms (fear, anxiety, or pleasure), psychic symptoms (derealization or depersonalization), dysmnestic symptoms (déjà vu or jamais vu), and visual symptoms as well as auditory phenomena. Motor symptoms may include a focal motor jerk that either remains localized or progresses to involve other parts of the body in sequence (Jacksonian march). A seizure of partial onset that progresses to a convulsion is referred to as a secondarily generalized seizure.

C. Generalized seizures may be convulsive or nonconvulsive. The latter can be diagnosed with EEG. In typical absence the EEG shows three cycles/second (3 Hz) spike and slow wave discharges. In atypical absence the EEG may show 4–6 Hz spike and slow wave discharges. Behaviorally, myoclonic jerks or automatisms may be seen. In atonic or astatic seizures, patients lose tone and "crumble" to the ground. In tonic seizures there is sudden generalized increase in tone resulting in falls. The EEG usually shows diffuse voltage suppression initially, followed by the usual background rhythm or diffuse slowing. Violent rhythmic clonic and tonic movements of the extremities occur in generalized clonic-tonic-clonic seizures.

D. Often, one may see seizures in which the clinical phenomena are atypical. Patients may have unusual or bizarre behavior akin to seizures. This type consists of an extremely wide range of events in which the EEG may be normal or unchanged from the preictal pattern during and after the episode. The patient may not respond to medical treatment and should be referred to an epilepsy center for video EEG monitoring.

E. An unprovoked seizure may occur in 10% of the population. Isolated seizures in which the neurologic examination, EEG, and imaging studies are normal may not require antiepileptic treatment. However, even under these circumstances, recurrence is possible. Warn patients of the potential risks of future seizures. Laws regarding driving, employability, and reporting requirements to traffic authorities vary among states, and patients should be advised accordingly.

F. The decision to use antiepileptic drugs is based on high risk. In a study of children from Halifax, Nova Scotia, three predictive factors were identified. With an abnormal neurologic examination, 73% had recurrence, as opposed to 47% of those with a normal neurologic examination. With complex partial seizures, 79% had recurrence, as opposed to 44% in tonic-clonic seizures. When EEG showed focal spikes, 68% had recurrence, as opposed to 60% of those with generalized spikes. In those with complex partial seizures and a focal EEG associated with an abnormal neurologic examination, the estimated recurrence was 96%. For a more recent and thorough review of the subject, please see the article by Cockerell et al. in the references.

References

Camfield PR, Camfield CS, Dooley JM, et al. Epilepsy after a first unprovoked seizure in childhood. Neurology 1985; 35:1657.

Cockerell OC, Johnson AL, Sander JWAS, et al. Prognosis of epilepsy: a review and further analysis of the first nine years of the British National General Practice Study of Epilepsy, a prospective population based study. Epilepsia 1997; 38:31.

Commission on Classification and Terminology of the International League Against Epilepsy. Proposal for revised clinical and EEG classification of epileptic seizures. Epilepsia 1981; 22:489.

Commission on Classification and Terminology of the International League Against Epilepsy. Proposal for the classification of the epilepsies and the epileptic syndromes. 1985; 26:268.

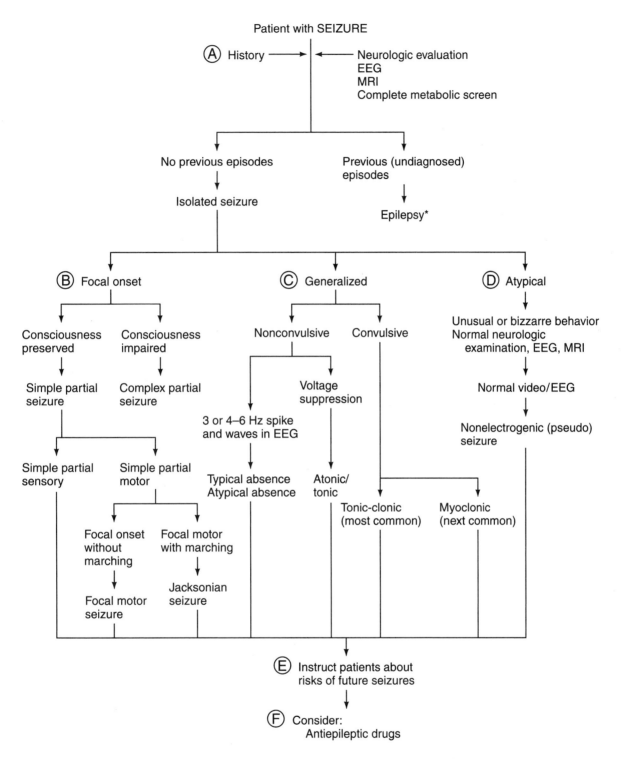

Patient with SEIZURE

(A) History → ← Neurologic evaluation
EEG
MRI
Complete metabolic screen

No previous episodes

Previous (undiagnosed) episodes

Isolated seizure

Epilepsy*

(B) Focal onset

(C) Generalized

(D) Atypical

Consciousness preserved

Consciousness impaired

Nonconvulsive

Convulsive

Unusual or bizzarre behavior
Normal neurologic examination, EEG, MRI

Simple partial seizure

Complex partial seizure

Voltage suppression

Normal video/EEG

Simple partial sensory

Simple partial motor

3 or 4–6 Hz spike and waves in EEG

Nonelectrogenic (pseudo) seizure

Focal onset without marching

Focal motor with marching

Typical absence
Atypical absence

Atonic/tonic

Focal motor seizure

Jacksonian seizure

Tonic-clonic (most common)

Myoclonic (next common)

(E) Instruct patients about risks of future seizures

(F) Consider:
Antiepileptic drugs

*See third and fourth references.

STATUS EPILEPTICUS

K.J. Oommen

Status epilepticus (SE) is continued seizures lasting at least 30 minutes without regaining of consciousness (except in simple partial SE) between individual attacks. Convulsive SE is an acute neurologic emergency that carries a high mortality risk if untreated. A duration of 30 minutes of uninterrupted seizures is required for diagnosis, but in view of the high mortality rate and possibility of complications, institute treatment in any patient with the potential for SE.

A. Consciousness is preserved in simple partial SE; awareness of surroundings is impaired in complex partial SE.

B. Generalized SE may be convulsive or nonconvulsive. The convulsive type includes both tonic-clonic and myoclonic status. The tonic-clonic form carries the gravest prognosis. In the myoclonic form there is continuous myoclonic activity, and consciousness is not completely lost; if the patient is unconscious, an underlying pathologic condition is often present. Myoclonic status may respond to clonazepam (Klonopin) 0.01–0.1 mg/kg/day in divided doses.

C. Assess cardiorespiratory function in the first 5 minutes, and monitor the ECG and ABGs. Administer oxygen, and suction oral secretions if necessary. Consider lorazepam (Ativan) 0.1 mg/kg IV at 2 mg/min for generalized seizures. Diazepam 0.2 mg/kg IV at 5 mg/min or Diastat rectally may stop partial or generalized seizures. The possibility of respiratory depression warrants caution in the use of benzodiazepines in patients with acute cerebral injury. These are best used for flurries in known seizure patients.

D. In both partial and generalized seizures, blood should be drawn for CBC, electrolytes, renal and liver functions, antiepileptic drug (AED) levels, and drug screen. In those with a history of chronic alcoholism, give 5% dextrose IV in normal saline (D_5NS) with B complex containing 100 mg of thiamine. Also, 2 ml of 20% magnesium sulfate may be given IM. Perform as thorough a neurologic examination as possible.

E. Correct any metabolic abnormality present. If there is no obvious metabolic derangement, start IV normal saline. In those with a history of diabetes and possible overdose, a Dextrostix test may provide quick results of serum glucose levels. Unless the patient is hyperglycemic, give an IV bolus of 25 g of glucose with B vitamins. If the seizures continue, start fosphenytoin (Cerebyx) 15–20 mg PE/kg, IV at rate not to exceed 150 mg PE/min. At that rate a dose of 1000 mg PE may be given in 7 minutes. It also may be given IM, giving it at two sites if the total volume is >20 ml. During administration of phosphenytoin, monitor the ECG and blood pressure. If the seizures do not stop within 10 minutes of phosphenytoin infusion, acute CNS injury is likely.

F. If the seizures stop, order a cranial CT scan to rule out a structural lesion. If this is negative, perform MRI and EEG electively.

G. If the seizures persist after phosphenytoin infusion, intubate the patient. Give phenobarbital 10 mg/kg at a rate of 100 mg/min. Additional doses at 10 mg/kg may be given as needed with monitoring of blood levels. A dose of 1 mg/kg should give a serum concentration of approximately 1 µg/ml of phenobarbital. The disadvantage is prolonged sedation. Sodium valproate (Depacon) 15 mg/kg/day IV in four divided doses each given over a 1-hour period has been shown to be effective in SE and may be used instead.

(Continued on page 354)

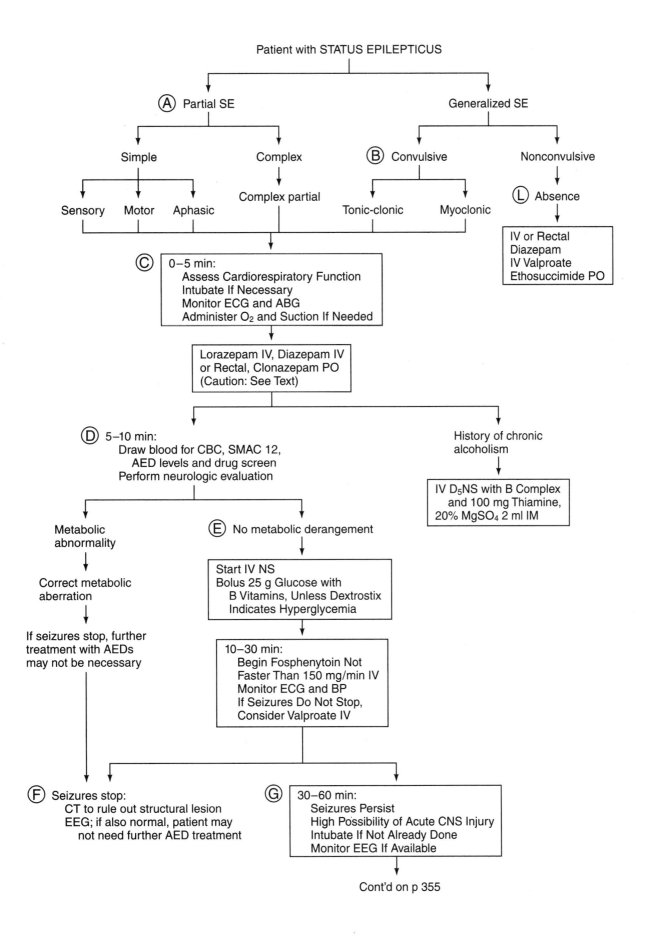

Patient with STATUS EPILEPTICUS

Ⓐ Partial SE

Generalized SE

Simple

Complex

Ⓑ Convulsive

Nonconvulsive

Sensory   Motor   Aphasic

Complex partial

Tonic-clonic   Myoclonic

Ⓛ Absence

IV or Rectal
Diazepam
IV Valproate
Ethosuccimide PO

Ⓒ 0–5 min:
    Assess Cardiorespiratory Function
    Intubate If Necessary
    Monitor ECG and ABG
    Administer O_2 and Suction If Needed

Lorazepam IV, Diazepam IV
or Rectal, Clonazepam PO
(Caution: See Text)

Ⓓ 5–10 min:
    Draw blood for CBC, SMAC 12,
    AED levels and drug screen
    Perform neurologic evaluation

History of chronic
alcoholism

IV D_5NS with B Complex
and 100 mg Thiamine,
20% $MgSO_4$ 2 ml IM

Metabolic
abnormality

Ⓔ No metabolic derangement

Correct metabolic
aberration

Start IV NS
Bolus 25 g Glucose with
    B Vitamins, Unless Dextrostix
    Indicates Hyperglycemia

If seizures stop, further
treatment with AEDs
may not be necessary

10–30 min:
    Begin Fosphenytoin Not
    Faster Than 150 mg/min IV
    Monitor ECG and BP
    If Seizures Do Not Stop,
    Consider Valproate IV

Ⓕ Seizures stop:
    CT to rule out structural lesion
    EEG; if also normal, patient may
        not need further AED treatment

Ⓖ 30–60 min:
    Seizures Persist
    High Possibility of Acute CNS Injury
    Intubate If Not Already Done
    Monitor EEG If Available

Cont'd on p 355

H. Alternatively, the patient may be placed in pentobarbital coma. Give a 5 mg/kg bolus of pentobarbital IV after intubation and artificial ventilation; 25–50 mg may be given every 2–5 minutes until the EEG shows burst suppression. Compressed spectral analysis (CSA), if available, may be used to monitor the electrical activity of the brain during pentobarbital coma. This has the advantage of reversal of sedation by reducing the dose.

I. Other choices include a 4% solution of paraldehyde 0.12–0.3 ml/kg IV over 15–30 minutes. The availability of paraldehyde is limited in the United States. Glass syringes and rubber tubing are necessary for administration. Other choices include lidocaine, 50 to 100 mg IV bolus, followed by 1 to 2 mg/min IV. However, high dosages of lidocaine itself can cause seizures. Because of this and the variability in its CNS distribution, it is best avoided.

J. If the status is broken, a cranial CT may be performed at this time. If this is abnormal (hemorrhage, abscess, or mass affect from tumor or traumatic lesions such as epidural or subdural hematomas), consult a neurosurgeon for appropriate management. If the CT is negative, a spinal tap may be performed to rule out an infectious process or, in some cases, subarachnoid hemorrhage. Manage these conditions appropriately if present.

K. If seizures continue despite these measures, general anesthesia should be instituted by a competent anesthesiologist. Neuromuscular blockade may be required to avoid musculoskeletal injuries.

L. The nonconvulsive generalized seizure of the absence variety may be indistinguishable from complex partial SE or a psychological fugue state except when myoclonic activity is present. EEG will help the diagnosis by showing the presence of 3/second spike and wave discharges as in classic absence, or 4–6 Hz discharges in atypical absence. Absence may respond to IV or rectal diazepam or IV valproate.

References

Status epilepticus in perspective: a symposium. Neurology 1990; 40(suppl 2):1.

Rashkin MC, Youngs C, Penovich P. Pentobarbital treatment of refractory status epilepticus. Neurology 1987; 37:500.

Working Group on Status Epilepticus, Epilepsy Foundation of America. Treatment of convulsive status epilepticus. JAMA 1993; 270:854.

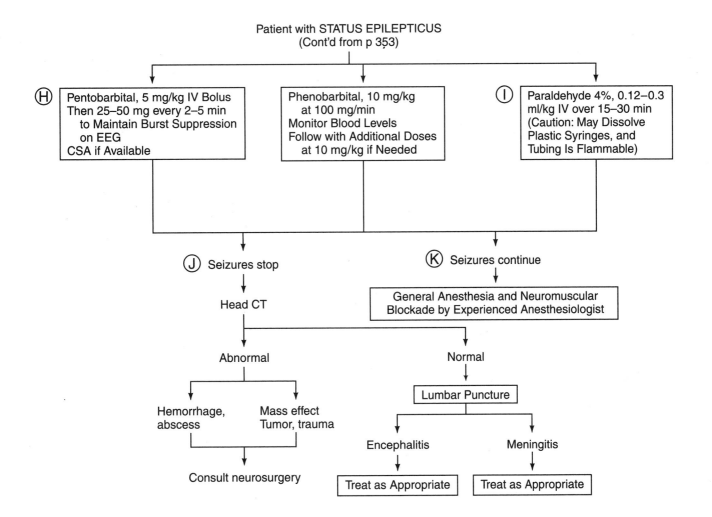

Patient with STATUS EPILEPTICUS
(Cont'd from p 353)

H Pentobarbital, 5 mg/kg IV Bolus
Then 25–50 mg every 2–5 min
to Maintain Burst Suppression
on EEG
CSA if Available

Phenobarbital, 10 mg/kg
at 100 mg/min
Monitor Blood Levels
Follow with Additional Doses
at 10 mg/kg if Needed

I Paraldehyde 4%, 0.12–0.3
ml/kg IV over 15–30 min
(Caution: May Dissolve
Plastic Syringes, and
Tubing Is Flammable)

J Seizures stop

Head CT

K Seizures continue

General Anesthesia and Neuromuscular
Blockade by Experienced Anesthesiologist

Abnormal

Normal

Hemorrhage,
abscess

Mass effect
Tumor, trauma

Consult neurosurgery

Lumbar Puncture

Encephalitis

Meningitis

Treat as Appropriate

Treat as Appropriate

WEAKNESS

Lynn M. Rankin

Weakness is a term used loosely by patients and physicians alike, ranging in meaning from stiffness to numbness to fatigue to true lack of strength. This discussion refers only to the last-named meaning.

A. Important historical facts include tempo of onset and time course, fluctuations, relation to exercise, distribution (e.g., hemiparesis, paraparesis, quadriparesis, proximal, distal, bulbar), involvement of facial musculature, family and medical history, and exposure to drugs or toxins. Also ask about associated symptoms such as cramps, pain, sensory loss, and myoglobinuria. The first step in the neuromuscular examination is to try to localize the lesion responsible for the weakness to the upper motor neuron (UMN), lower motor neuron (LMN), both, or neither. UMN signs include spasticity, hyperreflexia, clonus, and Babinski's sign; LMN signs include diminished muscle tone, atrophy, fasciculations, and hyporeflexia or areflexia.

B. UMN signs generally can be easily localized to above or below the foramen magnum (i.e., intracranial or spinal cord). Intracranial lesions typically cause a contralateral hemiparesis, often with associated signs such as aphasia, neglect, hemianopia, or hemisensory loss. An abrupt onset suggests a vascular event (stroke or hemorrhage), but occasionally tumors, abscesses, and multiple sclerosis (MS) present acutely. Investigation should include a brain CT or MRI scan and further tests, such as angiography, as indicated. In the acute setting when hemorrhage is suspected, a noncontrasted CT is preferred. When MS is suspected, MRI is superior.

C. In evaluating patients with potential spinal cord lesions, remember that with acute presentations, clear UMN signs may be initially lacking because of spinal shock. However, a clear sensory and motor level often is present. Lesions at the lower cervical level may be accompanied by LMN signs at the level of the lesion, with UMN signs below the level. Another unique spinal cord presentation is the Brown-Séquard hemisection, which causes ipsilateral weakness and loss of position and vibratory sense, with contralateral loss of pain and temperature sense. Spinal cord lesions can be further divided into compressive (extramedullary) and intramedullary lesions. Pain tends to be a more prominent feature of compressive cord lesions. Herniated disc, epidural hematoma, epidural abscess, and epidural metastasis usually present acutely; osteophytic ridges and dural-based tumors (meningioma, neurofibroma) have a slower onset. Intramedullary lesions tend to be painless but cause early urinary dysfunction. Transverse myelitis has a quick onset and may be of viral, demyelinating, or vasculitic origin. Myelopathies can result from vitamin deficiencies (B_{12}, E), radiation, or HIV infection. Tumors of the spinal cord include astrocytomas and ependymomas. Traumatic lesions include contusion, severed cord, and delayed syrinx. Examples of vascular cord lesions are anterior spinal artery infarct and ruptured arteriovenous malformation. Congenital malformations of the cord and vertebral column may not produce symptoms until adolescence or adulthood. Hereditary spastic paraparesis is the name given to a slow degeneration of the cord; it affects older family members. Spinal cord lesions should be investigated with MRI or CT-myelography, and further tests such as lumbar puncture as indicated. Rapid intervention often is necessary to preserve remaining neurologic function.

D. Although variable in presentation, some conditions can be associated with both UMN and LMN findings on examination. Classically, this is seen in amyotrophic lateral sclerosis (ALS) as a result of degeneration of motor neurons whose nuclei are located in the anterior horns and corticospinal tracts. ALS begins insidiously in middle or late life with bulbar or limb weakness and progresses to death within 2–10 years. Helpful clues on examination include diffuse muscle wasting, bulbar weakness, fasciculations, Babinski's sign, and preserved sensation. Nerve conduction studies (NCS) are normal early on, whereas EMG demonstrates widespread denervation. Because of the dismal prognosis, a diagnosis of ALS should be made only after serial examinations and exclusion of potentially treatable disorders such as syringomyelia, brainstem or high spinal cord tumor, myasthenia gravis, lead toxicity, and neuropathy (particularly multifocal motor neuropathy with conduction block). Subacute combined degeneration (vitamin B_{12} deficiency), Friedreich's ataxia, and tabes dorsalis involve the corticospinal tracts as well as the dorsal columns and peripheral nerves, thereby causing weakness and sensory loss. Lesions of the termination of the spinal cord, or conus, cause paraparesis and (classically) saddle anesthesia and early urinary retention.

E. By far the largest group of disorders with LMN signs falls under the category of peripheral neuropathy (p 366). Lesions restricted to the anterior horn of the spinal cord produce LMN weakness, atrophy, and fasciculations. Spinal muscular atrophy, aside from the severe infantile form, tends to cause slowly progressive weakness beginning in childhood or adolescence. It has an autosomal-recessive inheritance pattern. Poliovirus infection rarely is seen acutely anymore. However, a postpolio syndrome has emerged as the cause of renewed weakness, atrophy, and cramps 30–40 years after the original illness. Cauda equina lesions, although

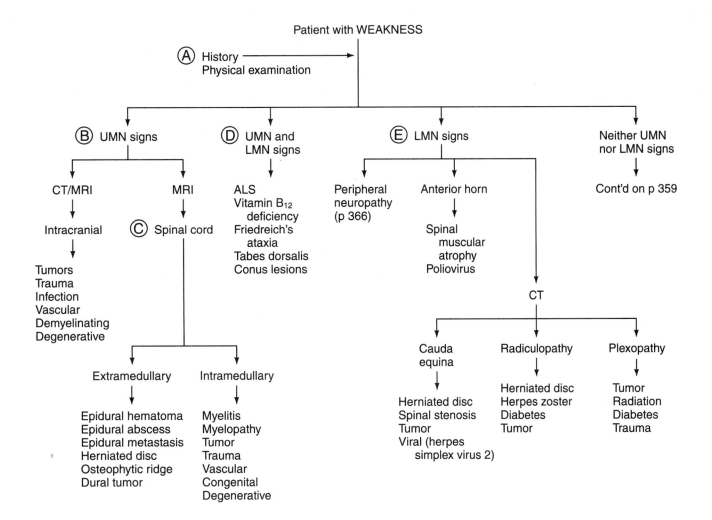

Patient with WEAKNESS

(A) History — Physical examination

(B) UMN signs

CT/MRI
- Intracranial
  - Tumors
  - Trauma
  - Infection
  - Vascular
  - Demyelinating
  - Degenerative

MRI
- (C) Spinal cord
  - Extramedullary
    - Epidural hematoma
    - Epidural abscess
    - Epidural metastasis
    - Herniated disc
    - Osteophytic ridge
    - Dural tumor
  - Intramedullary
    - Myelitis
    - Myelopathy
    - Tumor
    - Trauma
    - Vascular
    - Congenital
    - Degenerative

(D) UMN and LMN signs
- ALS
- Vitamin B$_{12}$ deficiency
- Friedreich's ataxia
- Tabes dorsalis
- Conus lesions

(E) LMN signs
- Peripheral neuropathy (p 366)
- Anterior horn
  - Spinal muscular atrophy
  - Poliovirus

CT
- Cauda equina
  - Herniated disc
  - Spinal stenosis
  - Tumor
  - Viral (herpes simplex virus 2)
- Radiculopathy
  - Herniated disc
  - Herpes zoster
  - Diabetes
  - Tumor
- Plexopathy
  - Tumor
  - Radiation
  - Diabetes
  - Trauma

Neither UMN nor LMN signs

Cont'd on p 359

often difficult to distinguish from conus lesions, usually are associated with pain and asymmetric paraparesis and sensory loss. Radiculopathies are characterized by loss of strength, sensation, and reflex in a dermatomal/ myotomal pattern. Plexopathies tend to cause widespread sensorimotor loss in one limb because of involvement of the brachial or lumbosacral plexus. Pain is common when a tumor is the cause of the plexopathy. Evaluate cauda equina lesions, radiculopathies, and plexopathies with CT or MRI. NCS/EMG can help differentiate a radiculopathy from a peripheral nerve lesion.

F. When weak patients lack clear UMN or LMN signs, have no sensory loss, and have normal to reduced tone and reflexes, the neuromuscular junction (NMJ) and muscle are possible sites of pathology.

G. By far the most common disease affecting the NMJ is myasthenia gravis (MG), in which autoantibodies attack the acetylcholine (ACh) receptor. A typical history is one of intermittent ptosis and diplopia. The muscles most often involved, in order, are the levator palpebrae; extraocular muscles; orbicularis oculi; facial muscles; muscles of mastication, swallowing, and phonation; and neck, shoulder, and hip muscles. The symptoms worsen with exercise and improve with rest. Ptosis can often be elicited by having the patient look up at the ceiling for 1–2 minutes. There is a female predominance in young-onset cases and a male-predominance in older-onset cases. The purely ocular form is more common in older-onset males. The course is progressive or fluctuating; spontaneous remissions occasionally occur. The risk of myasthenic crisis is highest in the first year after onset. Diagnosis can be confirmed with electrophysiologic testing (specifically, repetitive nerve stimulation), the Tensilon test, and an ACh receptor antibody assay. Seek associated conditions such as hyperthyroidism and thymoma. The Eaton-Lambert, or myasthenic, syndrome is a paraneoplastic condition most commonly seen in patients with small cell lung cancer. It can be differentiated from MG by an increase rather than decrease in strength with muscle activity and by electrophysiologic testing. Drugs that reduce neuromuscular transmission include penicillamine, aminoglycoside antibiotics such as gentamicin and kanamycin, magnesium salts, and antiarrhythmics such as quinidine, procainamide, and lidocaine. Botulism is characterized by GI upset followed by weakness, ophthalmoplegia, and pupillary abnormalities.

H. Diseases of muscle generally are termed *dystrophies* or *myopathies*. The dystrophies are inherited; the myopathies generally are acquired. However, the naming of some inherited disorders such as the mitochondrial myopathies and congenital myopathies fails to follow the general rule.

I. Acquired myopathies fall into three main groups: endocrine, infectious/inflammatory, and drugs and toxins. The hyperthyroid state can produce chronic thyrotoxic myopathy, thyroid ophthalmopathy, and thyrotoxic periodic paralysis. Diagnosis can be tricky. Chronic thyrotoxic myopathy most often is caused by a nodular goiter. The degree of atrophy may be striking, and classic signs of hyperthyroidism are sometimes absent. Thyroid ophthalmopathy typically causes limitation of upward gaze, with or without exophthalmos. Diagnosis is made by orbital CT or MRI rather than thyroid function tests (TFTs). Thyrotoxic periodic paralysis is a sporadic, not familial, disorder. It is associated with hypokalemia during attacks. Asian males are particularly predisposed. Hypothyroid myopathy is associated with increased muscle mass and slowed reflexes. It often is overlooked as a cause of elevated creatine kinase (CK). Hyperaldosteronism, acromegaly, Cushing's syndrome, hypophosphatemia, and hyperparathyroidism are other endocrinologic causes of myopathic weakness. Polymyositis (PM) and dermatomyositis (DM) are the prototype inflammatory myopathies. PM/DM typically begins in middle-aged individuals and has an acute to subacute onset. Early symptoms may be fatigue and difficulty in rising from a chair, climbing stairs, or combing hair. Myalgias are present in <50% of cases. The cervical and pharyngeal muscles may be involved, but unlike MG, the extraocular muscles are spared. In dermatomyositis, there is a characteristic violaceous rash involving the eyelids and knuckles. Diagnostic evaluation should include thyroid function tests and a Tensilon test in uncertain cases, plus ESR, ANA, rheumatoid factor, CK, EMG, and muscle biopsy. Look for malignancy in older-onset individuals. Other infectious and inflammatory causes of myopathy are inclusion body myositis, bacteria and viruses, sarcoidosis, toxoplasmosis, trichinosis, and cysticercosis. A CBC with differential, CK, ESR, and muscle biopsy are necessary for diagnosis. Of drugs and toxins, steroids and ethanol are the most important causes of proximal myopathy. Steroid myopathy appears to be more common in women, in patients receiving treatment for >1 month, and in those taking fluorinated steroids such as dexamethasone. Muscle toxicity from ethanol includes an acute, painful necrotizing myopathy; chronic myopathy; and cardiomyopathy. Other drugs to consider include guanethidine, chloroquine, hydroxychloroquine, clofibrate, lovastatin, gemfibrozil, colchicine, zidovudine, doxorubicin, emetine (in ipecac), pentazocine, potassium-lowering diuretics, and heroin. Of note, the risk of myopathy in patients taking lovastatin increases with simultaneous administration of gemfibrozil or cyclosporin A. Similarly, the risk of myopathy with clofibrate and with colchicine increases in patients with chronic renal insufficiency. Many drug-induced myopathies coexist with neuropathy or cardiomyopathy.

J. The inherited muscle disorders usually can be diagnosed clinically and then confirmed by CK, EMG, and muscle biopsy. The Duchenne and Becker forms of muscular dystrophy (MD) are X-linked and therefore primarily affect males. They are characterized by young age of onset, pseudohypertrophied muscles, cardiac involvement, severe proximal muscle weakness, and very high CK levels. The life span in Duchenne MD averages just two to three decades; in Becker MD the average is five decades. Definitive diagnosis can now be made by muscle biopsy showing deficiency of the protein dystrophin. Myotonic dystrophy is inherited in an autosomal-dominant pattern and is the most common form of MD. It is unique in its characteristic myotonia, "hatchet facies," distal predominance of weakness, and multisystem involvement. Facioscapulohumeral (and sometimes peroneal) MD has an adolescent onset and an unmistakeable pattern of weakness. The congenital myopathies (central core, nemaline, myotubular) generally are mildly progressive and show

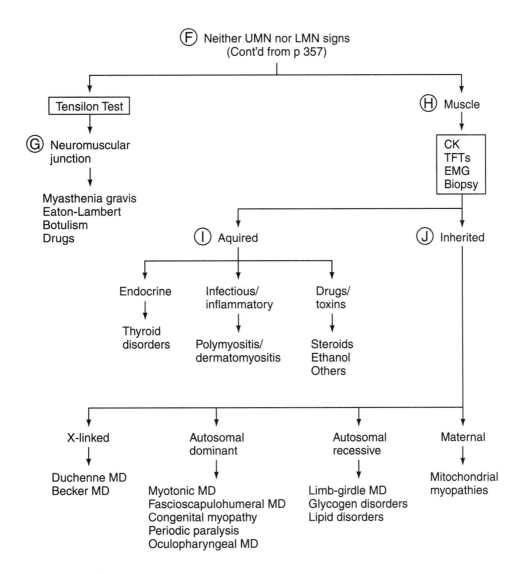

F Neither UMN nor LMN signs
(Cont'd from p 357)

Tensilon Test

G Neuromuscular
junction

Myasthenia gravis
Eaton-Lambert
Botulism
Drugs

H Muscle

CK
TFTs
EMG
Biopsy

I Aquired

Endocrine

Thyroid
disorders

Infectious/
inflammatory

Polymyositis/
dermatomyositis

Drugs/
toxins

Steroids
Ethanol
Others

J Inherited

X-linked

Duchenne MD
Becker MD

Autosomal
dominant

Myotonic MD
Fascioscapulohumeral MD
Congenital myopathy
Periodic paralysis
Oculopharyngeal MD

Autosomal
recessive

Limb-girdle MD
Glycogen disorders
Lipid disorders

Maternal

Mitochondrial
myopathies

distinct pathology on muscle biopsy. Familial hyper-/ hypo-/normokalemic periodic paralysis is episodic in nature, as the name suggests. Onset usually is in early adulthood. Last, oculopharyngeal dystrophy is a late-onset, focal form of MD. Autosomal-recessive muscle disorders include limb-girdle MD and disorders of glycogen and lipid metabolism. With improved classification of muscle disease, the category of limb-girdle MD has dwindled and consists of a heterogeneous group of patients. The juvenile form of spinal muscular atrophy must be considered in the differential diagnosis. McArdle's disease, phosphofructokinase deficiency, and carnitine palmitoyl transferase deficiency typically present with exercise-induced cramps and myoglobinuria. Measurement of low serum lactate in the ischemic lactate test suggests the diagnosis of McArdle's disease. Muscle biopsy with histochemical studies is necessary for definitive diagnosis of metabolic muscle disorders.

The mitochondrial myopathies are a growing group of disorders characterized by weakness, fatigability, and multisystem involvement. Diagnosis must be confirmed by muscle biopsy.

References

Amyotrophic lateral sclerosis. Neurol Clin 1987; 5:1.

Muscle disease. Neurol Clin 1988; 6:1.

Ross MA. Acquired motor neuron disorders. Neurol Clin 1997; 15:481.

Targoff IN. Diagnosis and treatment of polymyositis and dermatomyositis. Comp Ther 1990; 16:16.

Younger DS. Advances in the diagnosis, pathogenesis and treatment of myasthenia gravis. Neurology 1997; 48(suppl 5).

GAIT DISTURBANCES

William A. Sibley

This chapter emphasizes gait problems caused by neurologic or neuromuscular disease, rather than those caused by orthopedic problems.

A. In very early gait disorders it often is difficult even for experienced observers to be sure of the cause simply from inspection of the gait. Associated findings on neurologic examination may be crucial.

B. Bilateral Babinski's signs and very active deep tendon reflexes (DTRs) in the legs suggest an early paraparesis caused by spinal cord disease, even though reduced strength in the legs may not be evident on direct muscle testing. In more advanced stages the paraparetic gait is a slow, labored, stiff process, and muscle weakness (especially in hip flexors and foot dorsiflexors) is easier to detect on examination.

C. Bilateral grasp reflexes and dementia suggest an apractic gait. Gait apraxia, when fully developed, resembles the first efforts of a toddler just learning to walk. There is a loss of the "blueprint" for walking; often the base is slightly widened and only a few difficult steps are possible. It is seen in bifrontal brain dysfunction such as that produced by bifrontal infarcts, advanced hydrocephalus, frontal tumors, Pick's disease, and very advanced Alzheimer's disease.

D. A steppage gait (exaggerated lifting of the knee with each step) suggests distal weakness of the leg, as might be seen in generalized peripheral neuropathy or peroneal nerve mononeuropathy (if unilateral). With generalized peripheral neuropathy, DTRs are absent or reduced, and weakness and sensory changes are greatest distally. With peroneal mononeuropathy, commonly caused by nerve trauma at the fibular head, DTRs are normal.

E. An absent or reduced arm swing on one side suggests parkinsonism or early hemiparesis. Micrographia, cogwheel rigidity and flexion of the limbs and trunk, difficulty rolling over in bed, aching shoulders, facial seborrhea, reduced voice volume, and poor facial expression are other features of parkinsonism. In advanced parkinsonism there is a disturbance of postural reflexes; the standing patient, when pushed, cannot make appropriate corrective movements to avoid falling. The gait may also become propulsive or retropulsive in advanced cases. Circumduction of the leg, increased tendon reflexes, and Babinski sign on one side suggest a hemiparetic gait, usually indicating some diseases of the contralateral cerebral hemisphere.

F. Any widening of the gait base or abnormality on heel-shin coordination testing suggests an ataxic gait. There are at least three types of gait ataxia: truncal, sensory, and gait-and-extremity ataxia.

G. Truncal ataxia is an unsteady gait with normal finger-to-nose and heel-shin coordination tests. Tandem walking is difficult, if not impossible. In severe cases patients cannot even stand with one foot directly in front of the other. Truncal ataxia is seen with vestibular disorders, and thus in anyone having vertigo (p 348); it also is seen in some patients with drug-induced vestibular damage who do not have vertigo. Truncal ataxia also occurs with disease of the cerebellar vermis (e.g., medulloblastoma, alcoholic cerebellar degeneration).

H. Sensory ataxia is an unsteady gait caused by loss of position sense in the toes. Many diseases associated with absent DTRs can be associated with this type of gait disorder. Unilateral loss of position sense usually does not produce a gait disorder.

I. Gait-and-extremity ataxia can occur with various types of drug intoxication that affect cerebellar function (e.g., alcohol, phenytoin, various sedatives and tranquilizers); it also may be seen in hypothyroidism. Such ataxia also is seen with diseases of the cerebellum and brainstem, including various types of cerebellar degeneration, multiple sclerosis (MS), strokes, and tumors.

References

Gilman S. Gait disorders. In: Rowland LP, ed. Merritt's textbook of neurology. 9th ed. Baltimore: Williams & Wilkins, 1995.

Masden JC, Sudarsky L, Wolfson L. Gait disorders of aging: falls and therapeutic strategies. Philadelphia: Lippincott-Raven, 1997.

Spillane J, Bickerstaff ER. Bickerstaff's neurological examination in clinical practice. 6th ed. Boston: Blackwell Science, 1996.

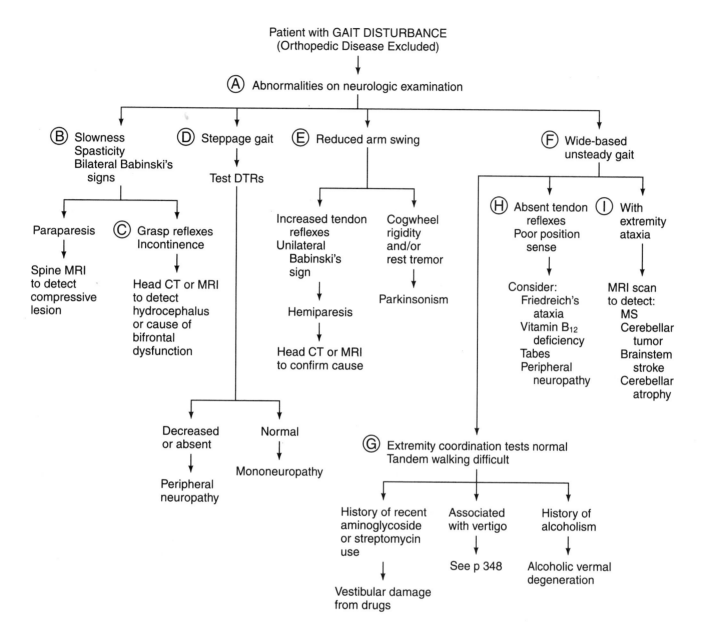

Patient with GAIT DISTURBANCE
(Orthopedic Disease Excluded)

Ⓐ Abnormalities on neurologic examination

Ⓑ Slowness
Spasticity
Bilateral Babinski's
signs

Paraparesis

Spine MRI
to detect
compressive
lesion

Ⓒ Grasp reflexes
Incontinence

Head CT or MRI
to detect
hydrocephalus
or cause of
bifrontal
dysfunction

Ⓓ Steppage gait

Test DTRs

Decreased
or absent

Peripheral
neuropathy

Normal

Mononeuropathy

Ⓔ Reduced arm swing

Increased tendon
reflexes
Unilateral
Babinski's
sign

Hemiparesis

Head CT or MRI
to confirm cause

Cogwheel
rigidity
and/or
rest tremor

Parkinsonism

Ⓕ Wide-based
unsteady gait

Ⓗ Absent tendon
reflexes
Poor position
sense

Consider:
Friedreich's
ataxia
Vitamin B$_{12}$
deficiency
Tabes
Peripheral
neuropathy

Ⓘ With
extremity
ataxia

MRI scan
to detect:
MS
Cerebellar
tumor
Brainstem
stroke
Cerebellar
atrophy

Ⓖ Extremity coordination tests normal
Tandem walking difficult

History of recent
aminoglycoside
or streptomycin
use

Vestibular damage
from drugs

Associated
with vertigo

See p 348

History of
alcoholism

Alcoholic vermal
degeneration

TREMOR

Erwin B. Montgomery, Jr.

Tremor is an involuntary movement that is regular in its rhythm. This distinguishes tremor from other involuntary movements such as myoclonus, chorea, atheotosis, and ballismus. Tremor is characterized by the situations in which it occurs, including resting, with movement (action) or when a posture is maintained. Some forms of tremor are present in more than one situation.

A. The signs of dysdiadochokinesia (impaired rapidly alternating movements), ataxia, rebound (secondary to decreased muscle tone), and decomposition of movement (complex single movements broken down into sequence of simple movements) are often called *cerebellar signs*. This is a misnomer because these signs can be associated with lesions elsewhere in the nervous system. Syndromes associated with cerebellar signs can be organized into precerebellar, cerebellar, and postcerebellar. *Precerebellar* refers to lesions of the sensory systems that ultimately project to the cerebellum. The cerebellum requires sensory information to adequately program movement. *Postcerebellar* refers to lesions that affect pathways from the cerebellum to motor cortex. These lesions prevent information regarding motor programming necessary for the normal execution of movement from reaching the motor cortex.

B. Flapping tremor is manifested by attempts to maintain a posture against resistance that is periodically interrupted by reduced muscular activity. This type of tremor is called *asterixis*. Typically, when testing, the arms are held outstretched with the wrists bent back. Initially the subject is able to hold the position, but periodically the muscles relax and the posture is lost. Next the posture is regained. This cycle continues, producing a flapping tremor.

C. A coarse tremor is tested by having the patient hold the arms outstretched. A tremor appears and increases in amplitude as the patient attempts to maintain the posture. This is called a *wing-beating tremor*.

References

Anouti A, Koller WC. Tremor disorders: diagnosis and management. West J Med 1995; 162:510.

Britton TC. Essential tremor and its variants. Curr Opin Neurol 1995; 8:314.

Findley LJ. The pharmacology of essential tremor. In: Marsden CD, Fahn S, eds. Movement disorders 1 and 2. London: Butterworth-Heinemann, 1995.

Gilman S, Bloedel JR, Lechtenberg R. Disorders of the cerebellum. Philadelphia: FA Davis, 1981.

Koller WC, Busenbark K, Miner K. The relationship of essential tremor to other movement disorder: report on 678 patients. Essential Tremor Group. Ann Neurol 1994; 35:717.

Montgomery EB Jr. Signs and symptoms suggesting cerebellar dysfunction resulting from a cerebral lesion. Arch Neurol 1983; 40:422.

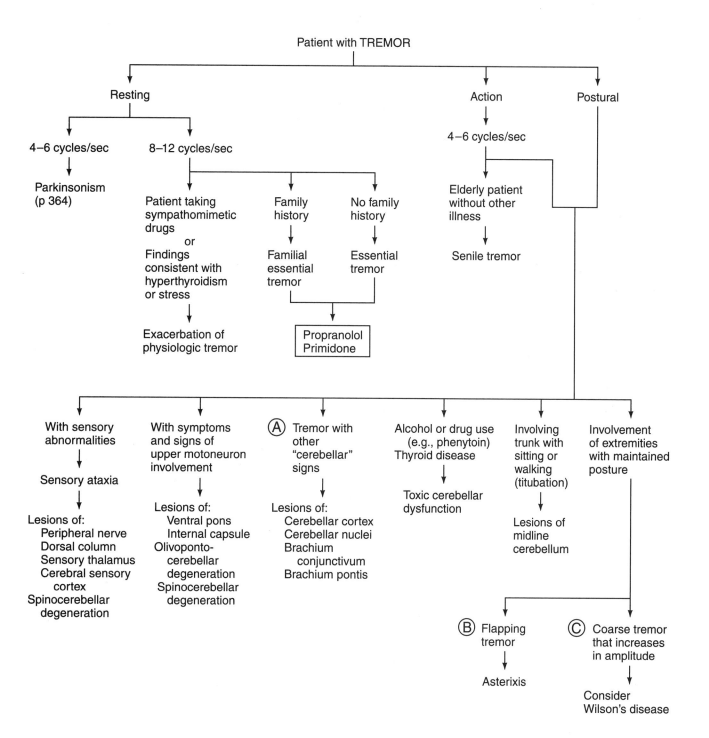

Patient with TREMOR

Resting

4–6 cycles/sec → Parkinsonism (p 364)

8–12 cycles/sec

Patient taking sympathomimetic drugs
or
Findings consistent with hyperthyroidism or stress
→ Exacerbation of physiologic tremor

Family history → Familial essential tremor

No family history → Essential tremor

Propranolol
Primidone

Action

4–6 cycles/sec

Elderly patient without other illness → Senile tremor

Postural

With sensory abnormalities → Sensory ataxia → Lesions of:
  Peripheral nerve
  Dorsal column
  Sensory thalamus
  Cerebral sensory cortex
  Spinocerebellar degeneration

With symptoms and signs of upper motoneuron involvement → Lesions of:
  Ventral pons
  Internal capsule
  Olivoponto-cerebellar degeneration
  Spinocerebellar degeneration

(A) Tremor with other "cerebellar" signs → Lesions of:
  Cerebellar cortex
  Cerebellar nuclei
  Brachium conjunctivum
  Brachium pontis

Alcohol or drug use (e.g., phenytoin)
Thyroid disease → Toxic cerebellar dysfunction

Involving trunk with sitting or walking (titubation) → Lesions of midline cerebellum

Involvement of extremities with maintained posture

(B) Flapping tremor → Asterixis

(C) Coarse tremor that increases in amplitude → Consider Wilson's disease

PARKINSON'S DISEASE

Erwin B. Montgomery, Jr.

Parkinson's disease is a common disorder of the elderly, affecting nearly 2% of the population >65 years of age. As the baby boom generation enters the age of greatest risk, there may be a marked increase in Parkinson's disease. In the past, treatment provided only symptomatic relief; if symptoms did not cause disability or embarrassment, there was little reason for medical treatment. A new medication, selegiline (Eldepryl), that may slow progression of the disease has been introduced. This emphasizes the need for early diagnosis.

A. The diagnosis of Parkinson's disease requires the presence of at least three of the major symptoms: resting tremor, lead pipe or cogwheel rigidity, bradykinesia/akinesia, or abnormal posture. However, any of these symptoms may vary among and within individuals, which may cause diagnostic confusion. As many as 30% of parkinsonian patients may not have tremor. Although parkinsonism has its greatest onset in the sixth and seventh decades of life, it may occur in the young. In about 7% of patients, onset occurs before 40 years of age.

B. This decision requires adequate trial of levodopa. Titrate levodopa/carbidopa compounds until a satisfactory response or limiting side effect is encountered.

C. The use of selegiline as protective therapy is aimed at slowing the progression of the disease. Two placebo-controlled studies have shown that selegiline delays worsening of symptoms to the point where symptomatic therapy is necessary. These studies have been complicated because selegiline may have a symptomatic benefit. As such, this agent may have delayed reaching an end point independent of any effect on the natural history of the disease. However, both studies include wash-in and wash-out periods that either showed no symptomatic benefit or delayed progression in those who did have symptomatic benefit.

D. The division between young or mildly affected and older or more severely affected patients is based on two issues. First is the relative risk of significant side effects. Older patients generally do not tolerate anticholinergics, amantadine, or direct dopaminergic agonists (bromocriptine or pergolide) as well as levodopa/carbidopa compounds. The second issue is the long-term risks of complications such as involuntary movements (dyskinesias) or postures (dystonias) and marked fluctuations in clinical response. The controversy centers on whether these long-term complications are a consequence of the natural history of the disease or of exposure to levodopa. The controversy is further complicated by the nature of levodopa exposure. It may be that the pulsatile administration rather than a more continuous application increases the risk of long-term complications. The algorithm is based on the assumption that exposure to levodopa should be minimized and when levodopa is needed, more continuous application that is desired (as can be accomplished with Sinemet CR). However, because of the high incidence of side effects from anticholinergics, amantadine, bromocriptine, and pergolide relative to levodopa, the latter is the first choice in the elderly.

E. Amantadine can be added, but it has significant anticholinergic properties that could be synergistic with anticholinergics already used and thus increase the risk of side effects.

F. Rarely, patients may not respond to levodopa/carbidopa compounds but may respond to direct dopaminergic agonists. In elderly patients who fail to respond to levodopa/carbidopa, try direct dopaminergic agonists.

References

Aminoff MJ. Parkinson's disease and other extrapyramidal disorders. In: Fauci AS, Braunwald E, Isselbacher KJ, et al, eds. Harrison's principles of internal medicine. 14th ed. New York: McGraw-Hill, 1997:2356.

Hopfensperger K, Koller WC. Recognizing early Parkinson's disease. Postgrad Med 1991; 90:49.

Jankovic J, Marsden CD. Therapeutic strategies in Parkinson's disease. In: Jankovic J, Tolosa E, eds. Parkinson's disease and movement disorders. Baltimore: Williams & Wilkins, 1993:115.

Parkinson Study Group. Effect of deprenyl on the progression of disability in early Parkinson's disease. N Engl J Med 1989; 321:1364.

Quinn W. Parkinsonism: recognition and differential diagnosis. BMJ 1995; 310:447.

Patient with SYMPTOMS OF PARKINSONISM

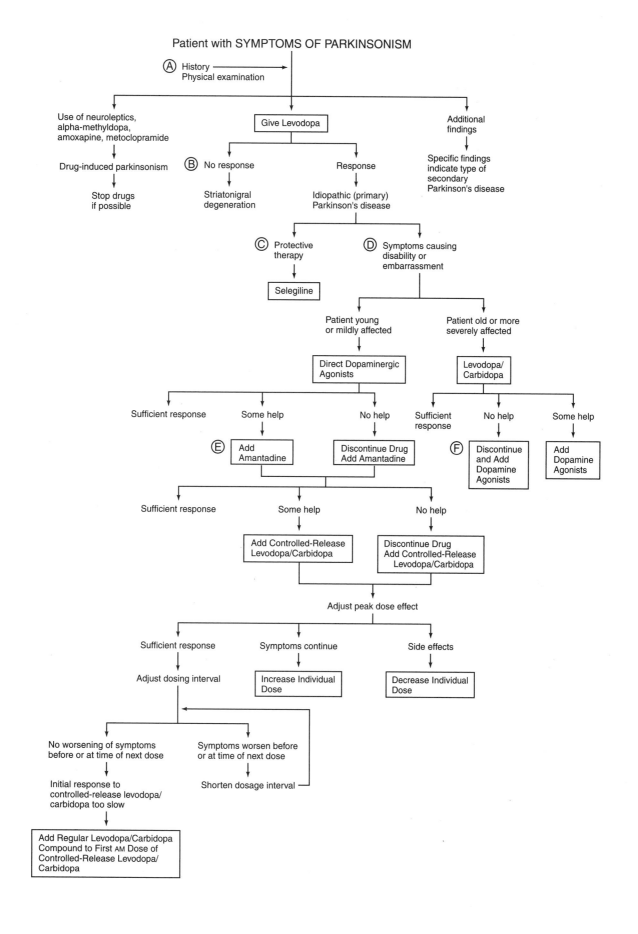

Ⓐ History ——————→
Physical examination

Use of neuroleptics,
alpha-methyldopa,
amoxapine, metoclopramide
↓
Drug-induced parkinsonism
↓
Stop drugs
if possible

Give Levodopa
↓
Ⓑ No response   Response
↓   ↓
Striatonigral   Idiopathic (primary)
degeneration   Parkinson's disease

Additional
findings
↓
Specific findings
indicate type of
secondary
Parkinson's disease

Ⓒ Protective
therapy
↓
Selegiline

Ⓓ Symptoms causing
disability or
embarrassment

Patient young
or mildly affected
↓
Direct Dopaminergic
Agonists

Patient old or more
severely affected
↓
Levodopa/
Carbidopa

Sufficient response   Some help   No help
↓   ↓
Ⓔ Add   Discontinue Drug
Amantadine   Add Amantadine

Sufficient
response   No help   Some help
↓   ↓
Ⓕ Discontinue   Add
and Add   Dopamine
Dopamine   Agonists
Agonists

Sufficient response   Some help   No help
↓   ↓
Add Controlled-Release   Discontinue Drug
Levodopa/Carbidopa   Add Controlled-Release
                          Levodopa/Carbidopa

Adjust peak dose effect

Sufficient response   Symptoms continue   Side effects
↓   ↓   ↓
Adjust dosing interval   Increase Individual   Decrease Individual
                          Dose   Dose

No worsening of symptoms
before or at time of next dose
↓
Initial response to
controlled-release levodopa/
carbidopa too slow
↓
Add Regular Levodopa/Carbidopa
Compound to First AM Dose of
Controlled-Release Levodopa/
Carbidopa

Symptoms worsen before
or at time of next dose
↓
Shorten dosage interval

PERIPHERAL NEUROPATHY

Lynn M. Rankin

A. Peripheral neuropathies (PNs) are disorders of the peripheral nerves and occasionally nerve roots or cranial nerves as well. They usually involve a mixture of motor, sensory, and autonomic dysfunction and rarely affect a single fiber type. The typical distribution of weakness and numbness is distal and symmetric, the feet being affected first in a stocking distribution followed by the hands in a glove distribution. The most distal deep tendon reflex, the Achilles, is the first to disappear. Spontaneous tingling sensations (paresthesias) or burning, unpleasant sensations (dysesthesias) also may occur distally. Atrophy may develop and usually is eventually proportional to the degree of weakness. The most common causes of PN are diabetes and alcoholism. When those risk factors are absent, obtain additional historical information, including occupation; family, medical, and travel history; drug and toxin exposure; nutritional status; and a review of systems. The next step is classification as symmetric PN, mononeuropathy, or multifocal mononeuropathy, also termed *mononeuritis multiplex*. This is accomplished by examination and electrophysiologic testing with nerve conduction studies (NCS) and electromyography (EMG).

B. NCS/EMG confirms mononeuropathy and rules out a more widespread peripheral nerve disorder. Consider conditions that predispose the patient to the development of a mononeuropathy, such as pregnancy, diabetes, collagen vascular disease, trauma, myxedema, and amyloid. Mechanisms of focal nerve damage include compression, entrapment, severance, infiltration, and ischemia. Common cranial neuropathies include idiopathic facial (Bell's) palsy and oculomotor palsy. The latter typically spares the pupil in diabetic or hypertensive patients. Common mononeuropathies of the upper extremity are radial (Saturday night) palsy, ulnar palsy, and median palsy (carpal tunnel syndrome). Nerves commonly affected in the lower extremity are the sciatic, femoral, lateral femoral cutaneous, and peroneal. Treatment depends on the nerve affected and the cause. For example, diabetic mononeuropathies and Bell's palsy tend to recover spontaneously; a short course of prednisone hastens recovery in the latter. Compression neuropathies often improve with removal of the offending behavior or underlying condition. Carpal tunnel syndrome is treated with rest and splinting. Surgery is reserved for refractory cases.

C. Multifocal mononeuropathy (MM) is suggested when two or more peripheral nerves are involved in an asymmetric manner. Confirm the pattern of involvement by NCS/EMG. Most cases are of the axonal type. Axonal damage results from various mechanisms, including ischemia, inflammation, compression, and infiltration. The two most important causes are diabetes and collagen vascular disease. Diabetes produces a painful MM that probably is ischemic in origin. Vasculitic neuropathies are seen in association with polyarteritis nodosa (PAN), rheumatoid arthritis (RA), systemic lupus erythematosus (SLE), allergic angiitis, and Wegener's granulomatosis. Leprosy is notable for its ability to cause widespread sensory loss without loss of reflexes. Sarcoid has a predilection for the facial and other cranial nerves. MM also has been reported in Lyme disease and AIDS. The multifocal variant of chronic inflammatory demyelinating polyradiculoneuropathy (CIDP) may be idiopathic or associated with myeloma, other malignancies, or dysproteinemias. Although similar in presentation to MM, multiple cranial nerve palsies and radiculopathies should alert one to the possibility of leptomeningeal metastases. The above-mentioned causes of MM have distinctive findings on nerve biopsy, making nerve biopsy extremely helpful in etiologic diagnosis. The importance of etiologic diagnosis is that treatment is available for most causes of MM. For example, both vasculitic neuropathies and CIDP may dramatically improve with steroid therapy.

D. Attempt to classify the type of PN, or polyneuropathy, and the cause in all cases. Electrical studies differentiate predominantly axonal from predominantly demyelinating neuropathies: The former are characterized by decreased amplitude and to a lesser extent slowing on NCS; the latter show more marked slowing of the nerve conduction velocity. The most common type of axonal PN, a distal, symmetric, and predominantly sensory type, is called a *dying-back* neuropathy.

(Continued on page 368)

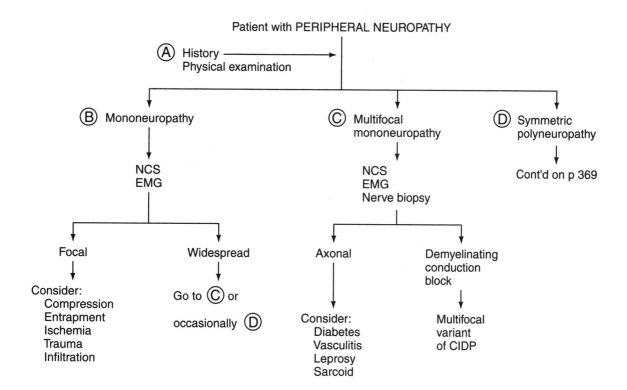

Patient with PERIPHERAL NEUROPATHY

(A) History ——————
Physical examination

(B) Mononeuropathy

NCS
EMG

Focal

Consider:
Compression
Entrapment
Ischemia
Trauma
Infiltration

Widespread

Go to (C) or

occasionally (D)

(C) Multifocal
mononeuropathy

NCS
EMG
Nerve biopsy

Axonal

Consider:
Diabetes
Vasculitis
Leprosy
Sarcoid

Demyelinating
conduction
block

Multifocal
variant
of CIDP

(D) Symmetric
polyneuropathy

Cont'd on p 369

E. Causes of acute axonal neuropathies include porphyria, tick paralysis, and certain toxins. Acute intermittent porphyria is autosomal-dominantly inherited with an adolescent onset. Attacks are characterized by abdominal pain, unusual behavior, seizures, sympathetic overactivity, and bibrachial weakness. They may be precipitated by drugs, particularly barbiturates, and alcohol. High urine porphobilinogen is diagnostic. Toxins causing acute axonal neuropathies include triorthocresylphosphate and thallium. There is considerable overlap between subacute and chronic axonal neuropathies. However, *subacute* generally refers to onset over weeks to months, whereas *chronic* neuropathies begin insidiously over years. The category of subacute axonal neuropathies is vast and is led by patients with underlying metabolic disease, including diabetes, renal failure, and hypothyroidism. Toxins known to cause axonal PN include alcohol, industrial solvents, organophosphates, and heavy metals (arsenic, thallium, mercury). Drugs known to cause PN include nitrofurantoin, isoniazid, hydralazine, vincristine, cisplatin, disulfiram, suramin, amiodarone, and dapsone. Nutritional deficiencies of thiamine and vitamins E, B_6, and B_{12} cause treatable neuropathies. (B_{12} deficiency may also cause myelopathy and dementia.) Vasculitic causes include SLE, PAN, RA, allergic angiitis, and Wegener's granulomatosis. Infectious causes include Lyme disease and AIDS. Neuropathies associated with dysproteinemias and paraproteinemias include multiple myeloma, macroglobulinemia, cryoglobulinemia, ataxia-telangiectasia, and benign monoclonal gammopathy. Amyloid may be inherited, sporadic, or associated with myeloma and has a characteristic appearance on biopsy. Carcinomas may cause PNs via paraneoplastic syndromes or in association with nutritional deficiencies or chemotherapy. Occasionally PN appears months to years before the tumor is found. Chronic axonal PNs include those entities listed under the subacute heading plus hereditary motor and sensory neuropathy (HMSN), type 2. Etiologic investigation of axonal PN includes vitamin B_{12} level, CBC, serum protein electrophoresis, ESR, ANA, rheumatoid factor, fasting glucose, BUN, thyroid-stimulating hormone, urine heavy metal screen, HIV titer, Lyme titer, and a chest film. Consider nerve biopsy if the etiology is difficult to determine.

F. Demyelinating neuropathies can be classified according to the pattern of slowing on NCS and mode of onset. Those of insidious onset generally are either hereditary neuropathies or inherited metabolic disorders affecting nerves. Nerves often are enlarged, and biopsy often is helpful. HMSN, type 1 known as Charcot-Marie-Tooth disease, familiarly is characterized by autosomal-dominant inheritance, pes cavus, distal atrophy, weakness and numbness, and profound slowing on NCS. A gene test is now commercially available. HMSN type 3, or Déjérine-Sottas, is characterized by autosomal-recessive inheritance, palpable nerves, severe weakness, and scoliosis. HMSN, type 4, or Refsum's disease, also is inherited in an autosomal-recessive pattern and causes elevated serum phytanic acid and multisystem dysfunction. Metachromatic leukodystrophy and abetalipoproteinemia are other inherited metabolic disorders affecting peripheral nerves. Acute segmental demyelinating neuropathies include the common Guillain-Barré syndrome and the now uncommon diphtheria. Guillain-Barré syndrome is preceded by a viral syndrome in 60–70% of cases. It begins with mild paresthesias followed by a rapid ascending paralysis and diffuse areflexia. Patients must be hospitalized or followed very closely because 10–25% require artificial ventilation. Autonomic and cranial nerve involvement are common. Consider plasmapheresis or intravenous immunoglobulin for patients with a rapid, severe course. Chronic or relapsing segmental demyelinating neuropathies include CIDP, dysproteinemias, osteosclerotic myeloma, and lead toxicity. CIDP may begin similarly to Guillain-Barré syndrome but has a more protracted and often relapsing course. Diagnosis is made clinically and with aid of lumbar puncture, NCS/EMG, and nerve biopsy. Current treatment is with steroids, plasmapheresis, and other forms of immunosuppressive therapy. Dysproteinemias and paraproteinemias may be isolated or may occur in the context of myeloma, Waldenström's macroglobulinemia, cryoglobulinemia, POEMS syndrome, or ataxia-telangiectasia. Lead toxicity in adults is characteristically manifested by a motor neuropathy, particularly bilateral wrist drop. It is uncertain whether lead exerts its toxic effect on myelin and/or the anterior horn cell.

References

Adams RD, Victor M, Ropper AH. Principles of neurology. 6th ed. New York: McGraw-Hill, 1996.

Dyck PJ, Dick JB, Grant IA, et al. Ten steps in characterizing and diagnosing patients with peripheral neuropathy. Neurology 1996; 47:10.

Dyck PJ, Thomas PK, Griffin JW, et al, eds. Peripheral neuropathy. 3rd ed. Philadelphia: WB Saunders, 1993.

Greene DA, et al. Diabetic neuropathy. Annu Rev Med 1990; 41:303.

McLeod JG. Investigation of peripheral neuropathy. J Neurol Neurosurg Psychiatry 1995; 58:274.

Ropper AH. The Guillain-Barré syndrome. N Engl J Med 1992; 326:1130.

Schaumburg HH, Berger AR, Thomas PK. Disorders of peripheral nerves. 2nd ed. Philadelphia: FA Davis, 1992.

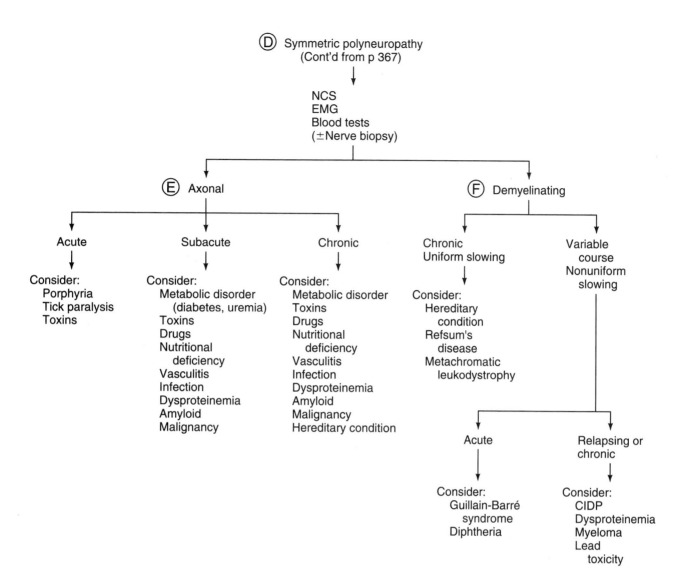

D Symmetric polyneuropathy
(Cont'd from p 367)

↓

NCS
EMG
Blood tests
(±Nerve biopsy)

E Axonal

F Demyelinating

Acute

Consider:
  Porphyria
  Tick paralysis
  Toxins

Subacute

Consider:
  Metabolic disorder
    (diabetes, uremia)
  Toxins
  Drugs
  Nutritional
    deficiency
  Vasculitis
  Infection
  Dysproteinemia
  Amyloid
  Malignancy

Chronic

Consider:
  Metabolic disorder
  Toxins
  Drugs
  Nutritional
    deficiency
  Vasculitis
  Infection
  Dysproteinemia
  Amyloid
  Malignancy
  Hereditary condition

**Chronic
Uniform slowing**

Consider:
  Hereditary
    condition
  Refsum's
    disease
  Metachromatic
    leukodystrophy

**Variable
course
Nonuniform
slowing**

Acute

Consider:
  Guillain-Barré
    syndrome
  Diphtheria

**Relapsing or
chronic**

Consider:
  CIDP
  Dysproteinemia
  Myeloma
  Lead
    toxicity

HYPERKINESIAS

Erwin B. Montgomery, Jr.

Hyperkinesias refer to a group of involuntary movements from which rhythmic movements such as tremor are excluded. Also generally excluded are myoclonic jerks, fasciculations, asterixis, restless leg syndrome, and seizures. The different entities that make up the hyperkinetic disorders are united by the association with disorders of the basal ganglia, whether documented or presumed. Akathisia also is generally excluded, although thought to be related to abnormal dopamine function in the basal ganglia. Akathisia is the subjective complaint of feeling the need to move to be comfortable. The manifestations of the hyperkinetic syndromes are divided into dystonia, chorea, athetosis, choreoathetosis, ballismus, tics, and mannerisms. Although the division gives the impression of discrete categories, they actually represent a continuum. The poles of the continuum are measured by coarseness versus gracefulness, proximal versus distal, and slow versus fast. There is not a one-to-one correspondence between the different hyperkinesias and disease entities. A single disease may be associated with a variety of hyperkinesias, and different types of hyperkinesias may coexist in the same individual.

A. Ballismus tends to be a coarse, rapid, violent, and proximal involuntary movement. Treat the underlying cause.

B. Athetosis tends to be a slow, graceful, and distal involuntary movement. Chorea is less graceful, faster, and more proximal than athetosis while more so than ballismus. Treatment of chorea, choreoathetosis, and athetosis is first directed at the underlying cause. Symptomatic benefit can be provided by use of drugs that deplete presynaptic dopamine stores (e.g., reserpine) or drugs that block postsynaptic dopamine receptors (e.g., phenothiazines, pimozide, haloperidol).

C. Levodopa in patients with Parkinson's disease can produce a dose-related hyperkinesia.

D. Any drug that blocks postsynaptic dopamine receptors or depletes presynaptic stores of dopamine can produce a tardive dyskinesia or dystonia. Treatment of tardive dyskinesia and dystonia is problematic because medications that can control the symptoms cause the disorder in the first place. Although many cases of tardive dyskinesias or dystonias do not improve, some may take years to resolve. Thus, make every effort to avoid drugs associated with tardive dyskinesias or dystonias. However, the symptoms of tardive dyskinesia and dystonia sometimes may be severe enough to warrant treatment.

E. Tics and mannerisms are distinguished from the remaining groups by the patient's ability to suppress or be distracted from having them.

(Continued on page 372)

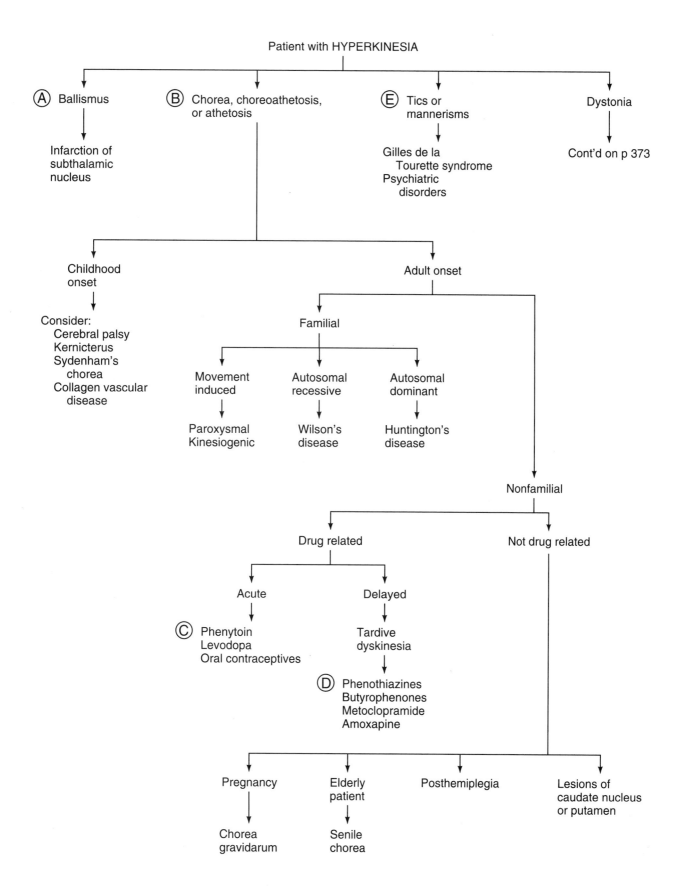

Patient with HYPERKINESIA

Ⓐ Ballismus

Ⓑ Chorea, choreoathetosis, or athetosis

Ⓔ Tics or mannerisms

Dystonia

Infarction of subthalamic nucleus

Gilles de la Tourette syndrome
Psychiatric disorders

Cont'd on p 373

Childhood onset

Adult onset

Consider:
    Cerebral palsy
    Kernicterus
    Sydenham's chorea
    Collagen vascular disease

Familial

Movement induced

Autosomal recessive

Autosomal dominant

Paroxysmal Kinesiogenic

Wilson's disease

Huntington's disease

Nonfamilial

Drug related

Not drug related

Acute

Delayed

Ⓒ Phenytoin
Levodopa
Oral contraceptives

Tardive dyskinesia

Ⓓ Phenothiazines
Butyrophenones
Metoclopramide
Amoxapine

Pregnancy

Elderly patient

Posthemiplegia

Lesions of caudate nucleus or putamen

Chorea gravidarum

Senile chorea

F. Dystonia tends to be the slowest of these types of involuntary movements, giving the appearance of an abnormal posture rather than an involuntary movement.

G. Treatment of dystonias is difficult. Many varied medications have been tried with varying success. High-dose anticholinergics generally have been the most successful, particularly in childhood generalized dystonia. Occasionally, levodopa may produce significant benefit, especially in childhood generalized dystonias.

H. Intramuscular injections of botulinum toxin may produce dramatic benefits in focal dystonias. The benefits may last for several months, and the injections may need to be repeated.

I. Surgical treatments in the past have included surgical ablations of thalamic nuclei. In torticollis, selective lesions of muscles or nerves may produce temporary benefit. However, dystonia is a dynamic process, and the pattern of muscular involvement changes. It may be possible to identify the muscles involved, cut them, and produce benefit. Later, other muscles become involved and the torticollis returns. The same phenomena may occur with botulinum injections, but the pattern of injections can be adjusted.

J. Early morning foot cramping or dystonia is common in parkinsonism.

References

Fahn S. Psychogenic movement disorders. In: Marsden CD, Fahn S, eds. Movement disorders. 3rd ed. London: Butterworth-Heinemann, 1994:359.

Fahn S, Marsden CD. The treatment of dystonia. In: Marsden CD, Fahn S, eds. Movement disorders 1 and 2. London: Butterworth-Heinemann, 1995.

Jankovic J. The neurology of tics. In: Marsden CD, Fahn S, eds. Movement disorders 1 and 2. London: Butterworth, 1995.

Jankovic J, Brin M. Therapeutic uses of botulinum toxin. N Engl J Med 1991; 324:1186.

Tsui JKD, Calnd DB, eds. Handbook of dystonia. New York: Marcel Dekker, 1995.

Wheeler AH. Therapeutic uses of botulinum toxin. Am Fam Physician 1997; 55:541.

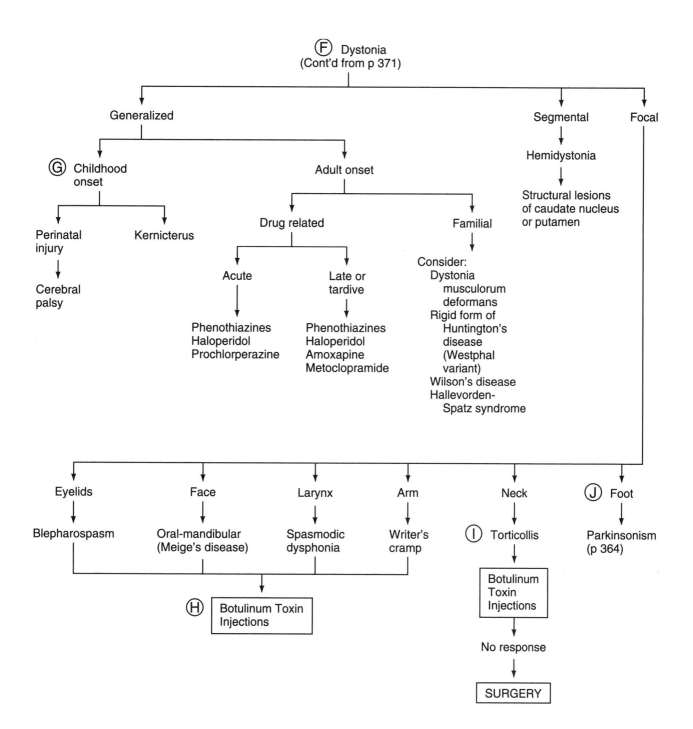

F Dystonia
(Cont'd from p 371)

Generalized

G Childhood onset
- Perinatal injury → Cerebral palsy
- Kernicterus

Adult onset

Drug related
- Acute → Phenothiazines, Haloperidol, Prochlorperazine
- Late or tardive → Phenothiazines, Haloperidol, Amoxapine, Metoclopramide

Familial → Consider:
Dystonia musculorum deformans
Rigid form of Huntington's disease (Westphal variant)
Wilson's disease
Hallevorden-Spatz syndrome

Segmental → Hemidystonia → Structural lesions of caudate nucleus or putamen

Focal
- Eyelids → Blepharospasm
- Face → Oral-mandibular (Meige's disease)
- Larynx → Spasmodic dysphonia
- Arm → Writer's cramp

H Botulinum Toxin Injections

- Neck → I Torticollis → Botulinum Toxin Injections → No response → SURGERY
- J Foot → Parkinsonism (p 364)

MUSCLE CRAMPS AND ACHES

Lawrence Z. Stern

Cramps are sudden, episodic, involuntary, painful contractions of a muscle or part of a muscle that last from seconds to several minutes. Ordinary cramps may occur spontaneously at rest, but more often they are precipitated by a brief muscle contraction. They are caused by a hyperexcitability of the motor neurons supplying the muscle. Such cramps are distinguished from those more correctly termed *contractures,* seen in certain metabolic myopathies such as phosphorylase deficiency (McArdle's disease). Contractures usually are associated with intense or ischemic exercise and are caused by depletion of muscle energy stores. They are often associated with myoglobinuria. In many cases the reason for recurrent cramps remains unclear even after a complete diagnostic evaluation. Treatment with quinine sulfate often is helpful in controlling nocturnal cramps. Frequent daytime cramps may respond to carbamazepine or amitryptyline. The initial history should elicit whether the cramps occur with exercise or at rest.

A. In children and pregnant women, leg cramps tend to occur at rest, often at night, after unusual daytime activity, and especially when the feet are cold. The neurologic examination and serum enzyme levels (creatine kinase and aldolase) are normal. These usually require no treatment.

B. Cramps occurring at rest or precipitated by minor exercise increase in frequency under certain conditions and in certain diseases. These should be excluded by appropriate inquiries and laboratory examinations. The cramps usually respond well to correction of the underlying problem.

C. Frequent cramps occurring during or after exercise require detailed investigation, including a complete history, neurologic examination, and serum enzyme level tests. Muscle biopsy should include histochemistry, electron microscopy, and appropriate biochemical studies. It should be preceded by electromyography (EMG) and a forearm ischemic exercise test, including determinations of serum lactate, pyruvate, and ammonia.

D. Exercise intolerance, along with cramps or myalgia, characterizes this group of hereditary disorders. All but the last two listed involve abnormalities of glycogen or glucose metabolism. Carnitine palmityl transferase deficiency results in a disorder of lipid metabolism more commonly associated with muscle soreness or aching than with cramps. With the exception of myoadenylate deaminase deficiency, all these disorders commonly result in myoglobinuria after especially strenuous exercise.

E. Cramps, and other entities that may be confused with cramps, occur in a variety of neurologic and neuromuscular disorders. Because investigations required to evaluate the diagnostic possibilities vary from patient to patient, such cases are usually best handled by a neurologist. Many of the conditions are treatable.

F. Leg pain and cramps in adults that are precipitated by exercise and promptly relieved by rest often are the result of peripheral vascular disease. When surgical treatment is feasible, results usually are excellent.

References

Joekes AM. Cramp: a review. J R Soc Med 1982; 75:546.

Layzer RB. Muscle pain, cramps, and fatigue. In: Engel AG, Franzini-Armstrong C, eds. Myology. 2nd ed. Vol 2. New York: McGraw-Hill, 1994:1754.

Layzer RB, Rowland LP. Cramps. N Engl J Med 1971; 285:31.

McGee SR. Muscle cramps. Arch Intern Med 1990; 150:511.

Sumi SM, Ruff RL, Swanson PD. Motor disturbances. In: Swanson PD, ed. Signs and symptoms in neurology. Philadelphia: JB Lippincott, 1984:168.

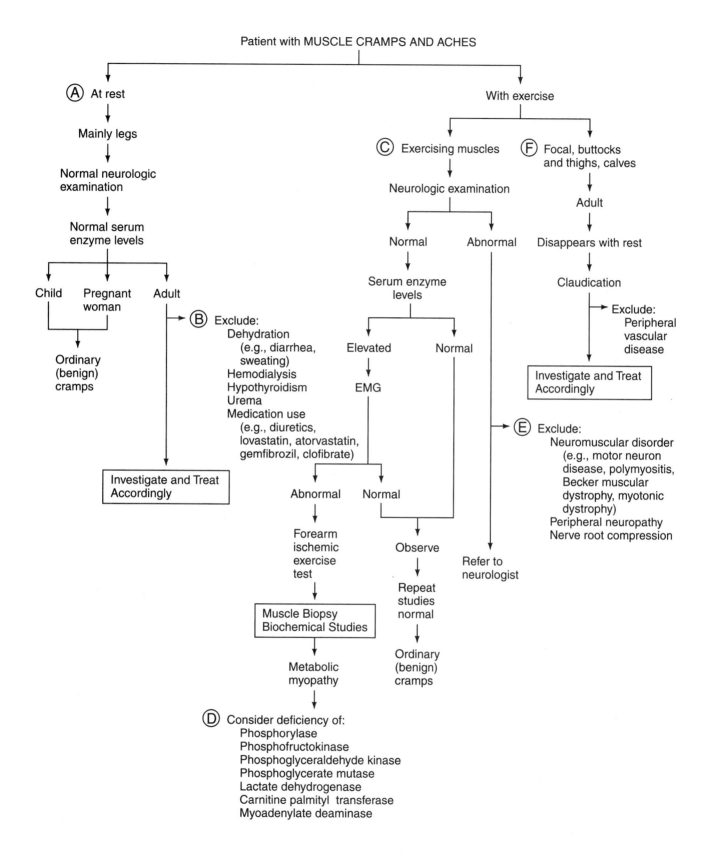

Patient with MUSCLE CRAMPS AND ACHES

Ⓐ At rest

Mainly legs

Normal neurologic
examination

Normal serum
enzyme levels

Child   Pregnant   Adult
         woman

Ordinary
(benign)
cramps

Ⓑ Exclude:
    Dehydration
       (e.g., diarrhea,
       sweating)
    Hemodialysis
    Hypothyroidism
    Urema
    Medication use
       (e.g., diuretics,
       lovastatin, atorvastatin,
       gemfibrozil, clofibrate)

Investigate and Treat
Accordingly

With exercise

Ⓒ Exercising muscles

Neurologic examination

Normal   Abnormal

Serum enzyme
levels

Elevated   Normal

EMG

Abnormal   Normal

Forearm
ischemic
exercise
test

Muscle Biopsy
Biochemical Studies

Metabolic
myopathy

Observe

Repeat
studies
normal

Ordinary
(benign)
cramps

Refer to
neurologist

Ⓓ Consider deficiency of:
    Phosphorylase
    Phosphofructokinase
    Phosphoglyceraldehyde kinase
    Phosphoglycerate mutase
    Lactate dehydrogenase
    Carnitine palmityl transferase
    Myoadenylate deaminase

Ⓕ Focal, buttocks
    and thighs, calves

Adult

Disappears with rest

Claudication

Exclude:
Peripheral
vascular
disease

Investigate and Treat
Accordingly

Ⓔ Exclude:
    Neuromuscular disorder
       (e.g., motor neuron
       disease, polymyositis,
       Becker muscular
       dystrophy, myotonic
       dystrophy)
    Peripheral neuropathy
    Nerve root compression

ACUTE BEHAVIOR CHANGE

Geoffrey L. Ahern

Acute behavior change is often considered synonymous with the term *acute confusional state*. Other labels include delirium, toxic-metabolic encephalopathy, and organic brain syndrome. The dominant feature of these states is a combination of confusion and inattention. Other higher-cortical functions also can be impaired. The most common causes of acute confusional states lie outside the CNS, such as metabolic derangements, toxins, and drugs or medications. Pathologic processes in the CNS also can produce the syndrome, as may primary psychiatric illnesses that impair higher-order attention and concentration.

A. Begin by taking a careful history, even though many patients are so confused that little or no useful information can be obtained. In this circumstance clinical examination and laboratory testing are crucial. The mental status examination should focus on the attentional matrix (e.g., digit span, reciting days of the week or months of the year forward and backward, word list generation). Particularly pertinent is an assessment for evidence of metabolic derangement such as asterixis, myoclonus, or exaggerated postural tremor. Findings such as hemiparesis, visual field defects, asymmetric reflexes, upgoing toes, or hemineglect may indicate focal CNS lesions, which may produce confusional states. When the history is virtually unobtainable and the clinical examination does not point to a clear precipitant, laboratory tests may have to be ordered.

B. Vascular disease may cause acute changes in mental status. Focal lesions in higher-order association cortex may result in confusion and agitation; specific sites of pathology include right frontal and parietal lobes, as well as mesial temporal-occipital lesions in either hemisphere; midbrain-diencephalic lesions may also cause acute behavior changes. Mass lesions of different types (e.g., tumors, subdural hematomas [SDHs], abscesses) may produce a picture similar to that of a cerebrovascular event. Also keep in mind the possibility of transient global amnesia (see p 344). In young patients migraine may present with confusion, with or without headache or other focal neurologic findings.

C. Patients with mild traumatic brain injury may have transient loss of consciousness (i.e., concussion), with or without residual problems with higher-order attention, concentration, and memory (postconcussion syndrome). When brain tissue has been damaged (i.e., contusion), more permanent deficits may occur; the profile of cognitive deficits depends on the areas involved. More severe cases may result in coma, and early intervention centers on intensive care issues. It cannot

be stressed enough that SDH may result from trivial injuries, especially in the elderly.

D. Exogenous substances may cause a toxic confusional state. Medications (particularly those with prominent anticholinergic effects) may adversely affect cognitive function. Consider street drugs in appropriate populations and/or circumstances. Alcohol's effects on mentation may result from chronic intoxication, alcoholic dementia, alcohol withdrawal, Wernicke's encephalopathy, and/or Korsakoff's psychosis. Eliminating alcoholic intake is important, but do not forget to administer thiamine and benzodiazepines in the acute period to prevent Wernicke-Korsakoff syndrome and alcohol withdrawal symptoms, respectively. Toxic agents include organic chemical substances (e.g., insecticides), heavy metals, and carbon monoxide. Reduction of further environmental exposure and of the body's burden of toxic agent is the therapeutic goal.

E. Confusional states may be secondary to metabolic derangements resulting from systemic illness. The potential causes are legion and include thyroid, hepatic, renal, and endocrine dysfunction. Any condition leading to hypoxia and/or ischemia also may lead to a confusional state. A chronic confusional state may result if the underlying illness cannot be brought under control. A related concept is "beclouded dementia," in which a patient with a known dementing illness becomes acutely worse during periods of intercurrent systemic illness. In both cases, vigorously attempt to find and treat the underlying cause.

F. Signs and symptoms compatible with systemic or CNS infection should prompt a search for the cause(s). Bacterial and viral agents are more likely to cause acute behavior changes than fungal agents. Also consider CNS abscesses and infected SDHs in certain instances. Order lumbar puncture when indicated.

G. Consider postictal confusion in a patient with a known seizure disorder who has confusion. Medication effects also may cause confusion. Alterations in consciousness may result from absence or complex partial seizures. In the extreme case (i.e., nonconvulsive status epilepticus), full consciousness may not be regained and a state resembling a fugue may result. If the diagnosis is in doubt, obtain an EEG.

H. Patients with known psychiatric disorders may have confusion or inattention as their main feature. Diagnoses such as anxiety, depression, and psychotic disorders, especially acute mania, may produce inattention. Appropriate consultation and treatment are indicated.

Patient with ACUTE BEHAVIOR CHANGE

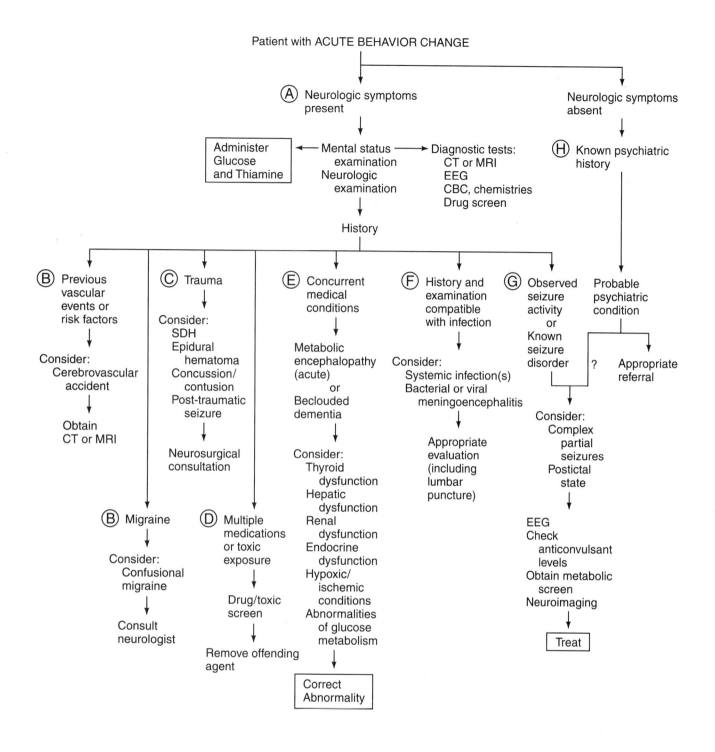

References

Jobe T, Gaviria M. Clinical neuropsychiatry. Boston: Blackwell Science, 1997.

Lipowski ZJ. Delirium: acute confusional states. New York: Oxford University Press, 1990.

Mesulam MM. Attentional, confusional states, and neglect. In: Mesulam MM, ed. Principles of behavioral neurology. Philadelphia: FA Davis, 1985:125.

CHRONIC BEHAVIOR CHANGE

Geoffrey L. Ahern

Many instances of chronic behavior change may be considered synonymous with dementia. Dementia itself may be defined as a progressive deterioration in mental function that interferes with activities of daily living appropriate for one's age and background. Any or all areas of mental function may be affected (e.g., language, memory, visuospatial skills, calculation, apraxia, agnosia, judgment, behavioral comportment). The persistence of the deficit(s) differentiates dementia from acute confusional state or delirium (see p 376). Although many of the dementias are progressive, some (e.g., post-traumatic and other static lesion etiologies, psychiatric causes) are not. The list of possible causes of chronic behavior change is long, but it is important to reach the correct diagnosis because some dementing illnesses are treatable. Intelligent use of the mental status and neurologic examinations, in conjunction with proper history taking and judicious use of laboratory tests, should permit a reasonably firm diagnosis in many cases.

A. Although considered separately in the decision tree, laboratory studies go hand in hand with the history and neurologic examination. Avoid a "shotgun" approach; instead, select tests on the basis of the most likely etiology(ies), given the history and examination. Nevertheless, the elements of what might constitute a dementia screening battery are presented here for the sake of completeness. Abnormalities in some of these tests may point to a potentially reversible cause of dementia. Although it is not a "test" for senile dementia of the Alzheimer type (SDAT), apolipoprotein E genotyping may help in estimating a patient's susceptibility to late-onset Alzheimer's disease.

B. If mental status testing reveals deficits in specific higher-cortical functions, the patient may have SDAT, the most commonly diagnosed form (about 50%) of dementia. It usually presents in the sixth to eighth decades with an insidious and steady progression, usually starting with problems in memory (especially short term), language (especially anomia), and orientation/judgment (e.g., getting lost, behaving inappropriately). It then progresses over 2–20 years, ultimately involving all aspects of mental function. The elemental neurologic examination is relatively preserved until late in the illness. Death usually results from intercurrent illness. The far less common Pick's disease may present with inappropriate and bizarre behavior or apathy in the presence of amnesia, aphasia, or agnosia. This presentation may lead to erroneous primary psychiatric diagnoses. The neuropathologic process in SDAT preferentially affects the parietotemporal regions (and the frontal lobes to a lesser extent), whereas in Pick's disease and the more general class of frontotemporal dementia, the frontal and temporal lobes bear the brunt of the damage. These changes may be reflected in atrophy of these regions shown on either CT or MRI scans. There is no cure for either of these entities, but low-dose neuroleptics, benzodiaz-

epines, and/or other psychopharmacologic agents may help control behavior. In SDAT modest improvements in cognitive function may be achieved with agents such as tacrine or donepezil.

C. When the clinical presentation is characterized by slowed mental processes, forgetfulness (rather than true amnesia), dilapidated cognition, hypophonic or dysarthric speech, and apathetic or depressed appearance, the two principal diagnoses to consider are depression and the dementia associated with one of the extrapyramidal syndromes such as Parkinson's disease (PD), Huntington's disease (HD), or progressive supranuclear palsy (PSP). Some differentiating points are a compatible history and clinical signs (e.g., vegetative signs) and a relatively nonfocal neurologic examination in depression, contrasted with characteristic motor system findings in the extrapyramidal syndromes (e.g., bradykinesia, rigidity, and tremor in PD; choreoathetosis in HD; eye movement abnormalities in PSP). In certain instances, however, differentiation may be difficult and one may have to resort to a trial of empiric therapy with antidepressants or drugs that affect the extrapyramidal system (e.g., amantadine, levodopa, bromocriptine, and selegiline in PD; neuroleptics in HD).

D. When elements of both B and C are present, the differential diagnosis includes a number of entities. In younger patients consider demyelinating disease (e.g., multiple sclerosis), degenerative diseases (usually genetic), and vasculitic syndromes (e.g., systemic lupus erythematosus). Appropriate laboratory studies, in conjunction with the clinical history and presentation, should permit a diagnosis. In older patients the neurologic examination may lead to the correct diagnosis. Multi-infarct dementia may show elements characteristic of SDAT and/or the extrapyramidal dementias, depending on the areas involved. Stepwise progression, a pseudobulbar syndrome, and focal neurologic deficits sometimes are found. Other entities that may be characterized by both higher-cortical and extrapyramidal dysfunction include diffuse Lewy body disease and corticobasal degeneration. Mass lesions may produce focal neurologic deficits and signs of decreased intracranial pressure (ICP). Myoclonus may suggest Creutzfeldt-Jakob disease, a slow viral infection; the EEG, which may demonstrate periodic discharges, may be useful in these cases. The triad of dementia, incontinence, and ataxic gait suggests normal-pressure hydrocephalus. Neuroimaging may demonstrate enlarged ventricles, whereas cisternography may show ventricular reflux and retarded clearance of the radioisotope. Removal of CSF by spinal tap may result in transient improvement of symptoms. Obtain neurosurgical consultation to determine whether a shunt procedure is indicated.

(Continued on page 380)

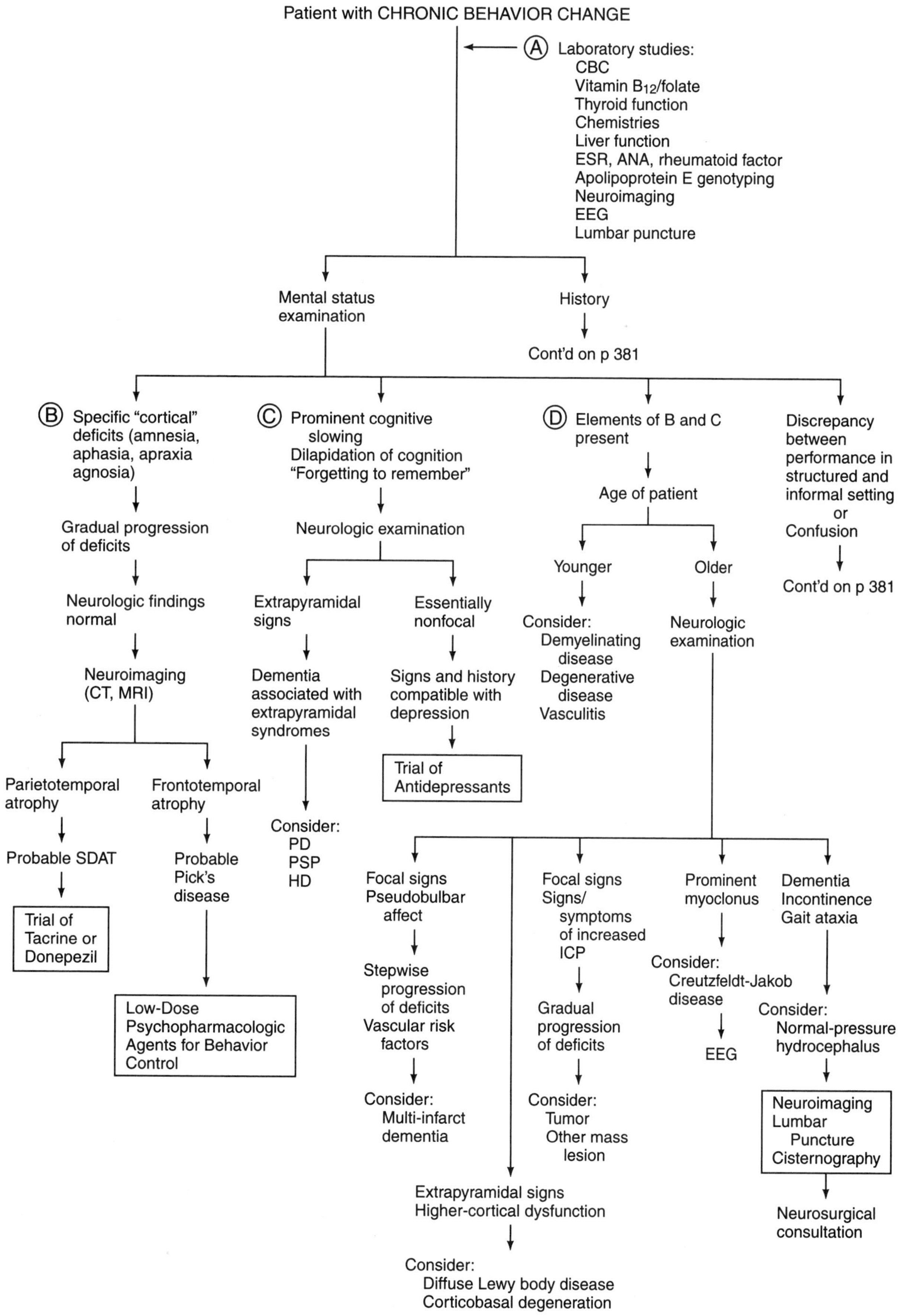
Patient with CHRONIC BEHAVIOR CHANGE
(A) Laboratory studies:
CBC
Vitamin B12/folate
Thyroid function
Chemistries
Liver function
ESR, ANA, rheumatoid factor
Apolipoprotein E genotyping
Neuroimaging
EEG
Lumbar puncture
Mental status examination
History
Cont'd on p 381
(B) Specific "cortical" deficits (amnesia, aphasia, apraxia agnosia)
Gradual progression of deficits
Neurologic findings normal
Neuroimaging (CT, MRI)
Parietotemporal atrophy
Probable SDAT
Trial of Tacrine or Donepezil
Frontotemporal atrophy
Probable Pick's disease
Low-Dose Psychopharmacologic Agents for Behavior Control
(C) Prominent cognitive slowing
Dilapidation of cognition
"Forgetting to remember"
Neurologic examination
Extrapyramidal signs
Dementia associated with extrapyramidal syndromes
Consider:
PD
PSP
HD
Essentially nonfocal
Signs and history compatible with depression
Trial of Antidepressants
(D) Elements of B and C present
Age of patient
Younger
Consider:
Demyelinating disease
Degenerative disease
Vasculitis
Older
Neurologic examination
Focal signs
Pseudobulbar affect
Stepwise progression of deficits
Vascular risk factors
Consider:
Multi-infarct dementia
Extrapyramidal signs
Higher-cortical dysfunction
Consider:
Diffuse Lewy body disease
Corticobasal degeneration
Focal signs
Signs/symptoms of increased ICP
Gradual progression of deficits
Consider:
Tumor
Other mass lesion
Prominent myoclonus
Consider:
Creutzfeldt-Jakob disease
EEG
Dementia
Incontinence
Gait ataxia
Consider:
Normal-pressure hydrocephalus
Neuroimaging
Lumbar Puncture
Cisternography
Neurosurgical consultation
Discrepancy between performance in structured and informal setting
or
Confusion
Cont'd on p 381

E. In hysterical dementia the examiner may observe a marked discrepancy between the patient's relatively normal performance in informal settings and poor performance in structured testing situations. Ganser's syndrome is a related variant in which patients may respond to questions with ridiculous or approximate answers. Make appropriate referral to a behavioral neurologist.

F. When the dominant clinical picture is confusion, look for signs of systemic illness or the ingestion of toxic substances. Confusional states may be secondary to systemic illness leading to metabolic derangements. The possible causes are legion (see p 344). A chronic confusional state may result if the underlying illness is not or cannot be controlled. A related concept is "beclouded dementia," in which a patient with a known dementing illness becomes acutely worse during periods of intercurrent systemic illness. In both cases make a vigorous attempt to find the underlying cause and treat it. Exogenous substances may also result in a toxic confusional state. Drugs (prescription or otherwise) commonly cause cognitive difficulties. If possible, eliminate from the patient's regimen any agents known to do this. Alcohol's effects on mentation may result from chronic intoxication, alcoholic dementia, alcohol withdrawal, Wernicke's encephalopathy, and/or Korsakoff's psychosis. Elimination of alcoholic intake is important, but do not forget to administer thiamine and benzodiazepine in the acute period to prevent Wernicke-Korsakoff syndrome and alcohol withdrawal symptoms, respectively. Do not overlook the effects of trauma (e.g., subdural hematoma [SDH], contusion, post-traumatic epilepsy) in this population. Other classes of agents capable of inducing cognitive changes include heavy metals (e.g., arsenic, lead, thallium, manganese, mercury), organic agents (e.g., solvents, organophosphate insecticides), and carbon monoxide. Reducing further environmental exposure and the body's burden of toxic agent is the therapeutic goal.

G. Elements of the history may be particularly useful in making a diagnosis. If trauma has occurred, consider SDH. Contusions of the brain substance may occur as a result of trauma; the frontal and temporal regions of the brain are most likely to be affected. Dementia pugilistica is a form of post-traumatic dementia seen in boxers. If history and examination are compatible with CNS infection, consider meningoencephalitis. Nonbacterial forms (e.g., cryptococcal, tuberculous, neurosyphilis) may have a relatively indolent course. Also consider the AIDS dementia complex if appropriate risk factors are present. Remember that HIV infection in the CNS may be accompanied by a number of "fellow travelers," including progressive multifocal leukoencephalopathy (PML), toxoplasmosis, and cryptococcosis.

References

Cummings JL, ed. Subcortical dementia. New York: Oxford University Press, 1990.

Cummings JL, Benson DF. Dementia: a clinical approach. 2nd ed. Boston: Butterworth-Heinemann, 1992.

Signoret JL. Memory and amnesias. In: Mesulam MM, ed. Principles of behavioral neurology. Philadelphia: FA Davis, 1985:169.

Strub RL, Black FW. The mental status examination in neurology. 3rd ed. Philadelphia: FA Davis, 1993.

Whitehouse PJ, Lerner A, Hedera P. Dementia. In: Heilman KM, Valenstein E, eds. Clinical neuropsychology. 3rd ed. New York: Oxford University Press, 1993:603.

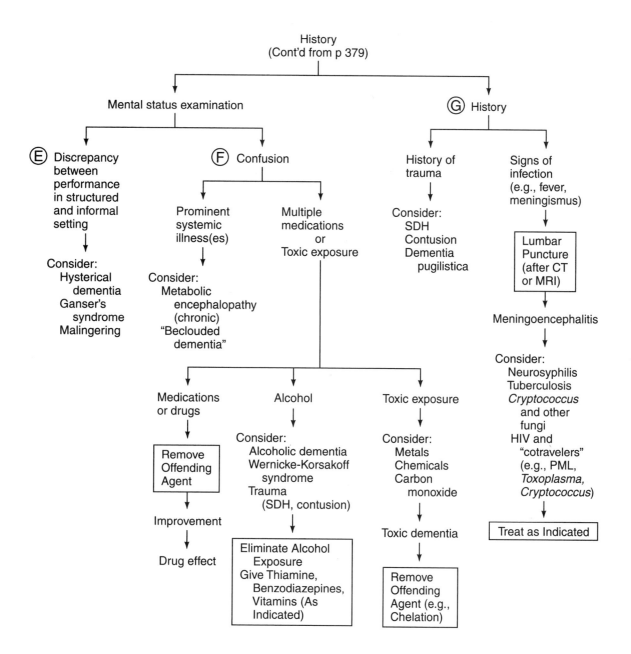

History
(Cont'd from p 379)

Mental status examination

Ⓔ Discrepancy between performance in structured and informal setting

Consider:
Hysterical dementia
Ganser's syndrome
Malingering

Ⓕ Confusion

Prominent systemic illness(es)

Consider:
Metabolic encephalopathy (chronic)
"Beclouded dementia"

Medications or drugs

Remove Offending Agent

Improvement

Drug effect

Alcohol

Consider:
Alcoholic dementia
Wernicke-Korsakoff syndrome
Trauma (SDH, contusion)

Eliminate Alcohol Exposure
Give Thiamine, Benzodiazepines, Vitamins (As Indicated)

Multiple medications or Toxic exposure

Toxic exposure

Consider:
Metals
Chemicals
Carbon monoxide

Toxic dementia

Remove Offending Agent (e.g., Chelation)

Ⓖ History

History of trauma

Consider:
SDH
Contusion
Dementia pugilistica

Signs of infection (e.g., fever, meningismus)

Lumbar Puncture (after CT or MRI)

Meningoencephalitis

Consider:
Neurosyphilis
Tuberculosis
Cryptococcus and other fungi
HIV and "cotravelers" (e.g., PML, *Toxoplasma*, *Cryptococcus*)

Treat as Indicated

DISTURBANCES OF SMELL AND TASTE

Eugenie A.M.T. Obbens

Dysfunction of smell or taste usually is not a disease entity in itself, but part of a disease process. Both are somewhat obscure symptoms; loss of taste often is not noticed by the patient, especially when the onset is gradual. Loss of smell, on the other hand, may be attributed to changes in taste. *Anosmia* is the absence of smell sensation; *dysosmia*, or *parosmia*, is a distorted smell perception, either with or without an odorant stimulus present. Abnormalities in taste sensation are classified into ageusia (absence of taste perception) and dysgeusia (distortion of taste resulting in a persistent metallic, bitter, sour, sweet, or salty taste).

A. Congenital anosmia appears to be caused by absence of olfactory epithelium. The most common congenital disorder is Kallmann's syndrome, in which there is agenesis of the olfactory bulbs in combination with hypogonadism and other developmental abnormalities.

B. Tumors implicated as a cause of anosmia are olfactory groove meningiomas, frontal lobe gliomas, and pituitary adenomas with suprasellar extension. Another cause is an aneurysm of the anterior cerebral or anterior communicating artery. Cigarette smoking has been demonstrated to cause progressive loss of smell in a dose-related manner, with a gradual restoration of smell perception once patients have stopped smoking. Medications affecting the sense of smell include opioid analgesics, β blockers, and some antithyroid medications. Diseases such as chronic rhinitis and sinusitis, or conditions leading to nasal obstruction, are a common cause of decreased smell. Anosmia caused by these conditions is most amenable to treatment; if untreated, it may steadily worsen.

C. Anosmia may occur after even mild head trauma, especially after a blow to the occiput. It is thought to be caused by shearing of the olfactory filaments as they course through the cribriform plate. Although there is no treatment for post-traumatic loss of smell, gradual recovery of smell function occurs in about one third of patients. The olfactory bulbs and its nerves can be damaged during subfrontal craniotomy or as the result of a subarachnoid hemorrhage, meningitis at the base of the skull, or a frontal lobe abscess. Sudden loss of smell, and sometimes also of taste, may occur after an upper respiratory infection. This is more common in older patients and is thought to result from viral damage of the olfactory mucosa. Recovery, if it occurs at all, may take years.

D. Uncinate fits, a form of temporal lobe seizures, consist of brief periods of unpleasant or foul odor perception, together with an alteration of consciousness. The diagnosis can be confirmed with EEG, and the seizures treated with anticonvulsant medication. Olfactory hallucinations also have been described with psychiatric illness such as endogenous depression, schizophrenia, Alzheimer's dementia, and alcohol withdrawal.

E. A unilateral loss of taste on the anterior two thirds of the tongue can be found in Bell's palsy and results from involvement of the chorda tympani. Loss of taste as a result of head injury is less common than loss of smell. It may be unilateral or bilateral, presumably caused by damage to the chorda tympani. Patients with diabetes mellitus often have a decreased sensation of sweet, bitter, and sour flavors. This is more common in patients with long-standing diabetes and in those with associated diabetic neuropathy.

F. Oral disorders causing taste disturbances include oral candidiasis, lichen planus, leukoplakia, carcinoma of the tongue, and other tongue afflictions; xerostomia and sialoadenitis; and palatal clefts and facial hypoplasia. Periodontal disease and other infectious processes may produce abnormal oral secretions, resulting in taste changes. Dental restorations or prostheses can give a metallic taste, whereas dentures may block taste reception. Numerous medications cause taste changes: antibiotics, antifungal agents, anti-inflammatory drugs, cytotoxic agents, and many cardiovascular drugs. Gustatory hallucinations may be part of a temporal lobe seizure, as well as manifestations of other temporoparietal dysfunctions.

References

Barwick MC. Neurological evaluation of taste and smell disorders. Ear Nose Throat J 1989; 68:354.

Downey LL, Jacobs JB, Lebowitz RA. Anosmia and chronic sinus disease. Otolaryngol Head Neck Surg 1996; 115:24.

Frye RE, Schwartz BS, Doty RL. Dose-related effects of cigarette smoking on olfactory function. JAMA 1990; 263:1233.

Henkin RI. Drug-induced taste and smell disorders. Drug Safety 1994; 11:318.

Jafek BW, Gordon ASD, Moran DT, Eller PM. Congenital anosmia. Ear Nose Throat J 1990; 69:331.

Le Floch J-P, Le Lievre G, Sadoun J, et al. Taste impairment and related factors in type I diabetes mellitus. Diabetes Care 1989; 12:173.

Osaki T, Ohshima M, Tomita Y, et al. Clinical and physiological investigations in patients with taste abnormality. J Oral Path Medic 1996; 25:38.

Scott AE. Medical management of taste and smell disorders. Ear Nose Throat J 1989; 68:386.

Patient with DISTURBANCE OF SMELL OR TASTE

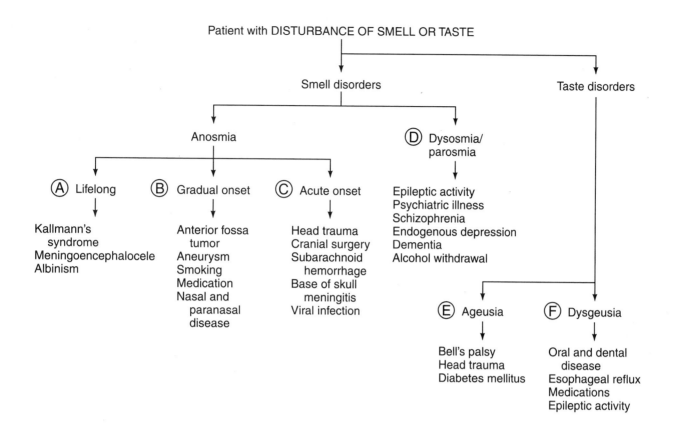

Smell disorders

Taste disorders

Anosmia

Ⓓ Dysosmia/ parosmia

Ⓐ Lifelong

Ⓑ Gradual onset

Ⓒ Acute onset

Kallmann's
   syndrome
Meningoencephalocele
Albinism

Anterior fossa
   tumor
Aneurysm
Smoking
Medication
Nasal and
   paranasal
   disease

Head trauma
Cranial surgery
Subarachnoid
   hemorrhage
Base of skull
   meningitis
Viral infection

Epileptic activity
Psychiatric illness
Schizophrenia
Endogenous depression
Dementia
Alcohol withdrawal

Ⓔ Ageusia

Ⓕ Dysgeusia

Bell's palsy
Head trauma
Diabetes mellitus

Oral and dental
   disease
Esophageal reflux
Medications
Epileptic activity

COMA

Geoffrey L. Ahern

The causes of coma may be broadly categorized into four main groups: (1) supratentorial lesions (including subarachnoid hemorrhage [SAH] and meningitis) that increase intracranial pressure (ICP) and thereby cause dysfunction of the reticular activating system, (2) infratentorial lesions that affect the reticular activating system directly, (3) toxic-metabolic encephalopathies that affect the neuraxis diffusely, and (4) status epilepticus. The roles of the primary care physician include stabilizing the patient's vital functions, initiating evaluation with the aim of being able to classify the coma into one of the four groups, and instituting appropriate treatment.

A. The primary goal is to stabilize the patient. This includes the ABCs (airway, breathing, circulation) of basic life support. Place IV, nasogastric, and urinary catheters. Endotracheal intubation probably will be necessary. Administer glucose (with thiamine) and naloxone after blood is drawn for CBC, chemistries, toxic screen, and blood gases.

B. The Glasgow Coma Scale (Table 1) provides a quick, systematic way to assess depth of coma. It most often is used in traumatic coma. These scores are useful in communicating to other professionals and in assessing progression.

C. Palpate the skull for hematomas, and look for Battle's sign (ecchymosis over the mastoid), raccoon eyes (ecchymosis around the eyes), hemotympanum, and CSF leaks from the nose or ears. Always consider the possibility of neck trauma and evaluate for it at first contact with the patient. This pertains not only to performing the examination but also to moving the patient during endotracheal intubation and performing other maneuvers. If trauma is present, order neuroimaging. CT may be preferable to MRI for its ability to detect acute blood and bone abnormalities. Also obtain neurosurgical consultation.

D. A nonfocal examination should raise suspicion of a toxic or metabolic etiology. Dysfunction in virtually any body system may lead to acute and chronic confusional states or even coma. Consider drug ingestion and toxic exposure. In most cases metabolic dysfunction does not cause nonreactive pupils or focal signs. However, atropine-like substances and glutethimide abolish pupillary reactivity; in opiate overdose the pupils may be so constricted that a very bright light and a magnifying glass may be needed for any reactivity to be observed. Toxic-metabolic insults also may result in seizures and lateralizing neurologic signs that may wax and wane or even shift from side to side. Extensor plantar responses also may be seen. On the other hand, metabolic causes of coma (especially intoxication) may obscure signs of an underlying focal lesion. Therefore, in practice, neuroimaging is performed in most patients with coma.

E. If a focal lesion is responsible for coma, it may be useful to try to localize the lesion to a supratentorial or infratentorial location. The examination should emphasize the following areas: appendicular movement (e.g., symmetric vs. asymmetric responses, decorticate/decerebrate posturing), stretch reflexes, pupillary response (size, asymmetry, reactivity), eye movement abnormalities (including doll's eyes), brainstem reflexes (e.g., corneal reflex), and respiratory pattern (e.g., Cheyne-Stokes, central neurogenic hyperventilation, ataxic and apneustic breathing, "fish mouthing"). Rostrocaudal deterioration of CNS function is reflected in a characteristic set of responses in each of these examination areas. A complete exposition of the abnormalities observed with lesions in different areas is beyond the scope of this chapter (any of the texts listed in the references provide the information needed to interpret these findings). The key is to have the examination information available for consultations with neurologists and/or neurosurgeons.

F. Signs of meningismus include nuchal rigidity and Kernig's and Brudzinski's signs. Such findings may accompany either a nonfocal or focal examination. In the former case they may reflect SAH or meningitis. In the latter case mass lesions may lead to meningismus either because of meningeal irritation per se (e.g., parenchymal hemorrhage with rupture into the subarachnoid space) or because of increased ICP, which may lead to herniation of the cerebellar tonsils (e.g.,

TABLE 1   Glasgow Coma Scale

Function	Score*
Motor response	
Obeys	6
Localizes	5
Withdraws	4
Abnormal flexion	3
Extensor response	2
No response	1
Verbal response	
Oriented	5
Confused conversation	4
Inappropriate words	3
Incomprehensible sounds	2
No response	1
Eye opening	
Spontaneous	4
To command	3
To pain	2
No response	1

*The best score from each of the three areas is summed. Scores can range from 15 (essentially a normal examination) to 3 (no response in any area).

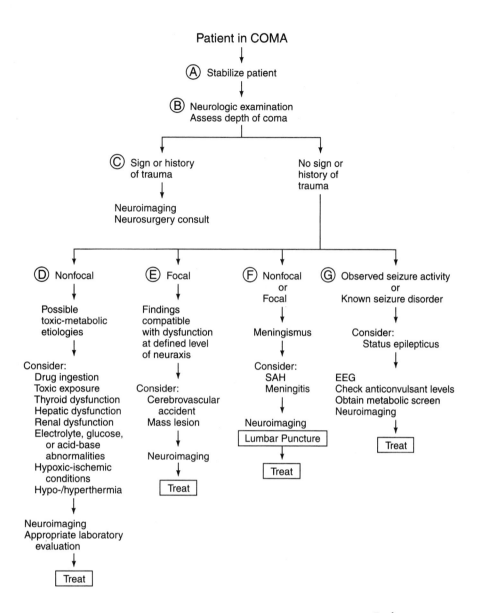

Patient in COMA

Ⓐ Stabilize patient

Ⓑ Neurologic examination
Assess depth of coma

Ⓒ Sign or history
of trauma

No sign or
history of
trauma

Neuroimaging
Neurosurgery consult

Ⓓ Nonfocal

Possible
toxic-metabolic
etiologies

Consider:
　Drug ingestion
　Toxic exposure
　Thyroid dysfunction
　Hepatic dysfunction
　Renal dysfunction
　Electrolyte, glucose,
　　or acid-base
　　abnormalities
　Hypoxic-ischemic
　　conditions
　Hypo-/hyperthermia

Neuroimaging
Appropriate laboratory
evaluation

Treat

Ⓔ Focal

Findings
compatible
with dysfunction
at defined level
of neuraxis

Consider:
　Cerebrovascular
　　accident
　Mass lesion

Neuroimaging

Treat

Ⓕ Nonfocal
or
Focal

Meningismus

Consider:
　SAH
　Meningitis

Neuroimaging
Lumbar Puncture

Treat

Ⓖ Observed seizure activity
or
Known seizure disorder

Consider:
　Status epilepticus

EEG
Check anticonvulsant levels
Obtain metabolic screen
Neuroimaging

Treat

References

Adams RD, Victor M, Ropper AH. Coma and related disorders of consciousness. In: Adams RD, Victor M, Ropper AH, eds. Principles of neurology. 6th ed. New York: McGraw-Hill, 1997:344.

Aquino TM, Samuels MA. Coma and other alterations in consciousness. In: Samuels MA, ed. Manual of neurologic therapeutics. 5th ed. Boston: Little, Brown, 1995.

Brust JCM. Coma. In: Rowland LP, ed. Merritt's textbook of neurology. 9th ed. Baltimore: Williams & Wilkins, 1995.

Gilroy J. Coma. In: Gilroy J. Basic neurology. 2nd ed. New York: Pergamon, 1990:48.

Plum F, Posner J. The diagnosis of stupor and coma. 3rd ed. Philadelphia: FA Davis, 1980.

Teasdale G, Jennett B. Assessment of coma and impaired consciousness: a practical scale. Lancet 1974; 2:81.

cerebellar hemorrhage). Order lumbar puncture (probably after a CT scan), looking for evidence of blood, xanthochromia, or infection. Up to 15% of SAHs are missed by CT scan. Furthermore, signs of meningismus may be absent in deep coma, so consider lumbar puncture if the history suggests an infectious etiology.

G. Prolonged or sustained seizure activity (i.e., status epilepticus) may lead to impaired consciousness. Seizures also may reflect an underlying process that itself leads to coma. Observe patients carefully for evidence of seizure activity. Focal seizures suggest a focal source. Generalized seizures or myoclonus may be caused by toxic-metabolic abnormalities. These rules are not absolute. Laboratory studies should consider anticonvulsant levels as well as metabolic parameters. An EEG may be useful not only to assess seizure activity but to look for abnormalities compatible with metabolic abnormalities or focal lesions. Neuroimaging is useful to look for underlying focal lesions. For treatment of status epilepticus, see p 352.

BRAIN DEATH

William M. Feinberg

Over the last 35 years the concept of brain death has become accepted by both medical and legal professions. In 1981 the President's Commission for the Study of Ethical Problems in Medicine and Biomedical and Behavioral Research issued a report on "Guidelines for the Determination of Death." This included a model statute called the *Uniform Determination of Death Act.* This states: "An individual who has sustained either (1) irreversible cessation of circulatory and respiratory functions, or (2) irreversible cessation of all functions of the entire brain, including the brain stem, is dead. A determination of death must be made in determination with accepted medical standards." Most states now have statutes or judicial decisions recognizing this concept. Criteria given in the decision tree are valid for adults >18 years of age.

A. Rule out reversible causes of cerebral depression. Body temperature must be >90° F (32.2° C). Profound metabolic or electrolyte disturbance cannot be present. Depressant drugs should not be present. Toxicology screens or measurement of serum drug levels may be required.

B. There should be no spontaneous respiration despite arterial Pco_2 >60 mm Hg. A suggested protocol for establishment of apnea follows: (1) The patient's hemodynamic and ventilatory status should be stable. The patient should have a systolic blood pressure >90 mm Hg. The arterial Pco_2 should be ≥40 mm Hg. The patient should be preoxygenated using an inspired oxygen tension of 100% to obtain an arterial Po_2 ≥200 mm Hg. (2) Disconnect the ventilator and place the patient on a t-piece with 6 L O_2/min via an endotracheal cannula at the level of the carina. (3) Observe carefully for respiration. If respiration occurs the test is negative. (4) After 8 minutes measure arterial Po_2, Pco_2, and pH and reconnect the ventilator. (5) If no respirations are present and the arterial Pco_2 is >60 mm Hg, the test is positive and supports a diagnosis of brain death. (6) If systolic blood pressure decreases below 90 mm Hg during the test, there is marked oxygen desaturation, or serious cardiac arrhythmias occur, the test should be terminated and ABG measured. If the Pco_2 is ≥60 mm Hg and respirations have not occurred, the apnea test is positive and supports brain death. If the Pco_2 is <60 mm Hg, the apnea test is indeterminate and additional confirmatory testing may be required.

C. Brain death is a clinical diagnosis and does not require ancillary testing. Ancillary studies such as EEG, radionuclide angiography, or transcranial Doppler ultrasonography may be confirmatory but are not required for the diagnosis.

References

Guidelines for the determination of death: report of the medical consultants on the diagnosis of death to the President's Commission for the Study of Ethical Problems in Medicine and Biomedical and Behavioral Research. JAMA 1981; 246:2184.

Joynt RJ. A new look at death. JAMA 1984; 252:680.

Quality Standards Subcommittee of the American Academy of Neurology. Practice parameters for determining brain death in adults (summary statement). Neurology 1995; 45:1012.

Wijdicks EFM. Determining brain death in adults. Neurology 1995; 45:1003.

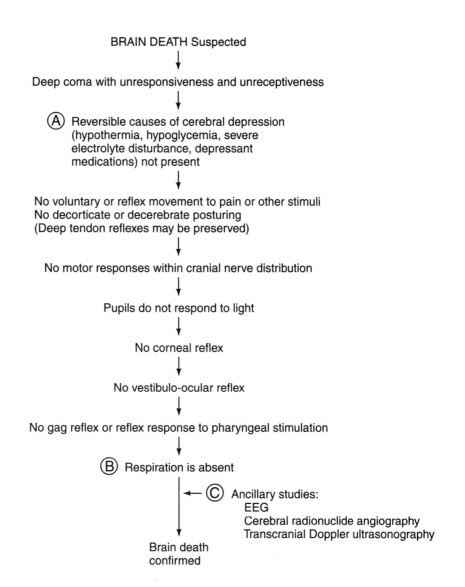

BRAIN DEATH Suspected

↓

Deep coma with unresponsiveness and unreceptiveness

↓

(A) Reversible causes of cerebral depression
(hypothermia, hypoglycemia, severe
electrolyte disturbance, depressant
medications) not present

↓

No voluntary or reflex movement to pain or other stimuli
No decorticate or decerebrate posturing
(Deep tendon reflexes may be preserved)

↓

No motor responses within cranial nerve distribution

↓

Pupils do not respond to light

↓

No corneal reflex

↓

No vestibulo-ocular reflex

↓

No gag reflex or reflex response to pharyngeal stimulation

↓

(B) Respiration is absent

← (C) Ancillary studies:
EEG
Cerebral radionuclide angiography
Transcranial Doppler ultrasonography

↓

Brain death
confirmed

PULMONARY DISEASE

HEMOPTYSIS

Anthony Camilli

Hemoptysis is the expectoration of blood from the tracheo-bronchial tree. It ranges from trivial to life threatening in severity and has numerous causes. Disease processes that may result in hemoptysis include those of the pulmonary parenchyma and the airways, and infectious, inflammatory, and malignant disorders.

A. The history may suggest likely causes of hemoptysis. Patients with known bronchiectasis may have a history of a recent infective exacerbation. A history of valvular heart disease may indicate elevated pulmonary capillary pressure as a likely cause. Hemoptysis in an older smoker suggests the likelihood of a malignant lesion.

B. The chest film provides two important pieces of information in this setting. First, it may strongly suggest the bleeding source by showing a lesion with bleeding potential, such as a cavitary mass in the lower left lobe. It also may show the amount of associated hemorrhage into the lung via associated infiltrate.

C. The basic approach to hemoptysis depends on prompt assessment of its severity; this can range from a medical emergency to a problem that can be handled on an outpatient basis. Mild intermittent hemoptysis such as blood-streaked sputum can be evaluated by bronchoscopy, which should include the entire respiratory tract. Patients with active bleeding but without impaired respiratory function can be treated for infection during quantitation of hemoptysis, reversal of coagulopathy, and optimizing the timing of bronchoscopy. Massive he-moptysis, usually defined as >600 ml in 24 hours, requires an emergent diagnostic/therapeutic approach. This may involve rigid bronchoscopy and protection of the nonhemorrhaging lung with a Fogarty catheter or endotracheal tube.

D. If hemoptysis is persistent despite treatment of presumed infection and supportive care, perform bronchial arteriography with embolization or resection of the involved segment or lobe if the source can be clearly identified. Bronchial artery embolization carries the risk of spinal cord infarction and the risk/benefit ratio must be weighed carefully.

References

Cahill BC, Ingbar DH. Massive hemoptysis: assessment and management. Clin Chest Med 1994; 15:147.

DiLeo MD, Amedee RG, Butcher RB. Hemoptysis and pseudohemoptysis: the patient expectorating blood. Ear Nose Throat J 1995; 74:822.

O'Neil KM, Lazarus AA. Hemoptysis: an indication for bronchoscopy. Arch Intern Med 1991; 151:171.

Poe RH, Isreal RH, Mari MG, et al. Utility of fiberoptic bronchoscopy in patient with hemoptysis and a nonlocalizing chest roentgenogram. Chest 1988; 93:70.

Thompson AB, Teschler H, Rennard SI. Pathogenesis, evaluation and therapy for massive hemoptysis. Clin Chest Med 1992; 13:69.

Patient with HEMOPTYSIS

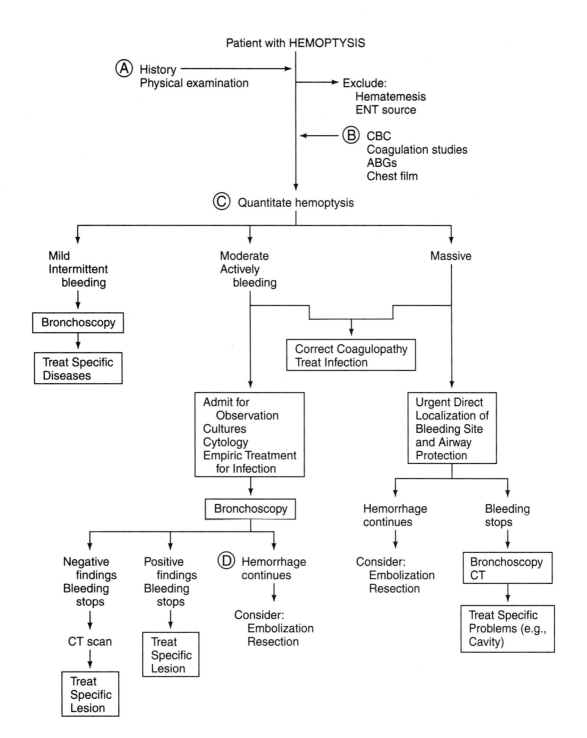

(A) History
Physical examination

Exclude:
Hematemesis
ENT source

(B) CBC
Coagulation studies
ABGs
Chest film

(C) Quantitate hemoptysis

Mild
Intermittent
bleeding

Moderate
Actively
bleeding

Massive

Bronchoscopy

Treat Specific
Diseases

Correct Coagulopathy
Treat Infection

Admit for
Observation
Cultures
Cytology
Empiric Treatment
for Infection

Urgent Direct
Localization of
Bleeding Site
and Airway
Protection

Bronchoscopy

Negative
findings
Bleeding
stops

Positive
findings
Bleeding
stops

(D) Hemorrhage
continues

Hemorrhage
continues

Bleeding
stops

CT scan

Treat
Specific
Lesion

Consider:
Embolization
Resection

Consider:
Embolization
Resection

Bronchoscopy
CT

Treat
Specific
Lesion

Treat Specific
Problems (e.g.,
Cavity)

389

STRIDOR

Neil C. Clements, Jr.

Stridor is a continuous, monophonic upper airway sound heard predominantly during inspiration. Because it indicates upper airway obstruction, expedient management is essential.

A. Initial history should elicit the duration (minutes, hours, or days) and the severity of symptoms. Clinical evidence of impending respiratory failure (fatigue, cyanosis, poor chest wall excursion, mental status changes) mandates intubation or tracheostomy (see D) before further diagnostic evaluation. All other patients with acute or subacute stridor also require constant observation in the ICU. Provide symptomatic relief in these patients by administering an inhaled mixture of helium and oxygen (heliox), during which specific diagnosis and treatment should be aggressively pursued.

B. Acute laryngospasm or laryngeal edema must be suspected after exposure to allergens; treat by subcutaneous injection of 0.5 ml of 0.1% epinephrine. Inhaled racemic epinephrine also may be useful and is indicated in inhalation airway injury, along with intubation and surgical repair. Tracheal stenosis (e.g., from previous airway intubation) may respond to racemic epinephrine if there is coexistent inflammation or edema.

C. Consider foreign body aspiration in alcoholics, in those with neuromuscular or cerebral disorders that impair swallowing or airway protective reflexes, and in children. Inspection of the oropharynx may reveal obstructions that can easily be removed with forceps or by suction. When it is determined that the patient is stable, soft tissue radiography and CT of the chest may complement the chest radiographic diagnosis.

D. In severe cases, laryngoscopy and bronchoscopy in the operating room or ICU may facilitate diagnosis. Intubation over the bronchoscope may be required when there is marked airway edema or when neck injury is suspected. Intubation by bronchoscopy, light wand, or laryngoscopy should always be performed by the most skilled available personnel.

E. Personnel skilled at tracheostomy should be present in case intubation cannot be successfully performed. Specific therapies include appropriate antibiotics or indicated surgery for infectious upper airway disorders. Achalasia may often be decompressed by nasogastric tube suction.

F. To localize the site of obstruction, stable patients may undergo chest and soft tissue neck radiography with continued cardiopulmonary monitoring, and a physician skilled in airway management in constant attendance.

References

Baughman RP, Loudon RG. Stridor: differentiation from asthma or upper airway noise. Am Rev Respir Dis 1989; 139:1407.

Hollingworth HM. Wheezing and stridor. Clin Chest Med 1987; 8:231.

Koster ME, Baughman RP, Loudon RG. Continuous adventitious lung sounds. J Asthma 1990; 27:237.

Miller RD, Hyatt RE. Evaluation of obstructing lesions of the trachea and larynx by flow volume loops. Am Rev Respir Dis 1973; 108:475.

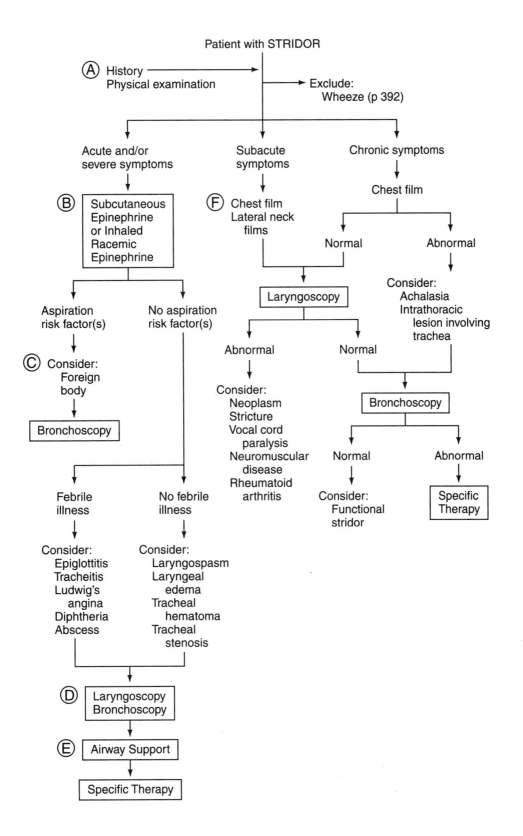

Patient with STRIDOR

Ⓐ History
Physical examination → Exclude:
Wheeze (p 392)

Acute and/or severe symptoms

Ⓑ Subcutaneous Epinephrine or Inhaled Racemic Epinephrine

Aspiration risk factor(s)

Ⓒ Consider: Foreign body

Bronchoscopy

No aspiration risk factor(s)

Febrile illness

Consider:
Epiglottitis
Tracheitis
Ludwig's angina
Diphtheria
Abscess

No febrile illness

Consider:
Laryngospasm
Laryngeal edema
Tracheal hematoma
Tracheal stenosis

Ⓓ Laryngoscopy Bronchoscopy

Ⓔ Airway Support

Specific Therapy

Subacute symptoms

Ⓕ Chest film Lateral neck films

Laryngoscopy

Abnormal

Consider:
Neoplasm
Stricture
Vocal cord paralysis
Neuromuscular disease
Rheumatoid arthritis

Normal

Chronic symptoms

Chest film

Normal

Abnormal

Consider:
Achalasia
Intrathoracic lesion involving trachea

Bronchoscopy

Normal

Consider:
Functional stridor

Abnormal

Specific Therapy

WHEEZING

Neil C. Clements, Jr.

Wheezes are continuous, high-pitched, mono- or polyphonic sounds that occur when airway caliber narrows sufficiently to produce oscillation of airway walls. Asthma is the most common cause. Nonasthmatic causes of wheezing also may produce stridor (p 390).

A. Initial evaluation of the wheezing patient should determine the degree of respiratory impairment (see B). Important diagnostic clues include a personal or family history of asthma, cigarette use, medical ailments predisposing to aspiration (e.g., alcoholism or neuromuscular or cerebral disorders that impair swallowing or airway protective reflexes), previous intubation or tracheostomy, or recent foreign travel. Seek signs and symptoms of infection, congestive heart failure (CHF), deep venous thrombosis, pulmonary embolism, or vasculitic or granulomatous disease (e.g., erythema nodosum or multiforme).

B. Endotracheal intubation is indicated emergently if there is clinical evidence of respiratory failure (e.g., refractory cyanosis, respiratory paradox) or refractory hypoxia and/or hypercarbia with acidosis. In patients with impending respiratory failure, give empiric antiasthmatic therapy with nebulized β agonists. IV steroids may require several hours to have a significant effect.

C. Drug-induced asthma may be caused by systemic or ophthalmic β blockers and NSAIDs. A trial of elimination of these should be made.

D. An obstructive spirometric pattern reversible by bronchodilators implies an asthmatic diathesis. Equivocal cases may be clarified by bronchoprovocation, exercise testing, or empiric courses of bronchodilators. Poorly reversible obstructive spirometric patterns suggest chronic obstructive pulmonary disease. Adjunctive diagnostic information may be provided by a history of excessive sputum (bronchitis, bronchiectasis), sweat chloride testing (cystic fibrosis), and CT scan (bronchiectasis, emphysema). An elevated urinary 5-hydroxyindoleacetic acid (5-HIAA) level in the pres-

ence of diarrhea, wheezing, and flushing may be found in carcinoid syndrome. Abnormally frequent and prolonged intraesophageal pH lowering often is present in reflux-associated bronchospasm. Large airway obstructions may be suggested by flattening of the inspiratory or expiratory limbs of the spirometric flow-volume loop.

E. Several atypical pneumonias, diffuse interstitial lung disease (DILD), autoimmune disorders, or vasculitis may present with wheezing. The optimal diagnostic approach depends on the clinical setting and specific x-ray findings. Rarely, pulmonary embolism presents with wheezing despite normal chest x-ray findings.

F. Previous chest radiographs are extremely useful in determining the duration and rapidity of evolution of existing abnormalities. Mass lesions and many infiltrates require invasive techniques of diagnosis (see D).

G. Invasive diagnostic techniques include bronchoscopy with bronchoalveolar lavage, Wang needle, or forceps bronchial biopsies; mediastinoscopy; transthoracic needle aspiration; and open lung biopsies. Determine the ideal approach by consultation with pulmonologists, radiologists, and surgeons. Decision making often is facilitated by CT scanning.

References

Holden DA, Mehta AC. Evaluation of wheezing in the nonasthmatic patient. Cleve Clin J Med 1990; 57:345.

Hollingsworth HM. Wheezing and stridor. Clin Chest Med 1987; 8:231.

Koster ME, Baughman RP, Loudon RG. Continuous adventitious lung sounds. J Asthma 1990; 27:237.

Miller RD, Hyatt RE. Evaluation of obstructing lesions of the trachea and larynx by flow-volume loops. Am Rev Respir Dis 1973; 108:475.

Teirstein AS. The differential diagnosis of asthma. Mt Sinai J Med 1991; 58:466.

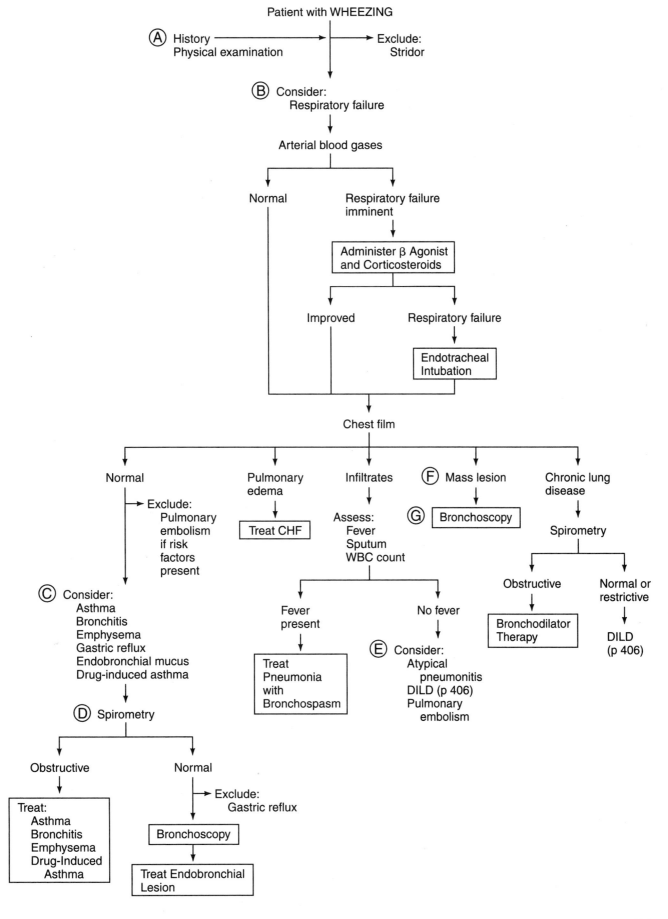

Patient with WHEEZING

Ⓐ History → Exclude:
Physical examination   Stridor

Ⓑ Consider:
Respiratory failure

Arterial blood gases

Normal   Respiratory failure
          imminent

Administer β Agonist
and Corticosteroids

Improved   Respiratory failure

Endotracheal
Intubation

Chest film

Normal   Pulmonary   Infiltrates   Ⓕ Mass lesion   Chronic lung
          edema   disease

→ Exclude: Treat CHF   Assess: Ⓖ Bronchoscopy   Spirometry
  Pulmonary   Fever
  embolism   Sputum
  if risk   WBC count
  factors
  present   Obstructive   Normal or
                                                                      restrictive

Ⓒ Consider: Fever   No fever   Bronchodilator   DILD
  Asthma   present   Therapy   (p 406)
  Bronchitis
  Emphysema   Treat   Ⓔ Consider:
  Gastric reflux Pneumonia   Atypical
  Endobronchial mucus with   pneumonitis
  Drug-induced asthma Bronchospasm DILD (p 406)
                                  Pulmonary
Ⓓ Spirometry   embolism

Obstructive   Normal

Treat: → Exclude:
  Asthma   Gastric reflux
  Bronchitis
  Emphysema   Bronchoscopy
  Drug-Induced
  Asthma   Treat Endobronchial
              Lesion

COUGH

Steven R. Knoper

In most instances, cough is beneficial. Generated by mechanical, thermal, or chemical stimulation of afferent receptors in the external auditory canal, paranasal sinuses, nose, pharynx, larynx, tracheobronchial tree, pleura, diaphragm, and stomach, cough acts as one of the main pulmonary defense mechanisms. Its importance increases when other defense mechanisms are impaired, such as in the absence of a gag reflex or the abnormal mucociliary clearance seen in chronic bronchitis. Nevertheless, in many patients it is either pathologic by itself or the manifestation of underlying disease that requires attention.

A. The history and physical examination assume overwhelming importance. Inquire about chronicity, frequency, whether it is productive and if so the quality and amount of phlegm, the existence or absence of sinusitis or rhinitis with attendant postnasal drip, heartburn, and smoking history. Factors that ameliorate or precipitate cough (e.g., positional or temporal) are important. Elicit concomitant signs such as hemoptysis (p 388). Chronic cough generally requires radiography; consider neoplastic, inflammatory, and immunologic causes. Acute cough usually is secondary to an infectious process, and if the history and physical are in concordance with this, radiography is not warranted unless symptoms persist or hemoptysis is present. Thick, discolored, purulent, and abundant phlegm is consistent with bronchiectasis, pulmonary abscess, acute bronchitis and pneumonia, or occasionally chronic bronchitis. The last-named often has a mucoid but noninfectious-appearing phlegm. The definition of chronic bronchitis is cough, with or without phlegm, for 3 months in two consecutive years. Positional change in cough occurs in pulmonary abscess, chronic bronchitis, bronchiectasis, postnasal drip, reflux esophagitis, and endobronchial tumor. If there is nocturnal cough, consider asthma, postnasal drip, or reflux esophagitis. Last, a medication history is important, especially in regard to angiotensin-converting enzyme inhibitors, which carry a high incidence of cough-related side effects.

B. Occasional patients with a presumed upper respiratory infection do not improve over time or after what is deemed appropriate therapy. This may be because there was no infection per se but rather an allergic or immunologic cause. Against the background of a now chronic process, new information may become available with a repeated history and physical examination. Chest radiography or a nasal smear for eosinophils may be helpful. Spirometry, with and without bronchodilators, may reveal occult asthma, or (rarely) bronchoprovocation with methacholine is necessary to yield the diagnosis. In the latter case, consider repeating the study in 2 to 3 months because postviral patients often have increased reaction to bronchoprovocation. Postviral cough may require both oral and inhaled steroids for prolonged periods.

C. Chest radiography is necessary in all patients in whom there is no clear etiology or who have a chronic cough, hemoptysis, or a new cough without an upper airway abnormality. Abnormalities may include pneumonia, pleural effusion, parenchymal mass such as neoplasm, bronchiectasis, interstitial lung disease, congestive heart failure (CHF), and signs of emphysema. The chest radiograph may be normal in the presence of a foreign body, endobronchial neoplasia, airway hyperresponsiveness, pulmonary hypertension, pulmonary embolic disease, and sinus problems.

D. If there are otolaryngologic symptoms such as hoarseness, referral is appropriate. The chest radiograph may have revealed hilar or aortopulmonary window fullness, suggesting recurrent laryngeal nerve paralysis. Chronic rhinitis or sinusitis, nasal or laryngeal polyposis, thyroiditis, laryngeal paralysis, cricoarytenoid arthritis, external auditory canal foreign bodies, or primary tumor may be discovered.

E. In patients with a normal chest radiograph, chronic cough, and a normal otolaryngologic examination, explore the possibility of occult asthma with pulmonary function testing. Usually this means spirometry, with and without bronchodilators, but in occasional patients bronchoprovocation, testing with methacholine or postexercise spirometry is necessary to confirm a diagnosis of airway hyperresponsiveness that is responsible for the cough. Examination of the inspiratory and expiratory flow loops may point to intra- or extrathoracic obstruction.

F. Patients in whom there is still no diagnosis after the above work-up may benefit from bronchoscopy. Endobronchial tumor, broncholith, tracheal web, or foreign body may be seen. In addition, if the preceding examination has suggested interstitial disease, transbronchial biopsies may be warranted. A negative work-up at this point should lead to patient reassurance, reanalysis over time, and symptomatic therapy.

References

Fitzgerald DJ, Speir WA, Callahan LA. Office evaluation of pulmonary function: beyond the numbers. Am Fam Physician 1996; 54:525.

Fuller RW, Jackson DM. Physiology and treatment of cough. Thorax 1990; 45:425.

Irwin RS, Carley FJ. The treatment of cough: a comprehensive review. Chest 1991; 99:1477.

Patrick H, Patrick F. Chronic cough. Med Clin North Am 1995; 79:361.

Rosenow EC 3rd. Persistent cough: causes and cures. Hosp Pract (Off Ed) 1996; 31:127.

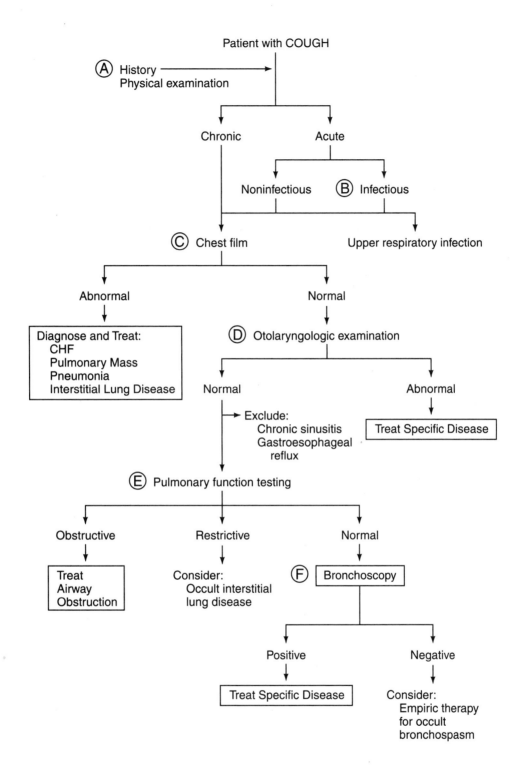

Patient with COUGH

A History
  Physical examination

Chronic   Acute

Noninfectious   B Infectious

C Chest film   Upper respiratory infection

Abnormal   Normal

Diagnose and Treat: D Otolaryngologic examination
  CHF
  Pulmonary Mass
  Pneumonia
  Interstitial Lung Disease

Normal   Abnormal

Exclude: Treat Specific Disease
  Chronic sinusitis
  Gastroesophageal
  reflux

E Pulmonary function testing

Obstructive   Restrictive   Normal

Treat   Consider: F Bronchoscopy
Airway   Occult interstitial
Obstruction   lung disease

                 Positive   Negative

                 Treat Specific Disease   Consider:
                                            Empiric therapy
                                            for occult
                                            bronchospasm

PULMONARY DYSPNEA

Anthony Camilli

Chronic dyspnea usually has a cardiac or pulmonary cause. Information elicited during the history and physical examination may strongly suggest a particular etiology, but laboratory studies often are required.

A. The chest film suggests an etiology not suspected by physical examination in some patients and will direct a specific work-up. Obvious congestive heart failure (CHF) can be treated while the etiology is clarified. A chest film showing chronic interstitial lung disease requires a specific diagnosis from sputum, bronchoscopy, or biopsy. A pleural effusion necessitates thoracentesis as the initial diagnostic test. Mass lesions of the mediastinum, pleura, and lung often require biopsy after further imaging.

B. Dyspnea in the context of a normal chest film suggests many pulmonary and cardiac causes. Airway obstructive disease may be easily detected with spirometry. ABGs may suggest neuromuscular problems or occult pulmonary interstitial disease by high P_{CO_2} or increased arterial-alveolar gradient.

C. Dyspnea in the context of a normal chest film, normal ABGs, and normal spirometry can be approached with exercise testing and echocardiography. Occult interstitial disease can be detected by arterial desaturation; an ischemic response would explain dyspnea on a cardiac basis.

References

Ingram RH Jr, Braunwald E. Dyspnea and pulmonary function. In: Fauci AS, Braunwald E, Isselbacher KJ, et al, eds. Harrison's principles of internal medicine. 14th ed. New York: McGraw-Hill, 1997:190.

Mahler DA. Dyspnea: diagnosis and management. Clin Chest Med 1987; 8:215.

Salzman GA. Evaluation of dyspnea. Hosp Pract (Off Ed) 1997; 32:195.

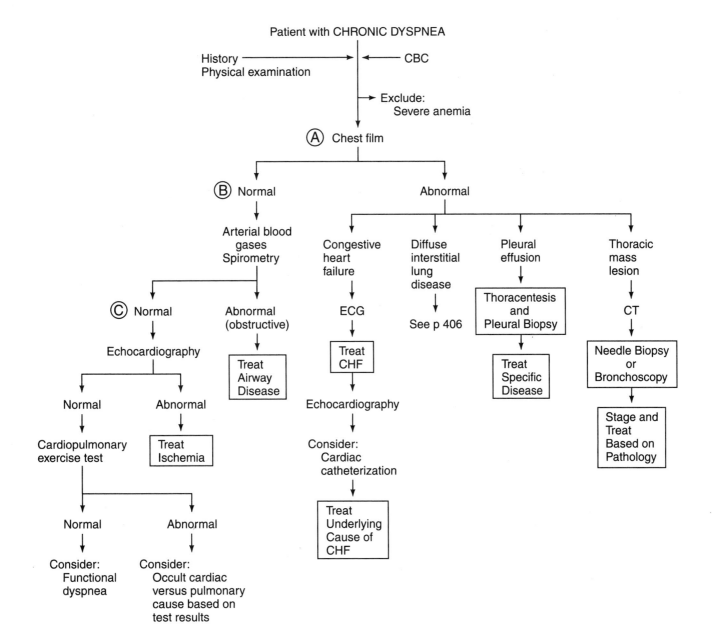

Patient with CHRONIC DYSPNEA

History ——————→ ←—— CBC
Physical examination

→ Exclude:
Severe anemia

(A) Chest film

(B) Normal   Abnormal

Arterial blood   Congestive   Diffuse   Pleural   Thoracic
gases   heart   interstitial   effusion   mass
Spirometry   failure   lung   lesion
                                   disease

(C) Normal   Abnormal   ECG   See p 406   Thoracentesis   CT
              (obstructive)   and
                                                 Pleural Biopsy

Echocardiography   Treat   Treat   Needle Biopsy
                   Airway   CHF   Treat   or
                   Disease   Specific   Bronchoscopy
                                                 Disease

Normal   Abnormal   Echocardiography   Stage and
                                                                   Treat
Cardiopulmonary   Treat   Consider: Based on
exercise test   Ischemia   Cardiac   Pathology
                             catheterization

Normal   Abnormal   Treat
                             Underlying
Consider: Consider: Cause of
Functional Occult cardiac   CHF
dyspnea   versus pulmonary
            cause based on
            test results

PLEURAL EFFUSION

Steven R. Knoper

An estimated 1 million patients per year in the United States develop a pleural effusion. Symptoms include dyspnea, cough, and/or pain. Many patients have no symptoms. In any one patient the symptoms usually reflect the causative disease. Radiographically, pleural effusions usually collect in dependent spaces, occasionally hide subpulmonically, and if loculated may appear as pseudotumors in the major fissure or as unusual pleural-based masses.

A. Examination of the thorax may reveal hemithoracic asymmetry, intercostal bulging or indentation, and occasionally subcutaneous edema as evidenced by pressure indentations. However, in many patients it is normal. Tactile fremitus over the effusion is reduced, percussion is dull, egophony at the superior margin often is elicited, and occasionally a pleural rub is heard on auscultation. Depending on the cause of the effusion, other organ systems may be abnormal; look for signs of pulmonary parenchymal disease, congestive heart failure (CHF), adenopathy, abdominal disease, arthritis, and other abnormalities.

B. The need for thoracentesis must be assessed individually and is guided by one's medical judgment. For instance, if the effusion occurs in the setting of pneumonia, thoracentesis is unnecessary if the height of freely flowing fluid on a lateral decubitus film is <1 cm because these rarely become complicated. Before attempting the procedure, ascertain the free-flowing nature with decubitus views. If the amount of fluid is small or loculated, aspiration with ultrasound guidance can be helpful.

C. The appearance is important. Most effusions are straw colored, but only 1 ml of blood per 0.5 L of effusion (assuming a normal hematocrit [Hct]) gives the fluid a bloody appearance. A pleural-to-blood Hct ratio <50% but a RBC count >100,000/mm^3 usually indicates pulmonary embolism, trauma, or malignancy—but not exclusively. If the fluid is purulent, an empyema is present and tube thoracostomy is indicated, although a chylous effusion can mimic a purulent appearance for those who have not seen one before. These can be differentiated by centrifugation or a fluid triglyceride level.

D. The effusion is considered an exudate if one of the following three conditions is met: (1) pleural-to-serum lactate dehydrogenase (LDH) ratio >0.6, (2) pleural LDH value more than two-thirds the upper normal value for the serum, and (3) the pleural-to-serum total protein ratio >0.5. Transudative effusions require no further workup; treat the underlying condition. Some diseases may appear in some patients as transudates and others as exudates; this is true of myxedema, and pulmonary embolism-effusion from the latter diagnosis occurs as a transudate 25% of the time.

E. The sensitivity of cytologic examination is 40–87%. Usually, if three samples are submitted from three different thoracenteses separated by a day or more, the sensitivity is about 80%. Add heparin to the collection container before obtaining the sample to prevent clotting. Occasionally, the pathologist can examine cell blocks cut from a centrifuged "button" specimen to increase the yield. Pleural biopsy usually only adds 10% additional sensitivity to that of cytology alone when the underlying cause is malignancy.

F. Most physicians do not proceed through the decision process outlined in this decision tree to decide that a parapneumonic effusion is present, but instead decide on the basis of the history and physical examination that pneumonia is present. Following Occam's razor, the effusion usually is a result of the pneumonia. The major decision in managing a parapneumonic effusion is whether to place a thoracostomy tube, and if so when. Gram stain, fluid pH (as measured from an iced, heparinized sample collected in the same fashion as that for ABG analysis), fluid glucose, and fluid LDH are the criteria by which the need for a thoracostomy tube is judged. In borderline pH values, for example, a low glucose or high LDH level indicates that the effusion is likely to become complicated over time and that earlier thoracostomy tube placement is appropriate.

G. Not all laboratories differentiate small lymphocytes from mononuclear cells, which consist of mesothelial cells, macrophages, plasma cells, malignant cells, and lymphocytes. Their presence in transudates has no significance. When seen in exudates, malignancy or tuberculosis was the diagnosis 94% of the time (90/96) when two series were added (present in 96/211 exudates). Because the ability to diagnose these two diseases is increased with pleural biopsy, consider this procedure when small lymphocytes are seen.

References

Light RW. Symposium on pleural effusion. Clin Chest Med 1985; 6:1.

Light RW. Pleural diseases. 3rd ed. Baltimore: Williams & Wilkins, 1995.

McElvein RB. Procedures in the evaluation of chest disease. Clin Chest Med 1992; 13:1.

Seibert AF, Haynes J Jr, Middleton R, Bass JB Jr. Tuberculous pleural effusion: twenty-year experience. Chest 1991; 99:883.

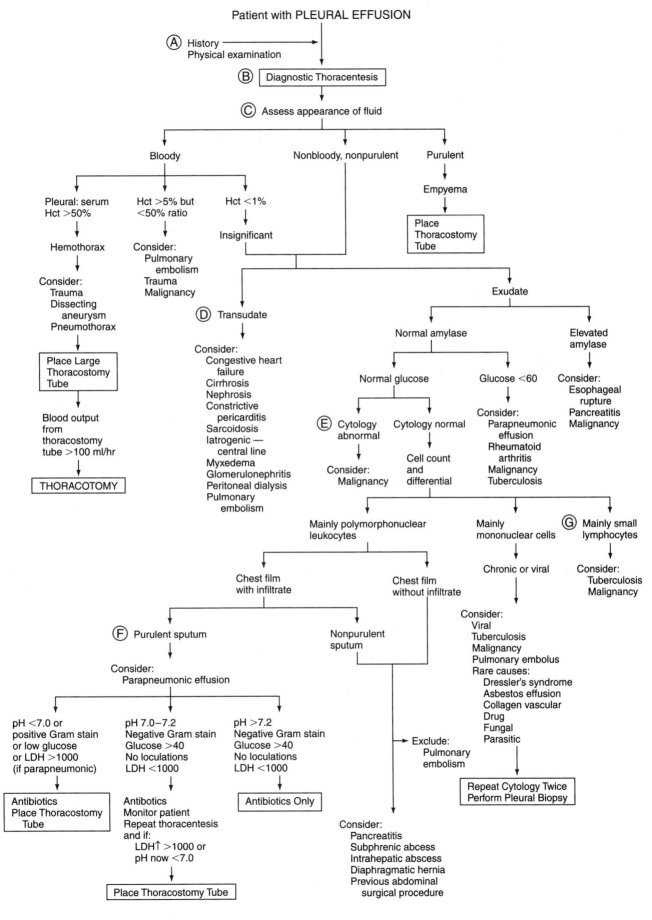

Patient with PLEURAL EFFUSION

(A) History — Physical examination

(B) Diagnostic Thoracentesis

(C) Assess appearance of fluid

Bloody

Pleural: serum Hct >50%
↓
Hemothorax
↓
Consider:
Trauma
Dissecting aneurysm
Pneumothorax
↓
Place Large Thoracostomy Tube
↓
Blood output from thoracostomy tube >100 ml/hr
↓
THORACOTOMY

Hct >5% but <50% ratio
↓
Consider:
Pulmonary embolism
Trauma
Malignancy

Hct <1%
↓
Insignificant

Nonbloody, nonpurulent

(D) Transudate
↓
Consider:
Congestive heart failure
Cirrhosis
Nephrosis
Constrictive pericarditis
Sarcoidosis
Iatrogenic — central line
Myxedema
Glomerulonephritis
Peritoneal dialysis
Pulmonary embolism

Purulent

Empyema
↓
Place Thoracostomy Tube

Exudate

Normal amylase

Normal glucose

(E) Cytology abnormal
↓
Consider:
Malignancy

Cytology normal
↓
Cell count and differential

Glucose <60
↓
Consider:
Parapneumonic effusion
Rheumatoid arthritis
Malignancy
Tuberculosis

Elevated amylase
↓
Consider:
Esophageal rupture
Pancreatitis
Malignancy

Mainly polymorphonuclear leukocytes

Chest film with infiltrate

(F) Purulent sputum
↓
Consider:
Parapneumonic effusion

pH <7.0 or positive Gram stain or low glucose or LDH >1000 (if parapneumonic)
↓
Antibiotics
Place Thoracostomy Tube

pH 7.0–7.2
Negative Gram stain
Glucose >40
No loculations
LDH <1000
↓
Antibiotics
Monitor patient
Repeat thoracentesis and if:
LDH↑ >1000 or pH now <7.0
↓
Place Thoracostomy Tube

pH >7.2
Negative Gram stain
Glucose >40
No loculations
LDH <1000
↓
Antibiotics Only

Chest film without infiltrate

Nonpurulent sputum

Exclude:
Pulmonary embolism
↓
Consider:
Pancreatitis
Subphrenic abcess
Intrahepatic abscess
Diaphragmatic hernia
Previous abdominal surgical procedure

Mainly mononuclear cells
↓
Chronic or viral
↓
Consider:
Viral
Tuberculosis
Malignancy
Pulmonary embolus
Rare causes:
Dressler's syndrome
Asbestos effusion
Collagen vascular
Drug
Fungal
Parasitic
↓
Repeat Cytology Twice
Perform Pleural Biopsy

(G) Mainly small lymphocytes
↓
Consider:
Tuberculosis
Malignancy

MEDIASTINAL ADENOPATHY

Anthony Camilli

The differential diagnosis of lesions causing mediastinal adenopathy includes malignancies (primary and secondary) and granulomatous disease.

A. Detection of peripheral adenopathy in a patient with suspected mediastinal adenopathy may provide a diagnosis by biopsy of the superficial lesion. Risk factors such as age, smoking history, or area of incidence may suggest malignant versus benign disease. A history of risk factors for HIV infection may suggest AIDS-related adenopathy.

B. The chest CT scan allows one to distinguish between masses, nodes, and vascular structures in the hilum and mediastinum. The diagnosis of vascular lesions such as thoracic aneurysms and enlarged pulmonary arteries can be easily confirmed by CT. CT more precisely defines the anatomic location and size of masses, or the distribution and size of nodes, and often shows more extensive adenopathy than revealed by chest radiography.

C. After exclusion of thromboembolism and other vascular lesions of the hilum, the principal differential diagnosis of unilateral hilar adenopathy is between fungal infection and carcinoma or lymphoma. Skin tests and fungal serologic studies may suggest a diagnosis of coccidio-idomycosis or histoplasmosis. Bronchoscopy often leads to a diagnosis with biopsy of an endobronchial lesion. If bronchoscopy is negative, attempt needle biopsy of the hilum with CT guidance. Thoracotomy is rarely required for diagnosis.

D. In patients with bilateral hilar adenopathy, the chest film or chest CT (particularly with thin-section technique) may confirm or demonstrate pulmonary parenchymal disease. Sarcoidosis often presents with bilateral hilar adenopathy and may include involvement of the lung parenchyma or airways. Bronchoscopy with transbronchial biopsy may confirm the diagnosis, particularly if there is evidence of parenchymal involvement.

References

Eisenberg RL. Chest and cardiovascular imaging: an atlas of differential diagnosis. New York: Raven Press, 1993.

Lillington GA. Bilateral hilar enlargement. In: Lillington GA, ed. A diagnostic approach to chest diseases. 3rd ed. Baltimore: Williams & Wilkins, 1987:283.

Lillington GA. Unilateral hilar enlargement. In: Lillington GA, ed. A diagnostic approach to chest diseases. 3rd ed. Baltimore: Williams & Wilkins, 1987:274.

THORACIC ADENOPATHY Suspected

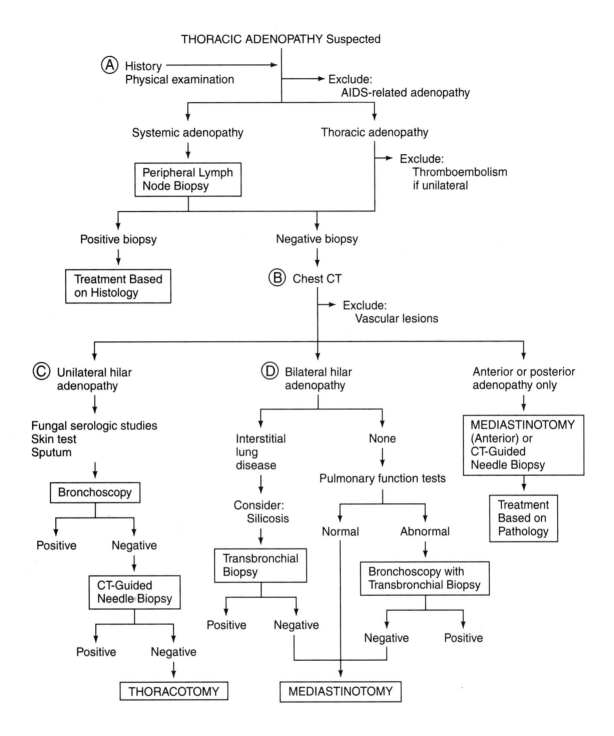

A History ────────→
Physical examination

Exclude:
AIDS-related adenopathy

Systemic adenopathy   Thoracic adenopathy

Peripheral Lymph
Node Biopsy

Exclude:
Thromboembolism
if unilateral

Positive biopsy   Negative biopsy

Treatment Based
on Histology

B Chest CT

Exclude:
Vascular lesions

C Unilateral hilar
adenopathy

D Bilateral hilar
adenopathy

Anterior or posterior
adenopathy only

Fungal serologic studies
Skin test
Sputum

Interstitial
lung
disease

None

MEDIASTINOTOMY
(Anterior) or
CT-Guided
Needle Biopsy

Bronchoscopy

Consider:
Silicosis

Pulmonary function tests

Treatment
Based on
Pathology

Positive   Negative

Normal   Abnormal

CT-Guided
Needle Biopsy

Transbronchial
Biopsy

Bronchoscopy with
Transbronchial Biopsy

Positive   Negative

Positive   Negative

Negative   Positive

THORACOTOMY

MEDIASTINOTOMY

401

SOLITARY PULMONARY NODULE

John W. Lace

A. A solitary pulmonary nodule is a common abnormality seen on radiography. It is a pulmonary opacity surrounded completely by lung, <4 cm in diameter, and without associated atelectasis or adenopathy. Malignant causes include primary lung neoplasms and metastases from distant primary tumors. Benign causes include infectious and noninfectious inflammatory lesions, as well as benign tumors such as hamartomas. Perform a physical examination with careful attention to the skin, lymphatic system, and upper respiratory tract in addition to the chest.

B. Exclude pseudonodules from intralobar fluid collections, nipple shadows, or other extrathoracic opacities.

C. Radiographic characteristics of solitary pulmonary nodules may suggest an underlying etiology. The presence of certain patterns of calcification is the most reliable radiographic criterion of benignity. A diligent search for old chest radiographs is warranted.

D. Pulmonary nodules usually show a constant growth rate throughout their clinical course unless altered by therapeutic intervention. The growth rate is expressed as a doubling time (the time it takes for the nodule to double in volume), which is determined on radiography to be an increase in diameter by a factor of 1.27. Malignant nodules usually show doubling times of 20–400 days. Nodules that show stability for >2 years do not require further follow-up.

E. CT of the chest is more sensitive in detection of calcification, multiple nodules, or mediastinal adenopathy. The type of calcification observed when present is useful in further risk stratification of patients.

F. The yield of fiberoptic bronchoscopy in the diagnosis of solitary pulmonary nodules is modest, and it is less effective in confirmatory diagnosis of benign lesions, which is the main goal of the procedure in avoiding unnecessary thoracotomy. Larger, more central lesions are more amenable to bronchoscopic diagnosis which also allows inspection of the central airways, and detection of endobronchial lesions as well as extrinsic compression from nodal enlargement. Risks of the procedure include pneumothorax and pulmonary hemorrhage. Always consider the preference and clinical status of the patient.

G. Transthoracic needle aspiration is simple to perform and has a low complication rate in experienced hands. Positive and negative predictive values >90% are achievable. Risks include pneumothorax and pulmonary hemorrhage. Chest tubes are required in 5–10% of patients. Again, always consider the preference and clinical status of the patient.

H. Mediastinoscopy is useful in the staging of malignancy once the diagnosis is established and there is radiographic evidence of hilar or mediastinal involvement.

I. Thoracotomy was often the first diagnostic procedure in the past, before the advent of less invasive means of obtaining tissue for examination. Thoracoscopy has now been developed as a technique for diagnosis and sometimes resection of pulmonary nodules. Immediate thoracotomy may yet be an appropriate choice in a patient with multiple risk factors that indicate a high probability of neoplasm. The pulmonary reserve of the patient is an important consideration when planning a pulmonary resection.

References

Lillington GA, Caskey CI. Evaluation and management of solitary and multiple pulmonary nodules. Clin Chest Med 1993; 14:111.

Salim A, Kathawalla , et al. Solitary pulmonary nodule. In: Bone R, ed. Pulmonary and critical care medicine on CD-ROM. St Louis: Mosby, 1996.

Santambrogio L, Nosotti M, Bellaviti N, Mezetti M. Videothoracoscopy versus thoracotomy for the diagnosis of the indeterminate solitary pulmonary nodule. Ann Thorac Surg 1995; 59:868.

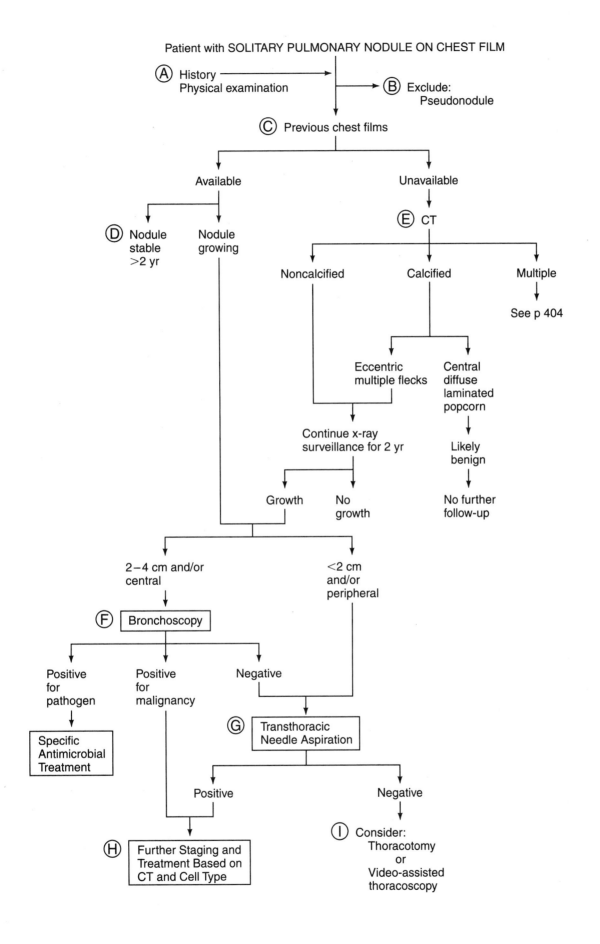

Patient with SOLITARY PULMONARY NODULE ON CHEST FILM

Ⓐ History
Physical examination → Ⓑ Exclude: Pseudonodule

Ⓒ Previous chest films

Available | Unavailable

Ⓓ Nodule stable >2 yr | Nodule growing

Ⓔ CT

Noncalcified | Calcified | Multiple

See p 404

Eccentric multiple flecks | Central diffuse laminated popcorn

Continue x-ray surveillance for 2 yr | Likely benign

Growth | No growth | No further follow-up

2–4 cm and/or central | <2 cm and/or peripheral

Ⓕ Bronchoscopy

Positive for pathogen | Positive for malignancy | Negative

Specific Antimicrobial Treatment

Ⓖ Transthoracic Needle Aspiration

Positive | Negative

Ⓗ Further Staging and Treatment Based on CT and Cell Type

Ⓘ Consider: Thoracotomy or Video-assisted thoracoscopy

MULTIPLE PULMONARY NODULES

John W. Lace

A. Multiple pulmonary nodules are usually defined as multiple discrete lesions discovered on chest radiography, at least two being >8 mm in diameter. Metastatic carcinoma to the lungs is a common cause of multiple pulmonary nodules. Others to consider include alveolar cell carcinoma; pulmonary lymphoma; multiple primary lung neoplasms; benign neoplasms; other benign conditions, including granulomas, both infectious and noninfectious; and arteriovenous malformations (AVMs). Combinations of lesions may occur and serial radiography may show that these lesions have appeared at different times. The presence of combinations is particularly important in the case of a potentially resectable lung carcinoma together with other benign nodular lesions. The history may reveal a geographic predisposition to histoplasmosis, coccidioidomycosis, or parasitic infestations. History indicating that the patient may be immunocompromised can be particularly important. Physical examination should include careful examination of the upper respiratory tract, eyes, skin, lymphatics, and in young males testicles. The radiographic appearance of the lesions on chest radiography, standard tomography, or CT scans can narrow the differential diagnosis. Additional imaging studies such as CT may demonstrate additional nodules more accessible by a particular diagnostic technique.

B. Patients are best classified into three groups: those with known extrapulmonary malignancy, those with extrapulmonary malignancy suggested by history, and those with no evidence of extrapulmonary malignancy. In the first group, the nodules are highly likely to be metastases. Obtaining a tissue diagnosis by invasive studies is warranted if the therapy would be changed or if there is doubt about the diagnosis.

C. When an extrapulmonary malignancy is suspected but not confirmed, make a vigorous search for the primary lesion. Transthoracic needle aspiration may assist in the search for the primary lesion and establish the pulmonary lesions as metastases.

D. Infections may at times be diagnosed by cultures of appropriate samples or by serologic studies. If septic emboli are suspected, start appropriate empiric antimicrobial therapy after cultures are taken. AVMs may be suggested by radiographic criteria and diagnosed by angiography.

E. Transthoracic needle aspiration is simple to perform and has a low complication rate in experienced hands. High positive predictive values are achievable. Risks include pneumothorax and pulmonary hemorrhage. Chest tubes are required in 5–10% of patients. Always consider the patient's clinical status.

F. The yield of fiberoptic bronchoscopy in the diagnosis of multiple pulmonary nodules is modest, and it is less effective in confirmatory diagnosis of benign lesions. Larger, more central lesions are more amenable to bronchoscopic diagnosis, which also allows inspection of the central airways. Risks of the procedure include pneumothorax and pulmonary hemorrhage. Always consider the patient's clinical status.

G. If only two nodules are present and there is evidence that one of these is old and stable, the second nodule may be a bronchogenic carcinoma that is potentially resectable for cure. The patient's pulmonary reserve is an important consideration when planning a pulmonary resection. Thoracoscopy may be used for diagnosis and sometimes resection of pulmonary nodules. Thoracotomy also may be indicated for localized hydatid cysts, for symptomatic multiple AVMs, and for diagnosis of opportunistic infections in immunocompromised hosts. Mediastinoscopy may be indicated before thoracotomy if there is evidence of mediastinal enlargement on imaging studies.

H. Miliary tuberculosis produces smaller nodules than the classic form. It usually presents as a diffuse pattern of 1- to 2-mm nodules throughout the lung fields. Diagnosis is made by examination of transbronchial, liver, or bone marrow biopsies.

References

Grodzin J, Bone C. Radiographic patterns of pulmonary disease. In: Bone R, ed. Pulmonary and critical care medicine on CD-ROM. St Louis: Mosby, 1996.

Lillington GA, Caskey CI. Evaluation and management of solitary and multiple pulmonary nodules. Clin Chest Med 1993; 14:111.

Patient with MULTIPLE PULMONARY NODULES ON CHEST FILM

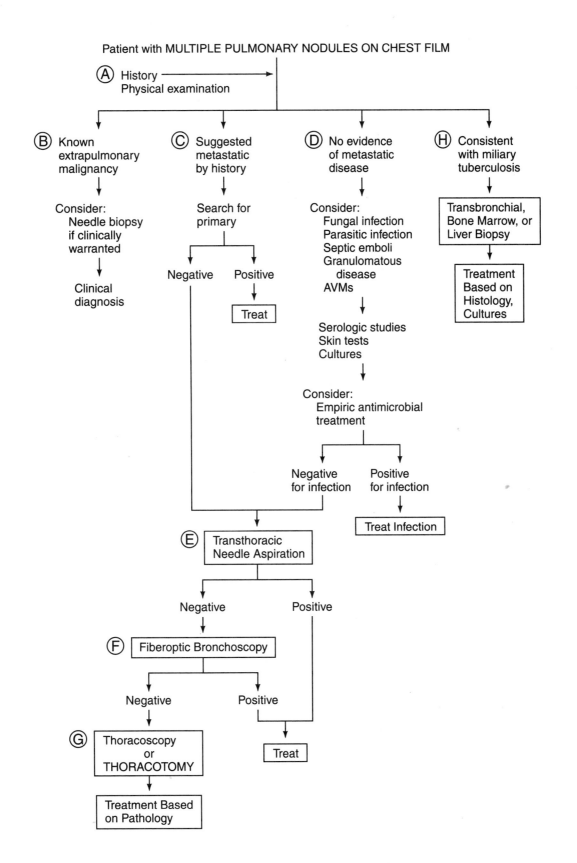

(A) History
Physical examination

(B) Known extrapulmonary malignancy

Consider:
Needle biopsy if clinically warranted

Clinical diagnosis

(C) Suggested metastatic by history

Search for primary

Negative

Positive

Treat

(D) No evidence of metastatic disease

Consider:
Fungal infection
Parasitic infection
Septic emboli
Granulomatous disease
AVMs

Serologic studies
Skin tests
Cultures

Consider:
Empiric antimicrobial treatment

Negative for infection

Positive for infection

Treat Infection

(H) Consistent with miliary tuberculosis

Transbronchial, Bone Marrow, or Liver Biopsy

Treatment Based on Histology, Cultures

(E) Transthoracic Needle Aspiration

Negative

Positive

(F) Fiberoptic Bronchoscopy

Negative

Positive

Treat

(G) Thoracoscopy or THORACOTOMY

Treatment Based on Pathology

DIFFUSE INTERSTITIAL LUNG DISEASE

Anthony Camilli

A. The clinical history (with attention to exposures), together with the chest film and other clinical findings, suggest a clinical diagnosis of diffuse interstitial lung disease in many cases. Such working diagnosis includes the pneumoconioses, congestive heart failure (CHF), post–adult respiratory distress syndrome, viral infections, and collagen vascular disease and may require further confirmation. Atypical findings or other considerations may require further tests, including biopsy.

B. Perform skin tests, sputum cultures, and where the diagnosis is not strongly suggested, serologic studies to establish diagnoses of mycobacterial and fungal disease. If these tests are negative, pulmonary function tests (PFTs) to assess obstructive versus restrictive physiology are helpful.

C. Many obstructive diseases (e.g., bronchitis, asthma, bronchiectasis) show changes on chest films representing fibrosis associated with the underlying disease. These diagnoses often can be made clinically. Biopsy confirmation in typical presentations of interstitial disease with airway obstruction may be necessary to diagnose conditions such as bronchiolitis obliterans or lymphangiomyomatosis.

D. Some patients with restrictive physiology may be diagnosed by bronchoscopy with bronchoalveolar lavage and transbronchial biopsy. Some of these require a more extensive tissue diagnosis with open lung biopsy. Careful consideration of clinical history, chest films, and bronchoscopic findings should determine the need for thoracotomy.

Reference

Reynolds HY. Interstitial lung diseases. In: Fauci AS, Braunwald E, Isselbacher KJ, et al, eds. Harrison's principles of internal medicine. 14th ed. New York: McGraw-Hill, 1997:1460.

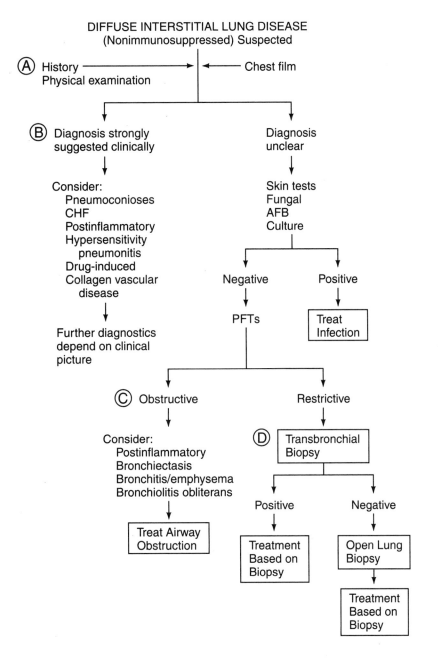

DIFFUSE INTERSTITIAL LUNG DISEASE
(Nonimmunosuppressed) Suspected

Ⓐ History ──────────→   ←────── Chest film
Physical examination

Ⓑ Diagnosis strongly
suggested clinically

Consider:
  Pneumoconioses
  CHF
  Postinflammatory
  Hypersensitivity
    pneumonitis
  Drug-induced
  Collagen vascular
    disease

Further diagnostics
depend on clinical
picture

Diagnosis
unclear

Skin tests
Fungal
AFB
Culture

Negative   Positive

PFTs   Treat
                            Infection

Ⓒ Obstructive   Restrictive

Consider: Ⓓ Transbronchial
  Postinflammatory   Biopsy
  Bronchiectasis
  Bronchitis/emphysema
  Bronchiolitis obliterans

                        Positive   Negative

Treat Airway   Treatment   Open Lung
Obstruction   Based on   Biopsy
                       Biopsy
                                          Treatment
                                          Based on
                                          Biopsy

POSITIVE TUBERCULIN SKIN TEST

Anthony Camilli

The tuberculin skin test is particularly useful to identify persons with infection from *Mycobacterium tuberculosis* who do not have clinical disease. The intradermal test (Mantoux) must be properly administered using 5 tuberculin units and properly interpreted at 48–72 hours to achieve best results. The American Thoracic Society and Centers for Disease Control and Prevention recommend that the criteria for positivity of the Mantoux test be based on risk group to improve sensitivity: 5-mm induration for those with HIV infection, close contact with an active case of tuberculosis (TB), and chest films showing healed TB; 10-mm induration for those from countries with a high prevalence of TB, IV drug abusers, medically underserved populations, residents of long-term care facilities, and those with comorbid medical conditions; and 15-mm induration for all others.

A. Chest films help determine whether the evidence of tuberculous infection is associated with active clinical disease, healed TB, or a normal chest film. Obtain multiple sputum smears and cultures if there are any x-ray abnormalities. Treat patients with active disease with at least two antituberculous drugs, and consider the possibility of isoniazid (INH) resistance when appropriate.

B. Prevention of tuberculous disease in those with tuberculous infection can be achieved by treatment with INH for 6–12 months. Patients with positive tuberculin tests and the highest risk of tuberculous disease include those (1) with close contact with infectious cases; (2) with a recent skin test conversion; (3) with previous TB who never received chemotherapy; (4) with stable radiographic changes of "healed" TB and negative sputum; (5) with silicosis, diabetes mellitus, hematologic or reticuloendothelial malignancy, HIV positivity, end-stage renal disease, or chronic undernutrition; and (6) who have received steroids, immunosuppressives, or gastrectomy.

C. The benefits of INH preventive therapy must be weighed against the risk of INH toxicity in the form of hepatitis. Studies show a clear relationship between age and INH hepatotoxicity and recommend that, in patients with no special risks, preventive therapy be limited to those <35 years of age.

D. In young people with no risk factors and those without comorbid conditions or other risks, those with adverse reactions to INH or active liver disease are excluded from preventive therapy.

E. Clinical monitoring at monthly intervals for liver damage or other adverse effects is essential. Those >35 years of age or with other risks of INH toxicity (possible drug interactions, continual alcohol use) should receive initial and subsequent monitoring of transaminase or other relevant clinical measures during preventive therapy. For those in whom resistant organisms are suspected (e.g., an INH-resistant source case) several alternatives have been proposed. Options include a different or additional drug, INH alone, or observation. Consider the risks of INH resistance, TB disease, and potential drug toxicity when deciding on alternatives.

References

American Thoracic Society. Diagnostic standards and classification of tuberculosis. Am Rev Respir Dis 1990; 142:725.

Bass JB Jr, Farer LS, Hopewell PC, et al. Treatment of tuberculosis and tuberculous infection in adults and children. American Thoracic Society and Centers for Disease Control and Prevention. Am J Respir Crit Care Med 1994; 149:1359.

Centers for Disease Control and Prevention. Initial therapy for tuberculosis in the era of multidrug resistance: recommendations of the Advisory Council for the Elimination of Tuberculosis. MMWR 1993; 42(RR-7).

Iseman MD. Treatment of multidrug-resistant tuberculosis. N Engl J Med 1993; 328:527.

McCollister P, Neff NE. Outpatient management of tuberculosis. Am Fam Physician 1996; 53:1579.

Telzak E, Sepkowitz K, Alpert P, et al. Multidrug-resistant tuberculosis in patients without HIV infection. N Engl J Med 1995; 333:907.

Weiss SE, Slocum PC, Blais FX, et al. The effect of directly observed therapy on the rates of drug resistance and relapse in tuberculosis. N Engl J Med 1994; 330:1179.

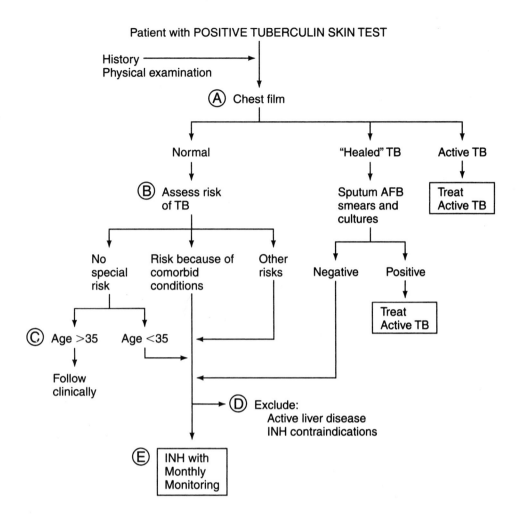

Patient with POSITIVE TUBERCULIN SKIN TEST

History ——————→
Physical examination

Ⓐ Chest film

Normal   "Healed" TB   Active TB

Ⓑ Assess risk of TB   Sputum AFB smears and cultures   Treat Active TB

No special risk   Risk because of comorbid conditions   Other risks   Negative   Positive

Ⓒ Age >35   Age <35   Treat Active TB

Follow clinically

Ⓓ Exclude:
Active liver disease
INH contraindications

Ⓔ INH with Monthly Monitoring

RESPIRATORY SYMPTOMS AND OCCUPATIONAL EXPOSURE TO ASBESTOS

Anthony Camilli

Asbestos-related disease of the thorax includes both benign and malignant disorders of the lung parenchyma and the pleura.

A. An occupational history of asbestos exposure may be described by the patient or may be suggested by specific work situations, including use of insulating materials, automotive brake repair, or shipyard employment.

B. A lung mass in an older asbestos-exposed smoker is likely to be malignant. The size and location of the lesion suggest needle biopsy or bronchoscopy as the initial diagnostic test. Staging for possible resection follows consideration of cell type, resectability, and operability.

C. Interstitial lung disease caused by asbestos is a diffuse process radiographically characterized by small, irregular opacities primarily in the bases. If exposure history, latency, physical and chest x-ray findings, and pulmonary function test changes are consistent, a clinical diagnosis of asbestosis can be made. Atypical presentations may require a tissue diagnosis.

D. Pleural lesions may show the characteristic shape, location, and calcification of plaques or may be otherwise. CT scanning may help identify noncalcified plaques from masses. Pleural mass lesions from mesothelioma are difficult to diagnose by needle biopsy and may require thoracotomy.

E. Pleural plaques are characteristically seen on the diaphragm and chest wall. The raised lesions of the parietal pleura are more easily identified when viewed tangentially. Oblique films or chest CT improve sensitivity.

F. Diffuse pleural thickening occurs as a sequence of asbestos exposure and may restrict lung function because of a "trapped lung." Lung volume tests help identify this restriction.

G. A pleural effusion in an asbestos-exposed person may be caused by occult malignancy (lung cancer or mesothelioma), a non–asbestos-related condition, or a benign asbestos effusion (a diagnosis of exclusion). Repeat radiography after thoracentesis; CT scans can help identify an associated mass.

References

Becklake MR. Asbestos-related diseases of the lung and other organs: their epidemiology and implications for clinical practice. Am Rev Respir Dis 1976; 114:187.

Frank AL. Medical and public health approaches to asbestos disease. Mt Sinai J Med 1995; 62:401.

Wagner GR. Asbestosis and silicosis. Lancet 1997; 349:1311.

Patient with RESPIRATORY SYMPTOMS AND OCCUPATIONAL EXPOSURE TO ASBESTOS

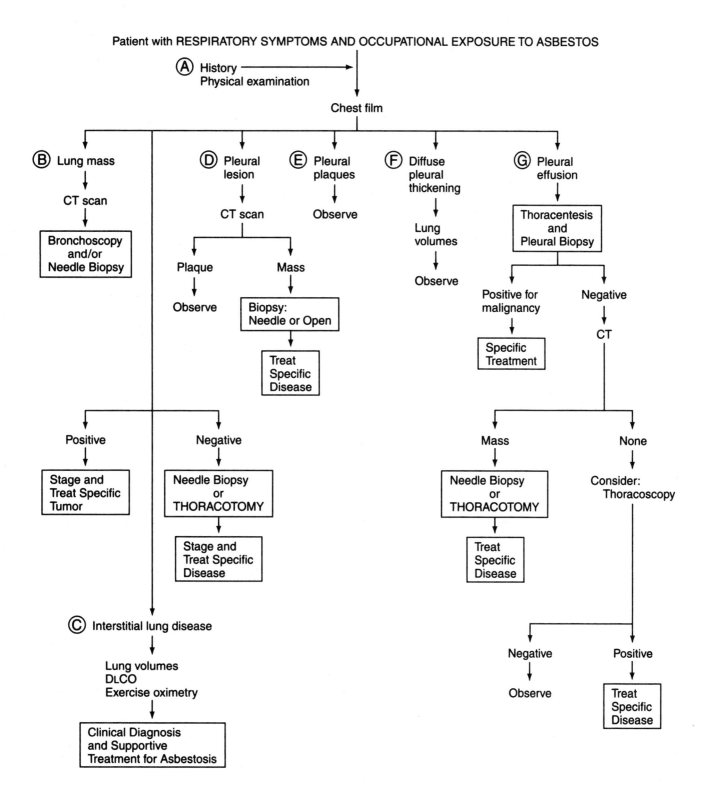

411

RHEUMATOLOGY

MONOARTICULAR ARTHRITIS

Deborah Doud

A. A complete history is vital. Monarthritis of acute onset usually indicates trauma, infection, or crystal-induced arthropathies. Monarthritis persisting >4–6 weeks suggests chronic conditions such as tuberculosis, fungal infection, osteoarthritis, or tumor. A complete physical examination is necessary to determine whether an articular or a periarticular disorder is present and whether a systemic process is involved.

B. Aspiration of the affected joint with subsequent synovial fluid analysis is always indicated in the evaluation of monarticular arthritis. The synovial fluid WBC count is the single most important quantitative measurement of synovial inflammation. If >5000, an inflammatory process is present; if <2000, the effusion is noninflammatory. Clinical correlation, however, is mandatory.

C. If analysis of fluid, including Gram stain, culture, sensitivity, and examination for crystals, does not reveal a diagnosis, perform radiography and a repeat synovial fluid analysis, including cultures and smears for acid-fast bacteria and fungus.

D. When chronic monarthritis persists for >4–6 weeks without a definite diagnosis, a synovial biopsy is indicated. This can reliably diagnose tuberculosis or fungal synovitis, amyloid (prevalent in dialysis patients), pigmented villonodular synovitis, and other tumors. If no diagnosis is obtained from synovial biopsy, follow the patient closely for development of new symptoms.

E. If analysis of fluid reveals monosodium urate crystals intracellularly, the diagnosis of gouty arthritis is established (p 442). Rhomboid-shaped, positively birefringent calcium pyrophosphate crystals indicate calcium pyrophosphate deposition disease (CPPD) or pseudogout. Consider disorders associated with CPPD, such as hyperparathyroidism, hemochromatosis, ochronosis, and Wilson's disease in a patient <60 years of age with pseudogout. Calcium hydroxyapatite crystals can be identified only by electron microscopy or alizarin red stain. Identification of crystals in joint fluid does not negate the possibility of coexistent infection, although this would be rare.

F. Acute bacterial arthritis is a true medical emergency. The most common cause of septic arthritis is disseminated gonococcal infection (DGI). Synovial fluid cultures from patients with DGI are positive <50% of the time. If DGI is suspected, other sites (blood, genitourinary, pharyngeal, rectal, and skin lesions) should be cultured. The most common nongonococcal infectious arthritis is due to *Staphylococcus aureus*. Two thirds of persons with nongonococcal infectious arthritis show evidence of a primary focus of infection elsewhere. Thus patients with an unexplained arthritis associated with pneumonia, genitourinary infection, or other infection should be presumed to have an infectious arthritis.

G. Hemarthrosis may result from trauma, excessive anticoagulant, inherited coagulopathies, or a neuropathic joint. It must be distinguished from a traumatic tap. The effusion of hemarthrosis is uniformly bloody throughout the aspiration, and the fluid will not spontaneously clot.

H. Persistent bloody effusions in the absence of trauma, anticoagulation, or a coagulopathy should lead to consideration of a tumor, particularly pigmented villonodular synovitis. In such cases, a synovial biopsy is indicated for accurate diagnosis.

I. Osteoarthritis may be present when there is little synovial inflammation in proportion to the degree of destruction of bone and cartilage, and the synovial fluid WBC count is <2000. In neuropathic arthropathy the loss of pain and proprioceptive responses allows joints to exceed normal ranges of motion and develop significant joint instability. Ultimately, dislocation and deformity occur. Diabetes mellitus is the most commonly associated disease, but neuropathic arthropathy may occur in a variety of neurologic diseases. Avascular necrosis is a common cause of monarthritis of the hip, shoulders, and knees in young people with systemic disease requiring corticosteroid therapy. It occurs in a variety of other conditions such as alcoholism, barotrauma, hemoglobinopathies, diabetes, hyperlipidemia, hyperuricemia, and systemic lupus erythematosus.

References

Canaso JJ. Rheumatology in primary care. Philadelphia: WB Saunders, 1997.

Schmid FR. Approach to monoarticular arthritis. In: Kelley WN, Harris ED, Ruddy S, Sledge CB, eds. Textbook of rheumatology. 5th ed. Philadelphia: WB Saunders, 1997.

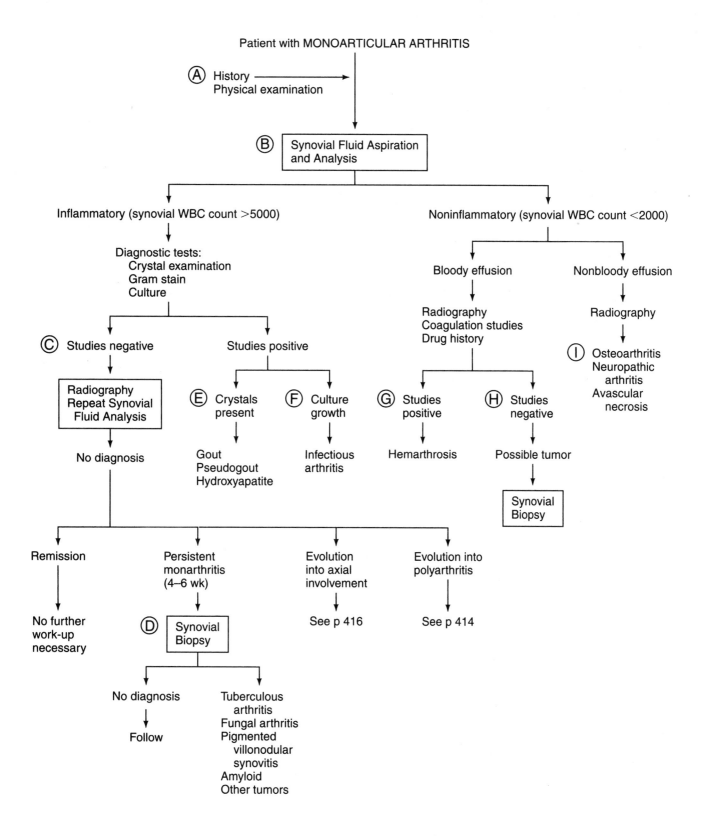

Patient with MONOARTICULAR ARTHRITIS

(A) History ———→
Physical examination

(B) Synovial Fluid Aspiration
and Analysis

Inflammatory (synovial WBC count >5000)

Noninflammatory (synovial WBC count <2000)

Diagnostic tests:
Crystal examination
Gram stain
Culture

Bloody effusion

Nonbloody effusion

Radiography
Coagulation studies
Drug history

Radiography

(C) Studies negative

Studies positive

(I) Osteoarthritis
Neuropathic
arthritis
Avascular
necrosis

Radiography
Repeat Synovial
Fluid Analysis

(E) Crystals
present

(F) Culture
growth

(G) Studies
positive

(H) Studies
negative

No diagnosis

Gout
Pseudogout
Hydroxyapatite

Infectious
arthritis

Hemarthrosis

Possible tumor

Synovial
Biopsy

Remission

Persistent
monarthritis
(4–6 wk)

Evolution
into axial
involvement

Evolution into
polyarthritis

No further
work-up
necessary

(D) Synovial
Biopsy

See p 416

See p 414

No diagnosis

Tuberculous
arthritis
Fungal arthritis
Pigmented
villonodular
synovitis
Amyloid
Other tumors

Follow

POLYARTICULAR ARTHRITIS

Deborah Doud

A. The history in polyarticular arthritis is crucial. Joint distribution, axial involvement, symmetry, and morning stiffness must be delineated. Because many systemic diseases present with polyarthritis, a complete physical examination is necessary.

B. Historical features supporting inflammation include prolonged morning stiffness, fever, weight loss, and spontaneous joint swelling. Physical examination may reveal local warmth, erythema, or effusions. Laboratory findings supporting inflammation include anemia and elevated ESR. Radiographs of affected joints may show uniform cartilage loss, periarticular osteopenia, or erosions of subchondral bone. If synovial fluid is present, evaluation may be helpful; reduced viscosity and an elevated WBC count (>2000) exist in most inflammatory conditions. Crystal examination also should be made to determine if a crystal-induced arthritis is present.

C. Inflammatory polyarthritis with axial involvement includes the seronegative spondyloarthropathies: ankylosing spondylitis, Reiter's syndrome, psoriatic arthritis, and enteropathic arthritis (p 416). Radiographs of the sacroiliac joints may detect the presence of early axial involvement.

D. Inflammatory polyarthritis without axial involvement includes polyarthritis limited to peripheral joints. One must then determine if the polyarthritis is symmetric or asymmetric.

E. Rheumatoid arthritis (RA) typically begins in multiple small joints in a symmetric pattern. The earliest involved joints are the small joints of the hands and feet, sparing the distal interphalangeal (DIP) joints. The arthritis of RA is typically additive and destructive. Systemic lupus erythematosus (SLE) often presents as a chronic polyarthritis and may be misdiagnosed as RA. This arthritis typically is mildly inflammatory and nondestructive. Subacute bacterial endocarditis (SBE) may cause a chronic polyarthritis resembling RA; positive rheumatoid factor often is found in SBE and can cause serious diagnostic errors. Psoriatic arthritis, typically pauciarticular and asymmetric, can present in a polyarticular fashion, resembling RA. Scleroderma often presents with painful swollen hands with early contractures.

F. Psoriatic arthritis may precede skin disease. There is a good correlation between nail involvement and psoriatic arthritis, but overall correlation with skin disease is not as strong. This condition usually begins as an asymmetric pauciarticular arthritis including the DIP joints, or it may include all the joints of a digit, producing a "sausage" digit. Reiter's syndrome may entirely spare the axial skeleton and present with an arthritis similar to psoriatic arthritis, but with greater predilection for lower extremity joints. Enteropathic arthritis may present with only peripheral pauciarticular arthritis. The arthritis usually involves the lower extremity joints and generally parallels the activity of the bowel disease. Ankylosing spondylitis may present initially without axial involvement, especially in juveniles. The most common peripheral joints involved are the knees and hips. Adult rheumatic fever is rare; it causes very painful pauciarticular disease, most prominent in the larger joints of the lower extremities. Carditis, chorea, rash, and subcutaneous nodules are rarely found. Gout may be misdiagnosed in its early stages and may progress to its polyarticular form, which can resemble RA (p 442). Polyarticular gout is common in the elderly. Calcium pyrophosphate deposition (CPPD, pseudogout) may present as polyarticular arthritis, mainly affecting the knees, wrists, and metacarpophalangeal (MCP) joints. Other rare causes of pauciarticular arthritis that may need to be considered include amyloidosis, sarcoidosis, Lyme disease, AIDS, relapsing polychondritis, polymyositis, and Behçet's disease.

G. If there is no clinical evidence of inflammation, and radiographs show changes such as bony hypertrophy and asymmetric cartilage loss, the patient may be presumed to have osteoarthritis (OA).

H. Secondary OA includes several polyarticular syndromes. Obesity causes a number of joint problems, the most characteristic being bilateral OA of the knees, especially in women. Chondromalacia of the patella has multiple causes but is usually seen in physically active young and middle-aged women. Hemophilia causes a severe destructive arthritis following repeated episodes of intra-articular hemorrhage.

I. Particular patterns of OA have been described in association with several metabolic disorders, including hemochromatosis, ochronosis, acromegaly, and hypothyroidism and hyperparathyroidism.

J. OA of the hands, a hereditary disease much more prevalent in women, typically develops within a few years of the menopause and often is associated with mild inflammation for the first year or two. The disease is symmetric and involves the proximal interphalangeal and DIP joints, with development of the typical osteophytes of Heberden's and Bouchard's nodes. This disease spares the MCP joints and the wrists except the first carpometacarpal joint. Primary generalized OA is a rare hereditary disease with a high frequency of OA of multiple joints. It usually begins in middle age and involves typical joints (hips, knees, hands) early; eventually it may involve other joints such as the shoulders and ankles.

Patient with POLYARTICULAR ARTHRITIS

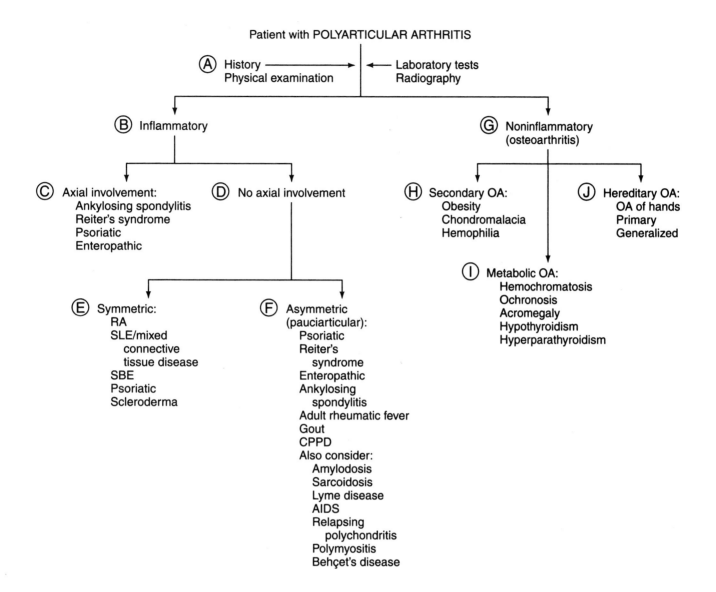

(A) History ⟶ ← Laboratory tests
Physical examination · Radiography

(B) Inflammatory

(G) Noninflammatory
(osteoarthritis)

(C) Axial involvement:
Ankylosing spondylitis
Reiter's syndrome
Psoriatic
Enteropathic

(D) No axial involvement

(H) Secondary OA:
Obesity
Chondromalacia
Hemophilia

(J) Hereditary OA:
OA of hands
Primary
Generalized

(E) Symmetric:
RA
SLE/mixed
connective
tissue disease
SBE
Psoriatic
Scleroderma

(F) Asymmetric
(pauciarticular):
Psoriatic
Reiter's
syndrome
Enteropathic
Ankylosing
spondylitis
Adult rheumatic fever
Gout
CPPD
Also consider:
Amylodosis
Sarcoidosis
Lyme disease
AIDS
Relapsing
polychondritis
Polymyositis
Behçet's disease

(I) Metabolic OA:
Hemochromatosis
Ochronosis
Acromegaly
Hypothyroidism
Hyperparathyroidism

References

Anderson RJ. Polyarticular arthritis. In: Kelley WN, Harris ED, Ruddy S, Sledge CB. Textbook of rheumatology. 5th ed. Philadelphia: WB Saunders, 1997.

McCarty DJ. Differential diagnosis of arthritis: analysis of signs and symptoms. In: McCarty DJ, ed. Arthritis and allied conditions. Philadelphia: Lea & Febiger, 1989.

SERONEGATIVE ARTHRITIS

Michael J. Maricic

A. The seronegative arthritides (ankylosing spondylitis, Reiter's disease, psoriatic arthritis, and arthritis associated with inflammatory bowel disease) may or may not involve the spine. When they do, they are commonly called the *seronegative spondyloarthropathies.*

B. Laboratory tests usually are not helpful. HLA-B27 is positive in >95% of cases of ankylosing spondylitis but usually is unnecessary. This test is neither specific nor sensitive enough to be useful for the other diseases. Consider AIDS in a patient with risk factors for HIV: In some patients, severe Reiter's disease has been reported as the initial manifestation.

C. Spinal involvement usually is categorized by inflammatory low back pain with morning stiffness and pain, improving with exercise. Physical examination should include Schober's test to examine lumbosacral mobility. This involves making two marks on the patient (one at the dimple of Venus and one 10 cm above the first) and asking the patient to flex at the waist. Normally, the marks should stretch to 15 cm apart. Thoracic expansion at the nipple line (normal, >3 cm) and occiput-to-wall distance (normal, 0) also should be measured.

D. Radiographic examination should begin with plain radiographs of the sacroiliac (SI) joints and lumbosacral spine. Technetium bone scans, CT, or MRI may be helpful in more subtle cases, depending on the need to establish a firm diagnosis. Ankylosing spondylitis usually involves both SI joints and ascends continuously up the spine, whereas the other diseases often involve only one SI joint and may skip areas of the spine.

E. Look for peripheral arthritis and determine the joint distribution. Common to all the seronegative arthritides is asymmetric involvement of the joints of the lower extremities. Involvement of two or more joints of the same digit (sausaging) may be found, especially in Reiter's disease or psoriatic arthritis.

F. Search meticulously for skin changes throughout the body and for clues to the type of arthritis. Nail changes such as pitting or onycholysis may be a clue to psoriatic arthritis or Reiter's disease. Psoriatic plaques may be subtle but may be the only clue to psoriatic arthritis. Keratoderma blennorrhagica, found in Reiter's disease, may be clinically and histologically indistinguishable from psoriasis, but it tends to occur more often on the palms and soles. Balanitis circumscripta, a circular, plaquelike lesion on the head of the penis, may be found in Reiter's disease. Pyoderma gangrenosum may be seen with either ulcerative colitis or Crohn's disease.

G. Other organ systems may be involved. Iritis or conjunctivitis, urethritis, prostatitis, and aortic or mitral regurgitation may be seen with any of the seronegative arthritides. Apical pulmonary fibrosis may be seen with ankylosing spondylitis.

References

Amor B, Dougados M, Khan MA. Management of refractory ankylosing spondylitis and related spondyloarthropathies. Rheum Dis Clin North Am 1995; 21:117.

Arnett FC. Seronegative spondylarthropathies. Bull Rheum Dis 1987; 37:1.

Keat A. Reiter's syndrome and reactive arthritis in perspective. N Engl J Med 1983; 309:1606.

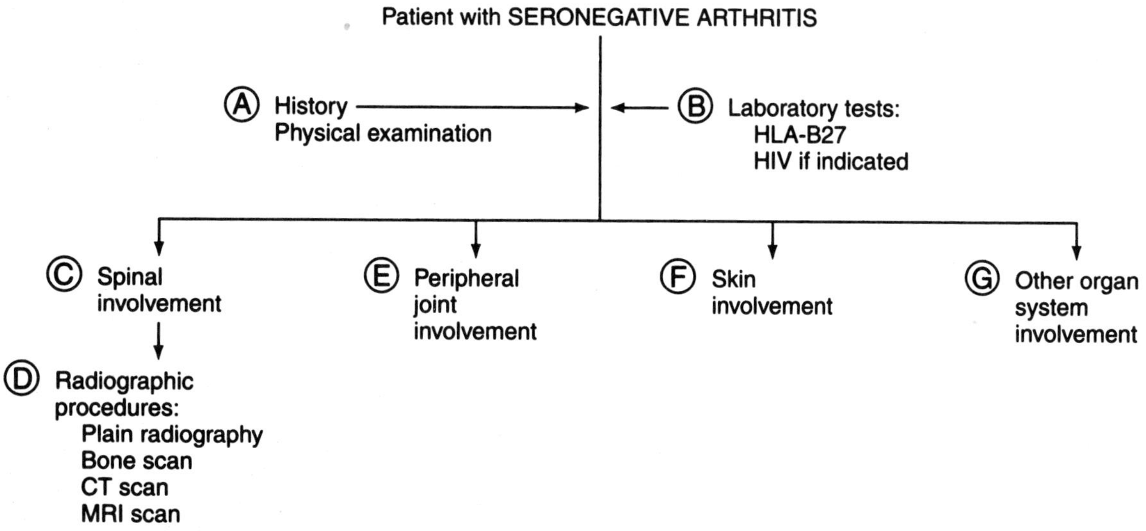

Patient with SERONEGATIVE ARTHRITIS

(A) History ——————→ ←—— (B) Laboratory tests:
    Physical examination   HLA-B27
                                      HIV if indicated

(C) Spinal   (E) Peripheral   (F) Skin   (G) Other organ
    involvement   joint   involvement   system
                        involvement   involvement

(D) Radiographic
    procedures:
      Plain radiography
      Bone scan
      CT scan
      MRI scan

SOFT TISSUE PAIN

Michael J. Maricic

A. Soft tissue pain (nonarticular rheumatism) is a common problem in patients with musculoskeletal symptoms. The history and physical examinations are vital in differentiating soft tissue pain from true arthritis. Although the suffix *-itis,* implying inflammation, is used with terms such as *tendinitis, bursitis,* and *fibrositis,* pain and tenderness usually are not accompanied by redness, heat, and swelling.

B. The first step is to determine whether the pain is intra- or extra-articular. This may be done by testing active and passive motion of the joint nearest the pain. Extra-articular problems cause pain on active but not passive movement of the joint. Intra-articular pain (true arthritis) is present on both active and passive motion.

C. If the pain is extra-articular, determine whether it is generalized or localized. If localized, the pain may be caused by inflammation of a number of different tendons, bursae, or soft tissue structures. Bicipital tendinitis (in the long head of the biceps within the bicipital groove of the humerus), subdeltoid bursitis (in the lateral aspect of the shoulder), lateral epicondylitis (at the proximal attachment of the brachioradialis muscle on the lateral epicondyle of the humerus), trochanteric bursitis (superior to the greater trochanter), and anserine bursitis (over the medial aspect of the knee) are some of the more common causes of localized soft tissue pain.

D. If pain is generalized, consider systemic disorders such as early rheumatoid arthritis, systemic lupus erythematosus, polymyalgia rheumatica, and hyper- or hypothyroidism. History and physical examination should exclude these. If they are suspected, confirmatory testing may be done with ANA, rheumatoid factor, ESR, and thyroid function tests. In general, these tests should not be conducted if the history and physical examination are otherwise normal. Also, question the patient about symptoms of depression, which may present as generalized pain.

E. If there is no evidence of another systemic disorder in patients with generalized soft tissue pain, consider fibrositis or fibromyalgia. Generalized aches and pains, stiffness, fatigue, and difficulty in staying asleep in a patient who usually is a young to middle-aged female suggest this diagnosis. The physical examination usually is remarkable only for multiple, symmetric tender points over the occiput, neck, trapezium, paraspinous muscles, elbows, shoulder, trochanters, and knees. Laboratory tests and radiographs are normal.

References

Bennett RM. The fibromyalgia syndrome. In: Kelley WN, Ruddy S, Harris ED Jr, eds: Textbook of rheumatology. 5th ed. Philadelphia: WB Saunders, 1997:511.

Campbell SM, Clark S, Tindall EA, et al. Clinical characteristics of fibrositis. Arthritis Rheum 1983; 26:817.

Fassbender K, Samborsky W, Kellner M, et al. Tender points, depressive and functional symptoms: comparison between fibromyalgia and major depression. Clin Rheumatol 1997; 16:76.

McCain GA. A cost-effective approach to the diagnosis and treatment of fibromyalgia. Rheum Dis Clin North Am 1996; 22:323.

Reveille JD. Soft tissue rheumatism: diagnosis and treatment. Am J Med 1997; 102(suppl):23S.

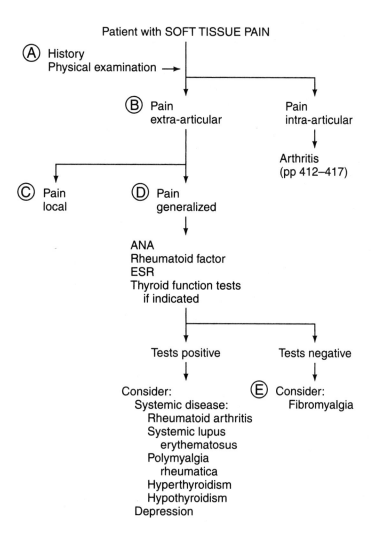

Patient with SOFT TISSUE PAIN

(A) History
Physical examination →

(B) Pain
extra-articular

Pain
intra-articular

Arthritis
(pp 412–417)

(C) Pain
local

(D) Pain
generalized

ANA
Rheumatoid factor
ESR
Thyroid function tests
if indicated

Tests positive

Tests negative

Consider:
Systemic disease:
Rheumatoid arthritis
Systemic lupus
erythematosus
Polymyalgia
rheumatica
Hyperthyroidism
Hypothyroidism
Depression

(E) Consider:
Fibromyalgia

NECK PAIN

Michael J. Maricic

The neck as a functional unit is composed of a variety of structures that may individually or in combination give rise to both local and radicular pain. These structures include the vertebrae, intervertebral discs, uncovertebral and apophyseal joints, spinal cord and nerve roots, paracervical muscles, and anterior and posterior longitudinal ligaments.

A. In taking a history, any recent trauma is of foremost importance. Fractures of the odontoid, C1, C2, and fracture dislocations of C3-C7 may occur and demand immediate neurologic and radiographic evaluation, immobilization, and orthopedic referral. A history of inflammatory arthritis such as rheumatoid arthritis, psoriatic arthritis, Reiter's syndrome, or ankylosing spondylitis may suggest that the pain is caused by synovitis (usually worse in the morning, relieved by motion). More important, a history of inflammatory arthritis should alert one to the possibility of a wide variety of axial and subaxial subluxations that may give rise to local pain, long tract symptoms, and vertebrobasilar symptoms (caused by compression of the vertebral arteries). Acute onset of neck pain may suggest nerve root irritation or muscle spasm. Chronic pain is more common with discogenic disease. Local pain may be caused by involvement of any of the structures listed above. Radicular pain is most commonly secondary to nerve root compression by foraminal encroachment or a herniated intervertebral disc. Neurologic symptoms may include paresthesias radiating to the arm and weakness of the arm, hand, or fingers secondary to nerve impingement. Paresthesias and weakness of the legs, with or without bladder or bowel symptoms, may indicate cord compression.

B. Local physical signs of spasm and tenderness may occur with involvement of any of the above structures. Weakness of the biceps and wrist extensors, decreased biceps reflex, and sensory loss in the thumb and index finger suggest C5-C6 root involvement. Weakness of the triceps muscle, wrist flexors, and finger extensors along with a decreased triceps reflex suggest a C6-C7 nerve root condition. Weakness of the intrinsic musculature of the hand and finger flexors and decreased triceps reflex suggests C7-C8 root involvement. Bilateral weakness, spasticity, and hyperreflexia in the lower extremities suggest cervical cord compression.

C. Order radiographs in the anteroposterior (AP), lateral, and oblique views. Open-mouth views of the odontoid may give information about odontoid fractures and also allow visualization of the C1-C2 facet joints. Flexion and extension views in the lateral projection are necessary when subluxation is suspected.

D. Electromyography may help document nerve root compression in cases of chronic radicular pain. Myelography may be performed in patients suspected of having cervical spinal stenosis or in those with intractable neck pain from nerve root compression. CT is useful for the same indications. MRI may be useful for the same indications as myelography and CT. It also is the procedure of choice in cases of suspected subluxation in inflammatory arthritis because soft tissue (including pannus) delineation is superior with this technique. Technetium bone scans may be helpful in cases of suspected infection when the radiograph is negative. MRI probably is superior where available.

References

Engstrom JW, Bradford DS. Back and neck pain. In: Fauci AS, Braunwald E, Isselbacher KJ, et al, eds. Harrison's principles of internal medicine. 14th ed. New York: McGraw-Hill, 1997: 73.

Jackson R. The cervical syndrome. 4th ed. Springfield, IL: Charles C. Thomas, 1979.

Patient with NECK PAIN

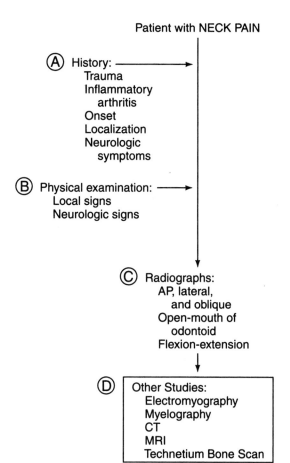

Ⓐ History: ⟶
   Trauma
   Inflammatory
     arthritis
   Onset
   Localization
   Neurologic
     symptoms

Ⓑ Physical examination: ⟶
   Local signs
   Neurologic signs

Ⓒ Radiographs:
   AP, lateral,
     and oblique
   Open-mouth of
     odontoid
   Flexion-extension

Ⓓ | Other Studies:
   Electromyography
   Myelography
   CT
   MRI
   Technetium Bone Scan

SHOULDER PAIN

James B. Benjamin

A. Standard radiographs should include an anteroposterior view of the shoulder with internal rotation and external rotation of the humerus, and an axillary view. A tangential "Y" view is often helpful in evaluating the position of the humeral head in relationship to the glenoid if an axillary view is unobtainable.

B. With a history of trauma, consider fracture of the humeral neck, distal clavicle, and scapula (decreasing incidence). Anterior dislocation of the glenohumeral joint is by far the most common (>90%) and usually is obvious on physical examination and radiography. Posterior dislocations often are missed radiographically if an axillary view is not obtained; these occur classically with seizures or electrical shocks and are the result of violent muscular contractions rather than direct trauma. The most salient physical finding with a posterior glenohumeral dislocation is the patient's inability to externally rotate the shoulder. Acromioclavicular separations usually result from a fall on the point of the shoulder with the arm adducted. Pain that is localized at the acromioclavicular joint can be severe even with minimal displacement of the clavicle. Standing views of the shoulder with the patient holding weights are of little additional value because muscle spasm can prevent displacement of the clavicle. Falls on the point of the shoulder also can result in tears of the rotator cuff that, if large enough, can prevent active shoulder abduction. Patients often can compensate with the deltoid, and physical findings are limited to pain and weakness with abduction. Although MRI is very sensitive in diagnosing rotator cuff tears, ultrasonography and shoulder arthrography are more cost-effective means of diagnosing this injury.

C. Inflammatory conditions about the shoulder often are precipitated by recreational or occupational overuse.

Although often diffuse, pain can be localized to specific tendons by careful palpation. Radiographs are most often unremarkable except with calcific rotator cuff tendinitis. In this case, calcium deposition in the supraspinatus tendon at its insertion into the greater tuberosity of the humerus is pathognomonic for this condition.

D. Most inflammatory conditions about the shoulder resolve with conservative care in 6–8 weeks. If symptoms persist beyond this time, consider rotator cuff tear and undertake further evaluation as in acute traumatic tears.

E. Rule out cervical radiculopathy in any patient with radiating upper extremity pain. If physical examination demonstrates evidence of cervical spine pathology, begin work-up with radiographic evaluation and proceed as indicated.

References

Belzer JP, Durkin RC. Common disorders of the shoulder. Prim Care 1996; 23:365.

Cuomo F. The value of the history and physical for shoulder pain. West J Med 1995; 63:389.

Donovan PJ, Paulos LE. Common injuries of the shoulder: diagnosis and treatment. West J Med 1995; 163:351.

Evancho AM, Stiles RG, Fajman WA, et al. MR imaging diagnosis of rotator cuff tears. AJR 1988; 151:751.

Norwood LA, Barrack R, Jacobson KE. Clinical presentation of complete tears of the rotator cuff. J Bone Joint Surg 1989; 21A:499.

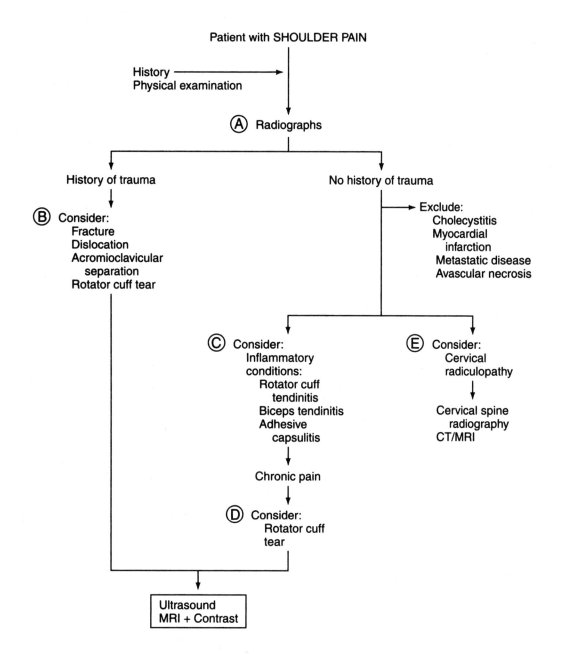

Patient with SHOULDER PAIN

History ———————→
Physical examination

Ⓐ Radiographs

History of trauma   No history of trauma

→ Exclude:
    Cholecystitis
    Myocardial
      infarction
    Metastatic disease
    Avascular necrosis

Ⓑ Consider:
    Fracture
    Dislocation
    Acromioclavicular
      separation
    Rotator cuff tear

Ⓒ Consider:
    Inflammatory
    conditions:
      Rotator cuff
        tendinitis
      Biceps tendinitis
      Adhesive
        capsulitis

Ⓔ Consider:
    Cervical
    radiculopathy

Cervical spine
    radiography
    CT/MRI

Chronic pain

Ⓓ Consider:
    Rotator cuff
      tear

Ultrasound
MRI + Contrast

LOW BACK PAIN

Barbara Bode

Low back pain accounts for about one third of rheumatic complaints and affects 80% of adults at some time during their life. It most commonly is self-limiting; even a herniated disc rarely requires surgery. Typically, diagnoses are non-specific; a precise pathoanatomic cause is identified in only 10–20% of patients. Consider this positive outcome in the evaluation and treatment of all patients with low back pain.

A. A thorough history and physical examination are crucial to obtain an accurate assessment of low back pain. History taking should fully characterize the pain to differentiate local from radicular or referred pain. The relationship of pain to activity associated with postural changes is important. The pain of spinal stenosis is exacerbated by walking and relieved by rest and spinal flexion. Sitting often worsens symptoms of disc herniation. Determine bowel, bladder, and sexual function because they may be involved in central midline herniations of the disc and spinal stenosis. Inspect the back for normal curvature and palpate it for local spasm, sacroiliac joint tenderness, or sciatic notch tenderness. Physical examination also should include evaluation of gait, back range of motion, leg length determination, straight leg raising, a thorough neurologic examination, chest expansion, and Schober's test.

B. About 1% of patients with low back pain have sciatica, which is pain in the distribution of a lumbar root, often associated with motor or sensory deficits. This often is the first indication of a herniated disc. Of lumbar disc herniations, 95% occur at the L4-L5 or L5-S1 levels. There is a 10% incidence of two-level herniations. Typically, L5 nerve root involvement results in extensor hallucis longus weakness with medial foot sensory loss, and there is no loss of reflex. S1 nerve root involvement causes loss of the ankle jerk, weakness of the plantar flexors of the foot, and sensory loss of the posterior calf and lateral foot. The knee reflex is lost with involvement at the L4-L5 level.

C. Multiple nerve root entrapment may result in symptoms of neurogenic claudication. Presentation typically occurs in the sixth decade. Spinal stenosis may be congenital or acquired secondary to degenerative changes, spondylolysis, or spondylolisthesis, and may be postsurgical or post-traumatic. It may involve either the lateral recesses or the central canal.

D. The inflammatory spondyloarthropathies affect 2% of the population. Patients often present before 40 years of age with insidious onset of low back pain relieved by exercise and associated with morning stiffness. These diseases are characterized by sacroiliitis, inflammatory peripheral arthritis, and enthesopathy. Evaluate these patients for ocular, pulmonary, and cardiovascular disease.

E. Target the early diagnostic work-up of low back pain toward identifying neurologic abnormalities, factors that may influence conservative treatment, and signs of systemic disease. Plain radiography is rarely useful in the definitive diagnosis of low back pain, although it can be important in identifying tumor, infection, fracture, spondylolisthesis, or sacroiliitis. Immediate additional imaging studies are indicated in patients with a cauda equina syndrome (bowel and bladder dysfunction with bilateral leg weakness and numbness), a progressive neurologic deficit, or evidence of tumor or infection. In patients with a suspected herniated disc, 1–2 weeks of conservative therapy before further diagnostic work-up is suggested. Disc herniation is common in asymptomatic persons, and this isolated test finding without the corresponding clinical signs may initiate unnecessary clinical interventions. In patients who have clinical signs to suggest a herniated disc and have failed conservative therapy, the diagnosis must be confirmed on CT scan, MRI, or myelography. The sensitivities and specificities of CT and myelography are similar (90–95% and 65–85%, respectively). It is as yet unknown how MRI compares with these. EMG may be useful in differentiating radicular pain from peripheral neuropathy. Bone scan may help in the diagnosis of tumor, infection, or early inflammatory disease. Depression, substance abuse, and excessive somatization are poor prognostic features that may warrant psychological testing.

F. If a patient is writhing in pain, suspect an intra-abdominal or vascular process. Suspect cancer or an infectious process, such as an epidural abscess or spinal osteomyelitis, in a patient with constant pain at rest or fever. Acute pain in a patient at risk for osteoporosis should suggest a vertebral compression fracture. Paget's disease is another metabolic bone condition that may give rise to low back pain.

References

Borenstein DG. Low back pain. In: Klippel JH, Dieppe PA, eds. Rheumatology. 2nd ed. London: Mosby, 1998:4.3.1–26.

Cherkin DC, Deyo RA, Wheeler K, Ciol MA. Physician variation in diagnostic testing for low back pain. Who you see is what you get. Arthritis Rheum 1994; 37:1.

Deyo RA, Loeser JD, Bigos SJ. Herniated lumbar intervertebral disc. Ann Intern Med 1990; 112:598.

Frymoyer JW. Back pain and sciatica. N Engl J Med 1988; 318:291.

Lipson SJ. Low back pain. In: Kelley WN, Ruddy S, Harris ED, eds. Textbook of rheumatology. 5th ed. Philadelphia: WB Saunders, 1997.

Patient with LOW BACK PAIN

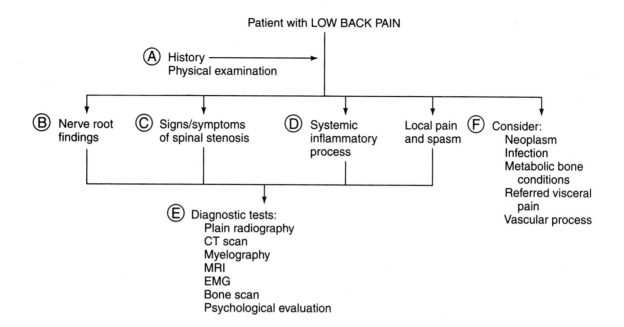

HIP PAIN

James B. Benjamin

A. For evaluation of hip pain, radiographs should include an anteroposterior (AP) view of the pelvis in addition to AP and lateral views of the hip. The pelvis view provides valuable additional information, including views of the sacroiliac joints, sacrum, and opposite hip for comparison.

B. In addition to the standard AP view of the pelvis, inlet and outlet views can be helpful in evaluating pelvic fractures. Judet or lateral oblique views are most useful in evaluating fractures about the acetabulum. The posterior elements of the pelvis can best be evaluated with CT.

C. Stress fractures of the proximal femur and pelvis can be difficult to diagnose on plain radiography. These injuries are commonly seen in patients who are long-distance runners or who do aerobic exercise with repetitive impact loading. A bone scan often assists the diagnosis.

D. Perform a joint aspirate if the diagnosis of inflammatory arthropathy is suspected. Often this procedure is diagnostic, as in cases of infectious etiology and crystalline arthropathy. Fluid should be analyzed for cell count with differential, the presence or absence of crystals, and Gram stain and culture if indicated. Glucose level is of benefit only if a serum glucose level is obtained at the same time for comparison.

E. Early avascular necrosis may not show any changes on plain radiography. MRI has evolved as the most sensitive tool in diagnosing this disorder.

F. Lumbar spine disorders can mimic hip pathology and should be considered if pain is localized to the buttock. Although osteoarthritic changes can be easily seen on routine radiography, nerve root compression and spinal stenosis are best evaluated with alternative imaging techniques.

G. Trochanteric bursitis is one of the most common problems in patients with "hip pain." The pain is classically localized to the lateral aspect of the hip over the greater trochanter.

References

Hauzeur JP, Pasteels JL, Schoutens A, et al. The diagnostic value of magnetic resonance imaging in nontraumatic osteonecrosis of the femoral head. J Bone Joint Surg 1989; 71A:641.

Kirkaldy-Willis WH, Wedge JH, Yong-Hing K, Reily J. Pathology and pathogenesis of lumbar spondylosis and stenosis. Spine 1978; 3:319.

Pavlov H, Nelson TL, Warren RF, et al. Stress fractures of the pubic ramus. J Bone Joint Surg 1982; 65A:1020.

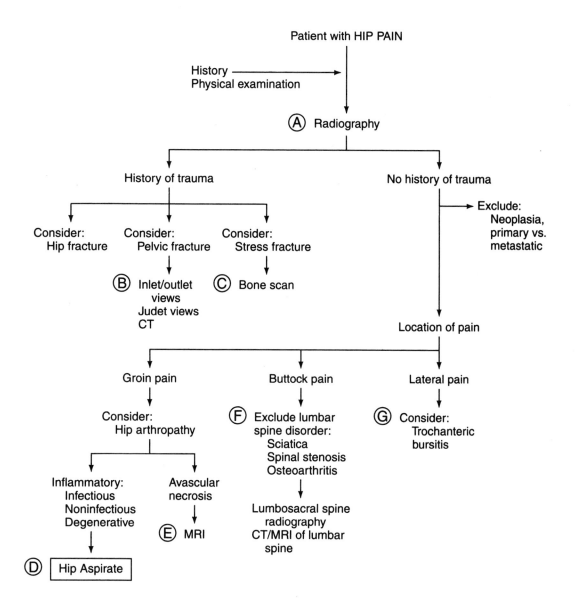

Patient with HIP PAIN

History ──────────►
Physical examination

Ⓐ Radiography

History of trauma

No history of trauma

→ Exclude:
Neoplasia,
primary vs.
metastatic

Consider:
Hip fracture

Consider:
Pelvic fracture

Consider:
Stress fracture

Ⓑ Inlet/outlet
views
Judet views
CT

Ⓒ Bone scan

Location of pain

Groin pain

Buttock pain

Lateral pain

Consider:
Hip arthropathy

Ⓕ Exclude lumbar
spine disorder:
Sciatica
Spinal stenosis
Osteoarthritis

Ⓖ Consider:
Trochanteric
bursitis

Inflammatory:
Infectious
Noninfectious
Degenerative

Avascular
necrosis

Ⓔ MRI

Lumbosacral spine
radiography
CT/MRI of lumbar
spine

Ⓓ Hip Aspirate

HAND AND WRIST PAIN

Michael J. Maricic

Pain in the hands or wrists may have a variety of causes. Pain may originate from the bones or joints or from extra-articular tissues such as the muscles or tendons, or it may be the result of vascular or neural compromise. The history and physical examination often provide the diagnosis without the need for further studies.

A. If the pain is articular (pain on active and passive motion of the joint), note symmetry and joint distribution. Degenerative joint disease (DJD) may be asymmetric but often affects the first carpometacarpal, distal interphalangeal (DIP), and proximal interphalangeal (PIP) joints in a symmetric fashion. There usually is a lack of inflammation. Gout or pseudogout (calcium pyrophosphate deposition disease [CPPD]) may involve any of the small joints of the hands or wrist in a symmetric or asymmetric fashion. CPPD has a predilection for the wrists and index and middle metacarpophalangeal (MCP) joints. Rheumatoid arthritis (RA) is always symmetric and involves the wrists and MCP and PIP joints.

B. Extra-articular causes of pain may be acute or chronic. Acute causes of pain include tenosynovitis, tendon rupture, and infection. The pain in De Quervain's tenosynovitis usually is near the anatomic snuffbox and is caused by inflammation of the abductor pollicis longus and extensor pollicis brevis. Adduction of the thumb while the wrist is held in ulnar deviation (Finkelstein's test) exacerbates the pain. Rupture of the extensor or flexor tendons may occur after trauma or in conditions such as RA. In RA, rupture of the ring and little finger extensors may result from dorsal subluxation and radial displacement of the ulnar styloid. Infections such as cellulitis, abscesses, felons (infections of the distal pulp of the fingertip), and paronychias (infections of the soft tissue around the nail) usually are obvious to the observer. Chronic soft tissue pain may be caused by ganglions (soft tissue tumors most commonly found over the dorsum of the wrist) or Dupuytren's contractures (thickening and contracture of the palmar aponeurosis). The latter is most commonly found in patients with diabetes, alcoholism, and a family history of these contractures.

C. Vascular problems in the hand are uncommon. Bilateral vascular spasm and discoloration suggest Raynaud's syndrome (p 438). Unilateral or digital problems suggest thoracic outlet syndrome, vasculitis, and thromboembolic disease. Doppler flow studies and angiography may be necessary in the latter disorders.

D. Neural pain may be caused by dysfunction of the radial, ulnar, or median nerves. Ulnar nerve dysfunction is suggested by weakness in the intrinsic muscles of the hand and numbness of the ulnar nerve distribution. Radial nerve dysfunction results in weakness of the wrist and finger extensors and numbness of the dorsum of the hand. The median nerve supplies innervation to the thenar muscles (except the adductor) and the lumbricales of the index and long fingers. It provides sensation to the palmar aspect of the thumb, index, and middle and radial half of the ring finger. Carpal tunnel syndrome is caused by compression of the median nerve at the wrist. It is commonly seen in diabetes, pregnancy, hypothyroidism, repetitive trauma, and any inflammatory arthropathy of the wrist (RA, gout, CPPD). Tinel's (tapping the median nerve over the wrist) and Phalen's (sustained hyperflexion of the wrists) signs may reproduce the symptoms. Nerve conduction velocities (NCVs) may document the involved nerves and sites of compression.

References

Kendall D. Aetiology, diagnosis and treatment of paraesthesiae in the hands. BMJ 1960; 2:1663.

Kuschner SH, Lane CS. Evaluation of the painful wrist. Am J Orthop 1997; 26:95.

Shipley M. ABC of rheumatology: pain in the hand and wrist. BMJ 1995; 310:239.

Zelouf DS, Posner MA. Hand and wrist disorders: how to manage pain and improve function. Geriatrics 1995; 50:22.

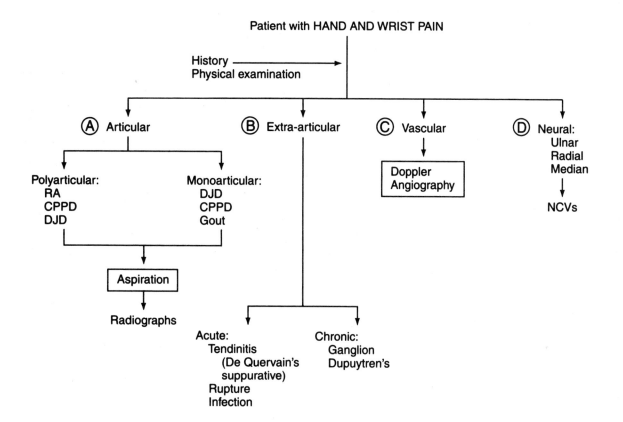

Patient with HAND AND WRIST PAIN

History ──────
Physical examination

Ⓐ Articular

Polyarticular:
RA
CPPD
DJD

Monoarticular:
DJD
CPPD
Gout

Aspiration

Radiographs

Ⓑ Extra-articular

Acute:
Tendinitis
(De Quervain's
suppurative)
Rupture
Infection

Chronic:
Ganglion
Dupuytren's

Ⓒ Vascular

Doppler
Angiography

Ⓓ Neural:
Ulnar
Radial
Median

NCVs

KNEE PAIN

Michael J. Maricic

A. The history and physical examination are crucial to establishing the proper diagnosis of knee pain. The first step is to determine whether the pain is intra-articular (which may involve any or all of the five joints in the knee: patellofemoral, fabellofemoral, medial tibiofemoral, lateral tibiofemoral, or tibiofibular) or extra-articular. Pain on both active and passive range of motion of the joint suggests intra-articular disease, whereas pain on active but not passive motion of the joint suggests extra-articular disease.

B. Pain that is worse in the morning, improves with motion, and is associated with signs of inflammation (redness, heat, swelling) suggests inflammatory arthritis. Bilateral inflammation of the knees associated with inflammation of the small joints of the hands and feet is consistent with rheumatoid arthritis (most common), psoriatic arthritis, and systemic lupus erythematosus. Unilateral inflammatory arthritis of the knee could be caused by crystals (gout, pseudogout), a seronegative spondyloarthropathy (Reiter's, psoriatic arthritis, ankylosing spondylitis), arthritis associated with inflammatory bowel disease, or infection (bacterial, mycobacterial, fungal). Also consider Lyme arthritis in endemic areas. A Baker's (popliteal) cyst may be present in any type of inflammatory arthritis. These sometimes rupture and simulate an acute deep venous thrombosis. Chronic pain that is worse on weight bearing and with activity and not associated with morning stiffness or signs of inflammation suggests degenerative arthritis. Consider avascular necrosis of the knee when there is acute onset of pain in a patient with predisposing factors (glucocorticoid use, alcoholism, sickle cell disease, infiltrative marrow disorders). Consider neoplastic disorders, especially in children or adolescents. Night pain and periarticular soft tissue swelling are diagnostic clues suggesting neoplasm. Meniscal tears often are preceded by a history of a twisting injury. Mild inflammation of the knee may be present. McMurray's test (internal and external rotation of the knee with the knee brought from full flexion into extension) may produce pain or an audible click. Chondromalacia patellae is suggested by the history of anterior knee pain that is worse during climbing or descending stairs or squatting. Physical examination may reveal crepitus of the patellofemoral joint or subluxation/dislocation of the patella.

C. In the case of monoarticular joint swelling, synovial fluid examination is mandatory (p 412).

D. Arthrography may be performed to demonstrate meniscal and cruciate tears or a popliteal cyst. Ultrasonography is a less invasive method for this purpose.

E. Technetium bone scanning may be useful for demonstrating infectious arthritis of avascular necrosis. MRI is preferable when available.

F. MRI is the procedure of choice when considering the diagnosis of meniscal or ligamentous tears, tumor, infection, or avascular necrosis.

G. The prepatellar bursa (anterior) and anserine bursa (medial) may cause localized pain and swelling. The pes anserinus tendons (sartorius, gracilis, semitendinous) located medially and the quadriceps and patellar tendons located anteriorly may be the source of localized pain. Osgood-Schlatter disease refers to pain at the insertion of the patellar tendon into the tibial tubercle in adolescents; it is believed to be caused by a mild avulsion. Ligamentous pain may arise from a strain of the medial collateral, lateral collateral, anterior cruciate, or posterior cruciate ligaments. Perform tests for valgus and varus stability and the anterior and posterior Drawer signs to test for laxity.

References

Hayes CW. MRI of the patellofemoral joint. Semin Ultrasound CT MR 1994; 15:383.

Johnson RP. Anterior knee pain in adolescents and young adults. Curr Opin Rheum 1997; 9:159.

Ruwe PA, McCarthy SM. Cost effectiveness of magnetic resonance imaging of the knee. Magn Reson Imaging Clin North Am 1994; 2:475.

Steere AC. Diagnosis and treatment of Lyme arthritis. Med Clin North Am 1997; 81:179.

Stoller DW, Genant HK. Magnetic resonance imaging of the knee and hip. Arthritis Rheum 1990; 33:441.

Patient with KNEE PAIN

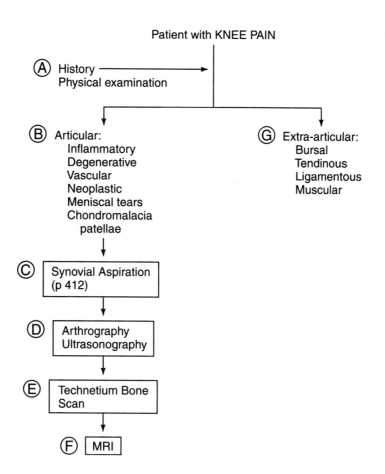

FOOT PAIN

Martin Snyder

A. A careful history and thorough physical examination provide many clues to the cause of foot pain. The onset of pain, aggravating and relieving factors, and the conditions in which pain occurs are important subjective information. Objective signs also are crucial. Radiography, laboratory values, muscle testing, vascular and neurologic examinations, ranges of motion, and comparison of one side with the other help in the differential diagnosis. Also consider simple skin patterns of discoloration, edema, warmth, and texture.

B. Trauma may be the result of a simple sprain, an athletic injury, or an accidental slip or fall while walking or running. There may be microtrauma, as seen in occupational injuries when a worker uses one foot to operate a lever or press. The mechanism of the injury should explain the trauma. Radiography is essential to rule out fractures. Edema and discoloration reflect the internal trauma to the vascular system. Pressure from the injured part on nerves and blood vessels must be reduced to prevent permanent damage. Trauma to the foot or toes also may result from improperly fitted footgear. Tight shoes may cause corns or toe contractures, with resultant metatarsal depression.

C. Systemic factors probably are the most common, and most disabling, cause of foot pain. These also may become the most chronic lesions of the foot because they encompass rheumatologic, vascular, and neurologic systems. Many systemic causes begin in areas remote from the feet. Because major systems are involved, consider such causes carefully in the differential diagnosis.

D. Rheumatologic causes are numerous. Some basic questions will help classify the pain as one of the many arthritides that affect the feet: Is the condition inflammatory (swollen, red, and warm)? Is the condition symmetric and bilateral? Is the pain greater at one time of day? How long does it take the patient to gain some relief from stiffness and aching? Because inflammatory arthritic changes are superimposed on a biomechanically weak structure, osseous articulations are destroyed and major digital deformities result. Even noninflammatory conditions affect weight distribution in the feet during the stance and propulsive phases of gait and cause pain and disability.

E. Vascular pain may be acute and potentially destructive. Arterial emboli may lead to limb-threatening situations. If the lesion is spastic, as in Raynaud's disease affecting the arterial trunk, the prognosis is not as devastating as organic clot or blockage. Temperature variations have a bearing on spasticity. Firm clots or emboli are not subject to outside temperature, although cold weather causes some vasoconstriction. Arteriography may be required to distinguish spastic from fixed stenosis. In venous problems, edema, ulcerations and phlebitis may be end results of venous failure or congestion. Varicose veins usually do not cause foot pain per se but reflect the inadequate return of the vascular system and can break down over bony prominences and ulcerate.

F. Neurologic pain generally falls within two major areas. Pain in the distal part of the foot, especially around the toes and commonly in the third intermetatarsal space, is common and may be caused by Morton's neuroma. Pain in the medial plantar portion of the heel is the result of a compression neuropathy in the tarsal tunnel. The pain from this condition may mimic other symptoms around the heel (e.g., plantar fasciitis, neuroma of the medial calcaneal nerve, or pain secondary to the seronegative arthritides such as in Reiter's disease, ankylosing spondylitis, or even psoriasis). Diabetes mellitus and the complication of peripheral neuropathy cause a burning pain that is greater when the foot is not weight bearing.

G. Biomechanical causes are not always evident to casual observation. Be attuned to both obvious and subtle variations in gait. Whether the primary complaint is in the forefoot or rear foot, the entire axial and appendicular skeleton must be observed and measurements obtained that detail any decrease in motion, strength, or size compared with the opposite side. Paddings, strapping, special shoes, orthoses made to casts, and physical medicine may alleviate symptoms and help re-establish normal foot function.

H. Infectious diseases that cause foot pain usually are related to trauma that permits the introduction of organisms into broken skin. A common infection is that of an ingrowing toenail that produces exudate and proud flesh and causes sharp, lancinating pain. The resultant paronychia, abscess, or even cellulitis may necessitate surgery. Other infections need not penetrate the skin but may lodge in the superficial cells and create the common verruca plantaris. Mycotic toenails with heavy deposits of subungual debris are uncomfortable with simple shoe pressure. Eventually, onychogryphotic nails develop from fungal infestation and neglect, and their very thickness may cause pain. Although tinea pedis in itself may not be especially painful, the use of very aggressive medications and delay in proper treatment may result in overlay infections secondary to loss of skin protection.

Patient with FOOT PAIN

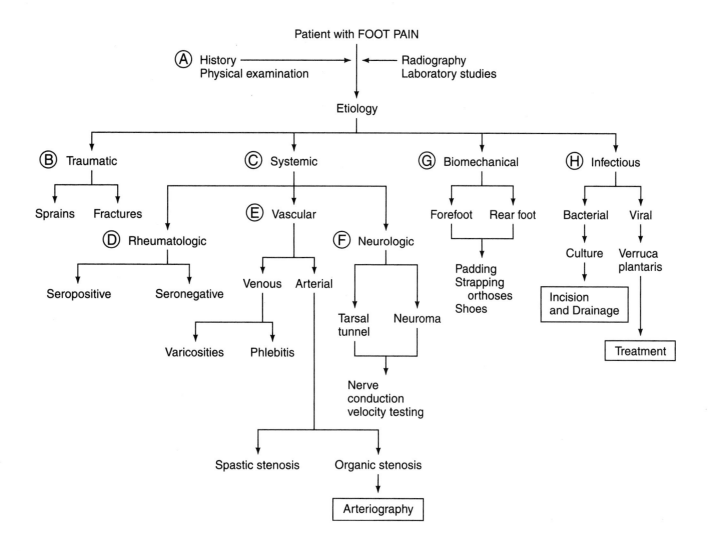

References

Cailliet R. Foot and ankle pain. 3rd ed. Philadelphia: FA Davis, 1997.
Hoppenfeld S. Physical examination of the foot by complaint. In: Jahss MH, ed. Disorders of the foot. Philadelphia: WB Saunders, 1982.

Joseph WS, Kosinski MA. Prophylaxis in lower-extremity infectious diseases. Clin Podiatr Med Surg, 1996; 13:647.
Synder M. Disorders of the foot. In: Riggs, Gall, eds. Rheumatic diseases: rehabilitation and management. Boston: Butterworth, 1994.
Young G. Evaluation of chronic foot pain. Clin Podiatr Med Surg 1994; 11:15.

SCLERODERMA

Barbara Bode

Scleroderma is a variable disease with several clinical presentations, each having differing prognoses. Progressive systemic sclerosis is considered the most severe and is characterized by diffuse inflammatory and proliferative vascular lesions with atrophy and fibrosis of skin, muscle, and involved organs (primarily GI tract, lung, and kidneys). The cause and pathogenesis are unknown. Disease onset is usually 30–50 years of age, with an increased incidence in women.

The sclerodermatous disorders often present with skin thickening. This usually involves the fingers and hands and may begin as painless swelling with pitting edema. The skin appears shiny and erythematous and eventually becomes indurated and "bound-down."

A. Patients with limited scleroderma typically have CREST syndrome (*c*alcinosis, *R*aynaud's phenomenon, *e*sophageal dysfunction, *s*clerodactyly, and *t*elangiectasia). Calcinosis most often is found over the hands and fingers or over the olecranon bursa. Sclerodactyly is defined as skin involvement distal to the metacarpophalangeal joints; telangiectasia is seen on the palms of the hands or over the face and lips. Patients with limited scleroderma and CREST syndrome also may have internal organ involvement, but this usually is delayed in comparison to diffuse scleroderma.

B. After the skin thickening of hands and fingers, the face and neck usually become involved next. The patient may develop pinched facies and pursed lips. The skin changes progress at variable rates to involve the arms, legs, and trunk. Hyper- and hypopigmentation commonly develop.

C. Patients with extensive skin involvement may develop digital skin ulcerations and joint contractures with inability to fully extend the fingers or form a fist. Skin tightening about the mouth may limit the oral aperture. In about 70% of patients, Raynaud's phenomenon is part of the initial presentation. GI complaints are the third most common symptom. Dysmotility of the lower two thirds of the esophagus may cause dysphagia and odynophagia as well as symptoms of reflux. Constipation and malabsorption may signify colonic dysmotility or small bowel involvement, respectively. Generalized arthralgias and morning stiffness often occur, although clinical synovitis is rare. Symptoms related to pulmonary involvement, such as progressive dyspnea on exertion, usually are insidious.

D. ANAs are present in >90% of patients with systemic sclerosis, usually with a nucleolar pattern. Anticentromere antibodies are present in most patients with CREST syndrome and in <10% of patients with systemic sclerosis. Chest radiographs may reveal increased bi-basilar interstitial markings but are relatively insensitive as a screening test. Pulmonary function testing reveals restriction with decreased vital capacity and compliance. The most common abnormality, however, is diminished diffusing capacity. Gallium lung scanning has proved relatively insensitive. Bronchoalveolar lavage has been used recently with increased frequency and reveals increased neutrophils and lymphocytes. Holter monitoring may detect atrial and ventricular tachyarrhythmias, which occur in 50% of patients. Skin biopsy may be helpful, but obviously the differentiation between the limited and diffuse forms of scleroderma is made clinically.

E. Eosinophilic fasciitis is a scleroderma-like disease characterized by inflammation and thickening of the deep fascia. The skin may have an "orange-peel" appearance. Raynaud's and internal organ involvement usually are absent. Eosinophilic myalgia syndrome is a recently described disease characterized by eosinophilia and myalgias. It has been associated with ingestion of the amino acid health food supplement tryptophan. In overlap syndromes, patients may have features of both scleroderma and systemic lupus erythematosus, inflammatory arthritis, or rheumatoid arthritis. Chronic graft-versus-host disease, a common complication of the allogeneic bone marrow transplant, may clinically appear similar to scleroderma, skin induration being the most common manifestation. Drugs that may induce skin thickening are bleomycin and pentazocine.

F. Localized scleroderma differs from systemic scleroderma in that there is no involvement of internal organs. Localized scleroderma may occur in at least two different clinical variants: morphea and linear scleroderma.

G. Morphea is characterized initially by well-circumscribed superficial plaques with subsequent development of ivory-colored centers and violaceous borders. Plaques may range in size from 1–30 cm; they may be few in number or multiple. Typically, they are asymmetric, although patients can have extensive involvement called *generalized morphea*. The disease course is variable, but there occasionally is spontaneous improvement or resolution over several months to years.

H. Linear scleroderma, unlike morphea, tends to involve deeper layers of the skin, often with fixation to underlying muscle and bone and occasionally causing fibrous contractures. It commonly occurs in a linear, bandlike distribution on the head, trunk, or extremities. When linear scleroderma involves the face and scalp, it may develop a depressed appearance and is called *en coup de sabre*.

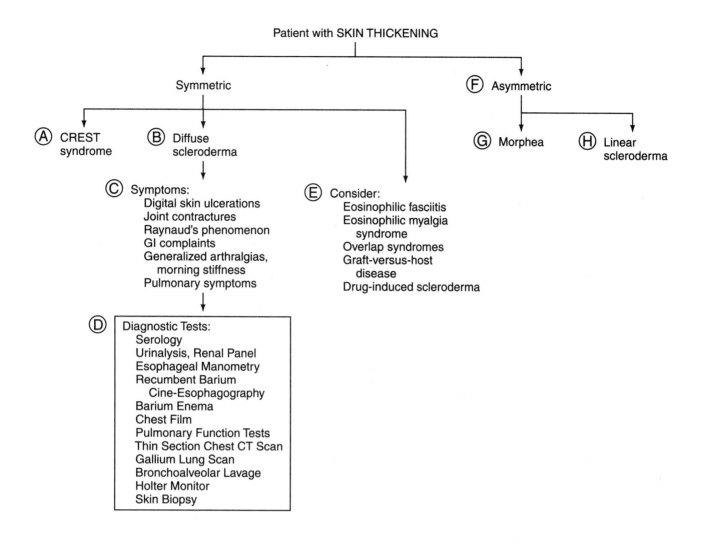

Patient with SKIN THICKENING

Symmetric

(F) Asymmetric

(A) CREST syndrome

(B) Diffuse scleroderma

(G) Morphea

(H) Linear scleroderma

(C) Symptoms:
    Digital skin ulcerations
    Joint contractures
    Raynaud's phenomenon
    GI complaints
    Generalized arthralgias,
      morning stiffness
    Pulmonary symptoms

(E) Consider:
    Eosinophilic fasciitis
    Eosinophilic myalgia
      syndrome
    Overlap syndromes
    Graft-versus-host
      disease
    Drug-induced scleroderma

(D) Diagnostic Tests:
    Serology
    Urinalysis, Renal Panel
    Esophageal Manometry
    Recumbent Barium
      Cine-Esophagography
    Barium Enema
    Chest Film
    Pulmonary Function Tests
    Thin Section Chest CT Scan
    Gallium Lung Scan
    Bronchoalveolar Lavage
    Holter Monitor
    Skin Biopsy

References

Black CM. Systemic sclerosis: management. In: Klippel JH, Dieppe PA, eds. Rheumatalogy. 2nd ed. London: Mosby, 1998:7.11.1.

Falanga V. Localized scleroderma. Med Clin North Am 1989; 73:1143.

Lally EV, Jimenez SA, Kaplan SR. Progressive systemic sclerosis: mode of presentation, rapidly progressive disease course, and mortality based on an analysis of 91 patients. Semin Arthritis Rheum 1988; 18:1.

Steen V. Systemic sclerosis. Rheum Dis Clin North Am 1990; 16:641.

Wigley FM. Systemic sclerosis: clinical features. In: Klippel JG, Dieppe PA, eds. Rheumatology. 2nd ed. London: Mosby, 1998:7.9.1.

KERATOCONJUNCTIVITIS SICCA (SJÖGREN'S SYNDROME)

Marcia Ko

A. Symptoms of keratoconjunctivitis sicca (KCS) result from decreased tear formation. Patients most often complain of gradual onset of "dry eyes" characterized as a foreign body sensation, grittiness, or sandy sensation, with or without visual changes or photophobia. Xerostomia or dry mouth secondary to salivary gland atrophy often is described as difficulty chewing or swallowing dry foods, such as crackers or bread, or difficulty talking secondary to dryness. There also may be a complaint of fissures or ulcers on mucosal surfaces or lips and the need to drink liquids to enable speech and eating. "Dryness" related to other exocrine gland dysfunction occurs (nose, tracheobronchial tree, skin).

B. Examination to confirm KCS may include a Schirmer test as a measure of tear formation. In this test, Schirmer filter paper is placed in the conjunctival sac. After 5 minutes the strips are removed to determine the extent of wetness (<15 mm of wetness is abnormal). A 1% rose bengal solution application and slit-lamp examination may demonstrate areas of corneal or conjunctival epithelial damage secondary to dryness. Another cause of diminished tear secretion is senile atrophy of the lacrimal glands.

C. Confirmation of dry mouth secondary to labial gland atrophy is difficult. Mild dryness may be normal or secondary to drugs such as anticholinergic medications. Salivary flow (volume) may be measured. Biopsy of minor salivary glands in the lip also has been used to support a clinical diagnosis because there is a characteristic histopathologic picture associated with Sjögren's syndrome characterized by a lymphocytic infiltration of the glands. Lack of salivary pooling in the floor of the mouth may be a sign of xerostomia.

D. Primary Sjögren's syndrome is diagnosed when other connective tissue disease is not present.

E. Other rheumatic diseases associated with Sjögren's syndrome ("secondary" Sjögren's) include rheumatoid arthritis, systemic lupus erythematosus, scleroderma, polyarteritis nodosa, and polymyositis.

F. Other clinical findings are related to exocrine gland dysfunction (mucous membrane dryness of the nose and upper airway, skin dryness, genital dryness). Pancreatic disease may also be seen. Atrophic gastritis has been described, but pernicious anemia is rare. Nonexocrine organs also may be involved, including peripheral nerves, joints, skin, and blood. Vasculitis and Raynaud's phenomenon may be found. Renal involvement is manifested most often as interstitial nephritis and type 2 renal tubular acidosis.

G. There are no specific laboratory tests for the diagnosis of Sjögren's syndrome. Rheumatoid factor is present in approximately 75–95% of patients; ANAs may be found in 50–80%. Anti-La (SS-B) and anti-Ro (SS-A) may be found. Other nonspecific laboratory tests include a normochromic, normocytic anemia; leukopenia; and elevated ESR. Serum protein electrophoresis may demonstrate diffuse elevation in all immunoglobulin classes. A fall in the rheumatoid factor may signify a malignant transformation to lymphoma, which has a 44-fold increased incidence in patients with primary Sjögren's syndrome.

References

Fox RI. Clinical features, pathogenesis and treatment of Sjögren's syndrome. Curr Opin Rheumatol 1996; 8:438.

Fox RI. Sjögren's syndrome. In: Kelley WN, Ruddy S, Harris ED Jr, eds. Textbook of rheumatology. 5th ed. Philadelphia: WB Saunders, 1997:955.

Price EJ, Venables EJ. The etiopathogenesis of Sjögren's syndrome. Semin Arthritis Rheum 1995; 25:117.

Talal N. Sjögren's syndrome. In: Schumacher HR, ed. Primer on rheumatic disease. 10th ed. Atlanta: Arthritis Foundation, 1993:132.

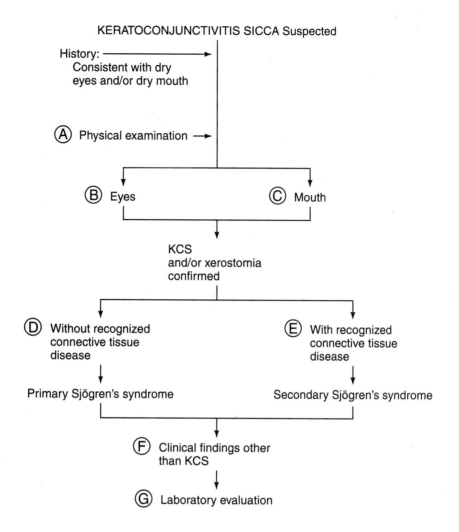

KERATOCONJUNCTIVITIS SICCA Suspected

History: ⟶
Consistent with dry
eyes and/or dry mouth

Ⓐ Physical examination ⟶

Ⓑ Eyes   Ⓒ Mouth

KCS
and/or xerostomia
confirmed

Ⓓ Without recognized   Ⓔ With recognized
connective tissue   connective tissue
disease   disease

Primary Sjögren's syndrome   Secondary Sjögren's syndrome

Ⓕ Clinical findings other
than KCS

Ⓖ Laboratory evaluation

RAYNAUD'S PHENOMENON

Patricia Mayer

Raynaud's phenomenon is characterized by intermittent vasoconstriction of the digits, usually triggered by cold or stress. Three classic stages are recognized: blanching, cyanotic, and ruborous. Raynaud's phenomenon may be mild and only minimally uncomfortable or may be severe, involving digital ulceration and/or gangrene. The phenomenon may be idiopathic (primary) or related to underlying abnormality (secondary).

A. A thorough history and a meticulous physical examination are essential to the evaluation and reveal most secondary causes.

B. Raynaud's phenomenon is almost always bilateral. Unilateral complaints should prompt an evaluation for neurogenic (thoracic outlet syndrome, carpal tunnel syndrome, reflex sympathetic dystrophy) or vascular (arteriosclerosis, embolic phenomenon, thromboangiitis obliterans) disease.

C. Raynaud's phenomenon may be seen in pneumatic hammer operators, in patients with repetitive wrist and finger motion (pianists, computer operators, typists), and after injury from trauma or cold. Environmental agents such as heavy metals and exposure to vinyl chloride monomer, used in the production of polyvinyl chloride, has been associated with Raynaud's phenomenon.

D. Multiple drugs and medications are associated with Raynaud's phenomenon. These include β-blocking agents, ergotamine preparations, various chemotherapeutic agents, oral contraceptives, nicotine, caffeine, and various antihistamines and decongestants.

E. Multiple underlying abnormalities may be associated with Raynaud's phenomenon, including most commonly any of the connective tissue disorders (e.g., systemic lupus erythematosus, Sjögren's syndrome, rheumatoid arthritis, dermatomyositis, scleroderma). If an underlying condition is suspected from the history and physical examination, further laboratory testing or other evaluations may be needed as the situation requires.

F. In patients in whom a thorough history and physical examination reveal no clues for further work-up or associated conditions, undertake a minimal laboratory work-up to rule out serious underlying causes, including occult malignancy, hematologic disease, and rheumatic disease. Raynaud's phenomenon may precede the development of connective tissue disease by months or years.

References

Coffman JD. The diagnosis of Raynaud's phenomenon. Clin Dermatol 1994; 12:283.

Langevitz P, Buskila D, Lee P, Urowitz MB. Treatment of refractory ischemic skin ulcers in patients with Raynaud's phenomenon with PGE infusions. J Rheumatol 1989; 16:1433.

Seibold JR, Allegar NE. The treatment of Raynaud's phenomenon. Clin Dermatol 1994; 12:317.

Patient with RAYNAUD'S PHENOMENON

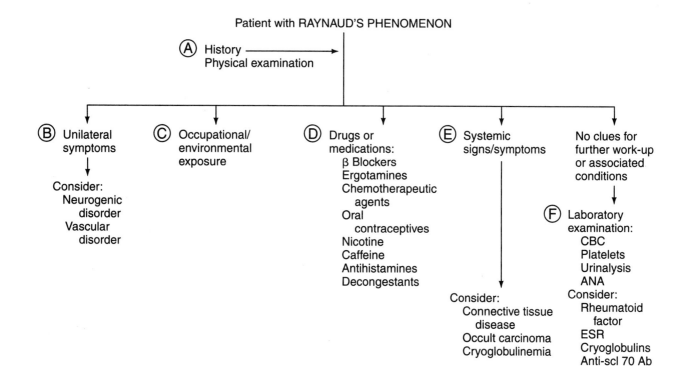

A History ——→ Physical examination

B Unilateral symptoms

↓

Consider:
Neurogenic
disorder
Vascular
disorder

C Occupational/
environmental
exposure

D Drugs or
medications:
β Blockers
Ergotamines
Chemotherapeutic
agents
Oral
contraceptives
Nicotine
Caffeine
Antihistamines
Decongestants

E Systemic
signs/symptoms

↓

Consider:
Connective tissue
disease
Occult carcinoma
Cryoglobulinemia

No clues for
further work-up
or associated
conditions

↓

F Laboratory
examination:
CBC
Platelets
Urinalysis
ANA
Consider:
Rheumatoid
factor
ESR
Cryoglobulins
Anti-scl 70 Ab

OSTEOPENIA

Michael J. Maricic

A. The initial evaluation of patients with osteopenia begins with evaluation of their risk factors. Risks for osteopenia include estrogen deficiency, family history, small body frame, calcium deficiency, inactivity, tobacco or alcohol abuse, or use of medications such as corticosteroids. A history of vitamin D deficiency, malabsorption, gastrectomy, anticonvulsant use, or renal disorders such as renal tubular acidosis should alert one to the possibility of osteomalacia.

B. Osteopenia, meaning "poverty of bone," is the radiographic appearance of diminished bone density. It is impossible to distinguish osteoporosis (decreased bone mass) from osteomalacia (decreased mineralization of bone) or osteitis fibrosa cystica (the bone lesion that occurs in hyperparathyroidism characterized by increased osteoclastic resorption and fibrosis) radiographically. Early radiographic signs of osteopenia may include preferential loss of horizontal striations in vertebral bodies or Schmorl's nodules (herniation of the nucleus pulposus into softened vertebral bodies). Often, 30% of bone density must be lost before osteopenia may be apparent on radiographs. Bone density scanning (e.g., dual energy x-ray absorptiometry) gives much more exact estimations of bone density and should be performed to confirm the diagnosis of low bone mass.

C. If osteopenia is present, perform screening laboratory tests for calcium, phosphorus, and alkaline phosphatase. A low phosphorus and high alkaline phosphatase level should alert one to the possibility of osteomalacia. Normal values do not exclude osteomalacia, however, and the vigor with which this is pursued depends on the presence of risk factors for osteomalacia previously mentioned. A dual-labeled tetracycline bone biopsy is necessary for the definitive diagnosis of osteomalacia. High calcium with low phosphorus and elevated alkaline phosphatase levels may be due to hyperparathyroidism.

D. Radiographically detected osteopenia most often is caused by osteoporosis. Genetics accounts for up to 75% of the variance in bone mass. Estrogen deficiency is the most common preventable cause of osteoporosis. Secondary causes of osteoporosis include neoplasia (multiple myeloma, lymphoma), drugs (corticosteroids), and endocrine disorders (hyperthyroidism, hyperparathyroidism, and secondary gonadal failure such as in prolactin-secreting tumors). Besides a detailed history and physical examination to seek these disorders, consider laboratory screening with serum calcium phosphate, alkaline phosphatase, CBC, thyroid function tests, ESR, and urinalysis.

References

Raiz LG. The osteoporosis revolution. Ann Intern Med 1997; 126:458.

Riggs BL, Melton LJ. Involutional osteoporosis. N Engl J Med 1986; 314:1676.

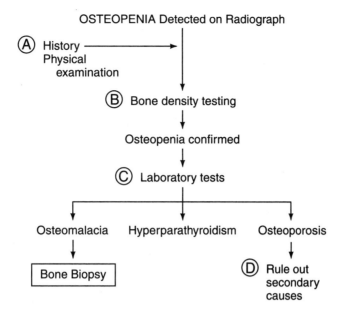

OSTEOPENIA Detected on Radiograph

(A) History
Physical
examination

(B) Bone density testing

Osteopenia confirmed

(C) Laboratory tests

Osteomalacia   Hyperparathyroidism   Osteoporosis

Bone Biopsy

(D) Rule out
secondary
causes

HYPERURICEMIA AND GOUT

Eric P. Gall

A. Hyperuricemia may be caused by many mechanisms, including overproduction of uric acid (20–25% of patients) and inability of the kidneys to excrete uric acid (75–80%). Overproduction may be caused by a congenital enzyme defect, but more often other clinical problems, including hemolytic anemia, myeloproliferative disease, and psoriasis, should be excluded. Underexcretion of uric acid may be caused by renal failure, drug action on the kidney, or in most cases, idiopathic mechanisms. Hyperuricemia generally is defined as a serum uric acid level >8 mg/dl. However, gout may occur even with a normal uric acid level because it is insoluble above 6 mg/dl.

B. The decision whether to treat asymptomatic hyperuricemia is controversial. Most physicians treat uric acid levels >10 mg/dl if the patient has only one kidney; hyperuricosuria (>1000 mg/day), placing the kidney at risk for stones; or extreme serum levels (>12–13 mg/dl). If these criteria are satisfied, treatment with allopurinol may begin. If these conditions are not present, observation of the patient will suffice.

C. The acute attack of gout can occur in any joint. Commonly, it occurs nocturnally in the first metatarsophalangeal (MTP) joint (podagra). The definitive diagnosis of gout is made by demonstration of sodium urate crystals under polarized light microscopy. The crystals are negatively birefringent and needle shaped. A polarizing microscope with a first-order red compensator is necessary. The definitive diagnosis is made when six or more of the following criteria are present: (1) more than one attack of arthritis, (2) development of maximum inflammation within 1 day, (3) oligoarthritis attack, (4) redness over the joint, (5) painful or swollen first MTP joint, (6) unilateral attack in the first MTP joint, (7) unilateral attack in the tarsal joint, (8) tophus, (9) hyperuricemia, (10) asymmetric swelling within a joint, and (11) termination of the attack with colchicine therapy.

D. The acute attack is treated before the underlying hyperuricemia. If there is no peptic ulcer disease or other contraindication to NSAIDs, these are the treatment of choice. A short-acting NSAID such as ibuprofen usually is chosen, but long-acting agents will work. The drugs should be started at relatively high dosage. Continue NSAID treatment until the acute arthritis is resolved. If peptic ulcer disease or other disease contraindicates the use of NSAIDs, alternative therapy is required.

E. If there is significant impairment of kidney, liver, or bone marrow function, give corticosteroids orally or parenterally at a dosage of 40–60 mg prednisone equivalent per day until the acute attack is resolved.

F. The use of alternative therapy depends on whether there is renal failure, hepatic insufficiency, or bone marrow depression. If none of these conditions is present, IV colchicine can be used in an initial dose of 2 mg in 50–100 ml of saline or glucose, infused by IV catheter over 15–30 minutes. It should not be pushed because it can cause cardiovascular collapse. Extravasation of colchicine can cause tissue necrosis. Doses of 1 mg may be repeated, if necessary, every 6 hours until a total daily dose of 4 mg is given. Because of the potential for toxicity, many physicians prefer the use of corticosteroids.

G. Before initiating chronic treatment for gout, measure serum and urine uric acid and creatinine levels. This should be done after the acute attack resolves. Patients are divided into overproducers of uric acid (24 hour uric acid >800 mg or a spot urinary uric acid/creatinine ratio >0.7) and underexcretors (24-hour urine uric acid <600 mg or a urinary uric acid/creatinine ratio <0.7).

H. In patients who overproduce uric acid, give allopurinol with colchicine. Begin with a single daily dose of 100–300 mg with 0.5 mg colchicine twice a day. If the patient has significant renal disease, use allopurinol as the drug of choice because uricosuric drugs will not be effective.

I. In patients who underexcrete uric acid and have no renal disease, uricosuric agents are the treatment of choice. The reason for using these drugs in this situation is because of allopurinol's significant toxicity, including skin rash and systemic vasculitis. Start probenecid 500 mg twice a day orally and adjust according to the serum uric acid. Adequate urinary volume with good fluid intake should be ensured. Patients who have had renal calculi should not take uricosuric agents. Those on probenecid should be given colchicine at a low dosage initially.

J. With either allopurinol or probenecid, adjust the serum uric acid level to < 6 mg/dl. This is done by instituting therapy and ensuring compliance. Gradual adjustments are made until the serum uric acid level drops to <6 mg/dl. Colchicine at a low dosage is maintained until 6 weeks after the required serum level is reached, until all recurrent acute attacks have resolved, or if the patient has tophaceous gout, until the tophi disappear. If acute attacks recur, treatment is similar to that mentioned earlier, without a change in uric acid–lowering drugs during the initial acute treatment.

References

Kelley WN, Wortman RL. Gout and hyperuricemia. In: Kelley WN, Harris E, Ruddy S, Sledge C, eds. Textbook of rheumatology. 5th ed. Philadelphia: WB Saunders, 1997:1313.

Siegel LB, Clark CL, Gall EP. Modern remedies for an age-old malady. Am J Therapeutics 1996; 3:468.

Patient with HYPERURICEMIA and GOUT

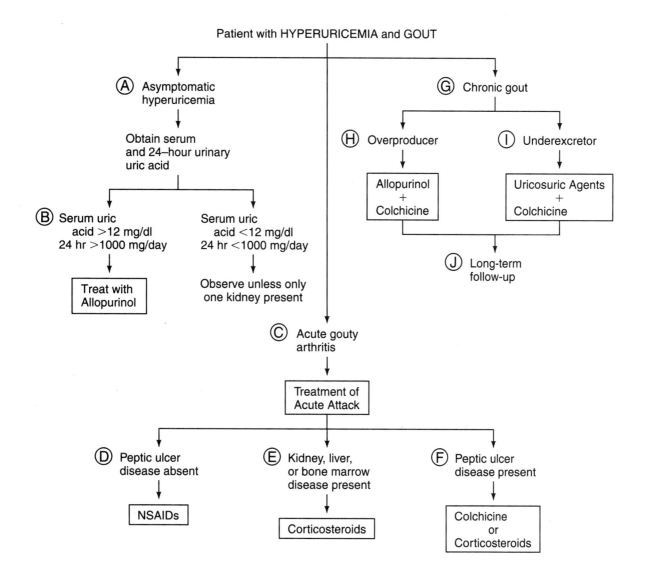

DIFFUSE MUSCLE PAIN AND STIFFNESS: POLYMYALGIA RHEUMATICA AND GIANT CELL ARTERITIS

Michael J. Maricic

A. Diffuse muscle pain and stiffness usually are manifestations of systemic disease and therefore necessitate a complete history and physical examination. It is important initially to determine whether myopathic weakness is present or absent (proximal weakness, e.g., inability to get out of a chair or to comb one's hair). Early in the disease, there may be mild overlap between the disorders that cause true weakness and those that do not.

B. If myopathic weakness is present, consider endocrine (hyper- or hypothyroid, hyperparathyroid, acromegaly, diabetes mellitus), electrolyte (hypophosphatemia, hypokalemia), neoplastic (Eaton-Lambert), drug-induced (alcohol, corticosteroids), inflammatory (poly- or dermatomyositis) disorders, and muscular dystrophy. Appropriate laboratory testing for the endocrine and electrolyte disorders, electromyographic (EMG) studies showing incremental response to repetitive muscle stimulation in the Eaton-Lambert syndrome, and characteristic rash, EMG, and biopsy findings in polydermatomyositis help lead to the appropriate diagnosis. A family history usually is present in the various types of muscular dystrophy.

C. If true muscle weakness is absent, yet the patient complains of severe pain and stiffness, consider polymyalgia rheumatica (PMR) (in patients >60 years old), viral syndromes, fibromyalgia, depression, and hypothyroidism as potential causes. Appropriate laboratory testing in such patients with chronic symptoms includes ESR and thyroid function tests.

D. PMR is most commonly seen in patients >60 years old with occasional onset in those >50. The onset is usually abrupt, with severe morning stiffness relieved by activity. True weakness of the muscles is absent, although patients may develop some disuse atrophy and flexion contractures of the shoulders over time because of severe pain. The ESR usually is greatly elevated, although a normal ESR does not rule out the diagnosis. Because 20% of patients with PMR have or will develop giant cell arteritis (GCA), once the diagnosis of PMR is entertained, question and examine them extensively for symptoms and signs of GCA. These include headache, visual changes, jaw claudication, scalp numbness, tender temporal arteries, and signs of ischemic retinopathy on funduscopic examination. Nonspecific systemic symptoms such as fever, night sweats, and weight loss should also alert one to the possibility of a systemic vasculitis.

E. If GCA is suspected, begin therapy with high-dose prednisone immediately and schedule the patient for temporal artery biopsy. If there are no signs or symptoms of GCA, low-dose prednisone may be started.

References

Hall S, Persellin S, Lie JT, et al. The therapeutic impact of temporal artery biopsy. Lancet 1983; 2:1217.

Huston KA, Hunder GG, Lie JT, et al. Temporal arteritis. A 25-year epidemiologic, clinical, and pathologic study. Ann Intern Med 1978; 88:162.

Swannell AJ. Polymyalgia rheumatica and temporal arteritis: diagnosis and management. BMJ 1997; 314:1329.

Patient with DIFFUSE MUSCLE PAIN AND STIFFNESS

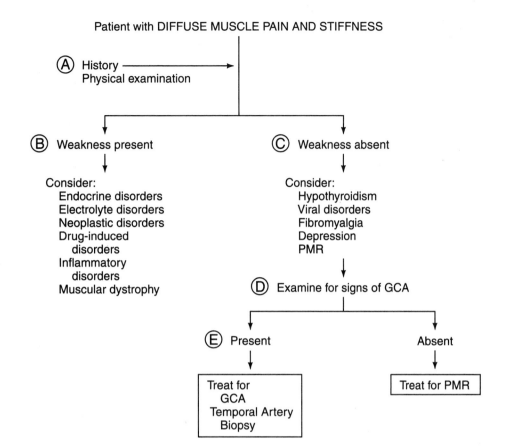

Ⓐ History ———————→
Physical examination

Ⓑ Weakness present

Consider:
    Endocrine disorders
    Electrolyte disorders
    Neoplastic disorders
    Drug-induced
      disorders
    Inflammatory
      disorders
    Muscular dystrophy

Ⓒ Weakness absent

Consider:
    Hypothyroidism
    Viral disorders
    Fibromyalgia
    Depression
    PMR

Ⓓ Examine for signs of GCA

Ⓔ Present

Treat for
  GCA
Temporal Artery
  Biopsy

Absent

Treat for PMR

JOINT HYPERMOBILITY

Patricia Mayer

A. The congenital disorders causing joint hypermobility usually can be diagnosed with a careful history and physical examination. Family history may provide a diagnosis, but spontaneous mutations do occur and are responsible for many cases. Because family history may be unhelpful or unavailable, the algorithm relies on clinical characteristics for diagnosis whenever possible. Patients with true joint hypermobility can perform at least four of the following maneuvers: hyperextend the elbow 10 degrees or more past neutral; extend the metacarpophalangeal (MCP) joints to 90 degrees or more; flex the thumb to touch the wrist, digits (hyperextension of the proximal interphalangeal with flexion of the distal interphalangeals); flex the trunk forward so that the palms rest on the floor.

B. Evaluate the patient for evidence of Marfan's syndrome. A patient with all the cardinal manifestations (ocular, skeletal, and cardiac) or two of the major manifestations in the presence of a positive family history can be considered to meet the criteria. The most common ocular manifestation is ectopia lentis with upward displacement of the lens. Cardiovascular involvement includes dilation of the ascending aorta, aortic dissection, aortic regurgitation, and mitral valve prolapse. Skeletal features include abnormally tall stature, dolichostenomelia, arachnodactyly, high arched palate, and anterior chest deformities.

C. If criteria are met, consider the differential diagnosis of Marfan's syndrome. It is especially important to consider the possibility of homocystinuria, a recessively inherited inborn error of metabolism that is treatable. Erdheim's disease (annuloaortic ectasia) and Stickler's syndrome (hereditary arthro-ophthalmopathy) also may mimic Marfan's syndrome.

D. An evaluation of skin texture allows categorization of most disorders into one of three groups: normal skin, hyperextensible skin with dystrophic scarring, or lax or wrinkled skin. A few disorders do not fit this classification (see R).

E. If the skin is normal, evaluate stature. Most patients with short stature have frank characteristics of dwarfism and are below the 5th percentile in height for their age and sex.

F. Abnormally short patients with joint hypermobility generally have one of the skeletal dysplasias associated with joint hypermobility. Prominent spinal involvement with malalignment and dislocation is a hallmark of spondyloepimetaphyseal dysplasia with joint laxity (SEMDJL). Larsen's syndrome (flattened nasal bridge and broad terminal phalanges) and Desbuquois' syndrome (prominent eyes, broad terminal phalanges, and supernumerary phalanges) generally lack features of spinal malalignment or dislocation.

G. Recurrent dislocations are the cardinal feature of familial joint hypermobility of the so-called dislocating type. Dislocations are most prominent at the knees, hips, and elbows. Larsen's syndrome also is characterized by recurrent dislocations and may be associated with normal, as well as short, stature.

H. Ehlers-Danlos syndrome (EDS) type X may show striae distensae or prominent bruising or petechiae on skin with otherwise normal texture and extensibility. Patients with joint hypermobility unrelated to skin or stature abnormalities, and without recurrent dislocations, may have either familial hypermobility, so-called uncomplicated type, or EDS III. Although EDS III usually has some skin hyperextensibility, it may be so mild that it is overlooked.

(Continued on page 448)

Patient with JOINT HYPERMOBILITY

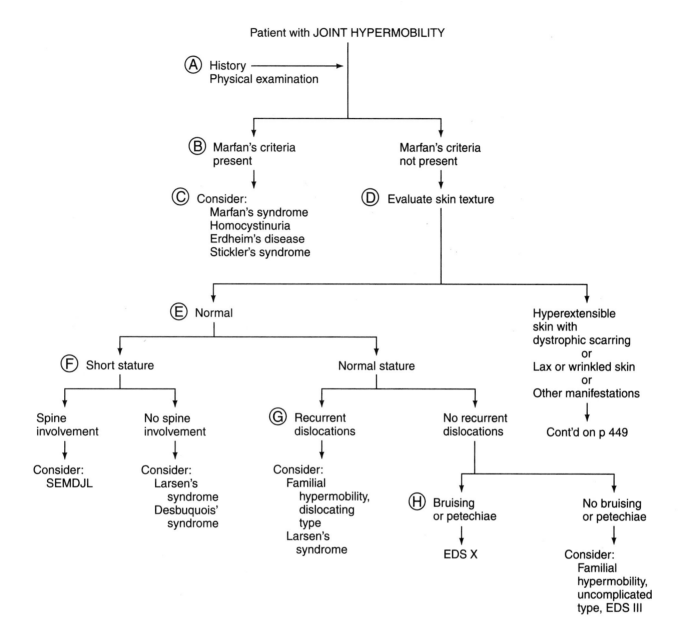

A. History
Physical examination

B. Marfan's criteria present

Marfan's criteria not present

C. Consider:
Marfan's syndrome
Homocystinuria
Erdheim's disease
Stickler's syndrome

D. Evaluate skin texture

E. Normal

Hyperextensible skin with dystrophic scarring
or
Lax or wrinkled skin
or
Other manifestations

F. Short stature

Normal stature

Cont'd on p 449

Spine involvement

No spine involvement

G. Recurrent dislocations

No recurrent dislocations

Consider:
SEMDJL

Consider:
Larsen's syndrome
Desbuquois' syndrome

Consider:
Familial hypermobility, dislocating type
Larsen's syndrome

H. Bruising or petechiae

No bruising or petechiae

EDS X

Consider:
Familial hypermobility, uncomplicated type, EDS III

I. Hyperextensible skin usually is associated with dystrophic scarring, as evidenced by the so-called cigarette paper scars, and also may be associated with tissue fragility and easy bruising. Such "loose skin" is a cardinal manifestation of several types of EDS.

J. Some of the Ehlers-Danlos syndromes are distinguished primarily by their dramatic extradermal/extra-articular involvement. EDS VIII is characterized by the early onset of severe periodontitis associated with gingival recession and early tooth loss. Short stature and micrognathia accompany severe skin and joint involvement in EDS VII. Ocular involvement and scoliosis are seen in EDS VI. Stickler's syndrome can mimic both EDS VI and Marfan's syndrome.

K. The severity of joint involvement in the EDS syndromes associated with characteristic hyperextensible skin with dystrophic scarring can be gauged as either severe to moderate or moderate to mild.

L. Severely affected skin and severely affected joints are seen in the X-linked EDS V as well as the autosomal-dominant EDS I, or gravis type.

M. EDS III, also called *benign hypermobility,* may have mild or even undetectable (see H) skin changes associated with severe joint hypermobility.

N. Both EDS II and EDS V may have moderate or mild joint involvement and are then distinguished by their inheritance. EDS II, or mitis type, is autosomal dominant; EDS V is X-linked.

O. The lax and wrinkled skin syndromes generally are not associated with hyperextensibility, scarring, or the fragility described above.

P. Menkes' syndrome, formerly called *Menkes' kinky hair syndrome,* is characterized by abnormal hair as well as vascular rupture and brain dysfunction. It is caused by an X-linked disorder of copper transport and can be seen in both classic (severe) and mild forms.

Q. Wrinkled skin over the hands and feet associated with low birth weight characterizes wrinkly skin syndrome. Diffuse wrinkly or lax skin is seen in both occipital horn syndrome and the variant of cutis laxa called *cutis laxa with joint hypermobility and developmental delay.* The classic form of cutis laxa is not associated with joint hypermobility.

R. Disorders with characteristic skin manifestations not described in other groups include the yellow infiltrated flexural lesions of pseudoxanthoma elasticum (PXE) and the striae distensae of EDS X.

References

Beighton P, dePaepe A, Danks D, et al. International nosology of heritable disorders of connective tissue, Berlin, 1986. Am J Med Genet 1988; 29:581.

Beighton P, McKusick VA, eds. McKusick's heritable disorders of connective tissue. 5th ed. St. Louis: Mosby, 1993.

Finsterbush A, Pogrund H. The hypermobility syndrome. Clin Orthop 1982; 168:124.

Pyeritz RE. The Marfan syndrome. Am Fam Physician 1986; 34:83.

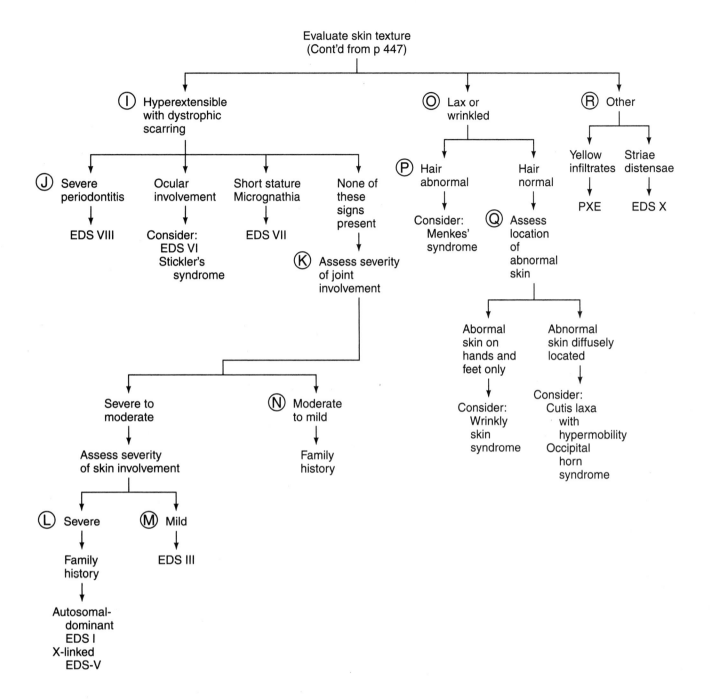

Evaluate skin texture
(Cont'd from p 447)

Ⓘ Hyperextensible with dystrophic scarring

Ⓙ Severe periodontitis → EDS VIII

Ocular involvement → Consider: EDS VI Stickler's syndrome

Short stature Micrognathia → EDS VII

None of these signs present → Ⓚ Assess severity of joint involvement

Severe to moderate → Assess severity of skin involvement

Ⓛ Severe → Family history → Autosomal-dominant EDS I X-linked EDS-V

Ⓜ Mild → EDS III

Ⓝ Moderate to mild → Family history

Ⓞ Lax or wrinkled

Ⓟ Hair abnormal → Consider: Menkes' syndrome

Hair normal → Ⓠ Assess location of abnormal skin

Abormal skin on hands and feet only → Consider: Wrinkly skin syndrome

Abnormal skin diffusely located → Consider: Cutis laxa with hypermobility Occipital horn syndrome

Ⓡ Other

Yellow infiltrates → PXE

Striae distensae → EDS X

449

TEMPOROMANDIBULAR PAIN

Michael J. Maricic

A. A thorough history and physical examination are required to exclude pain not originating in the temporomandibular joint (TMJ).

B. Plain radiographs should be taken in the panoramic and transcranial views in both open and closed positions. Tomography also may be helpful. Radiography may reveal roughened and irregular bony cortices and flattening and anterior lipping of the condyle in degenerative joint disease. Radiographs may be normal in internal derangement, and in this case arthrography and/or MRI may be needed to establish a definitive diagnosis.

C. Nonarticular causes of pain in the TMJ region include otitis, pain of dental origin, sinusitis, neuralgia, and temporal arteritis. Myofascial pain and dysfunction of the muscles of mastication may be the cause of the pain. Pain present on palpation of the muscle, no pain on palpation of the TMJ, and normal radiographs may be clues to this latter diagnosis.

D. Internal derangement of the TMJ occurs because of an abnormal relationship of the fibrous connective tissue disc with the condyle when the teeth are in maximal occlusion. Pain on palpation of the condyle and popping and clicking in the TMJ are common signs.

E. Degenerative joint disease generally has an insidious onset. Pain usually is continuous and increases with activity. Coarse crepitus may be present.

F. Other systemic arthritides such as rheumatoid arthritis and systemic lupus, as well as developmental deformities and neoplasia, also may affect the TMJ, necessitating a complete history and physical examination.

References

Dolwick MF, Katzberg RW, Helms CA, Bales DJ. Arthrotomographic evaluation of the temporomandibular joint. J Oral Surg 1979; 37:793.

Ryan DE. Painful temporomandibular joint. In: McCarty DJ, Koopman WJ, eds. Arthritis and allied conditions. 12th ed. Baltimore: Williams & Wilkins, 1993.

Stack BC Jr, Stack BC Sr. Temporomandibular joint disorder. Am Fam Physician 1992; 46:143.

Patient with TEMPOROMANDIBULAR PAIN

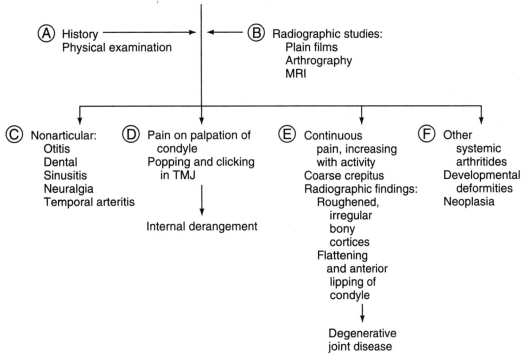

Ⓐ History
Physical examination

Ⓑ Radiographic studies:
Plain films
Arthrography
MRI

Ⓒ Nonarticular:
Otitis
Dental
Sinusitis
Neuralgia
Temporal arteritis

Ⓓ Pain on palpation of
condyle
Popping and clicking
in TMJ

Internal derangement

Ⓔ Continuous
pain, increasing
with activity
Coarse crepitus
Radiographic findings:
Roughened,
irregular
bony
cortices
Flattening
and anterior
lipping of
condyle

Degenerative
joint disease

Ⓕ Other
systemic
arthritides
Developmental
deformities
Neoplasia

POSITIVE ANTINUCLEAR ANTIBODY TEST

Marcia Ko

A. Order the ANA test only if there is a strong clinical suspicion of rheumatic disease based on history and physical examination. The ARA criteria may be helpful in focusing in an organized manner, specifically on clinical symptoms and signs suggesting systemic lupus erythematosus (SLE).

B. The titer of ANA may be helpful. Low titers of 1:40 may be seen in up to 5% of normal individuals and increase with age.

C. The pattern of ANAs may help direct further laboratory evaluation of ANA-related diseases. The four recognized patterns of ANA immunofluorescence are (1) homogeneous (suggests antibodies to nuclear proteins); (2) speckled (antibodies to nonhistone nuclear antigens, such as Smith [SM] and ribonucleoprotein [RNP]), (3) rim (antibodies to DNA) and (4) nucleolar (antibodies to nucleolar RNA). For example, the rim patterns may be seen in SLE and may suggest follow-up testing for antibody to double-stranded DNA. A speckled ANA immunofluorescence pattern may warrant further evaluation with testing for extractable nuclear antigens such as SM or RNP.

D. Antibodies to double-stranded DNA are measured via the Farr assay (radioimmunoassay) or using *Crithidia luciliae* as a substrate for indirect immunofluorescence. These antibodies are thought to be fairly specific for SLE and the titer may be used to follow disease activity.

E. Many extractable nuclear antigens are recognized. In clinical practice, the most commonly measured include anti-SM, anti-RNP, anti-RO (SSA), and anti-LA (SSB).

F. The SM antigen is saline extractable and, although not very sensitive (20–35% of patients with SLE), is considered very specific for SLE.

G. Antibody to RNP is nonspecific and found in many connective tissue diseases, including SLE, rheumatoid arthritis, Sjögren's syndrome, scleroderma, and polymyositis. The presence of high-titer anti-RNP in the absence of other ANA and typical clinical picture may suggest mixed connective tissue disease (MCTD).

H. Anti-RO and anti-LA are antibodies to the extractable nuclear antigens SS-A and SS-B. These antibodies may be detected in several rheumatic diseases, including Sjögren's syndrome (approximately 60–70%), SLE, and subacute cutaneous lupus. The neonatal lupus syndrome has been associated with the presence of RO or anti-SS-A in the mothers of affected infants.

I. The anticentromere antibody, directed against the centromere of chromosomes, appears as a speckled ANA and may be helpful if other clinical features of the CREST syndrome are not fully apparent. The test is reported to be 57–96% positive in patients with this diagnosis.

J. Antihistone antibodies have been reported to be a helpful adjunct in the diagnosis of drug-induced lupus syndromes. Multiple drugs have been incriminated, including sulfonamides, penicillin, procainamide, alpha-methyldopa, anticonvulsants, isoniazid, antithyroid agents, and quinidine.

K. A negative ANA does not completely exclude the diagnosis of SLE: 10–15% of SLE patients may have a negative ANA, depending on the methods used. A negative ANA also may be interpreted as unsupportive of a diagnosis of SLE if other criteria are absent.

References

Hietarinta M, Lassila O. Clinical significance of antinuclear antibodies in systemic rheumatic diseases. Ann Med 1996; 28:283.

Nakamura RM, Tan EM. Update on autoantibodies to intracellular antigens in systemic rheumatic diseases. Clin Lab Med 1992; 12:1.

Robin R. Drug-induced lupus. Clin Asp Autoimmun 1988; 2:16.

Schumacher HR, ed. Primer on rheumatic disease. 10th ed. Atlanta: Arthritis Foundation, 1993.

Tan EM. Antinuclear antibodies: diagnostic markers for autoimmune disease and probes for cell immunology. Adv Immunol 1989; 44:93.

Tan EM, Cohen AS, Fries JF, et al. The 1982 revised criteria for the classification of system lupus erythematosus. Arthritis Rheum 1982; 25:127.

Watson RM, Lane AT, Barnett NK, et al. Neonatal lupus erythematosus: a clinical, serological and immunogenetic study with review of the literature. Medicine 1984; 63:362.

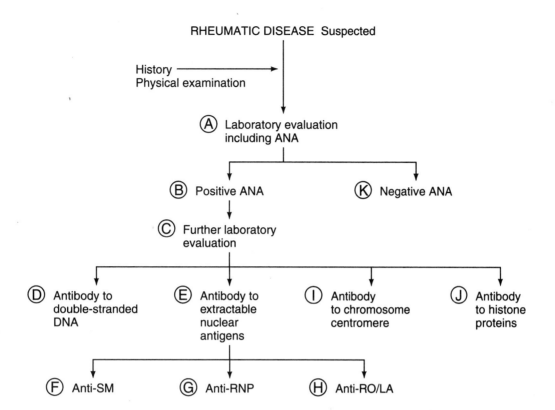

RHEUMATIC DISEASE Suspected

History
Physical examination

(A) Laboratory evaluation
including ANA

(B) Positive ANA

(K) Negative ANA

(C) Further laboratory
evaluation

(D) Antibody to
double-stranded
DNA

(E) Antibody to
extractable
nuclear
antigens

(I) Antibody
to chromosome
centromere

(J) Antibody
to histone
proteins

(F) Anti-SM

(G) Anti-RNP

(H) Anti-RO/LA

ELEVATED SERUM ALKALINE PHOSPHATASE LEVEL

Michael J. Maricic

A. An isolated elevated serum alkaline phosphatase level is a common finding with the widespread use of chemistry screening. A complete history and physical examination may point toward the cause of the elevation and preclude the need for further extensive evaluation. Although alkaline phosphatase may be derived from any organ, an elevation most commonly is seen in biliary tract and bone disease.

B. The first step in the laboratory work-up should be to obtain a serum gamma glutamyl transferase (GGPT) and other liver function tests (LFTs) to determine whether there is biliary tract or liver disease. The serum alkaline phosphatase may be fractionated, the heat-stable portion being derived from liver and the heat-labile portion from bone, or a serum bone-specific alkaline phosphatase may be obtained.

C. If these tests point toward a biliary origin, a work-up of liver and biliary tract disease, including ultrasonography, is indicated.

D. If the tests point toward bone as the source of the elevation, check serum calcium and phosphorus to screen for metabolic bone disease.

E. An elevated calcium and low phosphorus level may suggest hyperparathyroidism. Normal calcium, low phosphorus, and elevated alkaline phosphatase levels may be found in osteomalacia.

F. If the calcium and phosphorus are normal in an asymptomatic patient, Paget's disease of the bone is the most common cause of an elevated alkaline phosphatase from bone. Metastatic disease to bone, healing fractures, and inflammatory arthritis also may cause an elevated alkaline phosphatase level, but these conditions should be apparent clinically.

G. Direct plain radiographic evaluation toward areas of pain or deformity when present. When these are not evident, obtain radiographs of the skull and pelvis, which are areas of frequent involvement in Paget's disease. If these are negative, obtain a technetium bone scan, always correlating areas of increased uptake with plain radiographs.

References

Delmas PD, Memnier PJ. The management of Paget's disease of bone. N Engl J Med 1997; 336:558.

Resnick D. Paget disease of bone: current status and a look back to 1943 and earlier. AJR 1988; 150:249.

Patient with ELEVATED ALKALINE PHOSPHATASE LEVEL

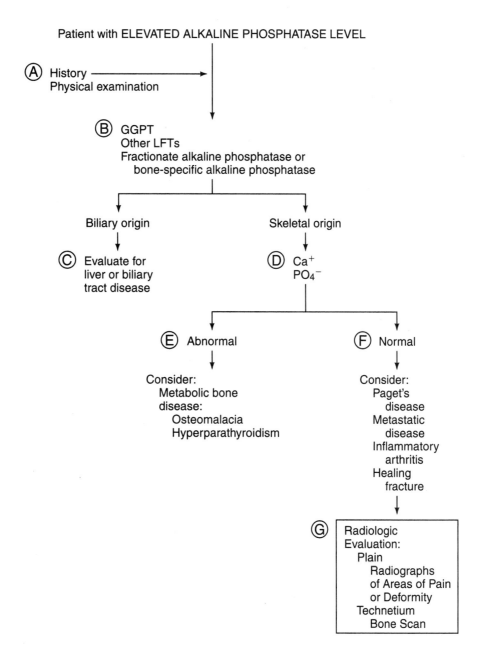

Ⓐ History ——————————→
  Physical examination

Ⓑ GGPT
  Other LFTs
  Fractionate alkaline phosphatase or
    bone-specific alkaline phosphatase

Biliary origin   Skeletal origin

Ⓒ Evaluate for   Ⓓ Ca$^+$
  liver or biliary   PO$_4^-$
  tract disease

                    Ⓔ Abnormal   Ⓕ Normal

                    Consider: Consider:
                      Metabolic bone   Paget's
                      disease: disease
                        Osteomalacia   Metastatic
                        Hyperparathyroidism   disease
                                                Inflammatory
                                                  arthritis
                                                Healing
                                                  fracture

                                        Ⓖ Radiologic
                                          Evaluation:
                                          Plain
                                            Radiographs
                                            of Areas of Pain
                                            or Deformity
                                          Technetium
                                            Bone Scan

ELEVATED CREATINE KINASE LEVEL

Patricia Mayer

A. An elevated creatine kinase (CK) level may be detected on routine panel testing or may be ordered in a variety of clinical settings, most commonly in the work-up of musculoskeletal or cardiac complaints. This chapter focuses on the elevated CK seen incidentally and in the work-up of musculoskeletal complaints. Several causes of elevated CK are obvious on presentation (malignant hyperthermia, severe hypo- or hyperthermia, acute crushing trauma causing rhabdomyolysis) and are not discussed here.

B. When assessing an elevated CK level, it is essential to first determine the origin of the enzyme: cardiac (represented by the MB isoenzyme fraction), brain (BB), or muscle (MM). This may be clinically apparent, as in a patient with acute chest pain and ECG changes, or with severe proximal muscle weakness. However, if the origin of the enzyme is in question, particularly if there is any suspicion of cardiac injury, perform isoenzyme tests on at least one occasion.

C. If the CK elevation is of cardiac origin, immediately undertake appropriate cardiac evaluation and therapy.

D. Occasionally, cerebral disease causes elevated CK levels, with a significant percentage of the BB isoenzyme. This situation is virtually always clinically apparent (acute cerebral trauma).

E. Most noncardiac elevations of CK are caused by enzyme release from muscle. The remainder of the decision tree is designed for use in distinguishing the various causes of muscle-related CK elevations.

F. A thorough history and detailed physical examination are essential and often reveal the cause of the CK elevation. The history should specifically cover family history (positive in the inherited myopathies), trauma history (including vigorous exercise, contusions, intramuscular injections, surgery, EMG studies, and ischemia), and drug/medication history (IV drugs, amphetamines, alcohol, cocaine, corticosteroids, cholesterol-lowering drugs, excessive licorice ingestion). Explore all musculoskeletal complaints, especially muscle weakness or tenderness, in detail. The physical examination must include a complete neurologic evaluation and musculoskeletal examination that includes muscle strength testing.

G. If there are musculoskeletal symptoms or findings, order CBC, electrolyte, and thyroid function studies before proceeding further. Again, treat underlying conditions.

H. If the preliminary examinations are unrevealing, perform specific muscle testing via EMG. This should distinguish normal muscle from muscle that exhibits either myopathic or neuropathic changes. Because most muscle diseases are bilateral and symmetric, a unilateral EMG is recommended.

I. If the EMG is completely normal when done on symptomatic muscle, the patient should be followed. If symptoms resolve, no further work-up is needed. If symptoms worsen or persist, consider a muscle biopsy.

J. If the EMG reveals myopathic changes, a muscle biopsy is performed to determine the underlying pathology.

K. A muscle biopsy should be done on clinically involved muscle on the side opposite the EMG site to avoid possible artifact in the biopsy from the EMG needle. In addition to routine histology, histochemical staining, ultrastructural studies, or other special tests may be required for a pathologic diagnosis.

L. If the muscle biopsy is normal, the patient may be followed. However, many muscle diseases are patchy and a single biopsy may miss the involved site. Therefore, if symptoms persist, consider repeat biopsy.

M. Treat inflammatory myopathies such as polymyositis primarily with corticosteroids.

N. The inherited and congenital myopathies are most often treated symptomatically. The muscular dystrophies in particular require appropriate neurologic follow-up.

O. A variety of other conditions may be revealed on biopsy, including other collagen vascular disorders, vasculitis, and steroid myopathy. Direct treatment specifically toward these entities.

P. If the EMG reveals neuropathic changes, consider motor neuron disease, peripheral neuropathies, or other neurologic disease. Further work-up of these conditions may be required (p 366).

Q. If the history and physical examination are completely normal, consider a minimal laboratory study, including a CBC (to evaluate possible occult infection), electrolytes (with special attention to potassium), and thyroid tests. If any of the tests are positive, the underlying abnormality should be corrected. If negative, no further work-up is recommended and the patient can be followed.

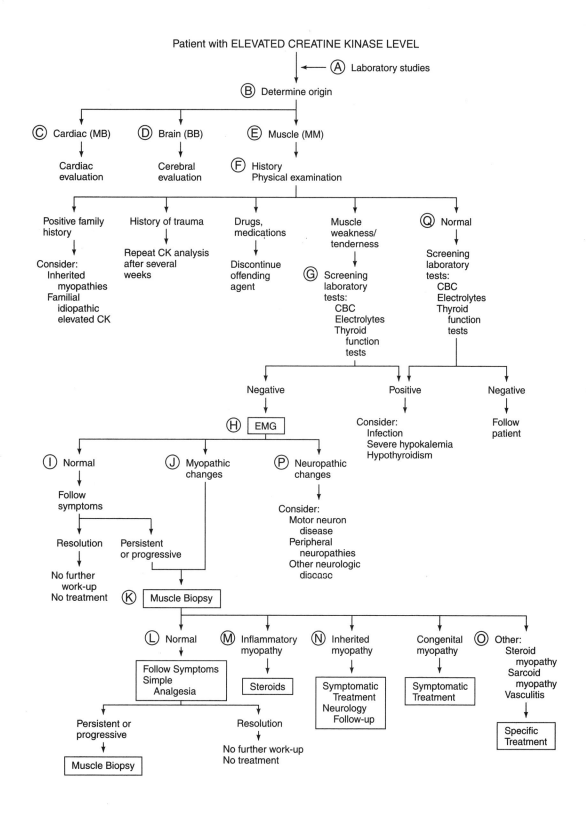

Patient with ELEVATED CREATINE KINASE LEVEL

Ⓐ Laboratory studies

Ⓑ Determine origin

Ⓒ Cardiac (MB) — Cardiac evaluation

Ⓓ Brain (BB) — Cerebral evaluation

Ⓔ Muscle (MM)

Ⓕ History / Physical examination

Positive family history
Consider:
Inherited myopathies
Familial idiopathic elevated CK

History of trauma
Repeat CK analysis after several weeks

Drugs, medications
Discontinue offending agent

Muscle weakness/tenderness
Ⓖ Screening laboratory tests:
CBC
Electrolytes
Thyroid function tests

Ⓠ **Normal**
Screening laboratory tests:
CBC
Electrolytes
Thyroid function tests

Negative
Ⓗ EMG

Positive
Consider:
Infection
Severe hypokalemia
Hypothyroidism

Negative
Follow patient

Ⓘ Normal
Follow symptoms

Resolution
No further work-up
No treatment

Persistent or progressive

Ⓙ Myopathic changes

Ⓟ Neuropathic changes
Consider:
Motor neuron disease
Peripheral neuropathies
Other neurologic disease

Ⓚ Muscle Biopsy

Ⓛ Normal
Follow Symptoms
Simple Analgesia

Persistent or progressive
Muscle Biopsy

Resolution
No further work-up
No treatment

Ⓜ Inflammatory myopathy
Steroids

Ⓝ Inherited myopathy
Symptomatic Treatment
Neurology Follow-up

Congenital myopathy
Symptomatic Treatment

Ⓞ Other:
Steroid myopathy
Sarcoid myopathy
Vasculitis
Specific Treatment

References

Bradley WG, Fries TJ. Neuromuscular testing. In: Kelley WN, Harris ED, Ruddy S, Sledge CG, eds. Textbook of rheumatology. 4th ed. Philadelphia: WB Saunders, 1995.

Chutkow JG. Diagnosis: muscular dystrophy. Hosp Med 1989; 138.

Kagen LJ. Approach to the patient with myopathy. Bull Rheum Dis 1983; 33:8.

Nanji AA. Serum creatine kinase isoenzymes: a review. Muscle Nerve 1983; 6:83.

Panteghini M. Enzymes and muscle diseases. Curr Opin Rheumatol 1995; 7:469.

WOMEN'S HEALTH

VAGINAL DISCHARGE

Amir Nasseri

A. Vulvovaginitis is the most common complaint necessitating a gynecologic examination. It commonly is defined as inflammation of the vulva and vagina. Upon initial evaluation, obtain a thorough history of previous episodes, possible sexual exposure, and color and consistency of the discharge. Pay particular attention to factors that can change vaginal flora, thus leading to vaginitis (recent antibiotic use, oral contraceptives, spermicides, douching). Also consider systemic conditions (poorly controlled diabetes, menopause, AIDS).

B. The cause of the vaginitis often can be determined at the time of speculum examination. Prepare two wet mounts using 10% KOH and normal saline, and view them under low and high power. Appearance of the discharge often can be helpful in diagnosis: Bacterial vaginosis gives a gray-white appearance; *Trichomonas vaginalis* a profuse, watery, white green or yellow appearance; and *Candida* a white cheesy discharge. Determining the pH of the vaginal discharge using pH indicator paper can be most useful. Normal physiologic discharge and yeast usually are <4.5; >5.0 may indicate *Trichomonas* or bacterial vaginosis.

C. If wet mount is nondiagnostic, consider allergic reaction to chemical or physical irritants. These possibilities are numerous and include tight clothing, deodorants, laundry detergent, soaps, tampons, and spermicides. Obtain culture for *Neisseria gonorrhoeae* and *Chlamydia trachomatis* in sexually active patients, and base treatment on subsequent results. Viral causes of vulvovaginitis include human papillomavirus (HPV) and herpes simplex virus (HSV). These often are diagnosed by appearance but can be confirmed by biopsy and culture. Aphthous ulcers can also occur on the vulva with an appearance similar to HSV.

D. The appearance of the unicellular protozoan *Trichomonas vaginalis* is diagnostic. Culture is not necessary for confirmation. The appearance under high power is of mobile flagellated organisms slightly larger than a WBC. The smear also may have many inflammatory cells and vaginal epithelial cells.

Both the patient and sexual partner must be treated with metronidazole given as a one-time 2-g dose or 500 mg bid for 7 days. Patients who are compliant, not reexposed to male partners, and fail initial therapy may be given 1 g metronidazole bid orally along with 500 mg metronidazole bid intravaginally for 7–14 days. (The 2-g dose is contraindicated in the first trimester of pregnancy.)

E. A thin gray-white discharge with an unpleasant odor ("musty" or "fishy") often is caused by *Gardnerella vaginalis,* a gram-variable coccobacillus. The normal saline wet mount often shows "clue cells": stippled epithelial cells (*Gardnerella* organisms adhered to the epithelial cells). Treatment consists of oral metronidazole 500 mg bid for 7 days or oral clindamycin 300 mg bid for 7 days. Local regimens provide similar response and are associated with fewer systemic side effects; these consist of 0.75% metronidazole gel inserted bid for 5 days, or 2% clindamycin cream nightly for 7 nights. In cases of recurrence, empirically switch to a different agent (e.g., from metronidazole to clindamycin). If recurrence persists, extended intravaginal therapy with either metronidazole or clindamycin daily for 3 weeks followed by intravaginal therapy every third day for an additional 3 weeks may be warranted, allowing lactobacilli to recolonize the vagina. Treatment of the partner is controversial.

F. Significant vulvar pruritus is the usual presenting symptom of vaginal yeast infections. The appearance of filamentous forms (pseudohyphae) and blastospores on KOH wet mount can confirm clinical suspicion. Many equally effective topical treatment regimens are available, including clotrimazole 1% cream, one applicator-full (5 g) per vagina qhs for 7 nights or miconazole, 200-mg suppositories qhs for 3 nights. The cream should also be applied to the vulva for pruritus. An alternative to topical therapy is a one-time dose of 150 mg oral fluconazole. Studies show single dose oral fluconazole to be as effective as intravaginal suppositories. Some patients prefer this single oral dose because of its low rate of side effects, route of administration, and cost-effectiveness.

G. Recurrent yeast infection can be frustrating for both practitioner and patient. Obtain culture of the discharge on Sabouraud's or Nickerson's medium to confirm the cause as yeast. Evaluate for other complicating factors, including evidence of diabetes, immunodeficiency (AIDS), or reinfection from partner (10–15% of male sexual partners of women with yeast infections have had positive oral, rectal, and seminal cultures). Treatment options are varied and include topical therapy for 30 days, and ketoconazole, 200 mg PO bid for 14 days. *Candida albicans* is the cause of monilial vulvovaginitis in >90% of cases, but occasionally *Torulopsis glabrata* can be a cause of resistant yeast. A 3- to 7-day course of terconazole often eliminates the organism.

In many cases, however, suppressive rather than curative therapy is in order. A daily 100-mg dose of Ketoconazole orally for 6 months may be used, but this must be weighed against the possibility of liver toxicity. Alternatively, topical therapy for 6–12 months using biweekly application of boric acid or an azole may

Patient with VAGINAL DISCHARGE

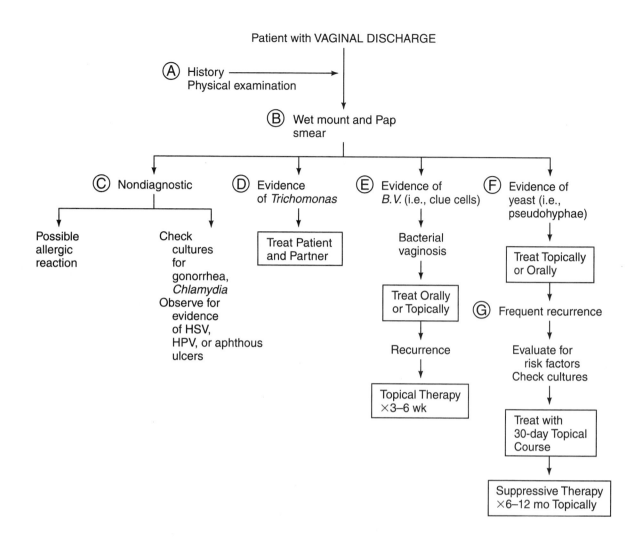

decrease the frequency of recurrence. (Boric acid, oral fluconazole, and ketoconazole should not be used during pregnancy.)

References

American College of Obstetricians and Gynecologists. Vulvovaginitis. ACOG Technical Bulletin No. 135. Washington, DC: American College of Obstetricians and Gynecologists, November 1989.

Sobel JD. Vaginal infections in adult women. Med Clin North Am 1990; 74:1573.

Sobel JD, Brooker D, Stein GE, et al. Single dose fluconazole compared with conventional clotrimazole topical therapy of *Candida* vaginitis. Am J Obstet Gynecol 1995; 172:1263.

Stenchever MA. Office gynecology. 2nd ed. St. Louis: Mosby, 1996.

Zuspan FP, Quilligan EJ. Current therapy in obstetrics and gynecology 4. Philadelphia: WB Saunders, 1994.

CERVICITIS

Hugh S. Miller

A. Although acute cervicitis can result from trauma, malignancy, or systemic collagen vascular conditions, it is most commonly caused by infectious agents, notably *Neisseria gonorrhoeae, Chlamydia trachomatis,* and to a lesser extent herpes simplex virus (HSV). The epidemiology of these pathogens is similar, and 25–45% of patients have concomitant infections. Assessing a patient's risk for cervical infection involves taking a careful history, including age at first sexual contact, number of sex partners, and history of previous STDs or pelvic inflammatory disease (PID). It is important to distinguish infections of the lower genital tract limited to the cervix (cervicitis) from those occurring in the vagina (vaginitis) or vulva (vulvitis), and from upper genital tract disease such as PID. When cervicitis is associated with signs or symptoms of systemic disease, including fever, lower abdominal pain, or pelvic pain, consider PID as an additional diagnosis. Cervicitis generally is associated with mucopurulent discharge collected from the cervix and posterior vaginal fornix. Because the vaginal discharge associated with vaginitis often appears similar, it is prudent to evaluate the discharge for the common vaginal pathogens (candidal vaginitis, bacterial vaginosis, and *Trichomonas vaginalis*). For patients with a confirmed diagnosis of cervicitis who are at risk for STDs, offer screening for other STDs, including syphilis, HIV, and human papillomavirus (HPV), and Pap smear, if not screened in the past year.

B. Too often, lower abdominal pain in sexually active women prompts the diagnosis of PID without application of criteria to substantiate the diagnosis. Hager's criteria for diagnosing acute salpingitis are listed in Table 1. The severity of the illness determines whether outpatient care or hospitalization is appropriate. Inpatient parenteral regimens combine a broad-spectrum cephalosporin (cefoxitin or cefotetan) with tetracycline (doxycycline) or clindamycin with an aminoglycoside. The preferred outpatient regimen combines ceftriaxone with tetracycline (doxycycline), but quinolones (ofloxacin) can be combined with either metronidazole (Flagyl) or clindamycin. If pregnancy is possible, avoid tetracyclines and quinolones.

TABLE 1   Criteria for Diagnosing Acute Salpingitis

History of lower abdominal pain or tenderness, cervical motion
    tenderness, and adnexal tenderness
Plus one of the following objective findings:
Fever (body temperature >38° C)
Leukocytosis (WBC >10,500/mm³)
Culdocentesis fluid containing WBCs or bacteria
Inflammatory mass on pelvic examination or sonography
ESR >20
Evidence of gonococcus or *Chlamydia* on cervical Gram stain

C. Cervical ulcerations often are accompanied by inguinal or vulvar adenopathy. Pain distinguishes HSV from syphilitic lesions in primary outbreaks. Primary genital HSV often involves the vulva, urethra, and cervix, progressing from multiple painful vesicles to ulcers in the presence of a systemic viremia. First episode nonprimary genital herpes, like recurrent HSV, occurs in the presence of circulating antibodies and is associated with an infection of muted duration and intensity. Acyclovir is the mainstay of treatment and is particularly effective in primary infections in which early intervention significantly reduces viral shedding, accelerates healing, and hastens recovery. Because acyclovir therapy has been changed to less-frequent dosing (400 mg tid) with proven efficacy, compliance is favored. Valacyclovir and famciclovir, two newer acyclic nucleoside derivatives, also may be considered for primary treatment of genital HSV. Syphilis, by contrast, usually manifests on the cervix in a primary infection; however, because it usually is asymptomatic, it is rarely diagnosed at this stage. Identification of the stage of infection plays a major role in determining the duration of treatment. Penicillin is the drug of choice, with almost no reported resistant strains.

D. When a growth is noted on the cervix in association with cervicitis and discharge, obtain a cervical biopsy specimen from the leading edge of the lesion to exclude endophytic cervical neoplasia. More commonly, a whitish exophytic lesion is associated with genital warts or HPV. These lesions by themselves usually represent an infectious process involving HPV serotypes 6 and 11. Many additional serotypes (16, 18, 31, 33, 35) are recognized for their contribution to the neoplastic transformation that can promote cervical cancer. Application of 3% acetic acid to the cervix, along with colposcopically directed biopsies, enables distinction between infectious and neoplastic lesions. This distinction influences the choice of treatment. In rare instances tuberculous cervicitis manifests as a mucopurulent discharge or fungating mass. Diagnosis is made by cervical biopsy demonstrating caseating granulomas and/or acid-fast bacilli stain or culture.

E. Gonococcal endocervicitis manifests symptoms, including mucopurulent vaginal discharge, uterine bleeding, and dysuria, in 40–60% of infections. The diagnosis traditionally is made by an endocervical culture plated on modified Thayer-Martin medium. More practical are newer rapid-assay techniques such as Gonozyme. Although procaine penicillin G, ampicillin, and amoxicillin continue to be effective, ceftriaxone, 250 mg IM, is preferred. The single treatment ensures compliance while simultaneously covering penicillinase-producing and chromosomally mediated resistant *N. gonorrhoeae*. Although *Chlamydia* is the most prevalent sexually transmitted organism in the United States, acute cervical

Patient with CERVICITIS

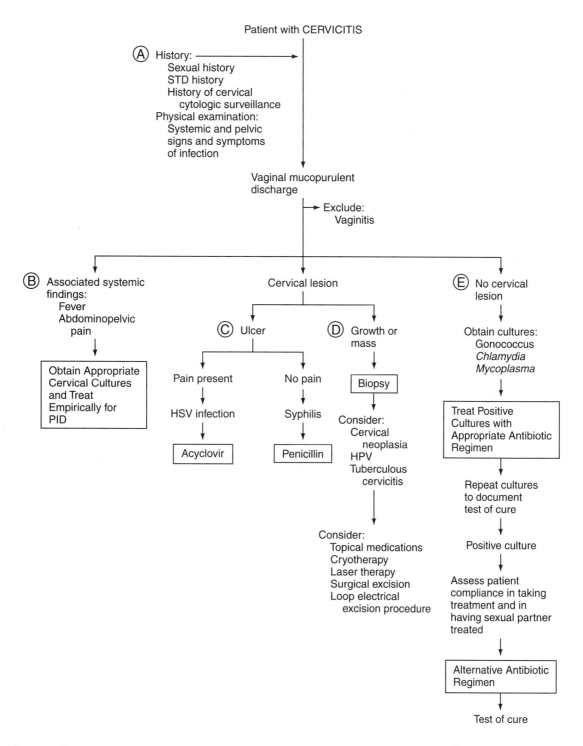

(A) History:
- Sexual history
- STD history
- History of cervical cytologic surveillance
- Physical examination:
  - Systemic and pelvic signs and symptoms of infection

Vaginal mucopurulent discharge

→ Exclude: Vaginitis

(B) Associated systemic findings:
- Fever
- Abdominopelvic pain

Obtain Appropriate Cervical Cultures and Treat Empirically for PID

Cervical lesion

(C) Ulcer

Pain present → HSV infection → Acyclovir

No pain → Syphilis → Penicillin

(D) Growth or mass

Biopsy

Consider:
- Cervical neoplasia
- HPV
- Tuberculous cervicitis

Consider:
- Topical medications
- Cryotherapy
- Laser therapy
- Surgical excision
- Loop electrical excision procedure

(E) No cervical lesion

Obtain cultures:
- Gonococcus
- *Chlamydia*
- *Mycoplasma*

Treat Positive Cultures with Appropriate Antibiotic Regimen

Repeat cultures to document test of cure

Positive culture

Assess patient compliance in taking treatment and in having sexual partner treated

Alternative Antibiotic Regimen

Test of cure

infection often is asymptomatic. *Chlamydia* is readily diagnosed by direct culture, fluorescent monoclonal antibody staining, or enzyme-linked immunoassay (ELISA). Doxycycline, 100 mg bid for 7 days, or azithromycin, 1 g as a single dose, are the therapeutic regimens of choice. When both *N. gonorrhoeae* and *Chlamydia* are present, azithromycin, 2 g as a single dose, can be used alone. Because both *N. gonorrhoeae* and *Chlamydia* are reportable STDs, encourage patients to facilitate the evaluation and treatment of their sex partners. In some cases it may be helpful to obtain a test of cure to verify both patient compliance and microbial sensitivity.

References

ACOG Technical Bulletin. Gonorrhea and chlamydial infections. No. 19a. March 1994.

Drugs for sexually transmitted diseases. Med Lett Drugs Ther 1995; 37:117.

Sweet RL, Gibbs RS. Infectious diseases of the female genital tract. 3rd ed. Baltimore: Williams & Wilkins, 1995.

SECONDARY AMENORRHEA

Nancy A. Curosh

Secondary amenorrhea is arbitrarily defined as the absence of menses for 6 months or the equivalent of three previous cycle intervals, whichever is longer, in women who previously had menses. Exclude physiologic amenorrheas such as pregnancy, the immediate postpartum state, lactation, and the menopause. It is helpful to consider secondary amenorrhea as an abnormality in one of four areas: the outflow tract, including the uterus, cervix, and vagina; the ovaries; the anterior pituitary; and the hypothalamus. Take a careful history, including questions concerning menstrual history, surgical procedures, medication use, changes in weight or diet, exercise patterns, and medical illnesses. On physical examination, pay attention to body habitus, secondary sexual characteristics, evidence of androgen excess, galactorrhea, visual fields, and evidence of endocrinopathies, and do a thorough pelvic examination. If localizing signs or symptoms are found, the investigation can be channeled as appropriate.

A. About 20% of cases of secondary amenorrhea are caused by hyperprolactinemia. Although galactorrhea may indicate this diagnosis, its absence is not reassuring, and all patients should be screened with a serum prolactin level. A number of physiologic and pharmacologic events can alter prolactin levels. Elevation can occur from any stress—physical or emotional. In fact, the stress of a blood draw may increase the level slightly. Levels should not be drawn after a recent breast examination because breast stimulation can increase prolactin. Prolactin also can be increased by many medications, including oral contraceptives, estrogens, phenothiazines, tricyclic antidepressants, metoclopramide, and benzodiazepines. The serum prolactin usually is <100 ng/ml if from one of these causes. If levels remain elevated after excluding these, investigate further.

B. The progestin challenge test is used to assess the endogenous estrogen level and the competence of the outflow tract; 10 mg medroxyprogesterone acetate (Provera) is given PO for 5 days. Withdrawal bleeding should occur within 2 days to 2 weeks if there is a sufficient estrogen level and a competent outflow tract. Any amount of bleeding is considered a positive test, but very mild spotting implies marginal estrogen levels, and periodic re-evaluation is wise. The presence of estrogen suggests that the major components of the hypothalamic, pituitary, ovarian, and uterine pathways are at least minimally functioning. The diagnosis of anovulation is made. Management of anovulation depends on whether the patient currently desires pregnancy or contraception. Because chronic unopposed estrogen can induce endometrial hyperplasia, endometrial shedding should be induced on a regular basis.

C. If there is no withdrawal bleeding after a progestin challenge, there is either an outflow tract problem or insufficient estrogen. An estrogen-progestin challenge test can help differentiate between these two problems. Orally active estrogen is given to stimulate endometrial proliferation. An appropriate dose is 2.5 mg of conjugated estrogens daily for 21–25 days. A progestational agent (10 mg Provera) is given for the last 5–10 days to induce withdrawal. If no withdrawal bleeding occurs, there is a problem with the outflow tract, such as Asherman's syndrome or active endometritis. In a patient with a normal pelvic examination and no history of pelvic infections or trauma, including curettage, the estrogen-progestin challenge test may be eliminated.

D. Hypothalamic amenorrhea is the most common cause of secondary amenorrhea, occurring in approximately 60% of cases. It is most likely caused by a defect in the pattern of pulsatile gonadotropin-releasing hormone (GnRH) secretion. Hypothalamic amenorrhea is a diagnosis of exclusion, but there are clearly groups in whom this occurs frequently, such as in patients with anorexia nervosa, strenuous exercisers, and patients under stress. If possible, the precipitating circumstances should be dealt with and eliminated. Often, reassurance and time is all that is needed. Follow these patients closely to ensure that nothing has been overlooked. Consider estrogen replacement if the amenorrhea is not resolved in a reasonable time. If fertility is desired, clomiphene, Pergonal, and GnRH are often effective.

E. If luteinizing hormone (LH) and follicle-stimulating hormone (FSH) levels are high, ovarian failure is the most likely explanation. Patients <35 years old should undergo karyotyping. If a Y chromosome is found, the chance of a gonadal malignancy is greatly increased. In rare circumstances, LH and FSH are elevated but the ovaries contain follicles. However, in most cases, if the gonadotropins are elevated, premature ovarian failure can be diagnosed. Premature ovarian failure can be caused by autoimmune disease; consider and investigate this as appropriate. If there are no contraindications, hormonal replacement therapy should be used in premature ovarian failure to avoid the long-term sequelae of estrogen deficiency.

F. Hyperprolactinemia warrants MRI of the head. Various tumors such as craniopharyngiomas and meningiomas may cause hyperprolactinemia, but pituitary adenomas are the most common. Dopamine agonists, radiation therapy, and neurosurgery are therapeutic options for pituitary adenomas, depending on the size and extension of the tumor and the presence of symptoms. Excellent results usually are obtained with bromocriptine. Often, no tumor is found and careful observation is warranted. Consider a trial of bromocriptine, particularly if fertility is desired.

Patient with SECONDARY AMENORRHEA

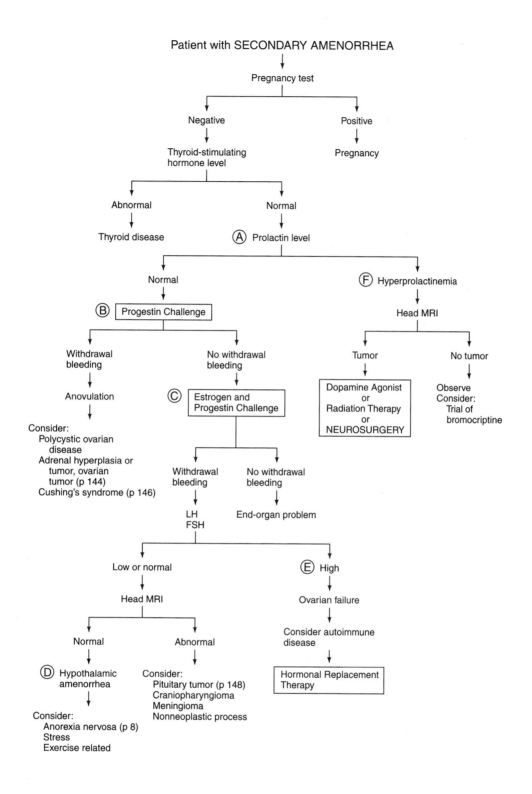

References

Malo JW, Bezdicek BJ. Secondary amenorrhea: a protocol for pinpointing the underlying cause. Postgrad Med 1986; 79:86.

Scommegna A, Carson SA. Secondary amenorrhea and the menopause. In: Gold JJ, Josimovich JB, eds. Gynecologic endocrinology. 4th ed. New York: Plenum, 1987:369.

Soulez B, DeWailly D, et al. Polycystic ovary syndrome: a multidisciplinary challenge. Endocrinologist 1996; 6:1.

Speroff L, Glass RH, Kase NG. Clinical gynecologic endocrinology and infertility. 5th ed. Baltimore: Williams & Wilkins, 1994.

Warren MP. Amenorrhea in endurance runners. J Clin Endocrinol Metab 1992; 75:6.

ABNORMAL VAGINAL BLEEDING

Hugh S. Miller

A. Significant abnormal vaginal bleeding not emanating from the uterus is uncommon and usually is discerned from a careful history and physical examination. The initial assessment should exclude genitourinary (hematuria) and GI (hematochezia) etiologies, allowing one to concentrate on genital etiologies, predominantly uterine. Abnormal perimenarchal and early perimenopausal bleeding usually is hormonally mediated, although bleeding characteristics may vary widely. Conversely, late peri- and postmenopausal bleeding is more likely to be related to a neoplastic process that is not necessarily malignant. Women at high risk for genital tract cancer can be identified through a detailed obstetric, gynecologic, and medical history (endocrine disorders, pituitary tumors, blood dyscrasias) that includes menstrual history, contraceptive use, exposure to STDs, history of premalignant conditions of the cervix or uterus, human papillomavirus infection, obesity, and pre-existing malignancy.

B. The complete physical examination permits exclusion of extragenital tract etiologies while lending further support to a potential endocrine or hematologic cause if thyromegaly or diffuse petechiae are present. Pelvic examination is essential to localize the source of bleeding through identification of lesions or other significant pathologic conditions (polyps, uterine fibroids, pelvic masses). The Pap smear, obtained before bimanual examination, is essential in screening for cervical cancer and occasionally suggests the presence of cervicitis or higher genital tract neoplasias. Collect appropriate cultures in patients identified by history to be at significant risk for STDs. Test all women of reproductive age for pregnancy, regardless of menstrual history, by urine human chorionic gonadotropin (hCG) testing. When bleeding is significant or persistent, obtain a CBC to determine anemia and rule out occult hematologic malignancies. Other testing is dictated by the history and physical examination, including various endocrine, coagulation, and imaging studies. Transvaginal ultrasound is invaluable in the evaluation and management of these patients. In addition to adnexal and ovarian assessment, evaluate the myometrium for fibroids and the endometrium for its thickness. In postmenopausal women, <5 mm generally is considered the upper limit of normal. In premenopausal women, endometrial thickness varies from 4–8 mm in the follicular phase and 7–14 mm in the secretory phase. Saline infusion sonohysterography, in which saline is infused into the endometrial cavity before sonography, has led to better definition of cavitary lesions (e.g., submucosal fibroids, uterine polyps) and is further expanding the indications for pelvic sonography.

C. Focus first on the source of the bleeding. The necessary equipment (including specula of various sizes and shapes), flexible lighting, and adequate assistance must be available. If a lesion is identified in the genital tract, obtain a biopsy regardless of the patient's age.

D. Abnormal bleeding in premenopausal women often is attributable to contraceptive methods. In addition to oral contraceptive pills, Norplant and Depo-Provera are associated with abnormal bleeding in the first 3–9 months of use. In the absence of an obvious cause, the etiology is most likely "dysfunctional uterine bleeding," a diagnosis of exclusion. The cause is likely to be anovulation with excess or insufficient estrogen or progesterone. Depending on the patient's wishes, therapeutic options include receiving no additional therapy, discontinuing or changing to a new contraceptive method, or adding some hormonal manipulation. Lack of an organic explanation for persistent abnormal bleeding refractory to hormonal manipulation should prompt further evaluation of the uterine cavity, in the form of transvaginal sonography with or without saline infusion, office hysteroscopy, or endometrial biopsy (EMB). In patients at risk for hyperplasia, EMB may be sufficient, although more and more physicians choose direct visualization by sonography or hysteroscopy.

E. The incidence of adenocarcinoma of the uterus in women <40 years old is about 5%. The incidence increases with age. Therefore abnormal bleeding in women ≥40 years old must be evaluated by EMB. Women at increased risk because of obesity, chronic anovulation, exogenous unopposed estrogen, or pre-existing cancer (particularly breast cancer) may warrant EMB regardless of age. With the increasing use of hormonal replacement therapy in postmenopausal women, reports of abnormal bleeding have likewise increased and require diligent evaluation to rule out occult carcinoma. When histopathologic study reveals hyperplasia with cellular atypia, medical or surgical treatment is necessary. Treatment of endometrial carcinoma should involve consultation with a gynecologist or oncologist to determine the best course of therapy. Re-evaluate patients diagnosed with hyperplasia with atypia for persistent or worsening hyperplasia within 3–6 months of treatment.

References

ACOG Technical Bulletin. Dysfunctional uterine bleeding. No. 134, October 1989.

ACOG Technical Bulletin. Gynecologic ultrasonography. No. 215, November 1995.

Mischell DR Jr. Abnormal uterine bleeding. In: Herbst AL, Mishell DR Jr, Stenchever MA, Droegemueller W, eds. Comprehensive gynecology. 3rd ed. St. Louis: Mosby, 1997:1025.

Wathen PI, Henderson MC, Witz CA. Abnormal uterine bleeding. Med Clin North Am 1995; 79:329.

Patient with ABNORMAL VAGINAL BLEEDING

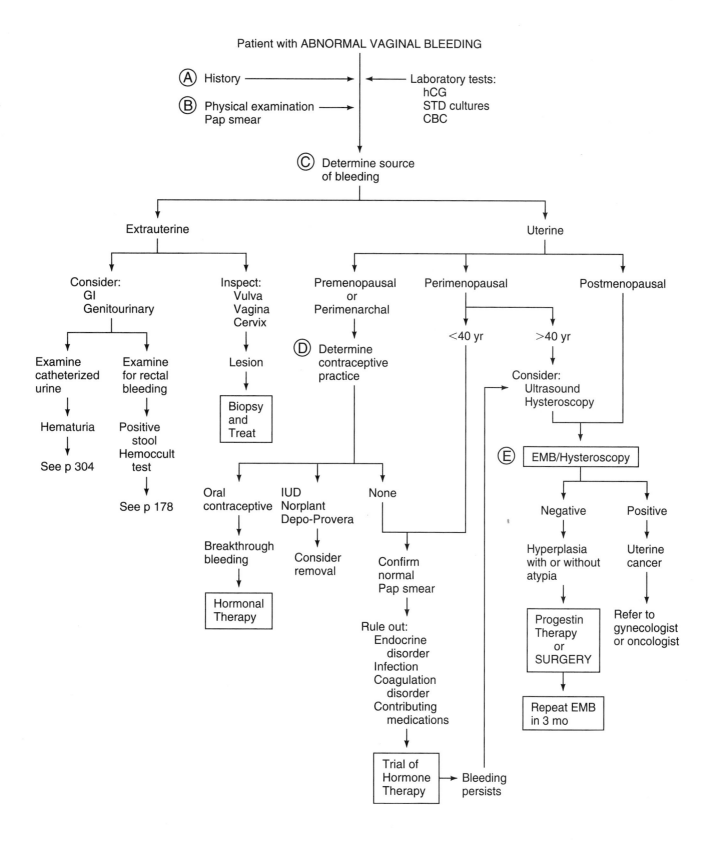

Ⓐ History ──────────────→ ←────── Laboratory tests:
                                          hCG
Ⓑ Physical examination ──→   STD cultures
   Pap smear   CBC

Ⓒ Determine source
  of bleeding

Extrauterine

Consider:
GI
Genitourinary

Examine   Examine
catheterized   for rectal
urine   bleeding

Hematuria   Positive
                     stool
See p 304   Hemoccult
                     test

                     See p 178

Inspect:
Vulva
Vagina
Cervix

Lesion

Biopsy
and
Treat

Uterine

Premenopausal
or
Perimenarchal

Ⓓ Determine
  contraceptive
  practice

Oral   IUD   None
contraceptive   Norplant
                  Depo-Provera

Breakthrough   Consider   Confirm
bleeding   removal   normal
                                    Pap smear
Hormonal
Therapy   Rule out:
                                      Endocrine
                                      disorder
                                      Infection
                                      Coagulation
                                      disorder
                                      Contributing
                                      medications

                                    Trial of   → Bleeding
                                    Hormone   persists
                                    Therapy

Perimenopausal

<40 yr   >40 yr

             Consider:
             Ultrasound
             Hysteroscopy

Ⓔ EMB/Hysteroscopy

Negative   Positive

Hyperplasia   Uterine
with or without   cancer
atypia
                  Refer to
Progestin   gynecologist
Therapy   or oncologist
or
SURGERY

Repeat EMB
in 3 mo

Postmenopausal

465

VAGINAL BLEEDING IN PREGNANCY

Janet Moore

Bleeding in pregnancy may have a number of causes, including obstetric, gynecologic, and nongynecologic causes. It is relatively common, complicating up to 5% of term pregnancies. Rapidly determining the cause is of utmost importance to ensure maternal and fetal well-being.

A. Initial management, regardless of gestational age, includes stabilization of the patient followed by thorough history and physical examination, with determination of the amount and rate of bleeding. Once the patient is hemodynamically stable, investigate the cause of the bleeding.

B. Gestational age can be estimated by date of last menstrual period, fundal height, or sonography. The main differential diagnosis for bleeding in early pregnancy is spontaneous abortion (SAb) and ectopic pregnancy. Proceed immediately to speculum examination.

C. SAb is termination of pregnancy before 20 weeks (< 500 g). Bleeding in SAb is caused by hemorrhage into the decidua basalis and necrotic changes in the tissue. If when the speculum is placed there is blood in the vagina but the os is closed, threatened abortion is the diagnosis. About half of women who bleed in the first trimester go on to abort. If the bleeding is associated with pain and cramping, the prognosis is worse. However, if fetal cardiac activity is demonstrated, only 10% proceed to abortion (fetal cardiac activity can be documented by transvaginal ultrasound [US] at 5 weeks). Management is complete pelvic rest; bed rest is not warranted.

D. Bleeding is the most common sign of a molar pregnancy and can be intermittent or continuous, lasting weeks to months. The bleeding usually is brown, rarely bright red. Other signs include uterine size greater than expected for gestational age, intractable nausea and vomiting, very highly elevated levels of β-human chorionic gonadotropin (β-hCG), or high blood pressure. The diagnosis is confirmed by US, which may show a complete mole or a partial mole with coexisting viable pregnancy. Treatment is evacuation, with serial β-hCG determinations until undetectable, and delaying conception for at least 1 year. Chemotherapy may be required if β-hCG remains elevated.

E. Cervicitis from chlamydial infection or gonorrhea can present with spotting and increased vaginal discharge. On speculum examination there are signs of inflammation and purulent discharge. Vaginitis most commonly is caused by bacterial vaginosis, trichomoniasis, or candidiasis. Vaginitis tends to present with serosanguinous discharge, especially after intercourse. Cervical polyps and cervical cancer also can present with bleeding. On speculum examination, polyps appear to be hanging out of the cervical canal and are smooth, soft, and red to purple. They bleed readily when touched. Cervical cancer often has a cauliflower-like, necrotic appearance. Both cause bleeding after intercourse or vaginal examination.

F. Nongynecologic causes include urinary tract infection, GI bleeding, lymphoma, and thrombocytopenia.

G. If on speculum examination the os is closed and there is no blood in the vagina but fetal cardiac activity is absent on US or fetal Doppler (present after about 10 weeks), a *missed abortion* has occurred; that is, the fetus has died but has been retained, often for weeks. Management generally is elective evacuation to decrease the risk of sepsis or disseminated intravascular coagulation (DIC).

H. In *ectopic pregnancy* implantation occurs at a site other than the endometrium, most commonly (96%) in the tubes. Bleeding is thought to be the result of the pregnancy outgrowing its blood supply, which leads to declining endocrine function of the placenta, resulting in inadequate endometrial support with subsequent breakthrough bleeding. Bleeding usually is scant and associated with abdominal pain, often unilateral. Diagnosis is made by serial β-hCG determinations and sonography. The β-hCG level doubles every 48 hours in a normal pregnancy. Ectopic pregnancies have impaired production of β-hCG and thus have a prolonged doubling time. Transvaginal US allows visualization of a gestational sac once the β-hCG is >1500 mIU/ml, whereas transabdominal US can detect the sac if β-hCG is >6000 mIU/ml. If no sac is seen in the uterus, ectopic pregnancy is presumed. Treatment is laparoscopic salpingostomy, laparotomy if the patient is hemodynamically unstable, or IM injection of methotrexate if the sac is <4 cm and unruptured. Regardless of treatment modality, β-hCG level is followed until undetectable.

I. If the os is open on speculum examination, *inevitable abortion* is the diagnosis. Bleeding in an inevitable abortion usually is associated with cramping. Management may be expectant or may consist of evacuation of the products of conception (POC).

J. An *incomplete abortion* has occurred when the os is open and there has been partial passage of the POC. Bleeding can be significant because the retained POC do not allow complete myometrial contraction and uterine involution. Evacuation is mandated to prevent significant hemorrhage and sepsis.

K. In *incompetent cervix* the os is open with symptoms of pelvis pressure, low back pain, and increased vaginal discharge. Risk factors include previous cervical laceration or surgery and exposure to diethylstilbestrol (DES). Treatment is attempted emergency cerclage in the existing pregnancy and elective cerclage in future pregnancies at 10–14 weeks.

(Continued on page 468)

Pregnant Patient with VAGINAL BLEEDING

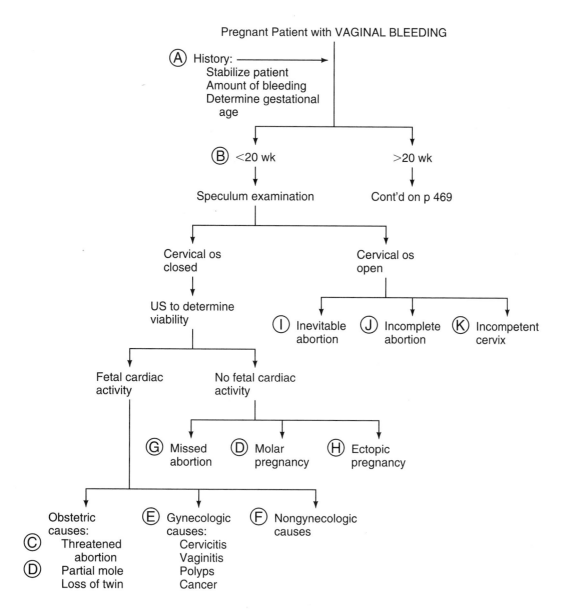

Cont'd on p 469

467

L. Vaginal bleeding in the third trimester is an absolute contraindication to pelvic examination until the location of the placenta can be determined. Therefore US must be performed to rule out placenta previa before further examination. Speculum or digital examination in the presence of placenta previa can lead to life-threatening obstetric hemorrhage.

M. Placenta previa is abnormal implantation of the placenta over the cervical os. *Complete* placenta previa covers the os; *partial* incompletely covers the os; *marginal* is directly adjacent to the os. Placenta previa complicates 1 of 200 term pregnancies and usually presents as painless vaginal bleeding. Incidence is increased with advanced maternal age, increased parity, and previous uterine surgery. Management from 24–36 weeks includes stabilization of the patient, fetal monitoring, blood typing and screening, and Rhogam injection if indicated. Once maternal and fetal well-being is ensured, the patient should remain hospitalized on bed rest with maintenance of hematocrit at ≥30% in case of future large hemorrhage. Twenty percent are complicated with uterine activity because blood acts as an irritant. However, cervical dilation cannot be determined directly, so tocolysis may be started empirically.

N. Placental abruption results from premature separation of the placenta before delivery. The cause in most cases is unknown, but there is an association with increased maternal age and parity, abdominal trauma, cocaine use, and smoking. Abruption presents with a clinical triad of bleeding, uterine hyperactivity/hypertonicity, and fetal distress. Diagnosis generally is clinical, although US may support the diagnosis in 50% of cases with evidence of retroplacental clot or other hemorrhage. Maternal complications include shock, DIC, and ischemic necrosis. Therefore, in addition to a hemoglobin and hematocrit and blood type and screen, evaluation for consumptive coagulopathy should include fibrinogen and fibrin split products, platelets, and prothrombin time/partial thromboplastin time. Rhogam should be given to the Rh(–) mother. A Kleihauer-Betke test will determine whether >30 ml of fetal blood has entered the maternal circulation, necessitating additional Rhogam therapy in the Rh(–) mother.

O. Rupture of a fetal blood vessel is a rare occurrence that can happen in association with a velamentous insertion of the umbilical cord. Fetal monitoring shows signs of fetal distress, most often alternating fetal tachycardia-bradycardia as the fetus attempts to compensate for acute blood loss.

P. In preterm labor with cervical dilation, cervical change can cause spotting secondary to dilation and effacement. Other symptoms include pelvic pressure, vaginal discharge, and backache, with or without frank contractions. Rule out premature rupture of membranes with sterile speculum examination looking for pooling of amniotic fluid in the vagina, positive nitrazine test, and ferning. If gestation is ≤34 weeks, management includes betamethasone injection for fetal lung maturity, antibiotic prophylaxis for group B streptococcus, and tocolysis. If >34 weeks, expectant management with bed rest and pelvic rest is recommended.

Q. Normal labor with bloody show is a final possibility.

References

Abortion. In: Cunningham FG, MacDonald PC, Leveno KJ, et al, eds. Williams obstetrics. 20th ed. Norwalk, CT: Appleton & Lange, 1996:579.

Benedetti T. Obstetric hemorrhage. In: Gabbe SG, Niebyl JR, Simpson JL, eds. Normal and problem pregnancies. 3rd ed. New York: Churchill Livingstone, 1996:499.

Droegemueller W. Benign gynecological lesions. In: Mishell DR Jr, Stenchever MA, Droegemueller W, Herbst AL, eds. Comprehensive gynecology. 3rd ed. St. Louis: Mosby, 1997:467.

Herbst AL. Malignant diseases of the cervix. In: Mishell DR Jr, Stenchever MA, Droegemueller W, Herbst AL, eds. Comprehensive gynecology. 3rd ed. St. Louis: Mosby, 1997:835.

Pregnant Patient with VAGINAL BLEEDING

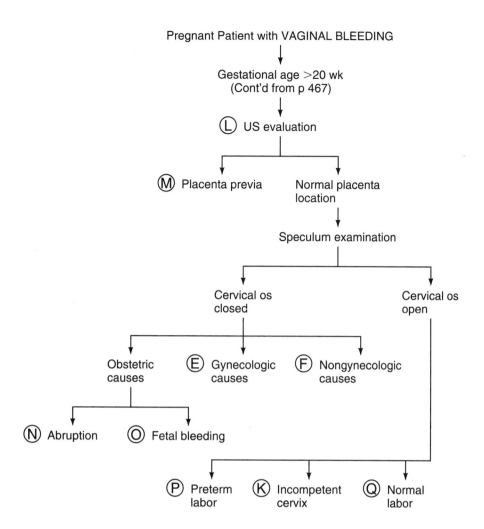

ACUTE ABDOMINAL PAIN IN WOMEN

Robert N. Samuelson

A. The acute abdomen refers to any condition requiring an "acute" medical decision. The potential causes of acute abdominal pain in women are multiple. A thorough history can quickly eliminate a number of these. Information about menstrual cycles, previous episodes of similar pain, sexual activity, contraception, vaginal discharge, and changes in bowel, bladder, or appetite can quickly narrow the differential diagnosis. Findings in the acute abdomen often include severe pain, which may be caused by infection, bleeding, infarction of tissue, or obstruction of a hollow viscus (bowel, fallopian tube, ureter). Any of these conditions can irritate and inflame the peritoneum, making it very sensitive to movement. Loss of appetite, nausea, and vomiting often accompany the pain and tenderness. Laboratory studies necessary for adequately evaluating an acute abdomen include a CBC with differential, ESR, pregnancy test (urine or serum), urinalysis, and occasionally an amylase or lipase. Obtain cervical cultures for *Neisseria gonorrhoeae* and *Chlamydia trachomatis* at initial evaluation if the history warrants.

B. If the pregnancy test is positive, the differential diagnosis can be narrowed considerably. It is important to recognize that conditions other than pregnancy can be the source of the pain. If gestational age is <10–12 weeks, consider ectopic pregnancy, rupture or torsion of ovarian cyst, or septic or threatened abortion. If gestational age is >12–14 weeks, ectopic pregnancy becomes less likely; consider other entities such as ruptured or torsed adnexa, appendicitis, septic abortion, ureteral colic, and pyelonephritis.

C. Ultrasonography continues to expand its role in the evaluation of obstetric and gynecologic patients with abdominal pain. Its use in conjunction with quantitative β-human chorionic gonadotropin (β-hCG) can be important. With normal pregnancy, a gestational sac often is seen at 5–6 weeks' gestation. When the β-hCG level reaches 6500 mIU/ml, an abdominal scan can visualize a gestational sac; at 1500 mIU/ml a transvaginal probe often visualizes the pregnancy. If, on the basis of sonographic findings and quantitative β-hCG values, the possibility of an ectopic pregnancy still exists, the patient needs referral for possible surgical management (laparoscopy/laparotomy) or medical management (e.g., methotrexate) for an ectopic pregnancy. If an early intrauterine pregnancy is confirmed by sonography, other sources for the pain must be determined. Ruptured or torsed ovarian cysts, appendicitis, or an infected abortion also can present with abdominal pain.

D. If the pregnancy test is negative, history again plays an important role. Patients with a history of recurrent cyclic pain related to menses and who now have an acute exacerbation may have a ruptured endometrioma. Patients with a history of fever, chills, and vaginal discharge with a recent change in sexual partners are at risk for pelvic inflammatory disease (PID). (Patients taking oral contraceptives are at decreased risk for ovarian cyst formation.) If an infectious cause is determined, admit the patient for IV antibiotics; if no improvement is seen in 24–48 hours, consider laparoscopy. The determination of PID versus appendicitis often is not resolved until laparoscopy or laparotomy is performed. Other entities that must always be considered are adnexal torsion, ovarian cyst rupture, exacerbation of endometriosis, degenerating fibroid, renal calculi, and mesenteric lymphadenitis.

E. Although many imaging modalities are available to the practitioner, the choice may need to be made in concert with the radiologist. A thin pregnant patient can be evaluated well with ultrasound; in obese postmenopausal patients more information may be obtained by CT. The need for surgical exploration often takes precedence over imaging studies. Many of the disorders in premenopausal patients apply also to postmenopausal patients. Cyst formation occurs infrequently in elderly patients, but its appearance must be evaluated carefully for the possibility of malignancy. Other processes that can cause acute pain include colonic diverticulitis (75% of these resolve with proper attention and antibiotics), bowel obstruction (most of these need exploration), and vascular lesions (mesenteric thrombosis), dissecting or leaking aneurysm, and acute cholecystitis or pancreatitis.

References

Epstein FB. Acute abdominal pain in pregnancy. Emerg Med Clin North Am 1994; 12:151.

Jeffrey RB, Ralls PW. CT and sonography of the acute abdomen. 2nd ed. Philadelphia: Lippincott-Raven, 1996.

Kiernan GV, Cales RH. Acute abdominal disorders. Emerg Med Clin North Am 1989; 7:30.

Merrell RC. Gastroenterological emergencies. Gastroenterol Clin North Am 1988; 17:75.

Wagner JM, McKinney WP, Carpenter JL. Does this patient have appendicitis? JAMA 1996; 276:1589.

Female Patient with ACUTE ABDOMINAL PAIN

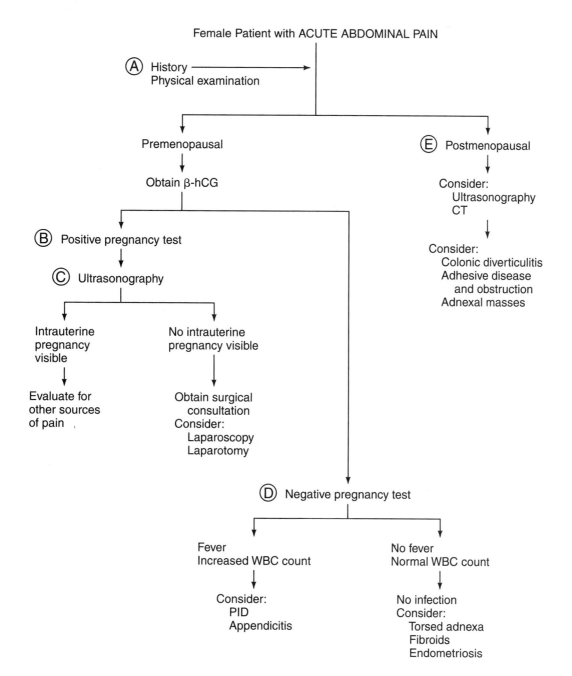

(A) History ⎯⎯⎯⎯⎯⎯⎯
Physical examination

Premenopausal

Obtain β-hCG

(B) Positive pregnancy test

(C) Ultrasonography

Intrauterine
pregnancy
visible

Evaluate for
other sources
of pain

No intrauterine
pregnancy visible

Obtain surgical
consultation
Consider:
Laparoscopy
Laparotomy

(E) Postmenopausal

Consider:
Ultrasonography
CT

Consider:
Colonic diverticulitis
Adhesive disease
and obstruction
Adnexal masses

(D) Negative pregnancy test

Fever
Increased WBC count

Consider:
PID
Appendicitis

No fever
Normal WBC count

No infection
Consider:
Torsed adnexa
Fibroids
Endometriosis

CHEST PAIN IN WOMEN

Dawn Lemcke

The evaluation of chest pain in women is an important step in the diagnosis of coronary artery disease (CAD). The diagnosis of CAD in women is problematic because most of the diagnostic pathways and outcomes are based on research in men. Epidemiologic studies show that CAD is a significant cause of morbidity and mortality in women and that women have a worse prognosis than men with myocardial infarction. Improved diagnosis of CAD in early stages is critical to prevent complications in women. This chapter's decision tree includes not only the pretest likelihood of disease but also guidelines for choosing the best tests for women.

A. There are clear gender differences in presenting symptoms of chest pain and in risk factor stratification. Women may have more atypical sites of pain, such as neck, shoulder, and intrascapular pain, and may have more associated symptoms of exertional dyspnea or decreased exercise tolerance. It is thus important to ask not only the usual historical questions to try to determine whether the patient has angina but also to ask about atypical characteristics. Risk factor assessment can be divided into major, intermediate, and minor determinants (Table 1). These, along with the character of the pain, can be used to place women in categories of likelihood of CAD. This stratification makes testing for CAD more cost-effective and informative. Risk factor assessment is more likely to predict CAD in women (54.5% of cases, compared with 39.3% of cases in men). Stronger predictive value exists, particularly in younger women with risk factors.

B. Evaluate a baseline ECG before conducting other tests in women. Because exercise tolerance testing (ETT) in women may be flawed by false-positive results, having a normal resting ECG improves the diagnostic yield of testing. If the resting ECG is abnormal, with left ventricular hypertrophy, bundle branch block, or an early J point elevation, it may increase the likelihood of a false-positive result, and therefore an imaging ETT may be the most cost-effective test in this group. The use of stress echocardiography as an initial test in all women with chest pain has been proposed as a very cost-effective approach, achieving a diagnostic accuracy similar to stress thallium ETT. Stress echocardiography is less costly than stress thallium ETT but is technically demanding for the average echo laboratory and thus may not be widely available.

C. High likelihood of disease or definite angina is predicted by two or more major determinants or by one major plus more than one intermediate or minor determinant. This group of women has a pretest likelihood of CAD of 80%. In this group, ETT without imaging is the initial test of choice (unless the patient has clinical characteristics other than being female that necessitate imaging). Studies show that 60–75% of women in this group had significant CAD at angiography, and 29–53% had multivessel disease. The specificity of ETT in this setting is 57%, with a sensitivity of 80%. Women with single-vessel disease may be missed by ETT; only 43% of them will have abnormal findings. When following women with characteristics suggestive of angina, remember that single-vessel disease is more common in women than in men. Nonetheless, despite its limitations, a maximal negative ETT should not be overlooked because it largely rules out exercise-induced ischemia associated with multivessel disease. If symptoms persist despite a negative maximal ETT, raising concern of single-vessel disease, stress echocardiography or pharmacologic stress echocardiography may be appropriate. This technique has a sensitivity and specificity of 80–90% for single-vessel disease in women.

D. The most cost-effective approach in women with typical angina and a normal baseline ECG is ETT. Women in this group are unlikely to have false-positive results, and the likelihood of false-negative results is much less than in their male counterparts if they achieve maximal heart rate. Imaging ETT increases the cost of this test and adds little clinically useful information.

E. If the ETT is negative, the patient can be followed closely. A decision about management may be difficult for the woman with a positive test result. The literature holds convincing evidence of the gender differences in further testing after a positive ETT result. It is unclear whether this gender difference represents patient preference (women perceive their risk of heart disease as low); physician perception of the "benign" nature of CAD in women, based on the Framingham and CASS studies; or overtreatment of men. A woman should be referred for

---

TABLE 1 Risk Factor Determinants of CAD in Women with Chest Pain

Major
  Typical angina
  Postmenopausal without hormone replacement therapy (HRT decreases risk of CAD by 50%)
  Diabetes (twice the risk of CAD of male diabetic patients)
  Peripheral vascular disease
Intermediate
  Hypertension
  Smoking, especially in premenopausal women
  Lipid abnormalities, including HDL <35 mg/dl and triglycerides >400 mg/dl
Minor
  Age >65 yr
  Central obesity (waist/hip ratio >0.85 increases risk of CAD over simple body mass index)
  Sedentary lifestyle
  Family history of CAD (2.8 times increase in RR of nonfatal myocardial infarction and 5 times increase in CAD)
  Other risk factors (hemostatic, psychosocial)

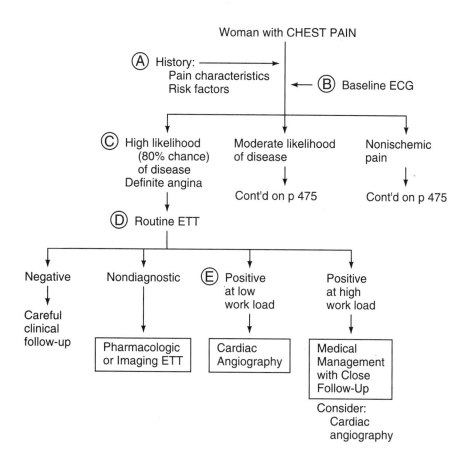

Woman with CHEST PAIN

(A) History:
Pain characteristics
Risk factors

(B) Baseline ECG

(C) High likelihood
(80% chance)
of disease
Definite angina

Moderate likelihood
of disease

Cont'd on p 475

Nonischemic
pain

Cont'd on p 475

(D) Routine ETT

Negative

Careful
clinical
follow-up

Nondiagnostic

Pharmacologic
or Imaging ETT

(E) Positive
at low
work load

Cardiac
Angiography

Positive
at high
work load

Medical
Management
with Close
Follow-Up

Consider:
Cardiac
angiography

coronary angiography for the same reasons as her male counterpart (i.e., unstable angina or markedly positive ETT at low work load). Some advocate angiography for women with a positive ETT at high work load. Some studies show a higher incidence of cardiac events in women regardless of initial ETT response: 14.3% of women with an abnormal ETT result will have a cardiac event, versus 6% of men with a positive ETT. Because most of the coronary events occurred in patients who did not undergo revascularization procedures, one can make an excellent case for complete evaluation and treatment, including catheterization, for all women with positive tests. This strategy may actually be of greater benefit to women than similar care is to men.

F. Moderate likelihood of disease is predicted by one major or by multiple indeterminate and minor determinants. This group has the widest pretest probability of CAD, ranging from 20–80%. Most women in actual practice are in this category. The prevalence of CAD in this group is about 30–40%, with 4–22% having multivessel disease. These women clearly need further examination, but the best test to use is unclear. The sensitivity and specificity of routine ETT in this group are about 65%. Therefore a test result has a reasonable chance of being either a false positive or a false negative. Because this may not add to the diagnostic certainty, it may be more prudent to proceed with either a thallium/sestamibi ETT or stress echocardiography. Although the sensitivity of these tests does not add significantly to the ETT, the addition of imaging improves specificity in women to 80–90%. In particular, stress echocardiography may dramatically improve the sensitivity and specificity for single-vessel disease.

G. Women with nonischemic pain are in the lowest risk group, with <20% likelihood of CAD. This group is defined as those with no major determinants, no or one intermediate determinant, and two or fewer minor determinants. On further analysis, the nonischemic pain group will have a 2–7% incidence of CAD and virtually no multivessel disease. Because of the low prevalence of significant disease in this group, any test that might show an abnormality is of little value, or more likely a false positive. Look for noncardiac causes of pain in this group before proceeding with evaluation.

H. If the patient continues to have symptoms that limit her lifestyle, further evaluation with imaging, ETT, or even angiography may be needed to refute or confirm the existence of CAD, particularly in postmenopausal women.

References

DeSanctis R. Clinical manifestations of coronary artery disease: chest pain in women. In: Wenger N, Speroff L, Packard B, eds. Cardiovascular health and disease in women. Proceedings of an NHLBI Conference. LeJacq Communications, 1993.

Douglas P, Ginsburg G. The evaluation of chest pain in women. N Engl J Med 1996; 334:1311.

Gibbons EF. Evaluation of chest pain. In: Lemcke D, Pattison J, Marshall L, Cowley D, eds. Primary care of women. Norwalk, CT: Appleton-Lange, 1995.

Gibbons EF. Risk factors for coronary artery disease and their treatment. In: Lemcke D, Pattison J, Marshall L, Cowley D, eds. Primary care of women. Norwalk, CT: Appleton-Lange, 1995.

Judelson D. Coronary heart disease in women: risk factors and prevention. JAMA 1994; 49:186.

Wenger N. Coronary heart disease in women: gender differences in diagnostic evaluation. JAMA 1994; 49:181.

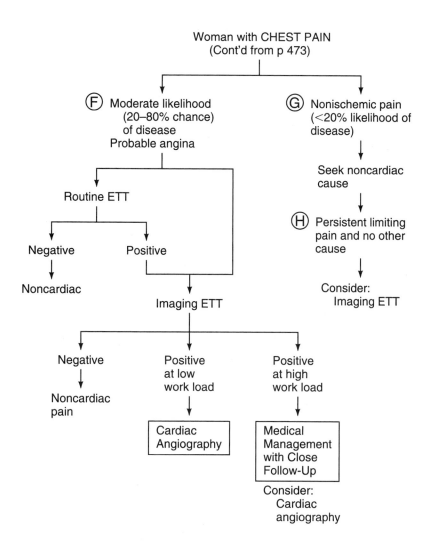

Woman with CHEST PAIN
(Cont'd from p 473)

(F) Moderate likelihood
(20–80% chance)
of disease
Probable angina

(G) Nonischemic pain
(<20% likelihood of
disease)

Seek noncardiac
cause

(H) Persistent limiting
pain and no other
cause

Consider:
Imaging ETT

Routine ETT

Negative

Positive

Noncardiac

Imaging ETT

Negative

Noncardiac
pain

Positive
at low
work load

Cardiac
Angiography

Positive
at high
work load

Medical
Management
with Close
Follow-Up

Consider:
Cardiac
angiography

URINARY TRACT INFECTION IN WOMEN

Michael D. Katz

A. Patients with lower urinary tract infection (UTI) or cystitis complain primarily of dysuria. Frequency, nocturia, urgency, and suprapubic tenderness also may be present. About one third of patients with only lower tract symptoms have an occult renal infection. Patients with overt upper tract infection or acute pyelonephritis usually have flank, low back, or abdominal pain; fevers; chills; malaise; and nausea and vomiting. Concomitant lower tract symptoms also may be present.

B. Individuals with pyelonephritis (PN) often can be successfully treated as outpatients. However, patients with nausea and vomiting who are unable to take oral fluids and medications should be hospitalized. Enterobacteriaceae are the most common pathogens associated with acute pyelonephritis. A wide variety of antimicrobial regimens are available. Initial outpatient therapy may include trimethoprim/sulfamethoxazole (TMP/SMX), a cephalosporin, or a fluoroquinolone. The conventional IV regimen of ampicillin and gentamicin is effective, although TMP/SMX, fluoroquinolones, and cephalosporins also may be considered. The initial choice of therapy must be based on the most likely organisms present and local susceptibility patterns. Definitive therapy must be guided by results of culture and sensitivity tests.

C. In patients with acute cystitis, certain risk factors increase the chance of an occult renal or complicated UTI. Such risk factors include nosocomial infection, pregnancy, known urinary tract abnormality or stone, indwelling catheter or recent instrumentation, previous relapse after therapy for UTI, previous UTI before 12 years of age, acute PN or more than three UTIs in the past year, symptoms for >7 days before therapy, recent antibiotic use, diabetes, and other immunosuppressing conditions. Treat patients with one or more of these risk factors as having an upper tract infection.

D. In acute, uncomplicated cystitis, 3-day antibiotic therapy can be given without obtaining a culture. Seven-day regimens are effective but are associated with a higher incidence of adverse drug reactions, noncompliance, and increased cost. Highly effective 3-day regimens include TMP/SMX 160 mg/800 mg bid, amoxicillin/clavulanate 500 mg/125 mg every 12 hours, ciprofloxacin 250 mg every 12 hours, and norfloxacin 400 mg every 12 hours. Because of widespread *Escherichia coli* resistance, ampicillin/amoxacillin alone may not be as effective as other regimens. Studies with cephalosporins in 3-day regimens have shown conflicting results. Post-therapy urine cultures are needed only in patients with persisting symptoms, complicating factors, or pregnancy.

E. Sexual intercourse and use of diaphragms or spermicide use alone have been associated with an increased risk of UTI. Urination after intercourse may reduce the frequency of relapse. Postcoital antibiotic therapy also is effective. Regimens include TMP/SMX ½ SS tablet, cephaloxin 250 mg or nitrofurantoin 50 mg within 2 hours after intercourse. Discontinuing use of a diaphragm for contraception also may reduce the frequency of relapse.

F. In patients with dysuria, a positive urine culture is considered to be >10^2 CFU/ml growth. Treat patients with a positive culture for 7–14 days. In acute cystitis, >90% of cases are caused by *Escherichia coli* and other Enterobacteriaceae, *Staphylococcus saprophyticus*, and *Enterococcus*. Unless a highly resistant pathogen is present, an inexpensive agent such as TMP/SMX should be adequate. Reserve more expensive agents such as the fluoroquinolones, cephalosporins, and amoxicillin/clavulanate for resistant infections.

G. In patients with frequent recurrences, chronic suppression can reduce this frequency by 95%. Many regimens have been evaluated. If possible, choose the least toxic, least expensive agent. Effective daily regimens include nitrofurantoin 50–100 mg, TMP/SMX 40–80 mg/200–400 mg, and trimethoprim 100 mg. Thrice-weekly administration of TMP/SMX 40 mg/200 mg also has proved effective. Cranberry juice, 300 ml/day, has significantly reduced bacteriuria in postmenopausal women.

References

Bacheller CD, Bernstein JM. Urinary tract infections. Med Clin North Am 1997; 81:719.

Hooton TM, Stamm WE. Diagnosis and treatment of uncomplicated urinary tract infection. Infect Dis Clin North Am 1997; 11:551.

Stapleton A, Stamm WE. Prevention of urinary tract infection. Infect Dis Clin North Am 1997; 11:719.

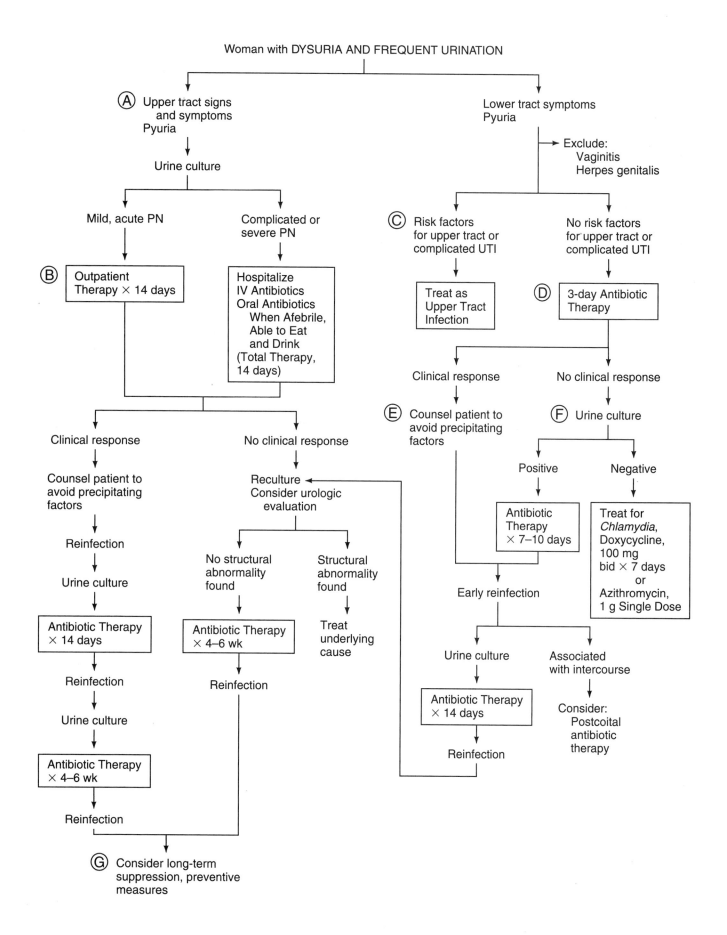

Woman with DYSURIA AND FREQUENT URINATION

A. Upper tract signs and symptoms Pyuria

Urine culture

Mild, acute PN

Complicated or severe PN

B. Outpatient Therapy × 14 days

Hospitalize
IV Antibiotics
Oral Antibiotics
When Afebrile,
Able to Eat
and Drink
(Total Therapy,
14 days)

Clinical response

No clinical response

Counsel patient to avoid precipitating factors

Reculture
Consider urologic evaluation

Reinfection

Urine culture

No structural abnormality found

Structural abnormality found

Antibiotic Therapy × 14 days

Antibiotic Therapy × 4–6 wk

Treat underlying cause

Reinfection

Reinfection

Urine culture

Antibiotic Therapy × 4–6 wk

Reinfection

G. Consider long-term suppression, preventive measures

Lower tract symptoms Pyuria

Exclude:
Vaginitis
Herpes genitalis

C. Risk factors for upper tract or complicated UTI

No risk factors for upper tract or complicated UTI

Treat as Upper Tract Infection

D. 3-day Antibiotic Therapy

Clinical response

No clinical response

E. Counsel patient to avoid precipitating factors

F. Urine culture

Positive

Negative

Antibiotic Therapy × 7–10 days

Treat for
Chlamydia,
Doxycycline,
100 mg
bid × 7 days
or
Azithromycin,
1 g Single Dose

Early reinfection

Urine culture

Associated with intercourse

Antibiotic Therapy × 14 days

Consider:
Postcoital antibiotic therapy

Reinfection

477

BREAST MASS

Laurie L. Fajardo

Breast cancer is the most common malignancy and the second leading cause of cancer-related death among American women. The most effective means for diagnosing early breast cancer is screening mammography in combination with physical examination. Nonpalpable breast lesions (detectable only by mammography) may represent small, early, and potentially curable cancers. Mammography does not always provide a specific diagnosis of benign or malignancy. More than 1 million breast biopsies are performed in the United States annually; 11–36% of biopsies performed for mammographically identified nonpalpable abnormalities are positive. The use of percutaneous fine needle aspiration (FNA) or core needle biopsy (CNB) for palpable breast masses, or stereotactic- or sonography-guided CNB for non-palpable masses, may reduce the expense and morbidity associated with the diagnostic work-up of breast lesions and decrease the number of benign breast biopsies performed (see also Gynecomastia, p 484).

A. Needle aspiration of breast masses that feel benign should be a routine part of the evaluation of breast masses. It is safe, is cost-effective, and immediately helps distinguish cystic from solid masses. It can be performed with an 18- to 22-gauge needle with local anesthesia. Nonbloody fluid can be discarded without being sent to the laboratory for pathologic study. A persistent mass or bloody fluid mandates excisional biopsy to rule out malignancy.

B. Diagnostic mammography is indicated (1) for breast signs or symptoms (pain, mass, discharge, thickening, skin or nipple retraction, nipple eczema), (2) before breast surgery (biopsy, augmentation, reduction), (3) as routine follow-up of a patient with previous breast cancer (all remaining breast tissue), and (4) for metastatic cancer of unknown primary site. Preoperative mammography is performed (1) to characterize a lesion as obviously benign (lipoma, oil cyst, calcified fibroadenoma) or malignant (to plan the surgical approach), (2) to determine the size and extent of the lesion for adequate excision and treatment selection (especially important in a patient for whom conservative surgery and irradiation are being considered because multicentric disease in the affected breast is a contraindication to this procedure), (3) to detect additional lesions in the ipsilateral or contralateral breast, and (4) to obtain a baseline for comparison with follow-up mammography. It is important to recognize that mammograms may be negative even when breast cancer is obviously present. Thus a negative mammogram does not replace the need for biopsy of a palpable mass.

C. For palpable breast masses, percutaneous FNA or CNB can be performed with local anesthesia. To evaluate nonpalpable masses, CNB can be guided with stereotactic mammography or sonographic images. The accuracy of these procedures is >90%. If needle biopsy shows a breast mass to be benign, conservative follow-up with physical examination and mammography can be instituted, obviating the need for further surgical intervention. If a needle biopsy is positive, surgical excision can be planned to cure or stage the patient with a single surgical procedure.

D. Many authors have suggested that because of the possibility of a false negative FNA, *all* palpable masses should undergo excisional biopsy. In one study using physical examination, mammography, and FNA followed by excisional biopsy for confirmation of pathology, patients who had negative or benign findings on all three clinical tests (physical examination, mammography, FNA) also had benign surgical pathologic conditions. This has led to the recommendation for clinical and mammographic observation rather than surgical excision when these criteria are fulfilled.

E. When breast malignancy is confirmed histologically, a routine outpatient work-up to exclude distant metastasis is indicated. Complete physical examination, CBC, liver function tests (LFTs), and chest radiography are routinely performed. A preoperative bone scan is indicated only if the patient has symptoms that are suspicious for bony metastasis. CT of the liver is indicated only if the LFT results are abnormal. The AJC-UICC staging system for breast cancer has been modified recently. Clinical staging includes careful inspection and palpation of the skin, breast, and lymph nodes (axillary, supraclavicular, and cervical) as well as pathologic examination of the breast or other tissues to establish the diagnosis of breast carcinoma. Pathologic staging includes data used for clinical staging, surgical resection, and a pathologic examination of the primary carcinoma. Pathologic staging can now be performed if the primary tumor is removed with no growth tumor in the margins and, in addition, if at least the lowest level (1) of axillary lymph nodes is resected, rather than all three levels.

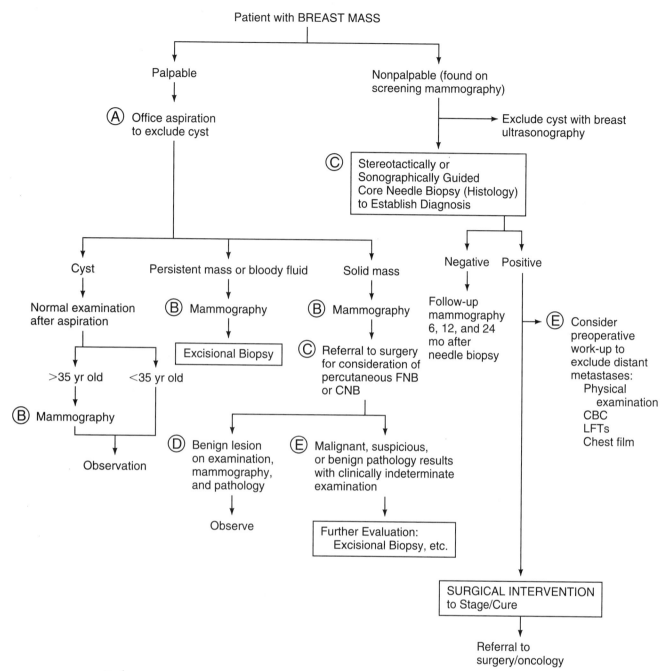

Patient with BREAST MASS

Palpable

Nonpalpable (found on screening mammography)

(A) Office aspiration to exclude cyst

Exclude cyst with breast ultrasonography

(C) Stereotactically or Sonographically Guided Core Needle Biopsy (Histology) to Establish Diagnosis

Cyst

Persistent mass or bloody fluid

Solid mass

Negative   Positive

Normal examination after aspiration

(B) Mammography

(B) Mammography

Follow-up mammography 6, 12, and 24 mo after needle biopsy

(E) Consider preoperative work-up to exclude distant metastases:
Physical examination
CBC
LFTs
Chest film

Excisional Biopsy

(C) Referral to surgery for consideration of percutaneous FNB or CNB

>35 yr old   <35 yr old

(B) Mammography

Observation

(D) Benign lesion on examination, mammography, and pathology

(E) Malignant, suspicious, or benign pathology results with clinically indeterminate examination

Observe

Further Evaluation:
Excisional Biopsy, etc.

SURGICAL INTERVENTION to Stage/Cure

Referral to surgery/oncology

References

Bigelow R, Smith R, Goodman PA, Wilson GS. Needle localization of nonpalpable breast masses. Arch Surg 1985; 120:565.

Brenner RJ, Fajardo LL, Fisher PR, et al. Percutaneous core biopsy of the breast: effect of operator experience and number of samples on diagnostic accuracy. AJR 1996; 166:341.

Donegan WL. Evaluation of a palpable breast mass. N Engl J Med 1992; 327:937.

Fajardo LL. Cost-effectiveness of stereotactic breast core needle biopsy. Acad Radiol 1996; 3(suppl 1):S21.

Fajardo LL, Davis JR, Wiens JL, Trego DC. Mammography-guided stereotactic fine needle aspiration cytology of nonpalpable breast lesions: prospective comparison with surgical biopsy results. AJR 1990; 155:977.

Fajardo LL, DeAngelis GA. The role of imaging guided breast biopsy in the evaluation of mammographically detected abnormalities. Surg Oncol Clin North Am 1997; 6(2):285.

Fleming ID. AJCC cancer staging manual. 5th ed. Philadelphia: Lippincott-Raven, 1997.

Hillner BE, Bear HD, Fajardo LL. Estimating the cost-effectiveness of stereotactic biopsy for nonpalpable breast abnormalities: a decision analysis model. Acad Radiol 1996; 3:351.

Howard J. Using mammography for cancer control: an unrealized potential. CA 1987; 37:33.

Silverberg E, Borring CC, Squires TS. Cancer statistics, 1990. Cancer J Clin 1990; 40:9.

ADJUVANT THERAPY CHOICES IN BREAST CANCER

Rita Blanchard

Breast cancer is the most common female cancer in industrialized nations. Fortunately, a third of all mammography detected tumors are noninvasive (carcinoma in situ [DCIS]), and most newly diagnosed invasive breast cancers (IBC) are limited to the breast and axilla. Even though IBC is apparently localized, early systemic spread is common, and extensive surgical treatment has not impacted survival (S). The benefit of adjuvant systemic therapy to eradicate potential micrometastases in all women with IBC has been established. The ideal management of patients with breast cancer includes a multidisciplinary team (surgeon, primary care physician, medical and radiation oncologists, plastic surgeon, nutritionist, and social service worker) to assess options and the risks and benefits of surgical and systemic therapies based on pathologic findings presented to the patient in a logical, coordinated, and expedited fashion. Therapy should be individualized and participation in clinical research trials stressed. Physicians play a delicate role in stressing benefits of therapy but must also be supportive of individual choices. Adequate time to discuss all options and presentation of local options before discussion of adjuvant therapy aids the patient in selecting therapy.

A. Local control of breast cancer is often done in two stages. Excisional biopsy assesses the pathologic type of cancer and whether the tumor is invasive, DCIS, or both. Tumor size, estrogen receptor (ER) status, grade, and margin involvement are standard parameters that should be reported. Even small tumors can have ER confirmed by histochemical means. Based on this information a decision about definitive surgery should be made. Because mastectomy shows no survival advantage over breast conservation surgery (BCS), BCS should be offered as an option to most women with tumors <5 cm. Women with multicentric disease, suboptimal location of tumor, breast size not conducive to good cosmesis, and certain skin disorders are not candidates for BCS. Even selected large tumors can be treated with BCS if good cosmesis and pathologically clean margins can be obtained. If BCS is desired but the tumor size is borderline, neoadjuvant chemotherapy can potentially shrink the primary tumor allowing subsequent BCS. Critical to local control in BCS are pathologically clear margins and subsequent radiation therapy to the breast. Even small IBCs have an unacceptably high rate of recurrence without breast irradiation.

B. Patients with only DCIS have litle risk of distant recurrence unless the tumor is large (adjusted survival rate 97.2%). With DCIS >4 cm, areas of microinvasion are more common. Axillary dissection is recommended for these patients. In patients with pure DCIS <4 cm, offer BCS without axillary dissection. Radiation therapy to the conserved breast reduces local recurrence for both DCIS and IBC. Controversy exists about whether subsets of patients with DCIS and favorable prognostic signs (small size, low grade, noncomedo necrosis) might be spared radiation after BCS. The benefit of adjuvant tamoxifen in DCIS is still under investigation.

C. Most IBCs are infiltrating ductal carcinoma. Invasive lobular carcinoma carries the same prognosis as infiltrating ductal. Pure tubular, mucinous, and papillary histologies are associated with better prognoses. The most important factor in predicting distant failure, however, is axillary lymph node involvement, followed by tumor size, nuclear grade, and degree of lymphatic invasion. ER status is important in determining response to hormonal therapy (ER – <10% response). Other tumor variables such as S-phase, oncogene overexpression, suppressor gene loss, ploidy, and cathepsin D appear promising as prognostic markers but are less important than axillary lymph node status and tumor size. Axillary dissection controls disease in the axilla, aids in the selection of further systemic therapy, and does not affect survival. Axillary dissection should be done routinely in all patients for whom adjuvant therapy options might change if spread to axillary lymph nodes is detected, or if there are clinically palpable axillary nodes. Sentinel node biopsy is a promising technique to avoid full axillary dissection, but it is still investigational. In summary, the current recommended approach to IBC is local excision with clear margins (either BCS or mastectomy) and level 1 to 2 axillary dissection. Patients with BCS should then have breast irradiation to 4500–5000 CGy with or without a boost to the area of primary tumor. Do not delay adjuvant systemic therapy for breast irradiation. Patients managed with BCS should have another baseline mammogram of the iradiated breast 6 months after radiation, then routine yearly follow-up. Patients with IBC who maintain an ideal body weight and low-fat diet have a better prognosis after diagnosis.

D. Adjuvant chemotherapy has been shown to improve both DFS and S in all patients with positive axillary nodes. Unless comorbid disease or limited life expectancy precludes chemotherapy, it should be considered standard of care in all patients regardless of ER status. Add tamoxifen in all postmenopausal patients whether ER– or ER+ and in all ER+ premenopausal patients. For patients with 0–3 positive nodes (DFS 60% at 5 years), chemotherapy given over 4–6 months is the standard of care. Patients with >3 positive nodes (DFS 40% at 5 years) should receive chemotherapy with a sequential regimen for a longer period or be seriously considered for a National Cancer Institute (NCI)–sponsored high risk protocol. All postmenopausal and ER(+) premenopausal patients should receive tamoxifen. Do not delay chemotherapy or hormonal therapy for breast radiation.

(Continued on page 482)

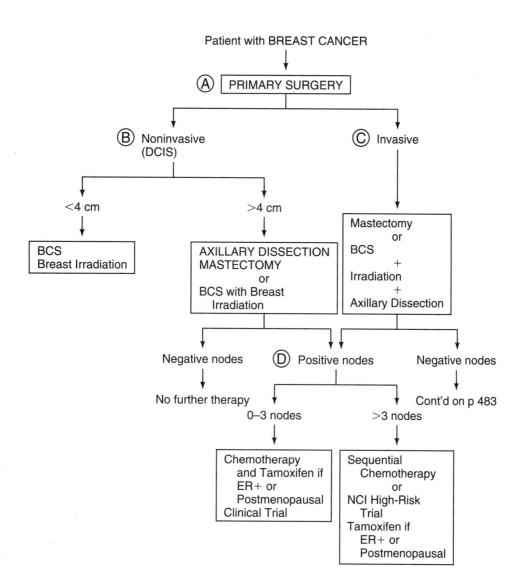

Patient with BREAST CANCER

(A) PRIMARY SURGERY

(B) Noninvasive (DCIS)

(C) Invasive

<4 cm

>4 cm

BCS
Breast Irradiation

AXILLARY DISSECTION
MASTECTOMY
or
BCS with Breast
Irradiation

Mastectomy
or
BCS
+
Irradiation
+
Axillary Dissection

Negative nodes

(D) Positive nodes

Negative nodes

No further therapy

Cont'd on p 483

0–3 nodes

>3 nodes

Chemotherapy
and Tamoxifen if
ER+ or
Postmenopausal
Clinical Trial

Sequential
Chemotherapy
or
NCI High-Risk
Trial
Tamoxifen if
ER+ or
Postmenopausal

E. Patients with negative axillary lymph nodes still have a risk of distant recurrence of 25–30%. Prediction of disease recurrence is based on tumor size with adjusted survival at 20 years of 90% for tumors <1 cm, 80.5% for 1–1.9 cm, 70% for 2.0–4.9 cm and 60.6% for tumors >5 cm. Adjuvant systemic therapy has been shown to improve disease-free survival (DFS) (about 25–30%) in all subsets of patients. Adjuvant tamoxifen has been shown to decrease contralateral and IBC recurrence in patients who are node negative and ER+. Chemotherapy added to adjuvant tamoxifen has been shown to improve DFS. Similarly, adjuvant chemotherapy improves DFS in node-negative, ER– patients. Whether adjuvant hormonal therapy adds to this benefit is currently under investigation. Given the prognosis with regard to tumor size and the patient's own prognosis independent of breast cancer, a therapeutic recommendation can be made. Patients who are otherwise healthy should receive adjuvant chemotherapy for all tumors >2 cm that are ER–, and chemotherapy should be offered in conjunction with tamoxifen in ER+ patients. Offer chemotherapy to patients with tumors of 1–1.9 cm that are ER–, and tamoxifen with chemotherapy to those with ER+ tumors who are in high-risk groups (younger patient, high grade, high S-phase, lymphatic invasion). Offer patients with ER+ tumors <1 cm tamoxifen, and those with high-risk ER– tumors chemotherapy.

References

Bonadonna G, Valagussa P, Moliterni A, et al. Adjuvant cyclophosphamide, methotrexate, and fluorouracil in node-positive breast cancer: the results of 20 years of follow-up. N Engl J Med 1995; 332:901.

Bonadonna G, Zambeti M, Valagussa P. Sequential or alternating doxorubicin and CMF regimens in breast cancer with more than three positive nodes: ten year results. JAMA 1995; 273:542.

Dhingra K, Hartobagyi GN. Critical evaluation of prognostic factors. Semin Oncol 1996; 23:436.

Hudis CA, Norton L. Adjuvant drug therapy for operable breast cancer. Semin Oncol 1996; 23:475.

Hughes KS, Lee AK, Rolfs A. Controversies in the treatment of ductal carcinoma in situ. Surg Clin North Am 1996; 76:243.

Recht A, Come SE, Henderson IC, et al. The sequencing of chemotherapy and radiation therapy after conservative surgery for early-stage breast cancer. N Engl J Med 1996; 334:1356.

Smart CR, Hendrick RE, Rutledge JH III, Smith RA. Benefit of mammography screening in women ages 40 to 49 years: current evidence from randomized controlled trials. Cancer 1995; 75:1619.

Zhang S, Folsom AR, Sellers TA, et al. Better breast cancer survival for postmenopausal women who are less overweight and eat less fat. The Iowa Women's Health Study. Cancer 1995; 76:275.

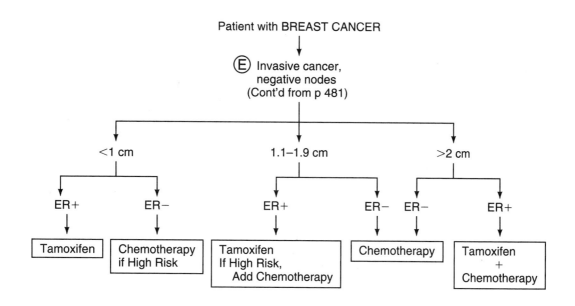

NIPPLE DISCHARGE

Homeira Baghdadi

A. Although nipple discharge is more commonly associated with benign than malignant lesions, cancer needs to be ruled out as the cause. As an initial step a careful medical history and examination is of paramount importance. To be significant, any type of nipple discharge should be true, spontaneous, persistent, and nonlactational. Question the patient for any medication, recent pregnancy, and evidence of amenorrhea. Pharmaceuticals that can cause galactorrhea include estrogens, phenothiazenes, opiates, tricyclic antidepressants, and many others by different mechanisms.

There are seven basic types of nipple discharge. Milky, multicolored, and purulent secretions are treated medically except for an abscess concomitant with a purulent discharge that requires surgical drainage. The remaining four types are yellow or serous, pink or serosanguineous, bloody or sanguineous, and clear or watery. These four types can be the result of cancer and often require surgery to obtain tissue for histologic study.

B. It is important to differentiate between galactorrheal and nongalactorrheal discharge. Galactorrhea may occur bilaterally or unilaterally. Secretions may be thick or thin, or pure white or close to colorless, or they may have a grayish or greenish hue. Fat stain is highly sensitive for determining presence of milk. Galactorrhea usually is of hormonal or pharmacologic origin. Measure serum prolactin and thyroid-stimulating hormone (TSH) in all patients with galactorrhea. If prolactin is elevated, obtain an MRI to determine whether the patient has a pituitary mass. If the prolactin and TSH are normal, follow the patient yearly or as indicated clinically. Human growth hormone (GH) binds to and activates prolactin receptors as well as GH receptors. Thus, galactorrhea may be an early sign of acromegaly. If clinically warranted, obtain a GH measurement. If the TSH is high, evaluate the patient for hypothyroidism. Patients with galactorrhea caused by hypothyroidism may have normal, high normal, or moderately elevated concentrations of prolactin. Galactorrhea itself rarely requires treatment unless the underlying cause does.

C. In patients with nongalactorrheal discharge, first perform a careful and thorough breast examination. Palpation of a mass requires immediate and complete evaluation to rule out a malignant process. If no mass is palpable, consider cytology and mammography. Although a mass usually is present when the discharge is caused by cancer, there is no palpable mass in 13% of cancers with nipple secretions. Do not rely solely on the cytology of the discharge. There is a reported 18% false-negative rate and 2.6% false-positive rate with standard cytology alone. Mammography has a 9.5% false-negative rate and 1.6% false-positive rate for detecting cancer in patients with a nipple discharge. The ability of soft tissue mammography to identify and localize intraductal papillomas is limited. A number of authors have suggested that galactography (a contrast mammogram obtained by injecting a radiopaque dye into the discharging duct) is the diagnostic procedure of choice for nipple discharge. It is better than soft tissue mammography in its ability to visualize and localize small intraductal papillomas. However, its ability to differentiate benign from malignant lesions is limited, and it is a time-consuming procedure that can be uncomfortable to the patients. Because diagnostic tests are not 100% accurate, surgically significant discharges should be evaluated with biopsy and histologic tissue examinations. Although rare, a watery discharge must be considered with concern. There is an increasing likelihood of cancer when the discharge is (in order of increasing frequency) serous, serosanguineous, sanguineous, or watery; when it is accompanied by a lump; when there are adverse cytologic and mammographic findings; and when the patient is >50 years of age.

References

Dickey, Richard P. Drugs that affect the breast and lactation. Clin Obstet Gynecol 1975; 18:95.

Fiorica JV, James V. Nipple discharge. Obstet Gynecol Clin North Am 1994; 21:453.

Gulay H, Bora S, Kilicturgay S, et al. Management of nipple discharge. J Am Coll Surg 1994; 178:471.

Haney AF. Galactorrhea. In: Bardin CW, ed. Current therapy in endocrinology and metabolism. 6th ed. St. Louis: Mosby, 1997:393.

Leis HP Jr. Management of nipple discharge. World J Surg 1989; 13:736.

Patient with NIPPLE DISCHARGE

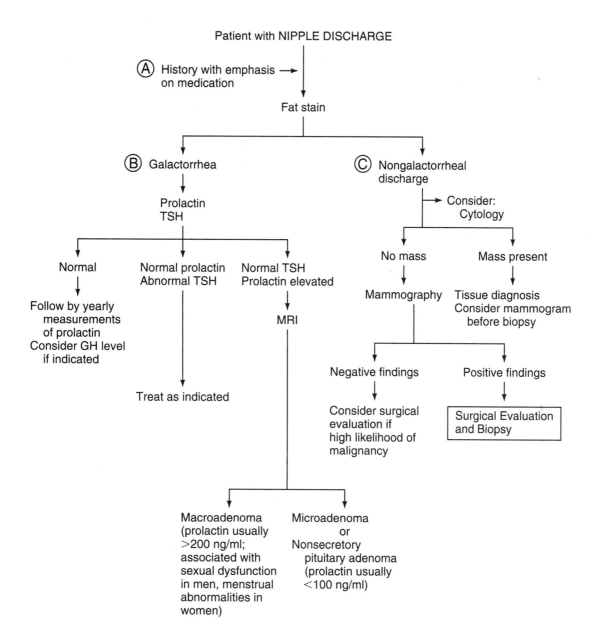

Ⓐ History with emphasis →
on medication

Fat stain

Ⓑ Galactorrhea

Prolactin
TSH

Normal

Follow by yearly
measurements
of prolactin
Consider GH level
if indicated

Normal prolactin
Abnormal TSH

Treat as indicated

Normal TSH
Prolactin elevated

MRI

Macroadenoma
(prolactin usually
>200 ng/ml;
associated with
sexual dysfunction
in men, menstrual
abnormalities in
women)

Microadenoma
or
Nonsecretory
pituitary adenoma
(prolactin usually
<100 ng/ml)

Ⓒ Nongalactorrheal
discharge

→ Consider:
Cytology

No mass

Mammography

Negative findings

Consider surgical
evaluation if
high likelihood of
malignancy

Mass present

Tissue diagnosis
Consider mammogram
before biopsy

Positive findings

Surgical Evaluation
and Biopsy

ABNORMAL PAP SMEAR

Hugh S. Miller

The decline in cervical cancer from the first to the seventh most common cancer among women in the United States is directly attributable to the use of screening Pap smears. The Pap smear is both sensitive and specific for pathology of the genital tract including the vagina, cervix, uterus, and occasionally even fallopian tubes and ovaries. The Bethesda System (TBS) was adopted in 1988 (revised in 1991) in an attempt to establish national standards for an industry that had been heavily criticized for its lack of standards and inadequate quality assurance. Its creation established the cytopathology report as a medical consultation and displaced the former Papanicolaou classification. With TBS cytopathologists must first determine the adequacy of the sample and then distinguish among inflammatory, infectious, and neoplastic processes. TBS adopted two new terms, *low-* and *high-grade squamous intraepithelial lesions* (SIL), to replace the previous terminology, exclusive of invasive carcinoma. Some cytopathologists may still use the former classifications of dysplasia, cervical intraepithelial neoplasia (CIN) 1-3. The new descriptive nomenclature, which includes the classifications of atypical squamous cells of undetermined significance (ASCUS) and low-grade squamous intraepithelial lesion (LSIL), has caused management controversy equal to that of the previous system.

A. Cervical cytopathology is strongly associated with sexual activity and human papillomavirus (HPV) infection, which is considered an STD. A complete gynecologic history, including STD history, age at first coitus, number of sexual partners, use of tobacco products, and previous abnormal cervical cytopathology with concomitant diagnostic procedures and treatment, is important in the evaluation of a patient with an abnormal Pap smear.

B. Evaluation of the female genital tract requires the best illumination and the proper size and shape of speculum to optimize visualization. Initially, examine the unprepared vulvar, vaginal, and cervical epithelium for whitish patches, growths, or ulcerations. Remember that the use of bactericidal or bacteriostatic lubricants compromises the culture and cytopathology results. Cervical friability, with or without an associated lesion, can represent an infectious condition or a neoplastic one. When a Pap smear is judged unsatisfactory, it usually is because of either the absence of endocervical cells or drying artifact. A properly obtained Pap smear contains exophytic and endophytic cervical cells to maximize the probability of sampling the transformation zone. A moistened cotton-tipped applicator and a spatula generally suffice. The endocervical brush collects a better endocervical sampling at an increased cost, with greater patient discomfort, and a higher risk of provoking bleeding that can obscure the cervical field. HPV DNA identification and cervicography are newer techniques developed to better identify patients at risk for invasive carcinoma by improving sensitivity and specificity. Papnet and the ThinPrep Pap Test are newer screening technologies that may replace the conventional Pap smear.

C. Consider the finding of ASCUS in a "satisfactory" Pap smear in the context of the patient's individual risk factors. For patients at risk or those with straightforward SIL, proceed with colposcopy and colposcopically directed biopsies. Loop electroexcision procedure (LEEP) has led some experienced colposcopists to collect a surgical specimen for diagnosis simultaneous with definitive surgical treatment. Patients exhibiting primary ASCUS associated with HPV derive minimal benefit from ablative therapy. Even many patients diagnosed with LSIL (60%) have spontaneous regression of their lesions without treatment. From the standpoint of infectious disease, patients with identifiable lesions benefit from ablative therapy, as do those with significant dysplasia. Cryoablation is preferred, but various topical preparations, laser therapy, LEEP, and cold-knife conization continue to be used. Management of patients with LSIL must be individualized to include the assessment of patient compliance with follow-up. After each specific intervention, reassess the cervix at 4- to 6-month intervals for 2 years, or until there have been three consecutive negative Pap smears. Annual surveillance may then resume.

D. Because abnormal Pap smears are strongly associated with HPV, consider other STDs in the evaluation of these patients. Cervicitis (see p 460) may be caused by more than one genital tract pathogen and may require collection of cultures and initiation of antibiotic therapy. Recurrent dysplasia should prompt further assessment of risk factors such as smoking, chronic disease, and HIV status.

E. The cervix regularly rests in the posterior vaginal fornix, contributing to its exfoliated cells as well as those arising from the upper genital tract (endocervix, uterus, fallopian tube, and rarely ovary). When normal endometrial or glandular cells are reported on the routine Pap smear, no further evaluation is needed. However, TBS allows a more precise characterization of the cell type and its morphology. In cases of atypical or neoplastic glandular cells, further evaluation and treatment of the upper genital tract is required.

Patient with ABNORMAL PAP SMEAR

(A) History ———→
    Physical examination

(B) "Unsatisfactory"   (C) "Satisfactory"
    Pap smear   abnormal Pap smear

    Repeat Pap smear

Normal   ASCUS   LSIL/HSIL   (D) Infection   (E) Glandular
                                                              cells

                                        Cervical
                                        culture and
                                        sensitivity

No risk factors   Risk factors   Normal   Abnormal
┌────────────┐   ┌────────────┐   cells   cells
│ Negative HPV│   │ Positive HPV│
│ Typing   │   │ Typing   │   ┌────────────┐
│ Negative   │   │ Positive   │   │ Appropriate │
│ Cervicogram│   │ Cervicogram│   │ Antibiotic │   ┌────────────┐
└────────────┘   └────────────┘   │ Therapy   │   │ Colposcopy │
                                         └────────────┘   │ ECC   │
  Repeat Pap smear   │ Endometrial │
                                                               │ Biopsy   │
                                    Abnormal   Normal   └────────────┘

Normal   Abnormal ———→ ┌────────────────┐   Normal   Abnormal
                         │ Colposcopy   │   findings   findings
                         │ Directed Cervical│◄─
                         │ Biopsies   │
                         │ Endocervical   │   ┌────────────┐
                         │ Curettage (ECC) │   │ Appropriate │
                         └────────────────┘   │ Therapy with│
                                                                     │ Follow-Up   │
                                                                     └────────────┘

Adequate assessment   Inadequate assessment
(limits of lesion seen)   (limits of lesion
                           not seen)
                          Positive carcinoma in situ (CIS)
                          Positive ECC

ASCUS/LSIL   HSIL/CIS

              ┌────────────┐
              │ Appropriate │
              │ Ablative Therapy│
              └────────────┘   ┌────────────┐
                                            │ Conization │
                                            └────────────┘

Follow-up 4–6 mo Pap smears ◄─
Continue 2–3 yr *or* three
consecutive normal Paps

References

American College of Obstetricians and Gynecologists. Cervical cytology: evaluation and management of abnormalities. Washington, DC: American College of Obstetricians and Gynecologists, ACOG Technical Bulletin No. 183, August 1993.

American College of Obstetricians and Gynecologists. Genital human papillomavirus infections. Washington, DC: American College of Obstetricians and Gynecologists, ACOG Technical Bulletin No. 193, June 1994.

Kurman RJ, Henson DE, Herbst AL, et al. Interim guidelines for management of abnormal cervical cytology. JAMA 1994; 271:1866.

PREMENSTRUAL DYSPHORIC DISORDER

Jessica Byron

A. More than 40% of women experiencing cyclic menstruation report premenstrual symptoms, ranging from negligible in many women to disabling in up to 15%. Many symptoms and signs have been described as part of PMS, including bloating, edema, weight gain, breast pain, acne, appetite changes, headaches, joint pain, diarrhea, constipation, anger or irritability, increased interpersonal conflicts, anxiety, aggression, depression, lethargy, fatigue, sleep disorder (hypersomnia, insomnia), difficulty concentrating, and restlessness. None of these symptoms is pathognomonic. It is the cyclic occurrence of symptoms beginning near or after ovulation and resolving soon after the onset of menses that is of diagnostic significance. In addition, the premenstrual changes must be significant enough to interfere with work, school, or usual social activities or relationships with others. The role of ovarian steroids, prolactin, prostaglandins, mineralocorticoids, neurotransmitters, endogenous opiates, vitamin and mineral deficiencies, and psychological factors is unclear.

B. Diagnostic evaluation of PMS involves clinical evaluation and review of the patient's prospective daily charting of the timing, type, and rating of severity of symptoms for at least two menstrual cycles. Take a medical history to rule out cardiac, renal, or thyroid disease; collagen vascular disease; and diabetes. Also exclude other problems, including anemia, breast disease, dysmenorrhea, endometriosis, perimenopausal changes, or premenstrual exacerbation of allergies, arthritis, asthma, diabetes, irritable bowel syndrome, migraine, and seizure disorders. Determine whether the patient has premenstrual dysphoric disorder (PMDD), which affects 5–10% of normally cycling women. Many women with severe PMS meet the diagnostic criteria for PMDD. PMS/PMDD must be differentiated from other psychiatric disorders (anxiety, depression, eating or personality disorders) because these disorders also cause symptoms in the follicular phase. Perform physical examination and laboratory testing as needed. Investigators have been unable to document specific changes in hormone levels, prolactin, aldosterone, endorphins, and glucose tolerance. There are no laboratory tests to diagnose PMS.

C. It is essential to review the patient's daily symptom chart, which has tracked symptoms for two complete menstrual cycles. A variety of forms are available. One way is to ask the patient to list the symptoms that affect her most. The checklist is started on the first day of the period and each evening the symptoms are rated on a scale of 0–4 (0 = symptom is absent; 4 = symptom is severe and patient cannot function). At least five symptom scores during the luteal phase must show a marked change from scores in the follicular phase for PMS to be diagnosed. For severe PMS and PMDD the questionnaire developed by Endicott and Harrison is helpful.

D. Review of treatment research fails to demonstrate consistently effective therapy, and the rate of response to placebo appears to be 50%. Numerous treatments have been advocated. Initial interventions are education and support, stress reduction, healthy nutrition, and regular exercise. Many women are reassured by chart review and can plan their schedules according to symptom severity, use relaxation exercises, join a support group, or participate in an exercise program to relieve stress. Eating complex carbohydrates (whole grains, beans, fresh fruits, vegetables) and low-protein foods, as well as tapering caffeine intake, especially during the luteal phase, may diminish symptoms but efficacy remains unproven. Neither natural progesterone (in suppository or micronized oral preparations) nor synthetic progestins are effective for PMS.

E. Offer medical treatment or referral to women who meet the diagnostic criteria for PMDD. Consider prescribing a selective serotonin reuptake inhibitor (SSRI) if there are symptoms of PMDD or if PMS is severe and symptoms include psychosocial difficulties. When SSRIs do not work, an anxiolytic agent may be the next choice. Anovulation therapy with oral contraceptives (OCPs), danazol, and GnRH agonists (goserelin acetate, leuprolide acetate, nafarelin acetate) can relieve symptoms of severe PMS, but unpleasant side effects are common and lead to discontinuance. OCPs appear to relieve PMS symptoms in about one third of women. Consider further evaluation or referral when the diagnosis is uncertain, another medical or psychiatric disorder is suspected, the patient is a risk to herself or others, or standard dosages of medications are ineffective in reducing symptoms.

References

Barnhart KT, Freeman EW, Sondheimer SJ. A clinician's guide to the premenstrual syndrome. Med Clin North Am 1995; 79:1457.

Endicott J, Freeman EW, Kielich A, Sondheimer SJ. PMS: new treatments that really work. Patient Care 1996; April:88.

Goodale IL, Domar AD, Benson H. Alleviation of premenstrual syndrome with the relaxation response. Obstet Gynecol 1990; 75:649.

Rubinow DR, Schmidt PJ. The treatment of premenstrual syndrome: forward into the past (editorial). N Engl J Med 1995; 332:1574.

Sayegh R, Schiff I, Wurtman J, et al. The effect of a carbohydrate-rich beverage on mood, appetite and cognitive function in women with premenstrual syndrome. Obstet Gynecol 1995; 86:520.

Severino SK, Moline ML. Premenstrual syndrome: identification and management. Drugs 1995; 49(1):71.

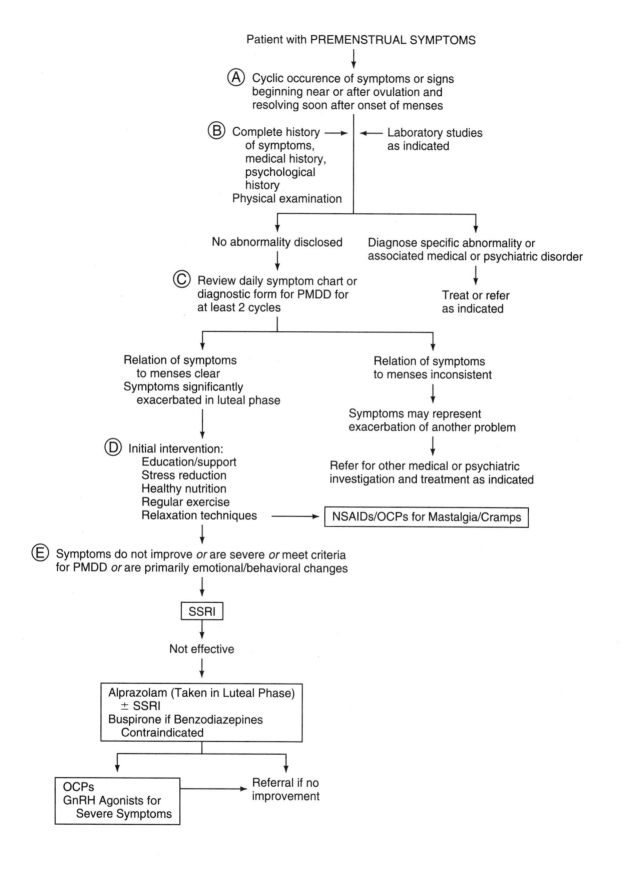

Patient with PREMENSTRUAL SYMPTOMS

(A) Cyclic occurence of symptoms or signs
beginning near or after ovulation and
resolving soon after onset of menses

(B) Complete history ——→ ←—— Laboratory studies
of symptoms,   as indicated
medical history,
psychological
history
Physical examination

No abnormality disclosed   Diagnose specific abnormality or
                                  associated medical or psychiatric disorder

(C) Review daily symptom chart or   Treat or refer
diagnostic form for PMDD for   as indicated
at least 2 cycles

Relation of symptoms   Relation of symptoms
to menses clear   to menses inconsistent
Symptoms significantly
exacerbated in luteal phase   Symptoms may represent
                                  exacerbation of another problem

(D) Initial intervention: Refer for other medical or psychiatric
Education/support   investigation and treatment as indicated
Stress reduction
Healthy nutrition
Regular exercise
Relaxation techniques ——→ NSAIDs/OCPs for Mastalgia/Cramps

(E) Symptoms do not improve *or* are severe *or* meet criteria
for PMDD *or* are primarily emotional/behavioral changes

SSRI

Not effective

Alprazolam (Taken in Luteal Phase)
± SSRI
Buspirone if Benzodiazepines
Contraindicated

OCPs   Referral if no
GnRH Agonists for   improvement
Severe Symptoms

CONTRACEPTIVE CHOICES

Ana Maria López

The decision to conceive or not to conceive is a complicated one dependent on multiple factors. It also is one in which many patients request physician participation. To facilitate this process, the physician must be well versed in biologic factors that may influence this decision and be sensitive to patient concerns. Biologic factors that affect contraceptive choice include age, tobacco use, history of pelvic inflammatory disease (PID), and history of cardiovascular disease. Important patient issues that must be clarified include plans for future fertility, current sexual lifestyle, impact of unplanned pregnancy, history of compliance, and role of partner in birth spacing. Patients often have questions about efficacy (Table 1), safety, cost, and noncontraceptive benefits as well as the need to access the health care system to obtain or continue use of a specific birth control method (BCM). By applying active listening skills to the patient-physician interaction, the clinician can help the patient make an informed choice.

TABLE 1   Contraceptive Effectiveness in First Year in the United States*

BCM	Effectiveness	
	Theoretical (%)†	Typical (%)‡
Vasectomy	99.9	99.85
BLTL	99.8	99.6
Norplant	99.96	99.96
Depo-Provera	99.7	99.7
Oral contraceptives		
Combined	99.1	97
Mini-pill	99.5	80
IUD		
Cu-T 380A	99.2	97
Progestasert	98.0	93
Condom	98	88
Diaphragm	96	82
Cervical cap	94	82
Sponge		
Parous patient	91	72
Multiparous patient	94	82
Spermicides	97	80
Fertility awareness method		
Calendar	90	80
With BBT, postovulation coitus only	98	97
Lactation		
Breast feeding on demand with amenorrhea, 1st 6 months post partum	99	96
Chance	15	15

*Based on data in Hatcher et al, Trussel et al (1987), and Trussel et al (1990).

†Theoretical effectiveness attempts to predict the percent of contraceptive failures expected among couples using the BCM perfectly, consistently and correctly, for an entire year.

‡Typical effectiveness attempts to predict the percent of contraceptive failures expected among typical couples using the BCM for an entire year.

A. Vasectomy is simple, inexpensive, and safe but does not confer immediate sterility. Sperm usually are not present after 25 ejaculations, but this can be confirmed only by microscopic examination of the semen. Although antibody formation to sperm has been noted after vasectomy, clinically adverse implications have not been fully elucidated. Bilateral tubal ligation (BLTL) is the most common BCM in the world. It is an outpatient procedure with a lower mortality rate than childbirth (3:100,000 vs. 14:100,000). If BLTL fails, the risk of ectopic pregnancy is increased. Vasectomy and BLTL may be reversed by microsurgical techniques. The success of reversals is inversely related to the amount of tissue originally damaged. Patients must be counseled that these are permanent BCMs and that their potential reversibility does not guarantee fertility.

B. Combination oral contraceptives (OCs) are second only to BLTL as the most common BCM in the world today. OCs were the first BCM to separate contraceptive use from sexual activity. They contain either estrogen and progesterone in fixed or variable combination or progesterone alone, the "mini-pill." The latter contains low-dose progesterone and is an option in women for whom estrogen is contraindicated (e.g., the older woman with cardiovascular risk factors). Its efficacy is less than that for the combination OCs. In the former, the estrogen and progesterone hormone combination may be fixed, monophasic, or variable, phasic. In phasic preparations, the pills within a pack contain variable doses of the progestin and occasionally of the estrogen to decrease the overall hormonal doses while maintaining contraceptive effects and decreasing metabolic side effects.

OCs act by preventing ovulation. If ovulation should occur, implantation is prevented by changes in the cervical mucus and endometrium.

Patients should be instructed to start the pack of pills at the onset of the menses or on the first Sunday after the start of menstruation. Contraceptive efficacy requires about 2–4 weeks to develop. During these initial first few weeks another BCM should also be used. In a 28-day pack, 21 pills contain active hormone preparation and 7 are placebo pills that serve to facilitate daily pill taking. 21-day packs without the placebo pills are available in some brands. If a pill is missed, the woman should take one pill every 12 hours until all the forgotten pills have been taken. A back-up BCM is advised for the remainder of the month. If three or more pills are missed repeatedly, another BCM should be considered. In the case of the "mini-pill," even a 3-hour delay in pill taking may result in compromised antifertility activity; therefore a back-up BCM is recommended for 48 hours for such a delay.

Absolute contraindications to OC use include history of thrombophlebitis or thromboembolic events, cigarette smoking (1 pack/day or more), and age >35 years; hypertension; history of estrogen-dependent

(Continued on page 492)

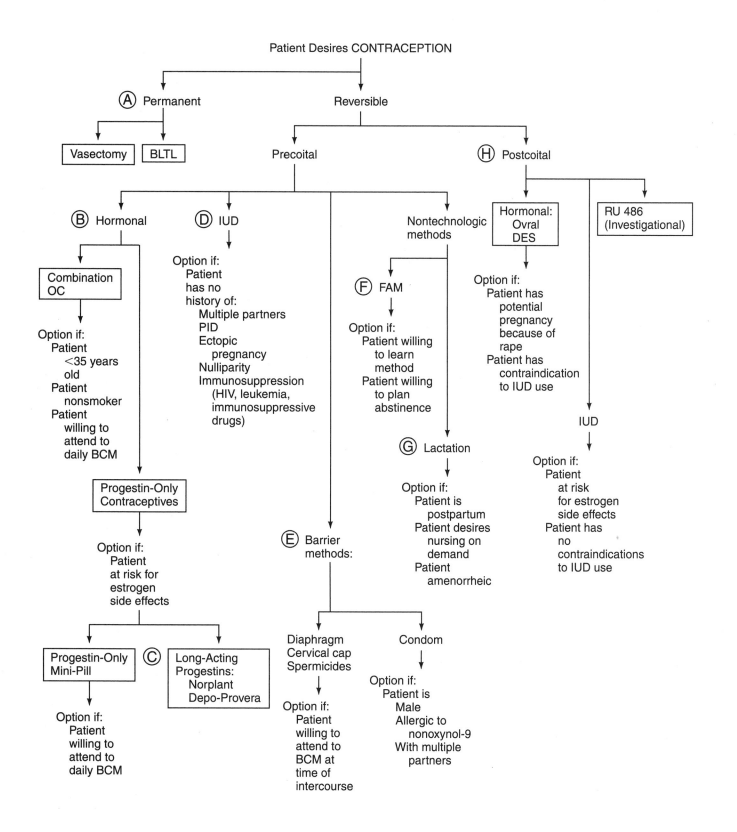

Patient Desires CONTRACEPTION

Ⓐ Permanent

Vasectomy   BLTL

Reversible

Precoital

Ⓑ Hormonal

Combination
OC

Option if:
Patient
<35 years
old
Patient
nonsmoker
Patient
willing to
attend to
daily BCM

Progestin-Only
Contraceptives

Option if:
Patient
at risk for
estrogen
side effects

Progestin-Only
Mini-Pill   Ⓒ

Long-Acting
Progestins:
Norplant
Depo-Provera

Option if:
Patient
willing to
attend to
daily BCM

Ⓓ IUD

Option if:
Patient
has no
history of:
Multiple partners
PID
Ectopic
pregnancy
Nulliparity
Immunosuppression
(HIV, leukemia,
immunosuppressive
drugs)

Ⓔ Barrier
methods:

Diaphragm
Cervical cap
Spermicides

Option if:
Patient
willing to
attend to
BCM at
time of
intercourse

Condom

Option if:
Patient is
Male
Allergic to
nonoxynol-9
With multiple
partners

Nontechnologic
methods

Ⓕ FAM

Option if:
Patient willing
to learn
method
Patient willing
to plan
abstinence

Ⓖ Lactation

Option if:
Patient is
postpartum
Patient desires
nursing on
demand
Patient
amenorrheic

Ⓗ Postcoital

Hormonal:
Ovral
DES

Option if:
Patient has
potential
pregnancy
because of
rape
Patient has
contraindication
to IUD use

RU 486
(Investigational)

IUD

Option if:
Patient
at risk
for estrogen
side effects
Patient has
no
contraindications
to IUD use

malignancy such as breast or endometrial cancer; undiagnosed abnormal vaginal bleeding; and impaired liver function with history of cholestatic jaundice with prior pill use or with pregnancy or history of hepatic adenomas or carcinomas. Relative contraindications to OC use: smoker (1 pack/day or more), and history of migraines, severe headaches, seizures, severe depression, hyperlipidemia, ovarian dysfunction, gallbladder disease, diabetes mellitus, gestational diabetes, melanoma, obesity (≥ 50% overweight), or lactation.

Estrogen-related side effects include nausea, breast tenderness, cyclic weight gain, thrombophlebitis and thromboembolic events particularly in smokers, leukorrhea, cervical ectopy, headaches, hypertension, and benign or malignant hepatic neoplasias. Progesterone-related side effects include weight gain, depression, fatigue, decreased libido, acne, carbohydrate intolerance, and hyperlipidemia. OCs should be prescribed after a thorough history and physical examination have been performed. Once the patient is placed on OC therapy, close follow-up is necessary.

C. Long-acting progestin-only contraceptives include Depo-Provera and Norplant. The advantage of these methods is that the estrogen-associated thromboembolic complications are avoided. Women most at risk for estrogen-related side effects are ≥ 35 years old, smokers, hypertensive patients, and those with a history of hypercoagulability. Progesterone-related side effects include increased low-density lipoprotein and decreased high-density lipoprotein with increased carbohydrate intolerance, possibly leading to diabetes. These methods act by inhibiting ovulation, maintaining thick cervical mucus inhospitable to sperm, and producing thin atrophic endometrium subject to premature luteolysis. Depo-Provera, "the shot," consists of 150 mg of medroxyprogesterone given IM every 3 months. Although women often experience irregular vaginal bleeding in the first 12 months, the most common side effect after the first year is amenorrhea. Norplant consists of six match-sized capsules surgically inserted subdermally in the woman's arm 7 days after the onset of menses. Slow hormonal release continues for the next 5 years; the failure rate is <0.57%. After 5 years the implants must be removed and a fresh set reinserted, if desired. Combination hormone monthly injectables are under development and are available outside the United States. They allow a normal menstrual pattern.

D. Intrauterine devices (IUDs) have a long history, but currently only two are available in the United States: Cu-T 380A and Progestasert, with the former being more widely used. Cu-T 380A is FDA approved for 10-year use; however, Progestasert must be replaced annually. IUDs are thought to act by inhibiting fertilization and implantation through local foreign body inflammation and because of the copper or progesterone effect of producing an atrophic endometrium. IUDs are contraindicated in patients with a known history of PID or ectopic pregnancy. They are inserted at the time of a woman's menses. Side effects include menorrhagia, which may result in anemia; dysmenorrhea; and uterine perforation secondary to a wandering IUD. Instruct the woman to ascertain IUD placement by checking for the IUD string.

E. Barrier methods require active patient participation. The diaphragm and cervical cap have been available for about 100 years and require fitting by a health care practitioner. Diaphragm use requires spermicide application before each episode of intercourse. It can be inserted up to 2 hours before intercourse and must remain in place 6–8 hours after coitus. Refitting must take place after pregnancy, pelvic surgery, or weight change of 10 pounds or more. In the United States, the Prentif cap is the only cervical cap available. It is inserted no less than 1/2 hour before intercourse with a small amount of spermicide within the dome and can remain in place for 72 hours. A 24-hour limit is recommended to decrease cervical irritation and risk of toxic shock syndrome (TSS). Repeated spermicide applications are not required. The cervical cap cannot be used during menses. The cervical sponge is no longer available in the United States but is available abroad. It does not require health practitioner fitting and contains 1 g nonoxynol-9. It is available without a prescription and can be used continuously for 24 hours after moistening with tap water. All the above methods carry the risk of TSS. Spermicides can be used alone, although their efficacy is greatest when used in combination with condoms. Noncontraceptive benefits of nonoxynol-9 include prevention of STD and PID. Condoms are the only male form of contraception. Problems with efficacy are associated with improper use (i.e., not leaving a 1/2-in. reservoir at the tip or not withdrawing carefully immediately after coitus). The Reality female condom has been developed and is commercially available. Recent studies in male contraception confirm the contraceptive efficacy of hormone-induced oligospermia.

F. Fertility awareness methods (FAMs) can be as effective as OCs in preventing pregnancy if used appropriately, with intercourse restricted to the postovulatory period. Efficacy is directly related to the use of multiple factors to detect fertility. Because of the complexity of these factors, formal instruction is advised before attempting use for either contraception or conception. Basal body temperature is recorded daily to detect a temperature rise of 0.4°–0.8° F, indicating ovulation. Cervical mucus also must be examined daily because wet, thin mucus (as opposed to thick, dry mucus) facilitates sperm mobility. A record of the length of the patient's cycles is maintained. From this historical information and awareness that ovulation usually takes place 14 days before the onset of menses, a period of high-risk days can be defined. Some patients also note changes in cervical position and texture throughout the menstrual cycle. Finally, mittelschmerz is a sign of ovulation that some women consistently recognize.

G. Worldwide, lactation is a successful BCM. Recent data reveal that breast-feeding on demand while remaining amenorrheic in the first 6 months postpartum is 98% effective as a BCM. Unfortunately, most U.S. patients are unable or do not desire to breast-feed on demand for 6 months.

H. Postcoital hormonal approaches include the use of Ovral or Lo-Ovral within 72 hours of the episode of unprotected intercourse: two tablets every 12 hours for a total of four tablets or four tablets every 12 hours for a total of eight tablets. Similarly, diethylstilbestrol (DES), 50 mg/day for 5 days, can be prescribed to prevent implantation; its most common side effect is nausea, and pregnancy termination is recommended if pregnancy does occur. Postcoital IUDs have also been used. The Cu-T may be inserted up to 5 days after intercourse; however, it is contraindicated in rape cases, in women with multiple partners, and in nulliparous patients. In prescribing postcoital OCs or IUDs, take care to screen for potential contraindications. Although these methods are part of clinical practice and are prescribed for postcoital contraception, the FDA has not approved their postcoital use. RU486, a progesterone antagonist, has been widely used in Europe to induce menses in the first 5 weeks of pregnancy and is under investigation in the United States.

References

Affandi B, Santoso SS, Djajadilaga, et al. Five-year experience with Norplant. Contraception 1987; 36:429.

Albertson BD, Zinaman MJ. The prediction of ovulation and monitoring of the fertile period. Adv Contracept 1987; 3:263.

Alderman P. The lurking sperm. JAMA 1988; 259:3142.

Burnhill MS. The rise and fall and rise of the IUD. Am J Gynecol Health 1989; III(3):6.

Choice of contraceptives. Med Lett Drugs Ther 1995; 37:9.

Gallen ME. Men—new focus on family planning. Pop Rep 1987; Series J:890.

Geerling JH. Natural family planning. Am Fam Physician 1995; 52:1749.

Haspels AA. Emergency contraception: a review. Contraception 1994; 50:101.

Hatcher RA, Stewart F, Trussell J, et al. Contraceptive technology. 16th ed. New York: Irvington, 1994.

Kaunitz AM, Illions EH, Jones HL, Sang LA. Contraception: a clinical review for the internist. Med Clin North Am 1995; 79:1377.

Kennedy KI, Rivera R, McNeilly AS. Consensus statement on the use of breastfeeding as a family planning method. Contraception 1989; 39:477.

Topical spermicides. Med Lett Drugs Ther 1980; 22:90.

Trussell J, Hatcher RA, Cates W Jr, et al. Contraceptive failure in the United States: an update. Stud Fam Plann 1990; 21:51.

Trussell J, Kost K. Contraceptive failure in the United States: a critical review of the literature. Stud Fam Plann 1987; 18:237.

USE OF ORAL CONTRACEPTIVES

Terra A. Robles

Early studies found that oral contraceptives (OCs), which had a greater amount of estrogen, were associated with serious adverse outcomes. Today's low-dose formulations retain efficacy while minimizing side effects and have an overall lower risk of cardiovascular disease. OCs contain synthetic estrogens and progestins. They differ in dosage, proportion of active ingredients, and prescribed regimens. Effectiveness, safety, and patient acceptability are important in selection of OC products. Provide a product that offers the lowest effective dose of both hormones and minimizes side effects. Data are not available for determining which OC is "better"; cost considerations should be included in product selection.

A. Before prescribing an OC, obtain a complete history, including history of previous contraceptive use and failures or adverse effects of previously used methods; menstrual history, focusing on patterns and problems; gynecologic and obstetric history; and general medical history. Perform a complete physical examination in which risk factors are assessed and contraindications to OC use determined. Order appropriate laboratory tests as necessary.

B. Monophasic pills contain a constant estrogen and progestin dose. Biphasic products contain a constant dose of estrogen, with a lower progestin dose on days 1–10 than on days 11–21. Triphasic pills have varied amounts of hormones; Ortho-Novum 777, Tri-Levelen, Tricyclen, and Triphasil have an increase of progestin at mid- and end-cycle; Tri-Norinyl has increased progestin only at midcycle. Ortho-Novum 777, Tricyclen, and Tri-Norinyl have fixed amounts of estrogen; Triphasil and Tri-Levelen have increased estrogen at midcycle. These differences in triphasic pills are generally insignificant in most women who do not have specific problems or menstrual irregularities.

Ethinyl estradiol (EE) and mestranol are the two estrogen agents used in OCs. EE is pharmacologically active and mestranol is hepatically converted to EE. Progestins used in OCs include norethindrone, norethindrone acetate, ethynodiol diacetate, dl-norgestrel, norethynodrel, levonorgestrel, desogestrel, and norgestimase. Norethindrone acetate and ethynodiol diacetate are metabolized to norethindrone and offer no significant advantage over norethindrone. dl-Norgestrel and levonorgestrel are isomers, levonorgestrel being the active component. Some studies suggest that dl-norgestrel has little pharmacologic activity, but others state that it prevents breakthrough bleeding (BTB) more effectively. Norgestrel, levonorgestrel, and desogestrel have the highest progestational effects. Norethynodrel has the highest estrogenic effects with all others having minimal to no estrogenic effects. The greatest androgenic effects are seen by norgestrel and levonorgestrel.

Estrogen is the major determinant for inducing increases in blood pressure (BP); however, progestins also may be associated. Carbohydrate and lipid alternations are caused by the progestin component in OCs.

Desogestrel, norgestimate, and low doses of norethindrone have little if any effects on carbohydrate metabolism. Progestins decrease high-density lipoproteins (HDLs) and increase low-density lipoproteins (LDLs); estrogens have the opposite effect.

A back-up method of birth control is recommended with the first cycle of OCs. Compliance is important for low-dose OCs because missed pills often lead to breakthrough ovulation.

C. The American College of Obstetricians and Gynecologists states that nonsmoking healthy women aged 35–44 years may continue using OCs. However, women with pre-existing diseases that affect the cardiovascular system should not use OCs. Use clinical judgment in deciding whether any woman with cardiovascular disease risk factors (e.g., hypertension, diabetes mellitus, hypercholesterolemia) should use OCs. Some studies of low-dose OCs show no increased risk of cardiovascular complications; however, OCs are currently considered synergistic in increased risk, and each patient must be carefully evaluated for OC use. Follow and monitor patients closely, and offer alternative contraceptive methods when indicated, especially for smokers >35 years old.

D. Progestin-only pills, or "mini-pills," have lower effectiveness than combination OCs (COCs) because ovulation is not consistently inhibited. Progestin-only pills are taken every day of the month, without a break for withdrawal bleeding. Up to two thirds of users experience menstrual irregularities, BTB, and amenorrhea. Mini-pills also are used in lactating women.

E. There is some concern about infant exposure to estrogens. Some believe this exposure is not clinically significant; others advocate waiting until an infant is weaned before instituting OC use. The pill may diminish the protein content and volume of breast milk. The FDA recommends deferring the use of OCs until a baby is weaned.

F. Diabetic patients whose diabetes is controlled may take low-dose OCs. Products with norethindrone, desogestrel, or norgestimate are least likely to alter glucose tolerance. Pregnancy prevention needs to be weighted against the risk of pregnancy.

G. ACHES is a mnemonic commonly used to help remember possible adverse effects of OCs: *A*, abdominal pain (gallbladder disease, hepatic adenoma, pancreatitis, blood clot); *C*, chest pain (pulmonary embolism, myocardial infarction); *H*, headaches (stroke, migraines, hypertension); *E*, eye problems (hypertension, stroke); *S*, severe leg pain (venous thromboembolism). COCs have relative estrogen dominance, and estrogen-related side effects can be expected to predominate. Familiarization with symptoms of estrogen/progestin excess/ deficiency will aid in OC adjustments. Symptoms of

494

(Continued on page 496)

Patient Desires ORAL CONTRACEPTIVE

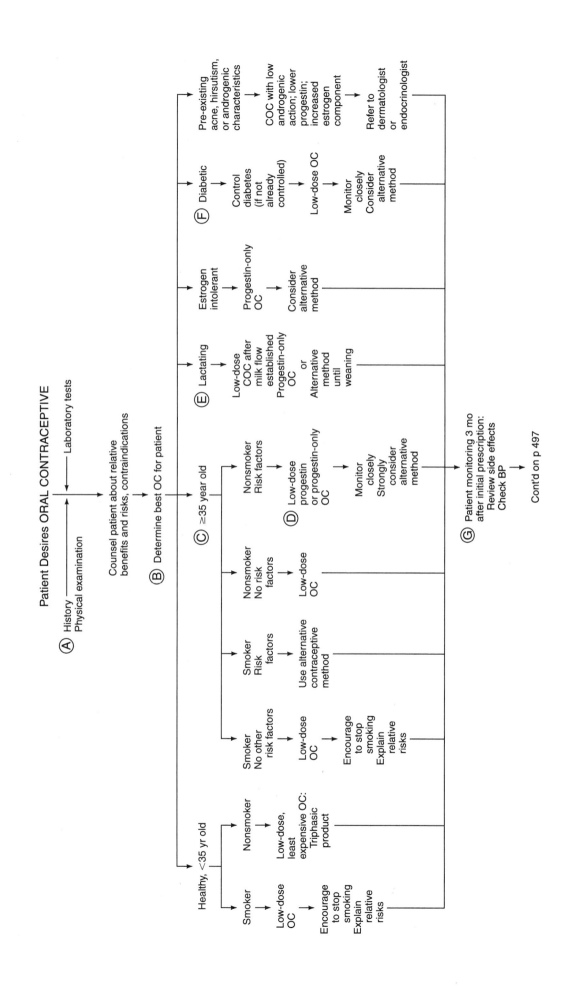

Cont'd on p 497

estrogen excess include nausea, breast tenderness, fluid retention, cervical mucorrhea, and cyclic headaches, whereas estrogen deficiency is suggested by early or midcycle BTB, increased spotting, and hypomenorrhea. Symptoms of progestin excess are increased appetite, depression, fatigue, acne, diabetogenic effects, and decreased libido; symptoms of progestin deficiency include late-cycle BTB, amenorrhea, and hypermenorrhea. An excess of both hormones can cause headaches, weight gain, and hypertension. Many symptoms occurring in the first cycle of OC use improve by the second or third cycle.

H. Lowering the potency of OCs for greater safety has led to an increased incidence of BTB. BTB is common in the first few cycles of OC use.

I. Estrogens are conjugated in the liver and hydrolyzed by intestinal bacteria. Any drug that affects these two systems may lead to decreased OC efficacy.

J. The absence of withdrawal bleeding may be the result of insufficient endometrial development. Switching to an OC with greater progestin content may resolve the problem.

K. An increase in BP may be seen even in normotensive patients. Increases can occur 1–36 months after initiation of the OC. The risk is lower with low-dose OCs. Patients who are started on OCs should be checked for BP changes within the first month. When hypertension is associated with an OC, it is reversible. Monitor any patient who develops hypertension while taking OCs closely for the development of OC-associated complications. A return to normal BP after discontinuation of OC may take 3–6 months.

L. Breast tenderness usually is caused by cyclic fluid retention or growth of breast tissue. An OC with lower estrogenic activity or greater progestational activity, or an OC with less estrogen *and* less progestin, may alleviate the tenderness. If tenderness persists, a progestin-only pill may be tried.

M. Nausea may occur often during the first few cycles of OC use or may occur with the first few pills of each cycle. Many patients can prevent nausea by taking the pill with food or at bedtime. If nausea persists, an OC with lower estrogenic activity (as little as 20 μg in severe cases) may bring relief. Vomiting is rare. If vomiting occurs within 2 hours after taking the OC, the dose should be repeated to ensure contraception.

N. Weight loss and gain occur with equal frequency in OC users. Most weight changes are unrelated to OC use. However, estrogen can cause cyclic weight gain as a result of fluid retention, and progestins can stimulate appetite and insulin release.

O. There is an increased risk of stroke in OC users with a history of migraine. Cerebrovascular accident (CVA) must be ruled out in all OC users who have migraine headaches. Vascular (migrainelike) headaches generally do not improve with a change in OC; these patients need to consider alternative contraceptive methods. Headaches accompanied by fluid retention (edema, breast enlargement, cyclic weight gain) may be caused by both estrogens and progestins. Prescribe an OC with lower estrogenic and/or progestational activity and follow the patient closely to ensure resolution of symptoms after one or two cycles.

P. Depression may be caused by an excess of estrogen and/or progestin or by a deficiency of estrogen. If switching to an OC with lower estrogenic and/or progestational activity does not alleviate the depression, the pill should be discontinued for three to six cycles and re-evaluation performed at that time.

References

Casper RF, Powell AM. Evaluation and therapy of breakthrough bleeding in women using a triphasic oral contraceptive. Fertil Steril 1991; 55:292.

Ellsworth AJ, Leversee JH. Oral contraceptives. Primary Care 1990; 17:603.

Hatcher RA, Stewart F, Trussell J, et al. Contraceptive technology. 16th ed. New York: Irvington, 1994.

Heath CB. Helping patients choose appropriate contraception. Am Fam Physician 1993; 48:1115.

Orife J. Benefits and risks of oral contraceptives. Adv Contracept 1990; 6(suppl):15.

Wall DM, Roos MP. Update on combination oral contraceptives. Am Fam Physician 1990; 42:1037.

Patient monitoring
(Cont'd from p 495)

Adjustments based on adverse effects

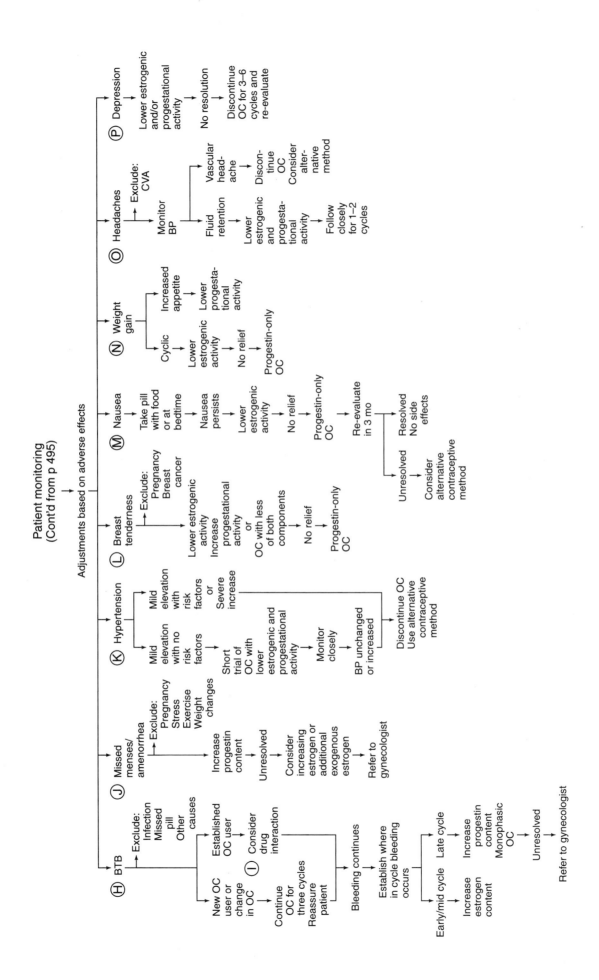

FEMALE INFERTILITY

Lorna A. Marshall

Infertility is failure to conceive after 1 year of unprotected intercourse. It is a common problem, estimated to affect 8–15% of married couples. Even before a couple is considered infertile, counseling should include a discussion of the menstrual cycle and appropriate timing of intercourse. In general, intercourse should occur about every 36–72 hours from 3–4 days before until 2 days after ovulation. It is important that sperm be available before ovulation. Ovulation usually occurs about 14 days before the subsequent menses or on about day 14 of a 28-day cycle. Encourage couples who wish to time intercourse more precisely to use prospective methods to detect ovulation such as home ovulation predictor kits that detect a surge in luteinizing hormone. Basal body temperature charts may identify the day of ovulation retrospectively, so they are not as useful in timing intercourse.

Considerable controversy remains about what constitutes a basic and complete fertility evaluation. Cost-effectiveness is an important part of the decision-making process because many insurance plans cover little or none of the evaluation and treatment of infertility. The current trend is to minimize testing and to move more quickly through a treatment plan. For example, laparoscopy was once a standard part of a fertility evaluation; now its considerable expense is often avoided in favor of using resources for treatments such as reproductive technologies. Often it is more cost-effective to refer the patient to a specialist before expensive testing is performed, so that the remainder of the evaluation can be integrated into the overall treatment plan.

A. The couple should be present for the initial fertility evaluation. Take a complete reproductive history of the female partner, including past and current menstrual pattern, contraceptive use, STDs, prior pregnancies, pelvic pain or dysmenorrhea, in utero exposure to diethylstilbestrol, and past gynecologic procedures. Review medical and family histories, use of medications, and coital pattern.

B. A complete physical examination includes body habitus, abnormal hair growth patterns, a careful thyroid examination, and exclusion of galactorrhea. Perform careful pelvic examination, ruling out pelvic masses. Tender nodularity in the posterior cul de sac or a fixed uterus suggests endometriosis.

C. Advanced age of the female partner (>35 years) is a strong risk factor for infertility. Initiate an evaluation after 6 months of unprotected intercourse and proceed more quickly than in younger women. Obtain a cycle day 3 follicle-stimulating hormone (FSH) level to provide information on the success of various therapies, and quickly perform a basic evaluation. Consider an early referral to a specialist. Many women >40 years old and those with elevated FSH levels may conceive only with eggs donated from younger women.

D. Ovulation may be evaluated in many ways. If the menstrual interval is >35 days, anovulation is likely. Obtain thyroid-stimulating hormone (TSH), FSH, and prolactin levels, and initiate treatment with clomiphene citrate. In women with normal menses, ovulation is likely if two to three cycles of basal body temperature charts are biphasic or if a luteinizing hormone (LH) surge is detected. A temperature elevation should be maintained for 11 days or longer. Ovulation can be confirmed with a midluteal (usually day 21) progesterone level of >5 ng/ml. Use other laboratory tests sparingly; many clinicians measure TSH and prolactin levels on all infertile women, regardless of ovulatory status. Serial ultrasound studies of ovulation add considerable expense and usually little information to a basic evaluation. A timed endometrial biopsy will document normal ovulation but adds expense and rarely influences decision making.

E. In general, a day 3 FSH level of >15 mIU/ml and estradiol >50 pg/ml predict a very low success rate with reproductive technologies, and probably with most other fertility treatments. These values may vary considerably between laboratories.

F. If the female partner is anovulatory or oligomenorrheic and laboratory test results are normal, clomiphene citrate may be prescribed for up to three ovulatory

(Continued on page 500)

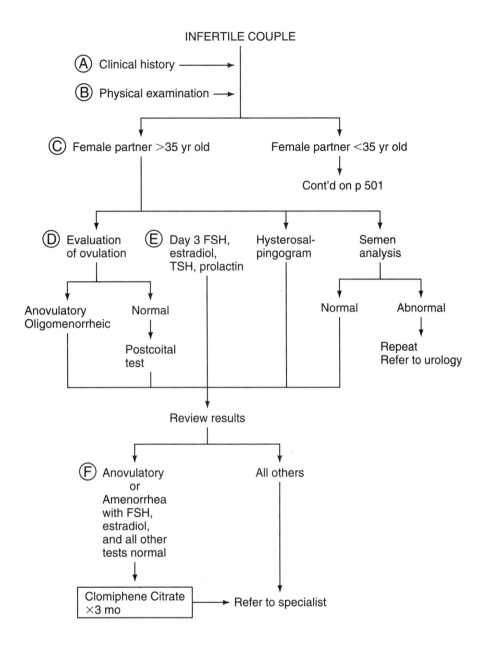

INFERTILE COUPLE

(A) Clinical history ⟶

(B) Physical examination ⟶

(C) Female partner >35 yr old   Female partner <35 yr old

Cont'd on p 501

(D) Evaluation of ovulation   (E) Day 3 FSH, estradiol, TSH, prolactin   Hysterosal-pingogram   Semen analysis

Anovulatory Oligomenorrheic   Normal   Normal   Abnormal

Postcoital test   Repeat Refer to urology

Review results

(F) Anovulatory or Amenorrhea with FSH, estradiol, and all other tests normal   All others

Clomiphene Citrate ×3 mo ⟶ Refer to specialist

cycles. After a spontaneous or progestin-induced menstrual cycle, the starting dosage is 50 mg for 5 days, starting on day 3, 4, or 5 of the cycle. Use basal body temperature charts to monitor ovulation. The dosage may be increased to 100 mg if anovulation persists, if basal body temperature rises after day 20, or if the luteal phase is <11 days. Of patients who will conceive, 80% do so within the first three ovulatory cycles.

References

Glatzstein IZ, Harlow BL, Hornstein MD. Practice patterns among reproductive endocrinologists: the infertility evaluation. Fertil Steril 1997; 67:443.

Jaffe SB, Jewelewicz R. The basic infertility investigation. Fertil Steril 1991; 56:599.

Marshall L. Infertility. In: Lemcke DP, Pattison J, Marshall LA, Cowley DS, eds. Primary care of women. Norwalk, CT: Appleton & Lange, 1995:499.

Speroff L, Glass RH, Kase NG. Clinical gynecologic endocrinology and infertility. 5th ed. Baltimore: Williams & Wilkins, 1994:809.

Toner JP, Hilput CB, Jones GS, Muasher SJ. Basal follicle-stimulating hormone level is a better predictor of in vitro fertilization performance than age. Fertil Steril 1991; 55:784.

Wilcox AJ, Weinberg CR, Baird DD. Timing of sexual intercourse in relation to ovulation: effects on the probability of conception, survival of the pregnancy, and sex of the baby. N Engl J Med 1995; 338:1517.

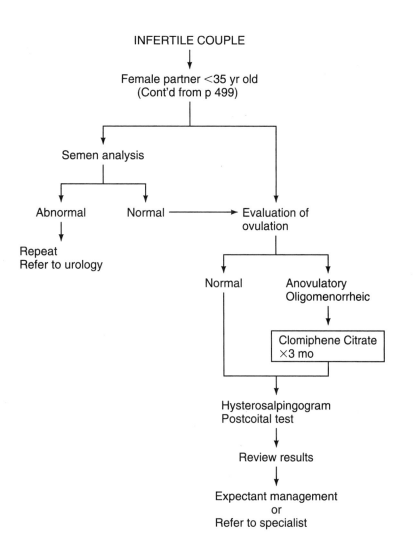

INFERTILE COUPLE

Female partner <35 yr old
(Cont'd from p 499)

Semen analysis

Abnormal

Normal

Repeat
Refer to urology

Evaluation of
ovulation

Normal

Anovulatory
Oligomenorrheic

Clomiphene Citrate
×3 mo

Hysterosalpingogram
Postcoital test

Review results

Expectant management
or
Refer to specialist

DOMESTIC VIOLENCE

Elaine J. Alpert

Domestic violence (DV) is a pattern of assaultive and coercive behaviors used in the context of dating or intimate relationships. This recently recognized problem in medicine affects 8–12% of American women per year, with lifetime prevalence approaching 30%. One in nine women seen for emergency care for any stated reason is actually there because of the acute or chronic effects of DV, and >50% of all women who seek emergency care have, at some time in their lives, been victims of DV. Fully one third of all women who visit emergency facilities for trauma are there for treatment of injuries caused by DV.

The spectrum of DV includes physical injury, sexual assault, social isolation, verbal abuse, threats, humiliation, economic deprivation, and restriction of access to transportation and other resources. DV has devastating short- and long-term effects on the life, health, and functioning of victims, their children, and other dependents. Of abused persons, 95% are adolescent or adult women in heterosexual relationships; however, DV also occurs in same-sex relationships and, in a small proportion of cases, by women perpetrators against male victims. Although women who are young, poor, and unmarried are most likely to experience DV, the condition affects every age, income level, and geographic area. Rates of DV are consistent across racial and ethnic categories when age, income, and education are controlled for.

Physicians in every specialty and practice setting have patients who are current, former, or potential victims of abuse. Asking questions about the possibility of DV must be done in a compassionate, nonjudgmental manner, preserving the patient's privacy and focusing on safety and empowerment. All patients should be routinely screened for DV in emergency, primary care, and specialty settings. Because of the prevalence, varied presentation, and consequences of DV, core competence in screening, assessment, and intervention is now part of the standard of care for all practicing physicians.

A. Taking a careful history is key to diagnosis and the first step toward assessment and intervention. Ask every patient about current or former abuse at the first visit and periodically thereafter. Because of the high prevalence of DV in the emergency setting, every patient should be screened at every visit. Ask questions in a respectful, nonjudgmental manner. Direct questions usually are best. You can ask, "At any time (or, since I last saw you) has your partner (or ex-partner) hit, kicked, or otherwise hurt or frightened you?" Even if your patient is being abused, she may choose not to disclose this to you at this time. If your index of suspicion is high, it is acceptable to follow your initial screening question with, "When I see a patient with an injury (or illness) such as yours, often it is because someone has hurt her. Has someone been hurting you?" Follow-up questions are indicated if the patient discloses (see E).

B. A careful physical examination with a high index of suspicion is key in diagnosing DV. Physical injuries often are multiple, bilateral, and occur over time; thus they may be in different stages of healing at the time of your evaluation. The explanation given for trauma may be inconsistent with the injury pattern. If this is the case, use the follow-up question in A. Other suspicious findings include psychological distress (including suicide attempts and substance abuse) and evidence of sexual assault.

(Continued on page 504)

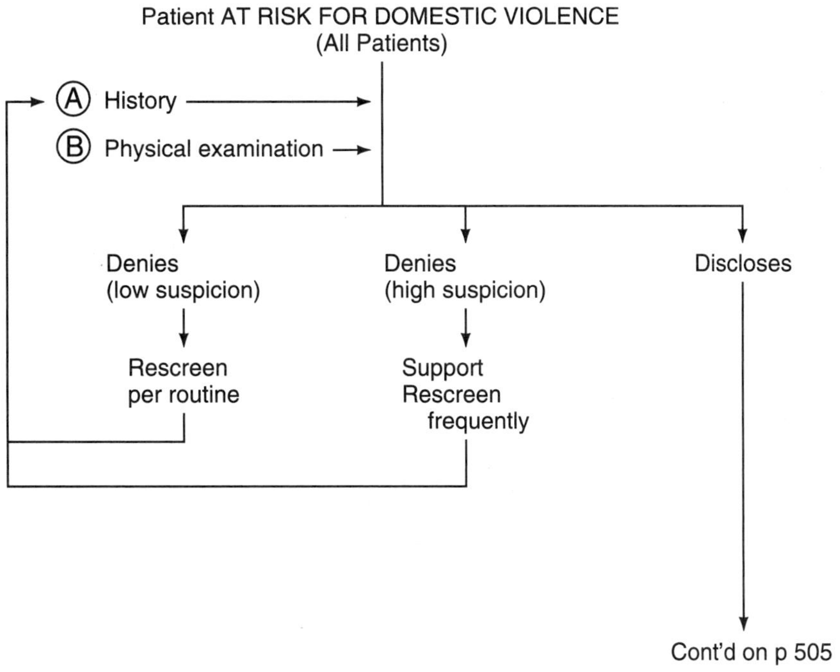

Patient AT RISK FOR DOMESTIC VIOLENCE
(All Patients)

(A) History ⟶

(B) Physical examination ⟶

Denies
(low suspicion)

Denies
(high suspicion)

Discloses

Rescreen
per routine

Support
Rescreen
frequently

Cont'd on p 505

C. Begin intervention as soon as the diagnosis of DV is established. It is crucial to validate and support the patient, who in all likelihood is fearful and ashamed. You can say, "I am glad you chose to share this difficult issue with me," "I am concerned for your safety and well-being," and "Help is available."

D. Careful documentation is key to appropriate care. Record the patient's statements without bias or judgment. After obtaining the patient's consent, sketch or photograph evidence of trauma and include it in the chart. Include the patient's face in at least one photo, as well as a notation of the exact date and time of the photo. Take follow-up photos if possible. Reporting requirements vary from state to state; thus all documentation should be undertaken with the patient's knowledge and consent and with the patient's immediate and long-term safety kept foremost in importance.

E. Risk assessment is also known as lethality assessment. Nationwide, approximately one third of all women murder victims whose assailant can be identified have been killed by a current or former intimate partner. Thus the patient's safety is the top priority in evaluation and intervention. Ask the patient, "Has your partner (or ex-partner) ever threatened or tried to kill you or your children?" "Do you feel you are in danger now?" "Is it safe for you to return home?" Indicators of potential lethality include an increase in the frequency or severity of the abuse, threats of homicide or suicide by the partner, the availability of a firearm, the abuser's knowledge of the victim's plan to leave or to get help, and a history of violent criminal behavior by the abuser.

F. Helping victims learn how to stay safe, defining and making accessible available resources, and providing options and referrals are the key interventions in DV. However, there is no medical magic to offer victims. Empowerment is key because disempowerment of victims is necessary for abusers to maintain the cycle of abuse. In addition to the validating and supporting statements suggested in C, convey to the patient that she deserves better and that the abuse is not her or his fault. Make the patient feel that choices and help are available. Offer information such as, "DV is common," "Physical violence is only one part of the spectrum of DV," "DV often increases in frequency and severity over time," and "Services for battered women include, in addition to shelter, support groups, community outreach, services for children, legal assistance, immigration assistance, and so on."

G. Necessary medical care, referrals, and follow-up can be provided in the office setting using posters, pamphlets, and a trusted office staff member or consultant (e.g., from social work or the local sheltering organization) to ensure follow-up for safety-related issues. Medical follow-up is also indicated to ensure improving physical and psychological health.

H. Initiate safety planning for every patient who is a victim of DV. Make the plan in concert with the patient according to the individual's resources and needs. Components of a safety plan include (1) a "crisis" plan to be followed in case of emergency, (2) identification of a safe place to go and a way to get there, and (3) logistical issues concerning finances, children, and housing. Life decisions should be made by the victim of DV. Physicians should provide information, support, resources, and follow-up, but they should not tell the patient what to do. The victim knows best what needs to take place to stay alive. The decision may be to remain in the house with the abuser still present, to remain in the house and obtain police or judicial assistance to have the abuser vacate the house, or to leave entirely, to a known or an undisclosed location. Regardless of the immediate decisions, the victim's situation will evolve over time, as will the readiness to change the situation and safety plan.

References

Abbott J, Johnson R, Koziol-McLain J, Lowenstein JR. Domestic violence against women: incidence and prevalence in an emergency department population. JAMA 1995; 273:1763.

Alpert EJ. Violence in intimate relationships and the practicing internist: new "disease" or new agenda? Ann Intern Med 1994; 123:774.

Bachman R, Saltzman L. Violence against women: estimates from the redesigned survey. Washington, DC: US Department of Justice, Office of Justice Programs, Bureau of Justice Statistics. NCJ-154348, August 1995.

Flitcraft A, Hadley S, et al. Diagnostic and treatment guidelines on domestic violence. Chicago: American Medical Association, 1992.

Ganley A. Understanding domestic violence. In: Ganley A, Warshaw C, Salber P, eds. Improving the health care response to domestic violence: a resource manual for health care providers. San Francisco: Family Violence Prevention Fund, 1995:15.

Wilt S, Olson S. Prevalence of domestic violence in the United States. J Am Med Women's Assoc 1996; 51:77.

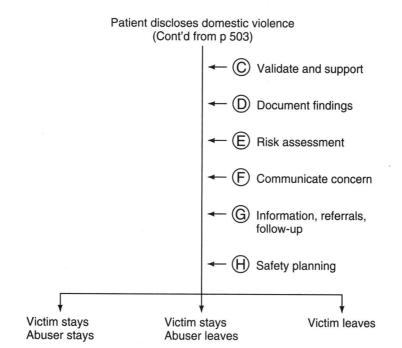

Patient discloses domestic violence
(Cont'd from p 503)

C Validate and support

D Document findings

E Risk assessment

F Communicate concern

G Information, referrals,
follow-up

H Safety planning

Victim stays
Abuser stays

Victim stays
Abuser leaves

Victim leaves

UROLOGY

ACUTE DYSURIA OR PYURIA IN MEN

Richard F. Hoffman

A. Dysuria is a sensation of discomfort with or after urination that often is accompanied by frequency, urgency, and nocturia. There are multiple causes, depending on the patient's age and sexual activity. Physical examination usually is unremarkable. Fever is uncommon but may be present in pyelonephritis, acute prostatitis, orchitis, or epididymitis. Inspect the genitals for evidence of urethral inflammation, discharge, and other penile lesions. Palpation may reveal swelling or tenderness of the testicles or epididymis and may elicit suprapubic or costovertebral tenderness. On rectal examination the prostate may be enlarged or tender or may have a palpable nodule.

B. A comprehensive sexual history is imperative. Sexual activity exposes a male to STDs, which are not a consideration in men who are sexually inactive or in a stable, monogamous relationship. Ask patients about the number and gender of partners, whether they consort with prostitutes, and whether they use condoms.

C. Microscopic examination of the urine is most commonly performed after the specimen is centrifuged for 5 minutes at 2000 rpm. The normal upper limits of WBCs per high-power field (hpf) is 5–10. The most widely accepted normal upper limit for RBCs is 3/hpf.

D. The most worrisome cause of dysuria and hematuria is urologic cancer, especially bladder cancer. Men >40 years old, tobacco users, analgesic abusers, those with a history of pelvic irradiation or cyclophosphamide chemotherapy, and men who work with dyestuffs and rubber compounds are at increased risk for malignancy. Other considerations are bladder calculi, which usually occur in the setting of benign prostatic hypertrophy (BPH), as well as BPH itself. Cystoscopy has a sensitivity of 87% in diagnosing bladder cancer and may directly visualize stones and confirm BPH. At the Mayo Clinic, urine cytology had a sensitivity of 67% and specificity of 96% in detecting bladder cancer.

E. When pyuria is present, perform culture and sensitivity tests. First-void specimens and clean-catch midstream voided specimens are equally sensitive for the detection of bacteruria. In men the growth of a single or predominant organism $\geq 10^3$ colony forming units (CFU)/ml indicates an infection; growth of $< 10^3$ CFU/ml or multiple organisms indicates contamination. Gram-negative bacilli, including *Escherichia coli, Proteus,* and *Providencia* species, cause about 75% of infections. Gram-positive bacteria, mainly enterococci and coagulase-negative staphylococci, cause most of the remaining infection. The presence of a urinary tract infection (UTI) in men has been assumed to warrant investigation for a structural abnormality of the urinary tract. Abnormalities often are found but usually do not alter treatment. The need for a diagnostic work-up in men with a first UTI has not been studied. Repeated infections or failure to respond to treatment requires further investigation. Sterile pyuria may be present in nephrolithiasis or urologic neoplasms and must be excluded. First morning urine cultures for acid-fast bacilli repeated three times are positive in 90% of men with renal tuberculosis.

F. The yield of a urethral smear depends on the timing of the collection. Highest yield is obtained by examining a smear collected early in the morning before micturition. Micturition decreases the number of WBCs seen on the smear. Obtain a smear by inserting a urethral swab 1–2 cm into the distal urethra and rotating it. If no discharge is apparent, stripping of the urethra or prostatic massage may produce a discharge. The urethral swab is smeared on a slide, heat fixed, and Gram-stained. A urethral smear in a symptomatic male showing gram-negative intracellular diplococci (GNID) has 98% sensitivity and 99% specificity in diagnosing gonococcal urethritis when compared with a single culture on Thayer-Martin media. Most patients with nongonococcal urethritis (NGU) have leukocytes on urethral smear (4 WBC/hpf), but 16–46% with culture-proved urethritis have <4 WBC/hpf.

G. In a recent national survey, 21% of gonococcal isolates showed resistance to penicillin, tetracycline, cefoxitin, and/or spectinomycin. All isolates were sensitive to ceftriaxone. Ceftriaxone, 125 mg IM, is recommended for all presumed cases of gonorrhea. Oral alternatives are cefixime 400 mg, ciprofloxacin 500 mg, or ofloxacin 400 mg one dose. Because up to 40% of patients with gonorrhea have a concomitant chlamydial infection, they should also be treated with azithromycin 1 g orally once or doxycycline 100 mg bid for 1 week.

H. The most common causes of acute NGU are *Chlamydia trachomatis* and *Ureaplasma urealyticum.* Bowie estimated that *C. trachomatis* causes 30–40% of acute cases and *U. urealyticum,* 15–25%. The role of *U. urealyticum* in urethritis is controversial because the organism has often been isolated from the urethra of asymptomatic men. Some authors consider that this represents colonization. *C. trachomatis* may be grown in tissue culture. It also can be diagnosed by tests using direct fluorescence antibody, enzyme linked immunoassay, and nucleic hybridization. *U. urealyticum* also may be grown on tissue culture. Both *C. trachomatis* and *U. urealyticum* can be treated with azithromycin, 1 g orally once, or doxycycline, 100 mg bid for 7 days. Tetracycline, 500 mg qid for 1 week, remains the cheapest regimen, but noncompliance is common be-

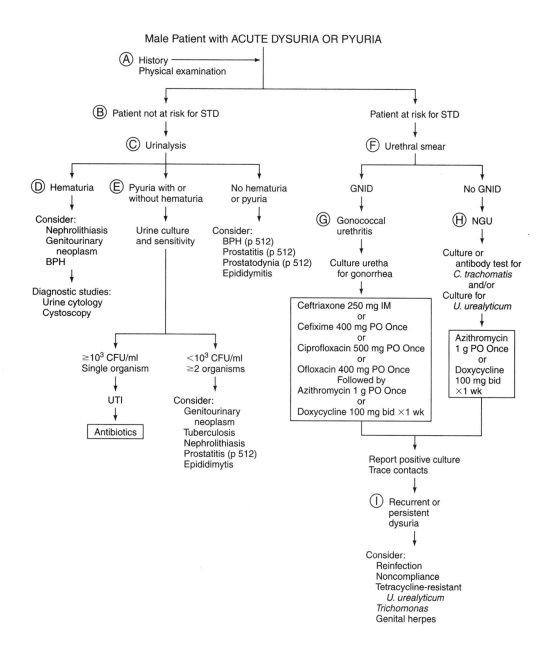

Male Patient with ACUTE DYSURIA OR PYURIA

(A) History — Physical examination

(B) Patient not at risk for STD

(C) Urinalysis

(D) Hematuria

Consider:
Nephrolithiasis
Genitourinary
neoplasm
BPH

Diagnostic studies:
Urine cytology
Cystoscopy

(E) Pyuria with or without hematuria

Urine culture and sensitivity

No hematuria or pyuria

Consider:
BPH (p 512)
Prostatitis (p 512)
Prostatodynia (p 512)
Epididymitis

$\geq 10^3$ CFU/ml Single organism

UTI

Antibiotics

$<10^3$ CFU/ml ≥ 2 organisms

Consider:
Genitourinary
neoplasm
Tuberculosis
Nephrolithiasis
Prostatitis (p 512)
Epididimytis

Patient at risk for STD

(F) Urethral smear

GNID

(G) Gonococcal urethritis

Culture uretha for gonorrhea

Ceftriaxone 250 mg IM
or
Cefixime 400 mg PO Once
or
Ciprofloxacin 500 mg PO Once
or
Ofloxacin 400 mg PO Once
Followed by
Azithromycin 1 g PO Once
or
Doxycycline 100 mg bid ×1 wk

No GNID

(H) NGU

Culture or antibody test for
C. trachomatis
and/or
Culture for
U. urealyticum

Azithromycin 1 g PO Once
or
Doxycycline 100 mg bid ×1 wk

Report positive culture
Trace contacts

(I) Recurrent or persistent dysuria

Consider:
Reinfection
Noncompliance
Tetracycline-resistant
U. urealyticum
Trichomonas
Genital herpes

cause of the need to avoid dairy products and calcium containing antacids and because of the frequency of dosing.

I. Reinfection from an untreated or new partner should be the first consideration. Noncompliance with treatment also is possible, especially in those treated with tetracycline regimens. *U. urealyticum* resistance to tetracycline has been reported, so patients may be given a 10-21-day course of erythromycin, 500 mg qid. *Trichomonas vaginalis* may cause urethritis in sexually active men. The diagnosis may be confirmed by microscopic examination of a urethral swab or by culture. Metronidazole is the drug of choice, and treatment of the sexual partner is important. Herpes simplex virus types 1 and 2 may cause urethritis, usually accompanied by external lesions on the genitalia. Herpes simplex may be isolated in tissue culture. Many other organisms may have a pathogenic role in NGU, including human papillomaviruses, *Mycoplasma hominis, Mycoplasma genitalium,*

and *Neisseria meningitidis.* In at least 20–30% of cases of NGU, no organism can be identified.

References

Bowie WR. Urethritis in males. In: Holmes KK, Mardh P-A, Sparling PF, Wiesner PJ, eds. Sexually transmitted diseases. 2nd ed. New York: McGraw-Hill, 1990:627.

Drugs for sexually transmitted diseases. Med Lett 1995; 37:117.

Hatton J. Management of bacterial urinary tract infections in adults. Ann Pharmacother 1994; 28:1264.

Lipsky BA. Urinary tract infections in men. Ann Intern Med 1989; 110:138.

Schwarcz SK. National surveillance of antimicrobial resistance in *Neisseria gonorrhoeae.* JAMA 1990; 264:1413.

Stamm WE. Azithromycin for empirical treatment of the nongonococcal urethritis syndrome in men. JAMA 1995; 274:545.

Sutton JM. Evaluation of hematuria in adults. JAMA 1990; 263:2475.

SCROTAL MASS

William P. Johnson

A. Palpation of an abnormal mass within the scrotal cavity often occurs during a careful examination of the male external genitalia. The importance of this finding depends on the establishment of an accurate diagnosis. Often, an accurate history and physical examination are all that are required to establish a diagnosis and determine subsequent management. The presence or absence of pain must be elicited. Ask the patient how long he has been aware of the mass, change in size, previous operative procedures, and the presence or absence of dysuria. During the physical examination the size, location, and consistency of the mass are precisely documented. Examine the patient in both the supine and erect positions. Finally, the examination must include transillumination of the scrotal mass, as nearly all benign conditions transilluminate easily; the notable benign exceptions are hematocele and varicocele. A urinalysis is routinely obtained looking for evidence of bacteriuria and pyuria. When the cause of the lesion remains in doubt, scrotal ultrasonography has proved an effective means of differentiation of intrascrotal masses.

B. In patients with a history of scrotal trauma, suspect a ruptured testicle. Remember that the degree of the traumatic blow must correlate with the extent of the injury. Testicular neoplasms are more prone to rupture and should be suspected in any patient who has a large scrotal mass after minimal trauma.

C. A painful scrotal mass usually is caused by an inflammatory process, but also consider testicular torsion or malignancy. Scrotal ultrasonography is a useful diagnostic tool in differentiating the above conditions.

D. Acute and chronic epididymitis are both extremely common clinical entities in adult males. The clinical presentation may range from an exquisitely tender scrotal mass (acute) to a low-grade process that the patient is barely aware of (chronic). In adults <40 years of age, *Chlamydia trachomatis* often is the initiating organism; in older men, gram-negative bacteria are the likely cause. Follow-up examination ensures that an underlying testicular tumor is not present after the acute inflammatory process subsides.

E. Testicular neoplasms are the most common solid tumor in males 20–39 years old. These patients usually have a mass within the substance of the testis. The masses usually are smooth or nodular, rock hard, and painless; they do not transilluminate. They often enlarge rapidly.

F. A hydrocele is the most common benign scrotal mass. It is of varying size and is located ventral, superior, and anterior to the testicle. It is nontender and transilluminates easily. It may be congenital or acquired. Because 10% of testicular tumors are associated with a hydrocele, perform aspiration or obtain scrotal ultrasound if the testicle is not palpable.

G. Primary tumors arising from the epididymis are rare and usually benign, adenomatoid tumors being the most common. A spermatocele is a cystic mass containing sperm that arises as a small diverticulum from the head of the epididymis.

H. Scrotal varicoceles are common (10–15% of the normal male population). This scrotal mass represents a dilated pampiniform plexus of the spermatic cord. It is usually asymptomatic but may reach a large size, resulting in a "dragging" or heavy sensation in the scrotum.

Reference

Blute RD Jr. Scrotal masses. In: Greene HL, ed. Clinical medicine. St Louis: Mosby, 1996:947.

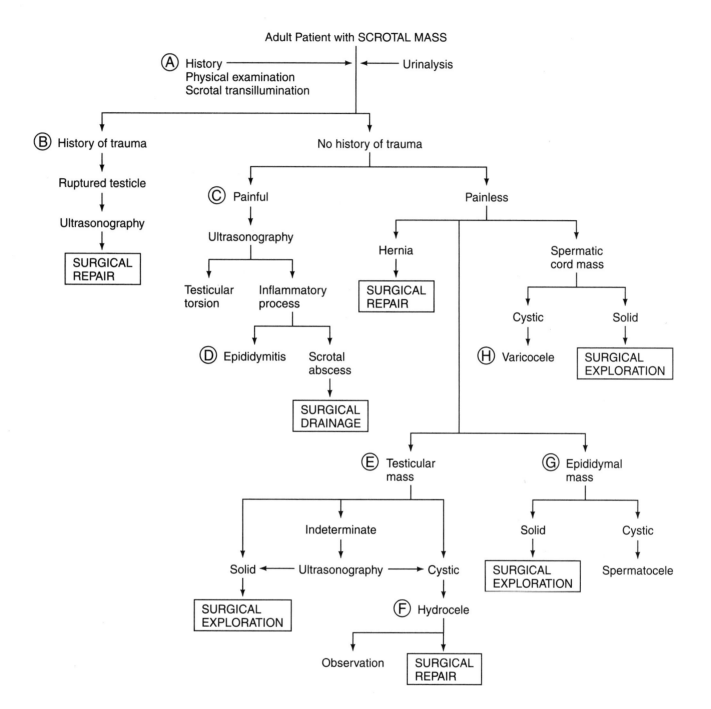

Adult Patient with SCROTAL MASS

Ⓐ History ——————→ ←—— Urinalysis
Physical examination
Scrotal transillumination

Ⓑ History of trauma   No history of trauma

Ruptured testicle   Ⓒ Painful   Painless

Ultrasonography   Ultrasonography   Hernia   Spermatic
                                                                                        cord mass
SURGICAL   Testicular   Inflammatory   SURGICAL   Cystic   Solid
REPAIR   torsion   process   REPAIR
                                                                    Ⓗ Varicocele   SURGICAL
                            Ⓓ Epididymitis   Scrotal   EXPLORATION
                                              abscess

                                              SURGICAL
                                              DRAINAGE

                        Ⓔ Testicular   Ⓖ Epididymal
                          mass   mass

                    Solid   Indeterminate   Cystic   Solid   Cystic

        SURGICAL   Solid ←— Ultrasonography —→ Cystic   SURGICAL   Spermatocele
        EXPLORATION   EXPLORATION

                    SURGICAL   Ⓕ Hydrocele
                    EXPLORATION

                                    Observation   SURGICAL
                                                   REPAIR

PROSTATE NODULE OR ENLARGEMENT

Jeffrey I. Miller
George W. Drach

Digital rectal examination to assess the size, shape, and texture of the prostate gland should be a part of every general physical examination. The normal prostate feels smooth and rubbery on palpation. Any firmness, nodularity, or induration should be considered abnormal. Anatomically, the gland is wider at its "base," near the bladder neck. The lateral sulci and the median furrow should be well defined. Note any irregularity of these landmarks. Assessment of prostatic size may be difficult: The normal average prostate triangle is about 4 cm on each side. Most men >50 years old have some degree of benign enlargement. As enlargement occurs, the lateral sulci become deeper and the gland becomes more prominent to rectal palpation. Benign enlargement becomes clinically significant in the presence of symptoms suggesting bladder outlet obstruction. If clinically significant benign prostatic hyperplasia (BPH) or a prostate nodule is detected, initiate the appropriate evaluation before urologic consultation.

A. Detection of a smooth, symmetrically enlarged prostate should prompt a thorough inquiry into symptoms suggestive of bladder outlet obstruction. Irritative symptoms include dysuria, frequency, urgency, and nocturia. Obstructive symptoms include hesitancy, straining, decreased force and caliber of the urinary stream, a sense of incomplete emptying, and stream interruption. Patients without significant symptoms are reassured and no further work-up is indicated. Patients with complete urinary retention should be catheterized and referred directly to a urologist. Remove obvious sources of retention (e.g., α-adrenergic agonists, antihistamines, anticholinergics) if possible.

B. Prostate-specific antigen (PSA) is a protein found only in prostatic epithelial cells. Serum levels can be elevated in a variety of prostatic disorders, including prostatitis, BPH, and prostate adenocarcinoma. Its usefulness in screening for prostate cancer in asymptomatic men has not been determined. PSA is not required for the evaluation and treatment of BPH. However, many investigators agree that a serum PSA level should be obtained in men with clinically significant symptoms suggestive of bladder outlet obstruction. Levels >4 ng/ml (Hybritech assay) suggest adenocarcinoma; however, a very large or infected benign gland may also produce elevated serum levels. Ideally, serum PSA levels should be drawn before or several weeks after prostatic manipulation (e.g., bladder catheterization) to avoid falsely elevated levels. A gentle rectal examination probably does not significantly influence serum levels.

C. A properly collected urinalysis and urine culture are crucial for detecting associated microhematuria and infection. The source of isolated microscopic hematuria may be an enlarged prostate. However, intravenous pyelography (IVP) is necessary to rule out upper tract disorders, including calculi or tumor. Even when IVP is normal, cystoscopic examination by a urologist is still required to exclude a bladder tumor or stone as the source of microhematuria. In the absence of microhematuria, IVP generally is not recommended.

D. Urinary tract infection in the older male should not simply be treated and dismissed. Residual urine may be the main contributor to infection, especially in someone with an enlarged prostate and symptoms suggestive of BPH. When there is high residual urine volume (>200–300 ml), leave a Foley catheter in place to help drain the infection. Obtain urologic consultation.

E. An elevated serum creatinine level may be the first indication of renal failure secondary to bladder outlet obstruction. Urinary symptoms may not be severe and patients often continue to void by overflow. Bilateral hydronephrosis on ultrasonography suggests bladder outlet obstruction as the source of the renal insufficiency. Residual urine volume is almost always elevated. Place a Foley catheter to decompress the bladder and upper tracts. The patient may need to be monitored for pathologic postobstructive diuresis, depending on the duration and severity of obstruction. Obtain a repeat serum creatinine level before urologic consultation.

F. The urologist rules out other causes of bladder outlet obstruction (e.g., urethral stricture, bladder tumor, neurogenic bladder) that may be contributing to the symptoms. A typical evaluation at this point might include urinary flow rate and office cystoscopy to assess the degree of apparent internal urethral obstruction. If the symptoms and physical examination suggest a neurogenic component, a urodynamic evaluation is indicated. When the patient desires treatment and the urologist is confident that the voiding symptoms are primarily related to BPH, he is offered a group of therapeutic options. These include standard transurethral resection of the prostate, transurethral prostatic incision for small prostates, open prostatic enucleation (for very large prostates), medical treatment with α-adrenergic blockers, 5α reductase inhibitors or, in rare instances, androgen ablation. Other options include prostatic hyperthermia or laser ablation to decrease prostatic size.

G. If a prostate nodule is palpated or there is induration of the gland on digital rectal examination, referral to a urologist is indicated. Obtain a serum PSA before referral; however, the result will have no bearing on the subsequent evaluation because normal PSA and prostatic carcinoma may coexist. There is no accurate means of detecting prostate adenocarcinoma other than by needle biopsy.

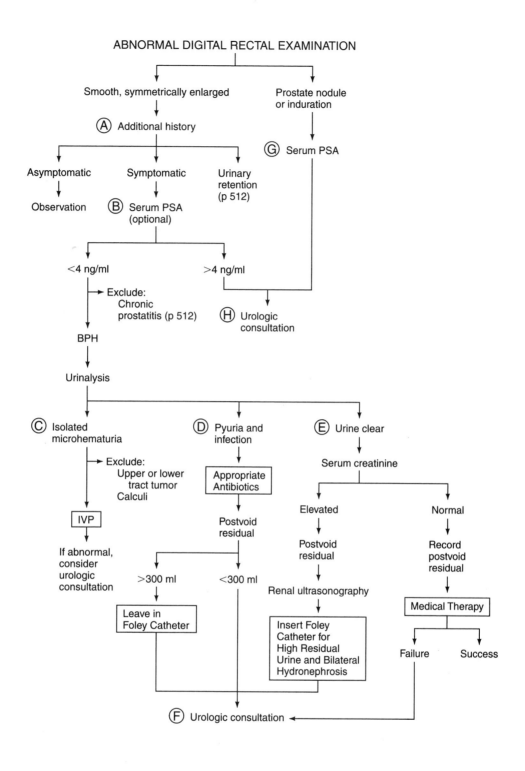

ABNORMAL DIGITAL RECTAL EXAMINATION

Smooth, symmetrically enlarged → (A) Additional history

Prostate nodule or induration → (G) Serum PSA

Additional history branches:
- Asymptomatic → Observation
- Symptomatic → (B) Serum PSA (optional)
- Urinary retention (p 512)

Serum PSA (optional):
- <4 ng/ml → Exclude: Chronic prostatitis (p 512) → BPH → Urinalysis
- >4 ng/ml → (H) Urologic consultation

Urinalysis branches:
- (C) Isolated microhematuria → Exclude: Upper or lower tract tumor / Calculi → IVP → If abnormal, consider urologic consultation
- (D) Pyuria and infection → Appropriate Antibiotics → Postvoid residual
  - >300 ml → Leave in Foley Catheter
  - <300 ml
- (E) Urine clear → Serum creatinine
  - Elevated → Postvoid residual → Renal ultrasonography → Insert Foley Catheter for High Residual Urine and Bilateral Hydronephrosis
  - Normal → Record postvoid residual → Medical Therapy
    - Failure
    - Success

(F) Urologic consultation

H. Perform a biopsy on all prostate nodules regardless of the serum PSA level or clinical symptoms. The urologist usually performs the biopsy under ultrasound guidance. A thin needle is passed transrectally or transperineally to obtain a small core of tissue for histologic analysis. Correct any bleeding diathesis or coagulopathy before prostate biopsy. In addition, give patients at risk for subacute bacterial endocarditis prophylactic antibiotics before and after the procedure.

References

Agency for Health Care Policy Research: BPH Clinical Practice Guidelines. AHCPR Pub. No. 94-0582: February 1994. (AHCPR Website: http://www.ahcpr.gov)

Coley CM, Barry MJ, Fleming C, et al. Early detection of prostate cancer. Part I: prior probability and effectiveness of tests. Ann Intern Med 1997; 126:394.

Hollander JB, Diokno AC. Prostatism: benign prostatic hyperplasia. Urol Clin North Am 1996; 23:75.

PROSTATITIS

Jeffrey I. Miller
George W. Drach

Prostatitis refers to a series of inflammatory diseases of differing causes affecting the prostate gland. It may be difficult to define a specific cause. Treatment is not always curative, and recurrence is common. Patients may be assigned to one of four prostatitis syndromes: acute or chronic bacterial prostatitis, nonbacterial prostatitis, or prostatodynia. The workup and treatment for each syndrome is different.

A. Acute bacterial prostatitis is a potentially serious process that can result in septicemia or abscess formation. Patients usually have acute onset of dysuria and irritative voiding symptoms. Obstructive voiding symptoms may occur. Low back pain, perineal discomfort, fever, chills, and malaise often are present. Patients with a chronic prostatitis syndrome have low-grade irritative voiding symptoms, ill-defined pelvic or perineal discomfort, and/or pain associated with ejaculation. They are not acutely ill. The hallmark of chronic bacterial prostatitis is a history of relapsing urinary tract infection.

B. Bacteriuria is always present in acute bacterial prostatitis; enteric pathogens usually are responsible. A culture before antibiotic treatment is mandatory.

C. Gentle rectal examination confirms the diagnosis of acute bacterial prostatitis. The prostate feels enlarged and edematous and is very tender. Never perform digital massage to obtain fluid for analysis in this situation, or bacteremia and septicemia may result.

D. In acute bacterial prostatitis the barrier to drug infusion into the prostate is not as prominent as in the chronically inflamed state. Therefore one may select any antibiotic to which the causative organism is sensitive and expect a favorable effect. Serial gentle rectal examinations, CT, or transrectal ultrasound imaging can rule out prostatic abscess (which requires surgical drainage). Suspect abscess when antibiotic treatment is unsuccessful. Urinary retention, caused by prostatic edema, may require urethral or suprapubic catheter drainage of the bladder. Hospitalization is commonly indicated. Continue antibiotic therapy for 4–6 weeks.

E. The urine culture usually is negative in chronic prostatitis. However, if present, bacteriuria should be treated first with a short course of an antibiotic that does not cross the blood-prostate barrier. Best drugs are nitrofurantoin, penicillin, or a cephalosporin. Bacterial cystitis treated in this way will not interfere with subsequent localizing studies to determine the cause of the prostatitis.

F. The prostate usually is normal to palpation in chronic prostatitis. Consider prostate carcinoma, however, if there is a nodule, induration, or asymmetry. Never attribute prostatic induration to chronic inflammation until carcinoma is ruled out by biopsy.

G. Perform digital massage to obtain expressed prostatic secretions (EPS), which should be microscopically examined under high power. In general, more than ten leukocytes/hpf and more than one or two lipid-laden macrophages suggest prostatic inflammation.

H. In the presence of prostatic inflammation, culture the EPS. Isolation of bacteria from the EPS is necessary to establish a diagnosis of chronic bacterial prostatitis. This is the first screening test.

I. To be certain that the source of the bacteriuria is the prostate, obtain divided quantitative urine cultures. A first-voided specimen (VB1) identifies the urethral flora that can contaminate subsequent specimens. Obtain a midstream urine culture (VB2) to rule out coexisting bacterial cystitis. These cultures are quantitatively compared with that of the EPS. Bacteriuria is localized to the prostate when the EPS colony count is proportionately greater (by a factor of 10) than that of the VB1 and VB2.

J. In patients with chronic bacterial prostatitis, there is an intact barrier to perfusion of many antibiotics into the prostatic fluid or tissue. Effective prostatic antibiotics include trimethoprim, doxycycline, and carbenicillin. The quinolones achieve excellent therapeutic concentrations in the prostatic parenchyma and are effective in eradicating chronic bacterial prostatitis.

K. Patients with chronic nonbacterial prostatitis have an inflammatory EPS with negative cultures. Causative agents, such as *Mycoplasma* or *Chlamydia,* cannot easily be demonstrated by present techniques. Thus empiric treatment with long-acting doxycycline or minocycline is indicated. Trichomoniasis also should be ruled out.

L. Patients with prostatodynia have complaints of prostatic pain but there is no evidence of prostatic inflammation and no bacterial cause is found. Patients may have mild prostatic tenderness upon rectal examination and also a mild to moderate decrease in voiding flow rate. Treatment options include low-dose diazepam, 2 mg tid to qid; this drug is used more for its smooth muscle-relaxing effect than for tranquilization. Antispasmodics such as hyoscyamine sometimes decrease the intensity of symptoms. Some patients seem to respond to α-adrenergic blocking agents; warn them of the side effects, including dizziness, hypotension, and loss of ejaculation.

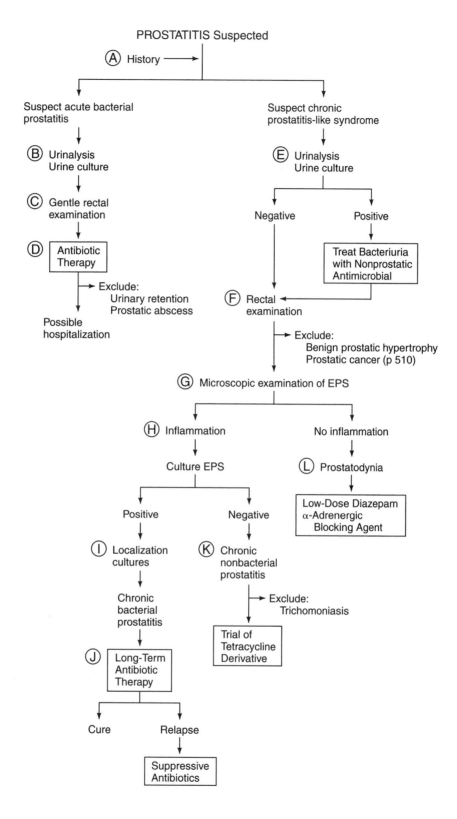

PROSTATITIS Suspected

(A) History

Suspect acute bacterial prostatitis

(B) Urinalysis
Urine culture

(C) Gentle rectal examination

(D) Antibiotic Therapy

→ Exclude:
Urinary retention
Prostatic abscess

Possible hospitalization

Suspect chronic prostatitis-like syndrome

(E) Urinalysis
Urine culture

Negative   Positive

Treat Bacteriuria with Nonprostatic Antimicrobial

(F) Rectal examination

→ Exclude:
Benign prostatic hypertrophy
Prostatic cancer (p 510)

(G) Microscopic examination of EPS

(H) Inflammation   No inflammation

Culture EPS   (L) Prostatodynia

Low-Dose Diazepam
α-Adrenergic
Blocking Agent

Positive   Negative

(I) Localization cultures

(K) Chronic nonbacterial prostatitis

Chronic bacterial prostatitis

→ Exclude: Trichomoniasis

(J) Long-Term Antibiotic Therapy

Trial of Tetracycline Derivative

Cure   Relapse

Suppressive Antibiotics

References

Drach GW, Mears EM Jr, Fair WR, et al. Classification of benign disease associated with prostatic pain: prostatitis or prostatodynia. J Urol 1978; 120:266.

Fowler JE Jr. Practical approach to bacteriologic investigation of chronic prostatitis. Urology 1985; 26:17.

Fowler JE Jr. Prostatitis. In: Gillenwater JY, Grayhack JT, Howards SS, Duckett JW, eds. Adult and pediatric urology. 3rd ed. St Louis: Mosby, 1991, 6:1715.

Moul JW. Prostatitis: sorting out the different causes. Postgrad Med 1993; 94:191.

URINARY INCONTINENCE

Hunter Wessells

Urinary incontinence is a major health care problem from both a clinical and an economic perspective. Billions of dollars are spent annually on managing incontinence. Increased public awareness and the aging of America necessitate a deeper understanding of the causes and treatments of incontinence.

Incontinence is the socially unacceptable loss of urine. The main categories of incontinence are stress (from increases in intra-abdominal pressure), urge (from uninhibited bladder contractions), reflex (from neurologic illness), functional, and overflow. Male and female incontinence are dissimilar in their pathophysiology and treatment. Common causes of male incontinence include benign prostatic hyperplasia (BPH), neurologic disease, and radical pelvic surgery. Female incontinence more commonly results from pelvic floor laxity, hormonal changes, and uninhibited bladder contractions associated with aging. A thorough urologic history and physical examination are of paramount importance in the initial evaluation of both male and female patients.

A. The initial evaluation of the incontinent female can be carried out in the ambulatory setting without extensive testing. A careful voiding history should address the nature of urinary leakage, onset, severity (number of pads or diapers used per day), frequency of accidents, association with physical activity, occurrence during daytime or overnight, and degree of inconvenience. Also note frequency, dysuria, straining, and nocturia. The use of a voiding diary can help document the frequency and timing of accidents and normal voiding. A sensation of vaginal fullness suggests prolapse. The history should focus on multiparity, obstetric trauma, gynecologic surgery, hormonal status, bowel function, and neurologic illnesses. Physical examination is key. Examination with the patient in the lithotomy position and a partially full bladder allows demonstration of urethral hypermobility and leakage with coughing (stress urinary incontinence). Note atrophic vaginal epithelium. Demonstration of anterior vaginal prolapse (cystocele) and posterior vaginal prolapse (rectocele) also is easy in this position. Perform urinalysis in all incontinent patients to exclude hematuria, which requires urologic evaluation with IVP and cystoscopy. Voided urine cytology is helpful in excluding carcinoma in situ of the bladder.

B. Detrusor instability in women increases in incidence with age. Women with suspected urge incontinence may be given a trial of antispasmodic drugs as long as hematuria has been excluded or evaluated. Bladder training to progressively increase the time between voids may allow the patient to suppress urge symptoms. Pharmacologic therapy may provide marked benefit in this population. Oxybutinin is the most commonly prescribed antispasmodic. An initial dosage of 2.5–5 mg bid or tid often improves the symptoms of urgency and urge incontinence. Dry mouth and constipation should be anticipated. Other agents may be better tolerated, but all agents in this class have similar anticholinergic side effects. Lack of improvement or presence of an underlying neuropathic process implies reflex incontinence. Consider neurologic evaluation to detect multiple sclerosis, spinal cord pathology, or disorders above the spinal cord; referral to a urologist for urodynamic evaluation and management of neurogenic bladder is indicated.

C. Stress incontinence may be anatomic (from hypermobility of the bladder neck and urethra) or less commonly a result of intrinsic sphincter deficiency (from prior operation, trauma, or loss of urethral vascularity after menopause). Most cases are anatomic: Change in bladder and urethral location as a result of pelvic floor laxity leads to incomplete compression and support of the urethra. Significant vaginal prolapse requires treatment with a pessary or surgery. In the absence of significant prolapse, a trial of conservative therapy is indicated. This would include pelvic floor (Kegel) exercises, hormone replacement in postmenopausal women, and pharmacologic therapy. α-Adrenergic agonists increase smooth muscle tone at the bladder neck and posterior urethra and may improve continence. Over-the-counter cold and diet preparations are effective and long acting. If an urge component exists, antispasmodics can be added. Imipramine, which has both anticholinergic and noradrenergic agonist properties, can be effective monotherapy in such situations (25 mg PO qhs). Newer modalities to treat stress incontinence include biofeedback programs and transvaginal electrical stimulation. Lack of improvement with conservative measures indicates a need for further urologic evaluation. Differentiation between anatomic stress incontinence and intrinsic sphincter deficiency is important in guiding appropriate surgical intervention. Correction of anatomic descensus by bladder neck suspension may cure anatomic stress incontinence, whereas intrinsic sphincter deficiency requires compression of the urethra.

D. Total incontinence is the continuous leakage of urine. If normal voiding also occurs, look for an ectopic ureteral orifice. Examination of the periurethral region may detect a steady drip of urine. IVP may detect abnormalities of the upper tracts suggestive of ureteral ectopia. Vesicovaginal fistulae from prior surgery or obstetric trauma may present with continuous leakage that prevents bladder filling. Urologic evaluation of such patients is mandatory.

(Continued on page 516)

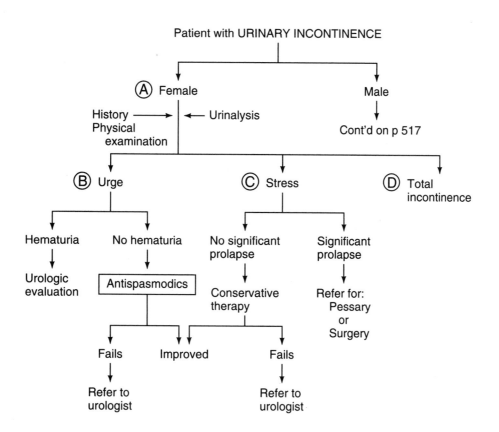

Patient with URINARY INCONTINENCE

Ⓐ Female

History
Physical
examination → ← Urinalysis

Male

Cont'd on p 517

Ⓑ Urge

Ⓒ Stress

Ⓓ Total
incontinence

Hematuria

No hematuria

No significant
prolapse

Significant
prolapse

Urologic
evaluation

Antispasmodics

Conservative
therapy

Refer for:
Pessary
or
Surgery

Fails

Improved

Fails

Refer to
urologist

Refer to
urologist

E. Evaluation of the incontinent male begins with a thorough voiding history. Frequency, urgency, decreased force of stream, nocturia, and the sensation of incomplete emptying suggest BPH but may be symptoms of other processes. The presence of diabetes mellitus, Parkinson's disease, multiple sclerosis, stroke, or spinal cord pathology indicates the need for a more in-depth evaluation. Surgical history may determine that radical pelvic surgery has led to stress incontinence. Over-the-counter and prescription medications may profoundly alter male micturition. Physical examination of the abdomen and genitalia will detect a distended bladder, abnormal perineal reflexes, or frank leakage of urine. Urinary retention may cause overflow incontinence and therefore a postvoid residual should be obtained (see prostate enlargement chapter, page 510). Bladder outlet obstruction may lead to bladder instability with urgency and urge incontinence. Urge symptoms in a male should be presumed to be caused by obstruction: Antispasmodics and anticholinergics are thus contraindicated before full urologic evaluation is done. Urinary tract infection or bladder carcinoma may cause urge incontinence; abnormal urinalysis findings should guide treatment. After retention and infection are ruled out, virtually all men with incontinence should be referred to a urologist.

References

Raz S, Sussman EM, Erickson DB, et al. The Raz bladder neck suspension: results in 206 patients. J Urol 1992; 148:845.

Resnick NM, Yalla SV. Management of urinary incontinence in the elderly. N Engl J Med 1985; 313:800.

Steers WD, Barrett DM, Wein AJ. Voiding dysfunction: diagnosis, classification, and management. In: Gillenwater JY, Grayhack JT, Howards SS, Duckett JW, eds. Adult and pediatric urology. St. Louis: Mosby, 1996:1220.

Stein M, Discippio W, Davia M, Taub H. Biofeedback for the treatment of stress and urge incontinence. J Urol 1995; 153:641.

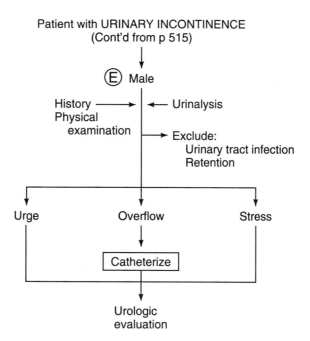

Patient with URINARY INCONTINENCE
(Cont'd from p 515)

Ⓔ Male

History ──────→ ←── Urinalysis
Physical
examination ──────→ Exclude:
                        Urinary tract infection
                        Retention

Urge   Overflow   Stress

Catheterize

Urologic
evaluation

MALE INFERTILITY

Hunter Wessells

Male factor infertility is involved in up to 50% of infertile couples. Evaluation should begin when the couple seeks advice. Potentially correctable causes of infertility can be identified with history, physical examination, laboratory studies, and semen analysis (SA). SA serves as a starting point in the initial evaluation. Significant changes in reproductive endocrinology within the last several years have dramatically altered the options available to couples with male factor infertility.

A. Semen is best collected by masturbation after 2–3 days of abstinence. Parameters reported in most laboratories include volume, sperm density, motility, morphology, and presence or absence of agglutination, pyospermia, or hyperviscosity. Treatment should not be based on a single SA; repeat studies at least 1 week apart are advised when the initial SA is abnormal. Normal parameters are listed in Table 1.

B. History and physical examination are important in the evaluation of the infertile male. Note history of prior paternity, frequency and technique of sexual intercourse, and use of contraceptives and lubricants. Review sexual development, puberty, and sexual history. History including chemotherapy, radiation, medications, exposure to industrial toxins, recent febrile illness, and smoking are all pertinent. Surgical history of herniorrhaphy, cryptorchidism, testicular cancer, and bladder neck or retroperitoneal surgery may indicate likely causes of infertility. Elicit use of medications, anabolic steroids, and recreational drugs. Physical examination includes evaluation of secondary sex characteristics, prior surgical incisions, presence of penile anomalies such as hypospadias, size and consistency of the testes, presence of a varicocele (in the standing position), presence of the vas deferens, and palpation of the prostate to detect prostatitis. Routine laboratory studies in the infertile male include serum testosterone, luteinizing hormone, and follicle-stimulating hormone (FSH) levels.

C. Azoospermia may be caused by congenital or acquired obstruction, ejaculatory dysfunction, or testicular failure. Retrograde ejaculation may lead to azoospermia. Presence of sperm in postejaculate urine implies retrograde ejaculation, which is treated by urinary alkalinization and collection. Azoospermia may be caused by obstruction of the ejaculatory duct, in which case the SA will have low volume. Transrectal ultrasonography can detect dilated ejaculatory ducts and seminal vesicles suggestive of obstruction. Normal volume azoospermia may be caused by obstruction or testicular failure. FSH levels three times normal indicate failure; biopsy is not indicated and adoption or artificial insemination donor (AID) is recommended. If FSH levels are less than three times normal, testis biopsy can confirm the presence of normal spermatogenesis. In the presence of normal spermatogenesis, surgical reconstruction is the most cost-effective method to attempt pregnancy. In certain instances sperm can be obtained from the epididymis or testis itself and used for intracytoplasmic sperm injection (ICSI); only one viable spermatozoon is required to attempt fertilization of each egg. Embryo transfer than allows implantation of the fertilized egg.

D. Oligoasthenospermia (low counts, abnormal motility, and/or abnormal morphology) has numerous causes. A varicocele is the most common correctable cause of male factor infertility and should be treated before institution of other therapies. Pregnancy is attained in 30–40% of couples after varicocelectomy. Abnormal clumping of sperm on the SA may suggest antisperm antibodies from vasectomy or trauma. Diagnosis of this entity can identify couples who may benefit from sperm processing and intrauterine insemination. Couples with oligospermia but >10 million motile sperm may be able to achieve pregnancy via intrauterine insemination. Finally, couples with no identifiable cause of oligoasthenospermia may choose to try ICSI.

E. Men with secondary hypogonadism may benefit from hormonal replacement. Primary hypogonadism is more difficult to treat because exogenous testosterone replacement may not adequately stimulate spermatogenesis. Oral clomiphene and human chorionic gonadotropin have been attempted with limited success.

References

Greenberg SH, Lipshultz LI, Wein AJ. Experience with 425 subfertile male patients. J Urol 1978; 119:507.

Howards SS. Treatment of male infertility. N Engl J Med 1995; 332:312.

Nagy Z, Liu J, Cecile J, et al. Using ejaculated, fresh, and frozen-thawed epididymal and testicular spermatozoa gives rise to comparable results after intracytoplasmic sperm injection. Fertil Steril 1995; 63:808.

Wessells H, Van Arsdalen KN. Surgery of male infertility. Part I: varicocelectomy, testis biopsy, and vasography. AUA UPDATE XIII, 1994, Lesson 10.

TABLE 1 Normal Parameters in Semen Analysis

Volume 1.5–5 ml (<2.0 abnormal)	Motility >60%
	Morphology >60% normal
Sperm density >20 million/ml	Total sperm 60–70 million

MALE INFERTILITY Suspected

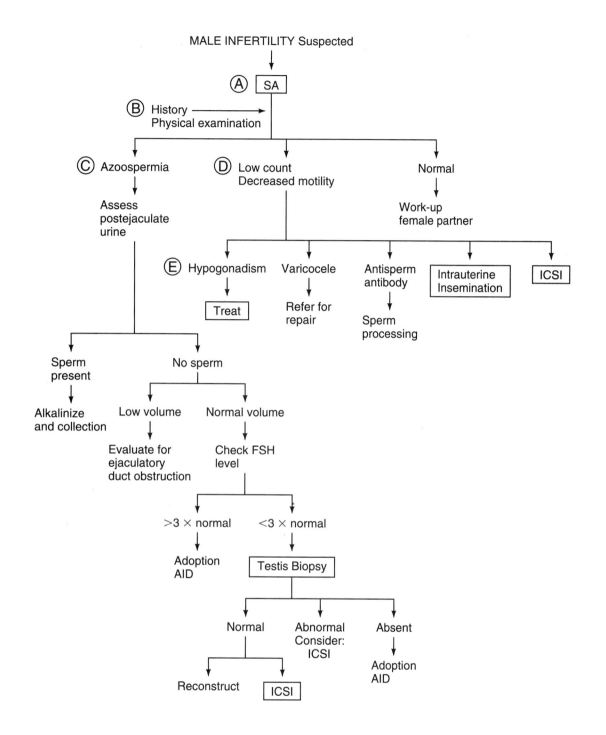

EMERGENCY MEDICINE

ACUTE PULSELESS EXTREMITY

Kenneth E. McIntyre, Jr.

A. The history and physical examination are of paramount importance. The onset is usually abrupt and may strike any time. Acute lower extremity ischemia may occur in patients with myocardial infarction, ventricular aneurysm, valvular heart disease, arrhythmia, or arterial occlusive disease. Inquire about the cardiac history. It is also important to establish whether previous vascular occlusive disease has been diagnosed or vascular reconstructive operations have been performed in the past.

B. Abrupt onset of severe unremitting pain is the classic symptom of acute ischemia. In patients with a known history of vascular occlusive disease of the lower extremities, pain may be less severe if there are abundant collaterals still open. Ischemic pain generally is not relieved by narcotics. There are no pulses below the level of obstruction, and the foot is generally white or pallorous.

C. The acute pulseless extremity may result from trauma that has injured an artery, thrombosis, or embolism. In patients who have previously undergone a vascular bypass operation, thrombosis of the bypass conduit may cause acute ischemia.

D. It may be difficult to differentiate thrombosis from embolism as the cause of an acute pulseless extremity. Thrombosis tends to occur in younger patients than in those with embolism and in patients with a known history of vascular occlusive disease or previous vascular surgery. Embolism usually occurs in patients with known heart disease (mitral stenosis or regurgitation, atrial fibrillation, acute myocardial infarction). Patients with embolism may have had an earlier embolic event but usually have no history of chronic circulatory impairment. Physical examination of the uninvolved extremity usually demonstrates normal pulses in patients with embolism.

E. Early heparinization helps preserve the patency of needed collateral blood vessels. Time is of the essence for salvage of the acutely ischemic extremity. Except in trauma, heparin is always indicated as soon as the diagnosis of acute circulatory impairment is made. Give heparin as an IV bolus of 10,000 U followed by a minimum dosage of 1000 U/hr to prolong the activated partial thromboplastin time to >2½ times control.

F. Arteriography is a luxury that may aid the vascular surgeon but should not be performed in any patient who has already developed paresthesia or paralysis. Monitor the patient during arteriography; if signs and symptoms of nerve ischemia develop, terminate the procedure and pursue operative intervention. Arteriography is especially helpful in patients with blunt injury who have an acute pulseless extremity, because an injury requiring repair can be differentiated from the arterial vasospasm often associated with fractures. Moreover, arteriography may help distinguish thrombosis from embolism. Patients who have sustained an embolism from a cardiac source often have normal peripheral vessels. Emboli tend to lodge where vessels taper or branch and are most commonly seen in the external iliac, superficial femoral, and popliteal arteries. With acute thrombosis, there usually is evidence of significant disease in other lower extremity arteries. During the angiographic contrast injection, late films are needed to demonstrate the patency of the distal circulation below the level of obstruction.

G. If the leg is viable, there is time to pursue intra-arterial thrombolysis using urokinase. The catheter is placed directly in the clot by the radiologist, and a bolus infusion of 500,000–1,000,000 U of urokinase is given directly into the clot. After this initial bolus, continue urokinase at 80,000–250,000 U/hr through the catheter. During thrombolytic therapy, the patient is monitored in the ICU and serum fibrinogen levels are drawn every 6 hours to monitor the systemic effect of the infusion. As long as the serum fibrinogen is >100 mg/dl and there are no signs of bleeding, the infusion may continue at the stated dosage. Also, monitor the perfusion of the foot and the status of pulses during the intra-arterial urokinase infusion. After several hours, perform repeat arteriography through the catheter to measure the amount of lysis. If thrombolysis is complete, continue giving the patient IV heparin until a definitive cause for the acute ischemia has been determined. If the cause is definitely cardiac embolism, institute warfarin. If the cause is thrombosis, the patient may be observed or considered for elective surgical revascularization. Intra-arterial urokinase usually is continued for a maximum of 2 days. If no or minimal thrombolysis has occurred and the foot remains viable, elective vascular surgery may be undertaken. If the leg deteriorates and becomes nonviable, an urgent operation must be performed for limb salvage.

H. If paresthesia or paralysis is present, the limb soon becomes unsalvageable without operative intervention. It is important to distinguish sensitivity to light touch from that of pressure, pain, and temperature. Pressure, pain, and temperature sensations are carried by larger nerves that are more resistant to ischemia and therefore may remain intact when sensation to light touch has diminished. If there are no sensory or motor deficits, a more elective work-up may proceed. After the abrupt onset of perfusion impairment, the clock begins ticking. If the collateral circulation is not well developed, one usually has <4–6 hours to restore the circulation. Attempts to provide revascularization after 8–12 hours are seldom successful.

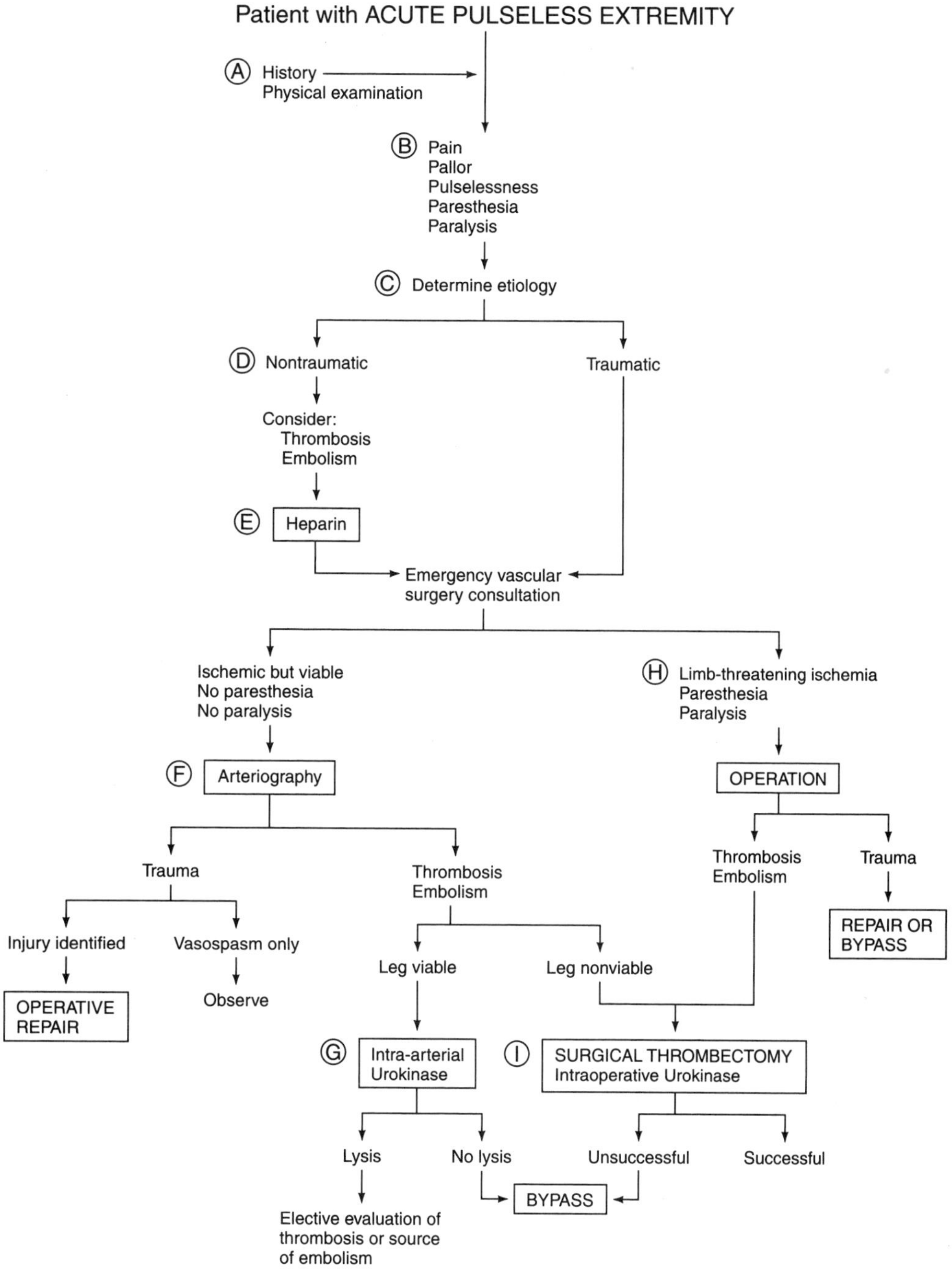

Patient with ACUTE PULSELESS EXTREMITY

Ⓐ History ——→
Physical examination

Ⓑ Pain
Pallor
Pulselessness
Paresthesia
Paralysis

Ⓒ Determine etiology

Ⓓ Nontraumatic · · · · · · Traumatic

Consider:
Thrombosis
Embolism

Ⓔ Heparin

Emergency vascular
surgery consultation

Ischemic but viable
No paresthesia
No paralysis

Ⓗ Limb-threatening ischemia
Paresthesia
Paralysis

Ⓕ Arteriography

OPERATION

Trauma   Thrombosis   Thrombosis   Trauma
                      Embolism   Embolism

Injury identified   Vasospasm only   REPAIR OR
                                                               BYPASS

OPERATIVE   Observe
REPAIR

                    Leg viable   Leg nonviable

Ⓖ Intra-arterial   Ⓘ SURGICAL THROMBECTOMY
Urokinase   Intraoperative Urokinase

Lysis   No lysis   Unsuccessful   Successful

Elective evaluation of   BYPASS
thrombosis or source
of embolism

I. When the leg is nonviable, as evidenced by paresthesia and/or paralysis, undertake an emergent operation to facilitate limb salvage. Surgical thrombectomy usually is performed through a groin incision overlying the common femoral artery. This enables the surgeon to pass balloon thrombectomy catheters proximally and distally to extract thrombus. Although the surgeon passes the balloon thrombectomy catheter until no clot is returned, distal clot remains in as many as 30% of patients. In addition, the balloon catheter may cause intimal injury to the arteries. Therefore intraoperative intra-arterial urokinase is used as an adjunct to facilitate the opening of arteries occluded by thrombus.

References

Abbott WM, Maloney RD, McCabe CC, et al. Arterial embolism: a 44 year perspective. Am J Surg 1982; 143:460.

Aufderheide TP. Peripheral arteriovascular disease. In: Rosen P, Barkin R, eds. Emergency medicine. St Louis: Mosby, 1998:1826.

Brewster DC, Chin AK, Fogarty TJ. Arterial thromboembolism. In: Rutherford RB, ed. Vascular surgery. 3rd ed. Philadelphia: WB Saunders, 1989.

Perry MO. Acute limb ischemia. In: Rutherford RB, ed. Vascular surgery. 3rd ed. Philadelphia: WB Saunders, 1989.

Quinones-Baldrich WJ, Zierler RE, Hiatt JC. Intraoperative fibrinolytic therapy: an adjunct to catheter thromboembolectomy. J Vasc Surg 1985; 2:319.

523

FOREIGN BODY INGESTION

Riemke Brakema

Most foreign body ingestions occur in children 6 months to 3 years of age. Among adults, those with psychiatric disorders, mental retardation, or dentures are likely to ingest objects. Children are most likely to ingest coins, balloons, buttons, tacks, marbles, beads, button batteries, and pins. In adults one might expect a food bolus (especially meat), chicken or fish bones, dentures, or toothpicks.

Of all foreign bodies ingested, >80% end up in the digestive tract. Any object lodged in the airway must be removed. Complications may include perforation with pneumothorax or hemorrhage, pneumonia, or lung abscess. A missed aspirated foreign body in a bronchus may present as recurrent or atypical pneumonia or asthma and may be extremely difficult to remove by bronchoscopy or surgery. In general, 80–85% of all foreign bodies in the GI tract pass spontaneously. Complications (usually related to perforations and/or obstruction) include mediastinitis, fistulas, aortic perforation, cardiac tamponade, and peritonitis.

A. The type of foreign body ingested and the site of obstruction determine the treatment approach. Try to determine what type of object was ingested. Obtain the history from the patient, family members, or bystanders. If a patient cannot talk because of airway obstruction, address that problem immediately.

   Certain foreign bodies deserve special mention. Button or disk batteries may contain the alkaline potassium hydroxide, as well as a number of heavy metals such as lithium, nickel, zinc, cadmium, or mercury. Most batteries are not biologically sealed. Batteries in the esophagus must be removed quickly because of the possibility of liquefaction necrosis from the alkaline solution and subsequent perforation and/or pressure necrosis of the esophageal wall. Once the battery passes into the stomach, spontaneous passage from the body is likely to follow and may be documented by repeat radiographs. Lack of passage from the stomach after 48 hours or lack of progression below the stomach after 72 hours may necessitate surgical intervention. If a radiograph shows the battery has come apart, obtain heavy-metal levels and follow up for consideration of chelation.

   Sharp objects (e.g., fish or chicken bones, pins, needles) lodged in the esophagus are a medical emergency. Above the cricopharyngeal muscle, direct laryngoscopy is the initial approach, while immediate esophagoscopy is applied for objects below this point. Most sharp objects that reach the stomach pass spontaneously through the rest of the digestive tract, but their complication rate is about 35%. Give careful consideration to expectant management versus surgical intervention in these cases.

   Physical examination generally is brief. The ABC approach determines general patient status. Make interventions as indicated by evaluation. Follow this with a detailed examination of the oral and nasal pharynx for erythema, edema, abrasions, and cuts. Evaluate the neck and soft tissues for subcutaneous emphysema. Auscultate and percuss the neck and chest for stridor, breath sounds, wheezing, hyperresonance, or dullness to percussion.

B. Use topical anesthesia for the mucosa to facilitate examination of the pharynx and hypopharynx with the indirect laryngoscope. If the foreign body cannot be visualized in this manner, use direct laryngoscopy after obtaining adequate sedation. If the object is visualized and no sharp or jagged edges are known to be present, remove it with Magill forceps.

C. Use radiologic studies to determine radiolucency (most objects are not) and the lodgement site of the foreign body. Soft tissue neck films may show air in the subcutaneous tissues, indicating perforation. Also look to see whether the foreign body is in the tracheal air column or the esophagus. Coins lodged in the trachea tend to align in the sagittal plane; those in the esophagus usually appear in the coronal alignment. An anteroposterior view of the chest may show a pneumothorax, the foreign body, a lung abscess, or lobar atelectasis. Finally, if indicated by the lack of findings on the first two radiographs, obtain a flat and upright plate of the abdomen to determine whether the foreign body is indeed radiolucent and has already passed beyond the pylorus. If the patient complains of abdominal pain, look for signs of obstruction or perforation such as free air under the diaphragm. If all these scouting x-ray studies are negative but there is a reliable history and/or the patient is symptomatic, continue to look for the foreign body.

D. If the foreign body was aspirated, symptoms may range from throat pain, cough, or stridor to episodes of cyanosis or apnea and acute respiratory distress or collapse. Direct interventions toward the patient's status before performing further evaluation. In case of complete airway obstruction, do an oropharyngeal sweep, Heimlich maneuver, and direct laryngoscopy as indicated, and have Magill forceps on hand to remove the object if it is visualized. If unsuccessful, prepare for cricothyrotomy.

E. If a foreign body acts as a one-way valve in a mainstem bronchus, air can get in but not out. Expiratory wheezes are present on physical examination, and the involved, partially obstructed lung may appear overexpanded and hyperlucent on an expiratory chest radiograph. The diaphragm may appear fixed and flat, and the heart and mediastinum may be shifted to the opposite, uninvolved side. When the obstruction becomes complete, air cannot get in or out, and the involved lung may appear atelectatic on radiographs, with the heart and mediastinum shifted to the involved side.

(Continued on page 526)

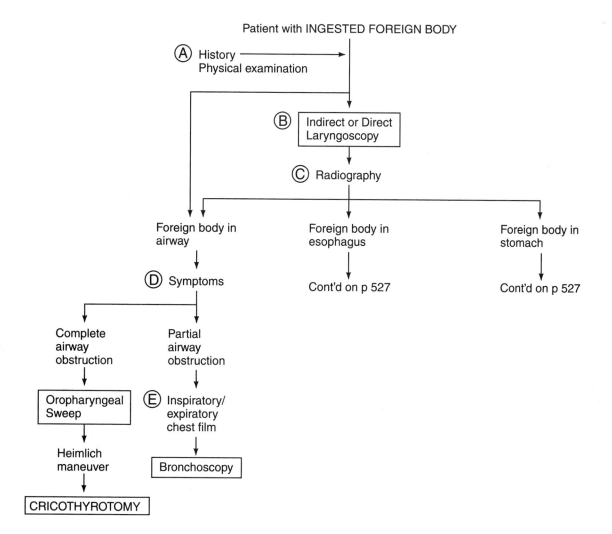

Patient with INGESTED FOREIGN BODY

(A) History
Physical examination

(B) Indirect or Direct Laryngoscopy

(C) Radiography

Foreign body in airway

Foreign body in esophagus

Foreign body in stomach

Cont'd on p 527

Cont'd on p 527

(D) Symptoms

Complete airway obstruction

Partial airway obstruction

Oropharyngeal Sweep

(E) Inspiratory/ expiratory chest film

Heimlich maneuver

Bronchoscopy

CRICOTHYROTOMY

F. Inability to swallow, trouble with secretions, and refusal to eat are common symptoms of a foreign body lodged in the esophagus. Patients also may be vomiting and gagging and may complain of neck, throat, or chest pain. They are often able to point exactly to the site of obstruction, although this is not a reliable sign. The most common sites of obstruction are those where physiologic narrowing occurs (e.g., the level of the cricopharyngeal muscle, the aortic arch, the gastroesophageal junction, Schatzki's ring).

G. A nasogastric tube may be placed gently just above the site of the obstruction to manage and control secretions.

H. After spontaneous passage of a known esophageal foreign body, perform nonemergent esophagoscopy to evaluate the esophagus for possible perforation and/or an underlying pathologic condition. No foreign body should remain in the esophagus for >24 hours because of the increased risk of perforation into the trachea or heart, fistula formation, and mediastinitis. Determining the exact lodgment site of the object in the esophagus by means of contrast studies such as barium or Gastrografin swallows has fallen out of favor because the contrast medium usually interferes with endoscopic visualization and removal of the foreign body.

I. The magnet tube was used in the past to remove pins, tacks, rings, and disk batteries from the upper esophagus, but few physicians still use this method. Patient cooperation and control of the foreign body are difficult to obtain, especially in children, and make this method prone to complications. Anticipate vomiting after the foreign body is dislodged; be prepared to deal with subsequent complications. Using a Foley catheter to remove an object from the esophagus also is considered controversial by many physicians, although those skilled in its use report few complications. The advantages are avoidance of general anesthesia and the complications of endoscopy. Significant disadvantages include complete or incomplete airway obstruction if the foreign body is dislodged in the oro- or nasopharynx, missed esophageal damage or perforation, and distress and pain to the patient. This method should be used only when endoscopy is not available and by physicians who are well versed in resuscitation and airway management. It is done as follows: Pass the Foley catheter orally past the foreign body with the patient in the upright position. Place the patient in prone Trendelenburg position and inflate the Foley balloon with contrast medium. Under fluoroscopic guidance, gently and steadily withdraw the catheter. Grasp the body with forceps in the hypopharynx. Referral for endoscopy should follow because the complications of a missed esophageal perforation can be severe.

J. Glucagon may be used to try to advance a food bolus lodged in the lower esophagus. Glucagon relaxes the smooth muscles and the lower gastroesophageal sphincter without inhibiting peristalsis. After a test dose to exclude hypersensitivity to the drug, give a 1-mg dose of IV glucagon with the patient in the upright position. Give it slowly; rapid IV administration may cause nausea and vomiting. Give a second dose of 2 mg if the patient experiences no relief 20 minutes after the first injection. Each dose should be followed with water. If the obstruction is relieved, perform esophagoscopy to evaluate for damage or an underlying pathologic condition. Papain is a digestive enzyme used in meat tenderizer. It was used in the past to dissolve meat boluses lodged in the esophagus but has fallen out of favor after a number of case reports described esophageal perforation after its use.

K. Consider esophagogastroscopic removal of sharp objects from the stomach. Objects thicker than 2–2.5 cm tend to get stuck at the pylorus, and those longer than 10 cm tend to get stuck at the duodenal sweep. Failure to progress as documented by radiographs is an indication to intervene and remove the object by endoscopic means.

L. Most foreign bodies that pass the pylorus are excreted per rectum in 24–72 hours without complications. Antacids and cathartics have not proved to be of value. Expectant observation may or may not include repeat radiographs to document advancement of the foreign body. If there is abdominal pain, nausea, or vomiting, obtain a radiograph to determine the presence of an obstruction or perforation. Surgical consultation and intervention may be indicated. Drug-filled condoms generally pass spontaneously without complications unless the condom perforates, in which case immediate intervention, including surgical and medical management, is necessary because of toxic exposure.

References

Gaasch WR, Barish RA. Swallowed foreign bodies. In: Tintanalli JE, et al, eds. Emergency medicine: a comprehensive study guide. 4th Ed. New York: McGraw-Hill, 1996:453.

Ginsberg GG. Management of ingested foreign objects and food bolus impaction. Gastro Endosc 1995; 41:33.

Halvorson DJ, Merritt RM, et al. Management of subglottic foreign bodies. Ann Otol Rhinol Laryngol 1996; 105:541.

Harnes RK 2nd, Strain JD, et al. Esophageal foreign bodies: safety and efficacy of foley catheter extraction of coins. AJR 1997; 168:443.

Kuhns D, Dire D. Button battery ingestions. Ann Emerg Med 1989; 18:293.

Leo PJ, Sachter JJ, Melrose M. Heroin body packing. J Accid Emerg Med 1995; 12:43.

Pons PT. Foreign bodies. In: Rosen P, Barkin R, eds. Emergency medicine: concepts and clinical practice. 4th Ed. St Louis: Mosby, 1998:861.

Schweich PJ. Management of coin ingestion: any change? Pediatr Emerg Care 1995; 11:37.

Suita S, et al. Management of pediatric patients who have swallowed foreign objects. Am Surg 1989; 55:585.

Taylor R. Esophageal foreign bodies. Emerg Med Clin North Am 1987; 5:301.

Velitchkov NG, Grigorov GI, et al. Ingested foreign bodies of the gastrointestinal tract: retrospective analysis of 542 cases. World J Surg 1996; 20:1001.

Webb WA. Management of foreign bodies of the upper gastrointestinal tract: update. Gastro Endosc 1995; 41:39.

Patient with INGESTED FOREIGN BODY

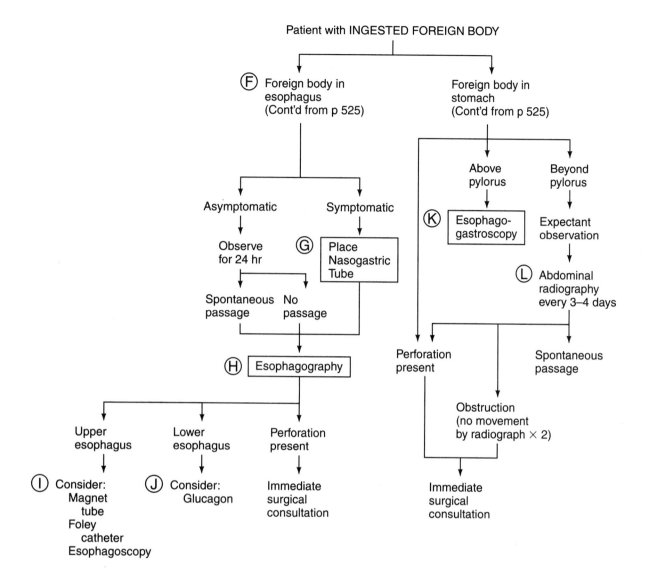

CAUSTIC INGESTION AND EXPOSURE

Cynthia Madden

Caustic exposure refers to all forms of chemical injury, alkali being more common than acid. Most exposures are in children (1–4 years old) and are accidental. Adult ingestions usually are from a suicide attempt.

A. Determine the patient's age, the time of ingestion in relation to the last meal, and the type, physical form, and concentration of material ingested. Alkaline chemicals are in lye, drain cleaners, oven cleaners, Clinitest tablets, and button batteries; acids are found in swimming pool cleaners, rust removers, and battery acid. Examine the oropharynx for ulcerations or eschar; however, up to 20% of patients without oropharyngeal burns show endoscopic esophageal wall damage. Be alert for signs of respiratory compromise: stridor, hoarseness, aphonia. Check for Hamman's sign (a crunchy sound synchronous with the heartbeat) on the chest examination and for subcutaneous emphysema when examining the neck. The pH of the patient's saliva can help determine whether an acid or alkali has been ingested.

B. Alkali burns cause liquefaction necrosis in the esophagus, involving the mucosa, submucosa, and longitudinal muscle. The stomach is affected in 20% of cases.

C. Alkali burns to the cornea are an ophthalmologic emergency and require continuous irrigation for at least 3 hours.

D. Symptoms of battery ingestion include vomiting, refusal to eat, increased salivation, and pain on swallowing. Emetics are contraindicated. Leave the patient NPO until radiographs of the entire GI tract have been obtained.

E. Cathartics may be administered to facilitate evacuation; emesis should not be attempted. Endoscopic removal is indicated if the battery does not pass in 36–48 hours or if the patient develops symptoms.

F. Acids cause coagulation necrosis with eschar formation and mainly affect the stomach, leading to pylorospasm and eventual full-thickness necrosis and perforation.

G. Patients without a reliable history and with no symptoms (e.g., oral burns, dysphagia, vomiting) can be monitored in the emergency room and discharged after 3–4 hours. Acid ingestion poses a higher risk of perforation and all such patients should be admitted.

H. First-degree burns cause hyperemia with superficial mucosal desquamation; second-degree burns cause blistering and shallow ulcers; third-degree burns suggest total loss of esophageal epithelium.

I. It generally is accepted that patients with first-degree burns rarely develop strictures; patients with third-degree burns develop strictures regardless of steroid treatment. Steroids may delay stricture development in those with second-degree burns and should be used with an antibiotic to offset the increase in infection rate caused by steroid use. The dose of methylprednisone is 2 mg/kg/day; 1 g ampicillin every 6 hours or 100 mg/kg every 24 hours in children may be used.

J. Hydrofluoric acid (HF) is a common agent in the home and industry and can produce life-threatening toxicity with minimal exposure. HF dissociates in tissue and affects metabolism in three ways: liquefaction necrosis, bone destruction, and production of insoluble salts. Inhalation exposures to concentrated HF for 5 minutes usually are fatal.

K. Initial management for HF burns includes deactivating the fluoride ion. For severe burns, inject intradermally 10% calcium gluconate into, and for a distance of 0.5 cm around, the burn. For mild to moderate burns, apply calcium gluconate gel locally.

L. For unknown amounts of HF ingestion, administer 300 ml magnesium citrate. If the concentration of HF is known, administer oral magnesium on a milliequivalent-for-milliequivalent basis.

M. Monitor the QT interval for signs of hypocalcemia, and make frequent evaluations of acid-base status, electrolytes, and calcium. Burn care includes cleansing and parenteral analgesics.

References

Crain EF, Gershel JC, Mezey AP. Caustic ingestions: symptoms as predictors of esophageal injury. Am J Dis Child 1984; 138:863.

Hoffman RS, Goldfrank LR, Howland MA. Caustics and batteries. In: Goldfrank LR, Flomenbaum NE, Lewin NA, et al, eds. Goldfrank's toxicologic emergencies. 4th ed. Norwalk, CT: Appleton & Lange, 1990.

Howell JM, Dalsey WC, Hartsell FW, Butzin CA. Steroids for the treatment of corrosive esophageal injury: a statistical analysis of past studies. Am J Emerg Med 1992; 10:421.

Karkal SS, ed, Wason S, consulting ed. Coping swiftly and effectively with caustic ingestions. Emerg Med Rep 1989; 10:25.

CAUSTIC INGESTION AND EXPOSURE Suspected

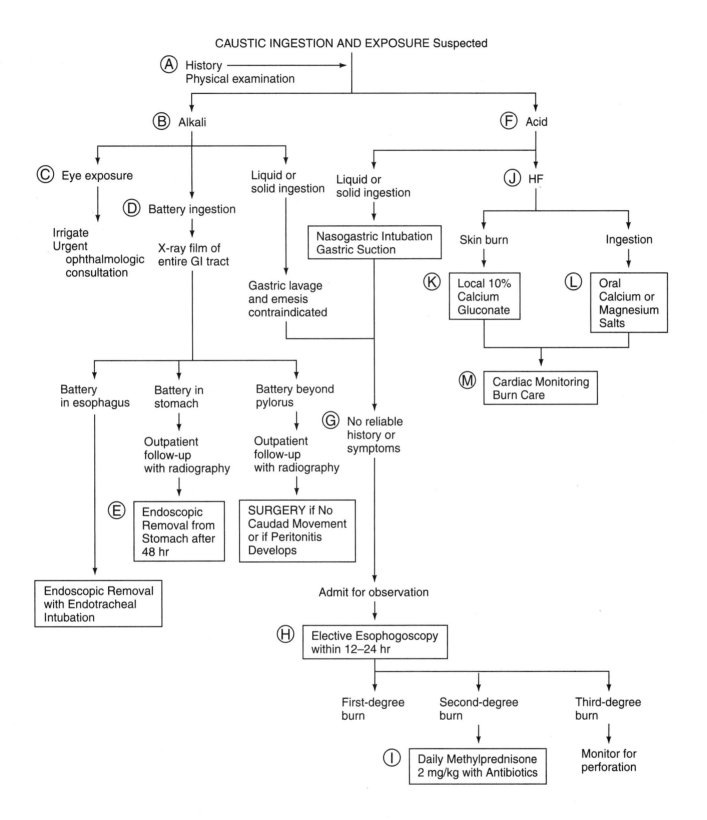

HUMAN AND ANIMAL BITES

Douglas Lindsey

Humans make up a subset of animals. Specificity of speciation notwithstanding, the boundary between humans and other animals is flexible when defined by value judgments of behavior. The only clinical distinction is in differences of dentition and musculature of mastication. The author is not aware of any valid data to support the common premise that anatomically comparable wounds require different management depending on species.

A. Every break of the skin demands attention to the prevention of tetanus. There is no such thing as a "clean minor wound": all wounds are tetanus prone.

B. With very rare exceptions, rabies is transmitted by the saliva of mammalian species. Humans are not excluded, but in many parts of the United States, rodents, squirrels, and rabbits are not a threat. Report all animal exposures to the local animal control authorities, follow their advice, and administer rabies prophylaxis exactly by CDC guidelines and those in the package insert.

C. Many patients have wounds that are already infected. Make a Gram stain, obtain a culture, and prescribe 4 days of an oral antimicrobial with the narrowest reasonable spectrum, most often a first-generation cephalosporin. Any cat bite, cat scratch, or dog bite that shows a sign of inflammation within 24 hours of the wounding is infected with *Pasteurella multocida* until proved otherwise, and the preferable agent is penicillin. Four days suffice for most simple wound infections and allows time for culture results to suggest a better choice if the patient is not improving.

D. If a patient steps on a nail or a similar object, any attempt to debride or irrigate the simple wound is unnecessary. The surface of the wound can be gently cleaned for aesthetic purposes.

E. Some puncture wounds require opening for visual inspection. The "knuckle sandwich" or "clenched fist injury" (CFI) is a prime example. Since the pre-antimicrobial days of Kanavel, the CFI has been recognized as a special problem, but it is one of human anatomy, not human oral flora. Tissue planes punctured in CFI do not permit drainage when the hand returns to its normal position of function. Return the hand to the clenched fist position, open the wound (with a transverse, not longitudinal, incision over the joint), and take a good look. If penetration of the joint capsule cannot be excluded, refer the patient to a specialist.

F. The canine tooth of canines is made for tearing meat, not for punching holes. Some canine tooth punctures are deeply undermined. The author has seen such punctures on the scalp of a child where the puncture into the cranium was 3 cm distant from the entrance wound. Probe punctures of bites by animals (nonhuman) larger than house cats. If the wound is undermined, irrigate and place a drain. A sterile rubber band is advisable. Remove the drain at 48 hours.

G. Repair bite wounds that are lacerations or avulsions in the same manner as comparable wounds from nonanimate instruments.

H. Although the profession of surgery has a sound database to support codified recommendations for perioperative prophylaxis, there is no such support for the use of systemic antimicrobial prophylaxis in accidental wounds. On the other hand, there is sound evidence to support the use of topical antimicrobials. For an undermined bite wound, flush the wound with a 10% solution of benzyl penicillin. A vial of 1 million units contains 0.6 g. Dilute with 6 ml water, not saline. Even if the wound edges are infiltrated with anesthetic, the instillation causes significant, but transient, aching pain.

References

Lindsey D. Tetanus prophylaxis—do our guidelines assure protection? J Trauma 1984; 24:1063.

Lindsey D, Christopher M, Hollenbach J, et al. Natural course of the human bite wound: incidence of infection and complications in 434 bites and 803 lacerations in the same group of patients. J Trauma 1987; 27:45.

Lindsey D, Nava C, Marti M. Effectiveness of penicillin irrigation in control of infection in sutured lacerations. J Trauma 1982; 22:186.

Mann JM. Systematic decision-making in rabies prophylaxis. Pediatr Infect Dis J 1983; 2:162.

Sacks T. Prophylactic antibiotics in traumatic wounds. J Hosp Infect 1988; 11(suppl A):251.

Vanhoof R, Costy F. Rabies prophylaxis. Acta Clin Belg 1996; 51:328.

Patient with HUMAN OR ANIMAL BITE

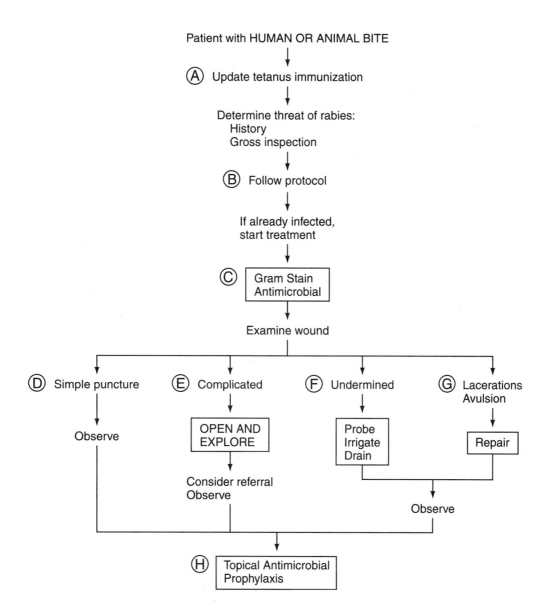

(A) Update tetanus immunization

Determine threat of rabies:
History
Gross inspection

(B) Follow protocol

If already infected,
start treatment

(C) Gram Stain
Antimicrobial

Examine wound

(D) Simple puncture

Observe

(E) Complicated

OPEN AND
EXPLORE

Consider referral
Observe

(F) Undermined

Probe
Irrigate
Drain

(G) Lacerations
Avulsion

Repair

Observe

(H) Topical Antimicrobial
Prophylaxis

SNAKE VENOM POISONING

William P. Johnson

Poisonous snakebites are caused by pit vipers (copperhead, cottonmouth, rattlesnakes) and by coral snakes. Pit viper bites are potentially lethal and require careful medical management. Rattlesnake bites are the most dangerous and account for about 60% of all bites, but all can cause life- or limb-threatening disease. The following management focuses on rattlesnake bites, but the algorithm can be used for all pit vipers. Coral snakebites are much rarer but can also cause life-threatening disease; their bites cause paralysis, which can be treated with antivenin and supportive care. Consult a regional poison control center for all envenomations.

A. In the United States the diagnosis of rattlesnake bite is primarily determined by a history of a bite followed by the development of symptoms. A snakebite may appear as one, two, or multiple puncture wounds or small lacerations. Pain, swelling, and ecchymosis usually become apparent during the first few hours. First aid to alter absorption with a Sawyer extractor or sling is indicated but should *not* delay transportation to the nearest medical facility. Oral suction, incision of fang marks, tourniquets, and other such methods are *not* recommended.

B. The grade of envenomation is established by evaluating local wound findings, the presence of a coagulopathy, and the severity of systemic symptoms. *Minimal* envenomation consists of local pain, edema and ecchymosis with normal blood coagulation tests, and normal mental status and vital signs. *Moderate* envenomation consists of spreading pain, edema, or ecchymosis; mild to moderately abnormal coagulation studies; mild to moderate thrombocytopenia; or hemolysis. The patient may appear sleepy or lethargic but can become alert and oriented on command. *Severe* envenomation is the rapid development of edema and ecchymosis, markedly abnormal coagulation studies, defibrination, disseminated intravascular coagulation–like syndromes, hemolysis, or depressed mentation. The worst findings are used to grade the envenomation. Thus, mild swelling with markedly abnormal coagulation studies or depressed mentation is classified as severe envenomation. The grade of envenomation is important because it determines whether antivenin is initially used and the amount used.

C. Several cases of delayed worsening of the envenomation have been reported. Observe patients for 6–8 hours with the bitten part elevated above heart level. The grade of envenomation should be changed if local or systemic symptoms signs appear or worsen.

D. Most deaths from snakebites are caused by the patient's failure to seek medical attention or the physician's failure to recognize the severity of the envenomation. If antivenin is not immediately available, give a rapid crystalloid infusion to maintain blood pressure and reduce heart rate. If bleeding is apparent, replace platelets or coagulation factors by infusing platelets or fresh frozen plasma until antivenin can be infused. After rapid evaluation of the patient, treat with antivenin.

E. Use skin test only when the decision to administer antivenin has been made. Administer antivenin (Crotalidae) polyvalent to patients with moderate or severe envenomations who demonstrate worsening of local or systemic findings. The skin test consists of 0.02 ml of a 1:10 dilution of the skin test material provided with the antivenin in one shoulder and 0.02 ml of normal saline (control) in the other shoulder. A positive skin test consists of a wheal and flare 10 mm at the site of injection. Strong reactions to the skin test indicate a high probability of a severe reaction to antivenin infusion.

F. Antivenin administration consists of infusion of 5–10 vials in 250–500 ml of dextrose and water over 1–2 hours except as noted in E. The initial infusion should be slow (60 ml/hr or 1 ml/min) in case an allergic reaction develops. If no reaction develops, the infusion rate can be increased to complete the infusion in 1–2 hours.

G. Up to 25% of patients develop some degree of reaction to antivenin infusion. If a reaction develops, stop the antivenin infusion immediately. Reactions take many forms, ranging from local erythema and itching to anaphylaxis. Give epinephrine, as well as H_1 and H_2 receptor blockers, to control the acute reaction. At this point, consult with a regional poison control center or medical toxicologist. The benefits of continued antivenin infusion must be compared with the risks of restarting the infusion. In general, the antivenin can be restarted after diluting the antivenin and infusing it more slowly.

References

Burgess JL, Dart RC. Snake venom coagulopathy: use and abuse of blood products in the treatment of pit viper envenomation. Ann Emerg Med 1991; 20:795.

Hardy DL. Fatal rattlesnake envenomation in Arizona: 1969–1984. Clin Toxicol 1986; 24:1.

Kunkel DB. Treating snakebites sensibly. Emerg Med 1988; 30 June: 51.

Norris RL, Oslund S, Auerbach PS. Disorders caused by reptile bites and marine animal envenomations. In: Fauci AS, Braunwald E, Isselbacher KJ, et al, eds. Harrison's principles of internal medicine. 14th ed. New York: McGraw-Hill, 1997:2544.

Wingert WA, Chan L. Rattlesnake bites in southern California and rationale for recommended treatment. West J Med 1988; 148:37.

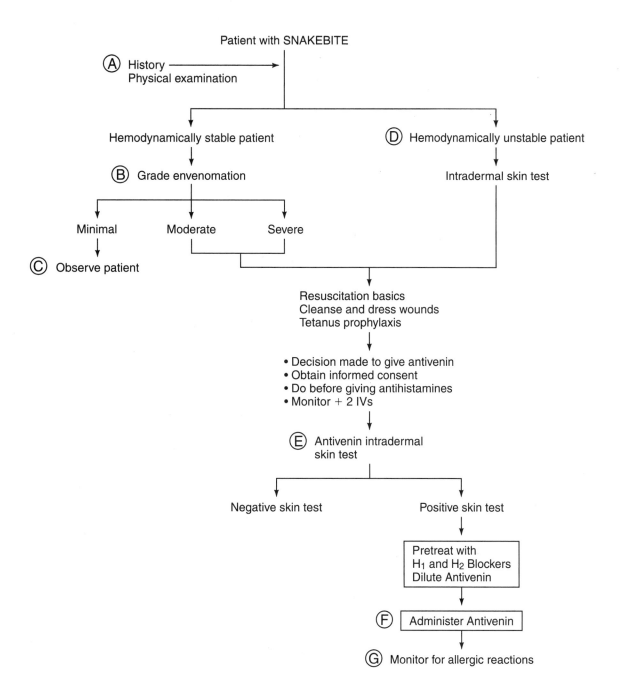

Patient with SNAKEBITE

(A) History
Physical examination

Hemodynamically stable patient

(B) Grade envenomation

Minimal   Moderate   Severe

(C) Observe patient

(D) Hemodynamically unstable patient

Intradermal skin test

Resuscitation basics
Cleanse and dress wounds
Tetanus prophylaxis

• Decision made to give antivenin
• Obtain informed consent
• Do before giving antihistamines
• Monitor + 2 IVs

(E) Antivenin intradermal
skin test

Negative skin test   Positive skin test

Pretreat with
H₁ and H₂ Blockers
Dilute Antivenin

(F) Administer Antivenin

(G) Monitor for allergic reactions

HYPOTHERMIA

Cynthia Madden

A. Establish an airway adequate to ensure proper ventilation. Administer warm, humidified 100% O_2. Gentle intubation after preoxygenation is safe in hypothermic patients.

B. Obtain blood specimens, including CBC, blood cultures, electrolytes, BUN, creatinine, and ABGs. Temperature correction of pH and P_{CO_2} is not necessary when interpreting ABGs. Establish IV access with warmed normal saline.

C. Patients with stable cardiac rhythm (including sinus bradycardia) and stable vital signs may undergo passive rewarming with blankets to prevent further heat loss. Noninvasive internal modalities may be used (warmed, humidified oxygen and warmed IV fluids).

D. Patients with cardiovascular instability need to be rapidly rewarmed using a combination of methods. Core warming (warming the heart before the extremities) must be used. Gastric/bladder/colon lavage or peritoneal lavage with warmed dialysate should be used. Severely hypothermic patients should receive extracorporeal blood warming with partial cardiopulmonary bypass if available. Continue warmed O_2, IV fluids, and blankets. For ventricular fibrillation or asystole, defibrillate once or twice, institute CPR, and rewarm rapidly. The hypothermic myocardium is refractory to atropine, pacing, and defibrillation. Prolonged resuscitation efforts are indicated.

E. Administer 50 ml $D_{50}W$, 2 mg naloxone (Narcan), and 100 mg thiamine IV. Obtain an ECG, which may reveal J-wave abnormalities. Continue to monitor the cardiac rhythm.

F. Assess environmental exposures, spinal cord or central neurologic injuries, shock (signs of trauma, hemorrhage, or sepsis), hepatic failure, sepsis, and burns. Consider exposure to drugs and toxins (organophosphates, ethanol, opioids, β blockers).

G. For frostbite, rapid rewarming by extremity immersion in 42° C water for 20 minutes is the most effective means of preserving tissue. Early surgical intervention is not indicated.

References

Danzl D, Pozos R. Accidental hypothermia. N Engl J Med 1994; 331:1756.

Delaney K, Howland MA, Vassallo S, Goldfrank LR. Assessment of acid-base disturbances in hypothermia and their physiologic consequences. Ann Emerg Med 1989; 18:72.

Weinberg AD. Hypothermia. Ann Emerg Med 1993; 22:370.

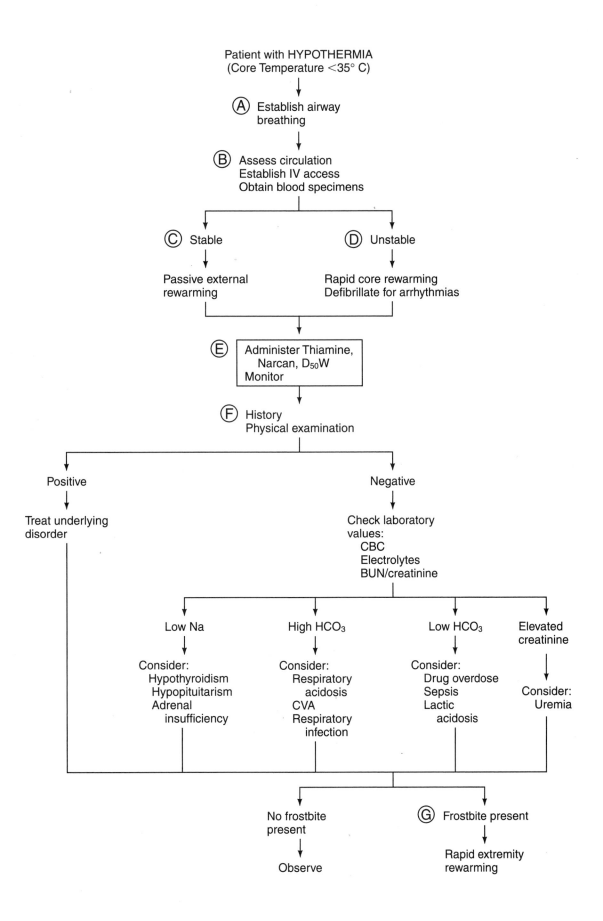

Patient with HYPOTHERMIA
(Core Temperature <35° C)

Ⓐ Establish airway
breathing

Ⓑ Assess circulation
Establish IV access
Obtain blood specimens

Ⓒ Stable

Ⓓ Unstable

Passive external
rewarming

Rapid core rewarming
Defibrillate for arrhythmias

Ⓔ Administer Thiamine,
Narcan, $D_{50}W$
Monitor

Ⓕ History
Physical examination

Positive

Negative

Treat underlying
disorder

Check laboratory
values:
CBC
Electrolytes
BUN/creatinine

Low Na

High HCO_3

Low HCO_3

Elevated
creatinine

Consider:
Hypothyroidism
Hypopituitarism
Adrenal
insufficiency

Consider:
Respiratory
acidosis
CVA
Respiratory
infection

Consider:
Drug overdose
Sepsis
Lactic
acidosis

Consider:
Uremia

No frostbite
present

Ⓖ Frostbite present

Observe

Rapid extremity
rewarming

DROWNING AND NEAR-DROWNING

Samuel M. Keim
Michael Loew

Drowning is death from suffocation as a result of submersion in a fluid. Near-drowning implies survival, at least temporarily, after such suffocation. About 10% of victims succumb to asphyxia while submerged, probably because of laryngospasm or breath holding. The other victims aspirate fluid: fresh water, salt water, contaminated water, or other liquids. The pathophysiology of drowning depends on the amount and type of fluid aspirated. Hypothermia decreases oxygen consumption and can thereby delay reversible cerebral damage. Unfortunately, hypothermia can produce lethal arrhythmias such as ventricular fibrillation. Neurologic injury and recovery depend on the duration and degree of hypoxia, the water temperature, and the patient's underlying physical condition.

A. Some victims of near-drowning do not aspirate water, have limited laryngospasm or breath holding, and regain effective ventilation before permanent damage occurs. These patients may appear sleepy or groggy, or completely alert. The first responder should not be lulled into a false sense of security by this presentation. Despite appearing stable, these patients may be severely hypoxic or become so quickly. Cervical spine (C-spine) precautions should be continued if neck injury is possible, and these patients should be transported with supplemental O_2 to the nearest emergency department (ED) or pediatric critical care center if < 18 years old and presenting with altered mental status or shock.

B. The fundamental goal for initial resuscitation of the apneic near-drowning victim is to restore Pa_{O_2} to normal as rapidly as possible. The victim should be extricated from the water as quickly as possible. If the victim is apneic and mouth-to-mouth ventilation in the water is possible, this should be initiated when the rescuer reaches the victim. Because chest compressions are not typically feasible in the water, they should be initiated when the victim can be removed. C-spine precaution should be followed during extrication if a fall or diving injury is suspected. The single most important factor related to a normal recovery is the prevention of irreversible hypoxia. This usually means that the first responder must know CPR and be able to use it when necessary.

C. If the initially apneic patient has a palpable pulse, the rescuer should continue providing assisted ventilation and activate the emergency medical system by asking another person to call 911 (or other local emergency number). The rescuer should continue assessing the victim's airway to ensure its patency. If necessary, the rescuer may use a Heimlich maneuver to clear the airway (with the awareness that gastric contents may be aspirated during this maneuver). The Heimlich maneuver should not be used in an attempt to empty the stomach. The apneic patient should be intubated by paramedic personnel as soon as possible and transported to the nearest ED or pediatric critical care center.

D. The apneic, pulseless patient should receive CPR (one- or two-rescuer) while C-spine precautions are maintained. The rescuer should have a bystander call 911. The patient should be intubated by paramedic personnel as soon as possible and transported with CPR and advanced cardiac life support (ACLS) in progress to the nearest ED or pediatric critical care center.

(Continued on page 538)

Victim of DROWNING or NEAR-DROWNING

Begin extrication

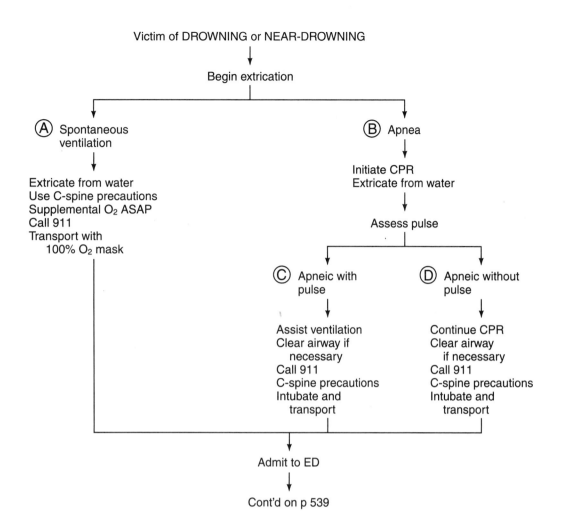

(A) Spontaneous ventilation

Extricate from water
Use C-spine precautions
Supplemental O_2 ASAP
Call 911
Transport with
    100% O_2 mask

(B) Apnea

Initiate CPR
Extricate from water

Assess pulse

(C) Apneic with pulse

Assist ventilation
Clear airway if
    necessary
Call 911
C-spine precautions
Intubate and
    transport

(D) Apneic without pulse

Continue CPR
Clear airway
    if necessary
Call 911
C-spine precautions
Intubate and
    transport

Admit to ED

Cont'd on p 539

E. In the ED the alert, yet hypoxic patient should be treated aggressively. If the patient is alert or easily arousable, the physician may try to use a mask for continuous positive alveolar pressure (CPAP) first. If CPAP is not readily available or cannot be implemented because of altered consciousness, the patient should be intubated via nasal or oral routes. The patient's oxygenation may then be augmented with positive end-expiratory pressure (PEEP). Place a nasogastric (NG) tube to aspirate stomach contents. If present, treat hypothermia, bronchospasm, and acidosis. Admit these patients to the ICU.

F. The spontaneously breathing patient who is extremely fortunate will have a normal Pa_{O_2}, Pa_{CO_2}, and pH. Check the C-spine for injuries. If the patient is normothermic and exhibits no other abnormalities, including bronchospasm or altered consciousness, he or she may be released to a strong social support system with strict precautionary advice. Treat the nonhypoxic hypothermic patient for hypothermia (see I). Admit patients exhibiting bronchospasm or acidosis for observation.

G. The initially apneic patient with an intact circulation will likely be hypoxic on arrival at the ED. If not yet intubated by prehospital personnel, intubate the patient on arrival. Occasionally, patients begin breathing spontaneously during the initial prehospital resuscitation and present without hypoxia. In this situation, they should be treated as in F. Intubated hypoxic patients benefit from PEEP. This can dramatically improve the ventilation-perfusion mismatch. Place an NG tube to aspirate gastric contents. If present, treat bronchospasm and acidosis (inhaled β_2-adrenergic agonists and sodium bicarbonate). Examine the patient for C-spine injuries, and obtain chest film. Treat hypothermia (see I). Admit these patients to the ICU.

H. The apneic and pulseless patient who arrives without previous intubation should be intubated on arrival. CPR and ACLS should be continued. Draw ABGs immediately, and treat acidosis. The evaluation of ABGs in hypothermia is controversial. In general, as temperature decreases, the oxygen-hemoglobin dissociation curve is shifted to the left, thereby decreasing the release of bound O_2. The acidosis (which shifts the curve to the right) may only partially compensate for this. Take care not to administer excessive sodium bicarbonate during resuscitation (alkalosis shifts the curve further to the left).

I. In the hypothermic patient, continue CPR until the core temperature is >32° C. In the severely hypothermic patient (core temperature <32° C), implement active core rewarming to prevent the phenomena of "afterdrop," which can occur when active external rewarming (e.g., warm immersion) used alone leads to reperfusion of cold peripheral tissues and subsequent cooling of the previously sequestered warm-core blood. Active core rewarming can include heated humidified O_2, heated peritoneal lavage, and cardiopulmonary bypass. Other methods include gastric and colonic irrigation, thoracostomy with pleural and mediastinal irrigation, and hemodialysis. Each of these techniques carries inherent risks and complications. Truncal active external rewarming may be added to augment core rewarming. For the patient with mild to moderate hypothermia (core temperature 32–37° C), passive external rewarming is appropriate. This includes the removal of wet clothing and prevention of further heat loss by applying blankets. The efficacy of ACLS medications is controversial in hypothermia. Bretylium has been reported to be effective in ventricular fibrillation. The efficacy of atropine in hypothermia-induced bradycardia is doubtful. The combination of hypoxia and hypothermia can lead to a marked decrease in tissue O_2 delivery. Although hypothermia may be protective via diminished metabolic rate, it is more often lethal. Nonetheless, the dictum "No one is dead until warm and dead" should be followed.

J. In the ICU, ventilatory management should be aggressive, including PEEP, frequent suctioning, and frequent monitoring of the ventilation-perfusion shunt. Acidosis and cardiac arrhythmias should also be treated aggressively. Although controversial, consider intracranial pressure (ICP) monitoring, pulmonary artery pressure monitoring, and barbiturate coma. These treatments contain risks and have questionable benefit. Ensure that no C-spine injury exists (if this is not already done). Treat hypothermia (see I). Treat bronchospasm and acidosis if present. Monitor electrolytes and fluid status closely. Steroids, barbiturates, and induced hypothermia have not been shown to improve survival. Address psychosocial issues with the family.

References

Bohn DJ, Biggar WD, Smith CR, et al. Influence of hypothermia, barbiturate therapy, and intracranial pressure monitoring on morbidity and mortality after near-drowning. Crit Care Med 1986; 14:529.

Boysen PG. Dispelling the myths and controversies of near-drowning. Emerg Med Rep 1984; 5:23.

Danzl DF, Sowers MB, Vicaria SJ, et al. Chemical ventricular defibrillation in severe accidental hypothermia. Ann Emerg Med 1982; 11:698.

Kunichika ET, Berman LS. Drowning and near-drowning. In: Civetta JM, ed. Critical care. 3rd ed. Philadelphia: Lippincott-Raven, 1997: 1875.

Marin TG. Near-drowning and cold-water immersion. Ann Emerg Med 1984; 13:263.

Modell JH. Drowning vs. near-drowning: a discussion of definition. Crit Care Med 1981; 9:301.

Rueler JB. Hypothermia. Ann Intern Med 1978; 89:519.

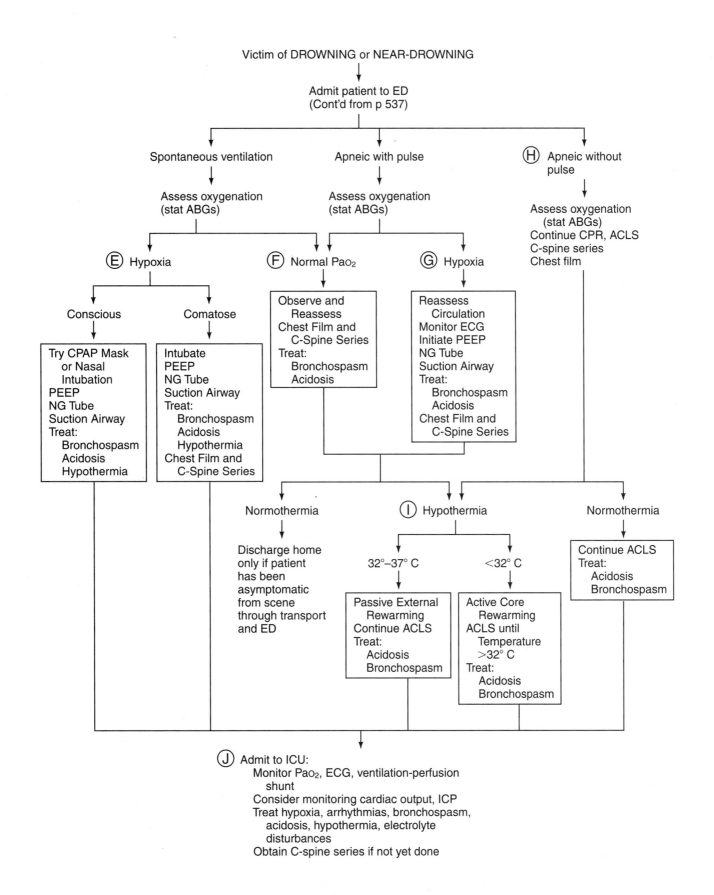

Victim of DROWNING or NEAR-DROWNING

Admit patient to ED
(Cont'd from p 537)

Spontaneous ventilation | Apneic with pulse | Ⓗ Apneic without pulse

Assess oxygenation
(stat ABGs) | Assess oxygenation
(stat ABGs) | Assess oxygenation
(stat ABGs)
Continue CPR, ACLS
C-spine series
Chest film

Ⓔ Hypoxia | Ⓕ Normal PaO₂ | Ⓖ Hypoxia

Conscious | Comatose

Try CPAP Mask
or Nasal
Intubation
PEEP
NG Tube
Suction Airway
Treat:
  Bronchospasm
  Acidosis
  Hypothermia

Intubate
PEEP
NG Tube
Suction Airway
Treat:
  Bronchospasm
  Acidosis
  Hypothermia
Chest Film and
  C-Spine Series

Observe and
Reassess
Chest Film and
  C-Spine Series
Treat:
  Bronchospasm
  Acidosis

Reassess
  Circulation
  Monitor ECG
  Initiate PEEP
  NG Tube
  Suction Airway
Treat:
  Bronchospasm
  Acidosis
Chest Film and
  C-Spine Series

Normothermia | Ⓘ Hypothermia | Normothermia

Discharge home
only if patient
has been
asymptomatic
from scene
through transport
and ED

32°–37° C | <32° C

Passive External
Rewarming
Continue ACLS
Treat:
  Acidosis
  Bronchospasm

Active Core
Rewarming
ACLS until
  Temperature
  >32° C
Treat:
  Acidosis
  Bronchospasm

Continue ACLS
Treat:
  Acidosis
  Bronchospasm

Ⓙ Admit to ICU:
  Monitor PaO₂, ECG, ventilation-perfusion
    shunt
  Consider monitoring cardiac output, ICP
  Treat hypoxia, arrhythmias, bronchospasm,
    acidosis, hypothermia, electrolyte
    disturbances
  Obtain C-spine series if not yet done

BEHAVIORAL MEDICINE

ALCOHOLISM

Michael E. Scott
Myra L. Muramoto

Patients with alcohol problems rarely present with a chief complaint of problem drinking. More commonly they exhibit various complications of alcohol abuse. Some are psychological in nature (fatigue, anxiety, depression, insomnia); others are somatic (palpitations, weakness, gastric upset, headaches). Emergency department physicians commonly encounter intoxicated patients brought in by police because of assaultive behavior, public intoxication, or drunk driving. Alcoholism is the primary diagnosis in 25% of suicides. The physician must maintain a *high index of suspicion* to avoid missing this common diagnosis. Consider alcohol-related problems in nearly every patient.

A. History is the key to a diagnosis of alcohol or drug abuse or dependence; however, patients often distort the history and minimize the problem. Denial is a strong defense in all alcohol and drug abusers. It often is necessary to interview family members to obtain accurate information. Review patients' alcohol and drug use history in detail. Look for problems in social (divorce, job loss, family arguments), legal (DUI), and medical (gastritis, peptic ulcer, hepatitis) areas of the patient's life. It is important to identify negative consequences that suggest loss of control and support a diagnosis of dependence. Compulsive use and preoccupation with drinking complete the criteria for dependence or addiction. The mnemonic *CPR* (compulsivity, preoccupation, relapse) is useful for recalling the essential features of dependence. Also review the family history because alcoholism shows strong family trends. Physiologic dependence often is present but not required for the diagnosis of alcohol dependence.

B. Physical examination should be detailed and thorough. Patients with cirrhosis, ascites, edema, rhinophyma, peripheral neuropathy, and jaundice characterize end-stage alcoholism. These patients usually have been drinking uncontrollably for >10 years. Physical complications of alcohol are late findings and may not be evident early in the disease.

C. Laboratory screening can be informative. Look for elevations in aspartate aminotransferase (AST), alanine aminotransferase (ALT), and gamma glutamyltransferase (GGT). Typically, the AST is greater than the ALT. The GGT is a more sensitive indicator of alcohol-induced liver damage. The CBC often shows elevated MCV and MCH with prolonged regular use of alcohol. Hypercholesterolemia and hyperlipidemia often are present. Blood alcohol level >300 mg/dl in an alert patient indicates significant tolerance.

D. Using the data thus far collected, the physician can usually make a diagnosis of alcohol abuse, dependence, or polysubstance dependence. The DSM IV lists the criteria for substance dependence as well as substance abuse. It has been modified and updated from the previous DSM III-R edition. There are now seven criteria for a diagnosis of substance dependence, three of the seven criteria being required for a formal diagnosis. In addition, there are now the categories of with and without physiologic dependence. There are also the addition of specifiers to further clarify the exact course of the illness. The criteria for substance abuse has also been modified from previous versions. There are now four criteria that are diagnostic for substance abuse. Only one of these criteria need be present for the formal diagnosis.

E. Dual diagnosis refers to substance abuse or dependence *plus* another major psychiatric diagnosis such as depression, bipolar disorder, schizophrenia, or anxiety disorder. These patients can be extremely difficult to diagnose and treat because substance abuse often causes many psychiatric syndromes. Psychiatric consultation is suggested. Successful treatment of alcohol problems requires identification and treatment of all other comorbid psychiatric problems.

F. Individualize treatment to the particular patient's needs. Merely telling the patient to quit drinking is futile and potentially dangerous. Consultation with an experienced psychiatrist or addictionist is strongly recommended. Referral to AA or other support group is an excellent place to begin but may not be enough for patients with advanced disease or comorbid psychiatric disorders.

References

Addiction medicine (special issue). Smith DE (special editor). West J Med 1990; 152:502.

American Psychiatric Association. Diagnostic and statistical manual of mental disorders. 4th ed. Washington, DC: American Psychiatric Association, 1994.

Hays JT, Spickard WA Jr. Alcoholism: early diagnosis and intervention. J Gen Intern Med 1987; 2:420.

Milhorn JT Jr. The diagnosis of alcoholism. Am Fam Physician 1988; 37:175.

Schorling JB, Buchsbaum D. Screening for alcohol and drug abuse. Med Clin North Am 1997; 81:845.

Patient with DRINKING PROBLEM

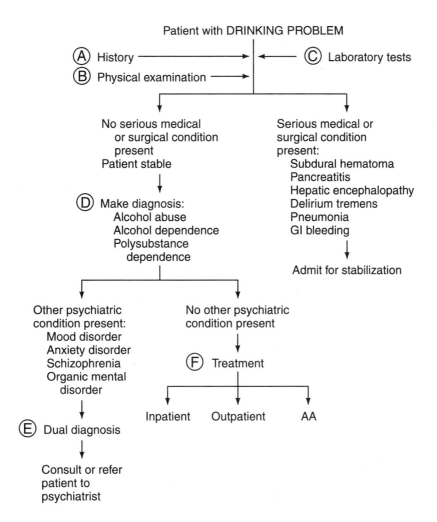

(A) History

(B) Physical examination

(C) Laboratory tests

No serious medical
or surgical condition
present
Patient stable

Serious medical or
surgical condition
present:
    Subdural hematoma
    Pancreatitis
    Hepatic encephalopathy
    Delirium tremens
    Pneumonia
    GI bleeding

(D) Make diagnosis:
    Alcohol abuse
    Alcohol dependence
    Polysubstance
      dependence

Admit for stabilization

Other psychiatric
condition present:
    Mood disorder
    Anxiety disorder
    Schizophrenia
    Organic mental
      disorder

No other psychiatric
condition present

(F) Treatment

(E) Dual diagnosis

Inpatient   Outpatient   AA

Consult or refer
patient to
psychiatrist

ANXIETY

Eric M. Reiman

A. Everyday stressors such as illness, injury, and loss can produce anxiety in patients and their families. Compassion, patience, and understanding can reduce feelings of helplessness and social isolation and increase patients' confidence and self-esteem. A benzodiazepine may be prescribed if patients understand that it is a temporary measure and if they have no history of a psychoactive substance use disorder.

B. Organic factors can produce symptoms of anxiety: for example, patients often experience anxiety during the initial stages of dementia (these patients may respond to sedative-hypnotics with increased anxiety and memory impairment). Diagnose and treat the underlying problem. However, the presence of a nonpsychiatric medical disorder does not always exclude the possibility of a concurrent anxiety disorder.

C. Anxiety is a feature of almost all psychiatric disorders; for example, it is a common symptom of major depression. Diagnose and treat the underlying problem.

D. Panic disorder is characterized by frequent panic attacks, at least some of which occur at unexpected times. Panic attacks are sudden episodes of severe apprehension or fear associated with at least four of the following symptoms: choking sensations, shortness of breath or smothering sensations, palpitations or tachycardia, chest discomfort, dizziness, trembling or shaking, numbness or tingling, hot flashes or chills, sweating, nausea or abdominal distress, feelings of unreality, a fear of dying, and a fear of going crazy or losing control. Look for abrupt onset (maximal intensity within 10 minutes of onset) and short duration (typically, 2–30 minutes). Many patients see cardiologists or emergency physicians seeking a medical explanation of the problem. Indeed, they account for >30% of patients with atypical or nonanginal chest pain. Several medications can block anxiety attacks, including selective serotonin reuptake inhibitors (SSRIs), such as paroxetine, and tricyclic antidepressants, such as imipramine (start low, go slow, warn the patient of an exacerbation in symptoms early in treatment); monoamine oxidase (MAO) inhibitors, such as phenelzine (provide a list of dietary and medication restrictions); and high-potency benzodiazepines, such as clonazepam (use standing doses to prevent attacks, warn patients about withdrawal symptoms and the related need for slow discontinuation, and avoid in patients with a history of a psychoactive substance use disorder). Recent evidence suggests that cognitive-behavioral therapy can prevent anxiety attacks as effectively as medication in patients with panic disorder. This standardized, short-term treatment should be administered by a well-trained professional; it is designed to help patients identify and revise the habit of responding to normally innocuous physical sensations as dangerous. Once the panic attacks are addressed, patients who have panic disorder with agoraphobia are encouraged to confront and learn to overcome their fears through repeated, frequent, intense exposures to the feared situations.

E. Phobias, irrational fears that are recognized by the individual as excessive, are extremely common. Agoraphobia is an irrational fear of situations from which it may be difficult or embarrassing to escape. Always consider the possibility of panic attacks in patients with this disorder. Social phobia is an excessive fear of being scrutinized in performance or social situations. Distinguish individuals who have the circumscribed type of social phobia (those who fear one particular performance situation, such as public speaking) from those who have generalized social phobia (excessively shy individuals who fear a variety of performance and social situations). Specific phobia is an irrational fear of particular objects or situations (e.g., animals, closed places, heights). Exposure therapy encourages patients to gradually confront and learn to overcome the feared object, activity, or situation; frequency, duration, and intensity of exposures are directly related to outcome. Prescribe a benzodiazepine if patients understand that it is a temporary measure and if there is no history of a psychoactive substance use disorder. Circumscribed social phobia may respond to adjunctive use of a β blocker or a benzodiazepine; the best established treatments for the generalized type of social phobia include SSRIs, MAO inhibitors, standing doses of the high-potency benzodiazepine clonazepam, and cognitive-behavioral group therapy.

(Continued on page 546)

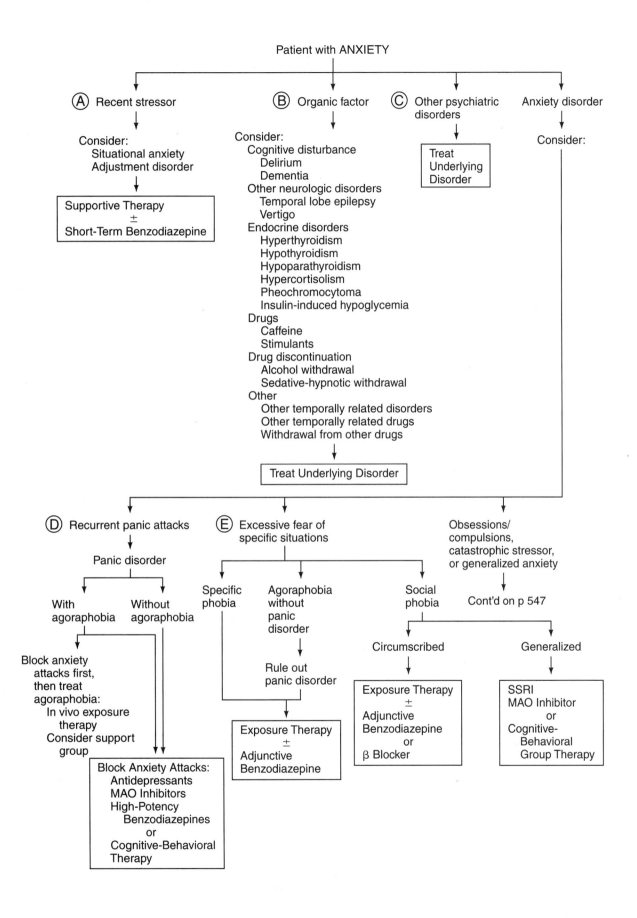

Patient with ANXIETY

(A) Recent stressor

Consider:
  Situational anxiety
  Adjustment disorder

Supportive Therapy
±
Short-Term Benzodiazepine

(B) Organic factor

Consider:
  Cognitive disturbance
    Delirium
    Dementia
  Other neurologic disorders
    Temporal lobe epilepsy
    Vertigo
  Endocrine disorders
    Hyperthyroidism
    Hypothyroidism
    Hypoparathyroidism
    Hypercortisolism
    Pheochromocytoma
    Insulin-induced hypoglycemia
  Drugs
    Caffeine
    Stimulants
  Drug discontinuation
    Alcohol withdrawal
    Sedative-hypnotic withdrawal
  Other
    Other temporally related disorders
    Other temporally related drugs
    Withdrawal from other drugs

Treat Underlying Disorder

(C) Other psychiatric disorders

Treat
Underlying
Disorder

Anxiety disorder

Consider:

(D) Recurrent panic attacks

Panic disorder

With agoraphobia

Without agoraphobia

Block anxiety attacks first, then treat agoraphobia:
  In vivo exposure therapy
  Consider support group

Block Anxiety Attacks:
  Antidepressants
  MAO Inhibitors
  High-Potency Benzodiazepines
  or
  Cognitive-Behavioral Therapy

(E) Excessive fear of specific situations

Specific phobia

Agoraphobia without panic disorder

Rule out panic disorder

Exposure Therapy
±
Adjunctive Benzodiazepine

Social phobia

Circumscribed

Exposure Therapy
±
Adjunctive Benzodiazepine
or
β Blocker

Obsessions/ compulsions, catastrophic stressor, or generalized anxiety

Cont'd on p 547

Generalized

SSRI
MAO Inhibitor
or
Cognitive-Behavioral Group Therapy

F. Obsessions are recurrent, intrusive, unwanted ideas that insistently enter the mind; they are distressing and typically recognized as senseless by the individual. Compulsions are repetitive, ritualistic behaviors typically performed to neutralize an obsession and reduce distress; most of these individuals recognize that their behaviors are unreasonable and excessive. The Yale-Brown Obsessive Compulsive Scale Symptom Checklist may help identify additional obsessions and compulsions in these patients. Many patients benefit from a trial of an SSRI or the non-SSRI clomipramine (often at higher dosages than that used to treat other disorders); behavioral therapy (e.g., a structured, short-term protocol that involves repeated exposure to the obsession-eliciting situation together with a mandate to suppress anxiety-reducing compulsions); or a combination of the two. Some patients benefit from participation in a support group. Rarely, consider stereotactic surgery, such as bilateral anterior cingulotomy, in patients with extremely disabling symptoms that are unresponsive to the arsenal of more conventional treatments.

G. Consider acute stress disorder (lasting <1 month) or post-traumatic stress disorder (PTSD, lasting >1 month) in individuals who have been exposed to traumatic events associated with a threat of injury or death to self or others and feelings of intense fear, helplessness, or horror (e.g., rape, accidental or natural disasters, military combat). Symptoms include reexperiences of the traumatic event (e.g., recurrent thoughts, nightmares, flashbacks, and distress in response to reminders of the event); avoidance behaviors (e.g., avoidance of thoughts, feelings, or situations associated with the event); restrictions in emotion and interpersonal relationships; and increased arousal (e.g., insomnia, irritability, or hypervigilance). Consider individual or group psychotherapy to increase self-esteem, decrease social isolation, and support coping resources; SSRIs, other antidepressants of PTSD or MAO inhibitors to reduce symptoms or associated depression; and referral for participation in a structured program of behavioral therapy, one that involves frequent imagined exposures to the stressor.

H. Generalized anxiety disorder is a diagnosis of exclusion. Ask, "Have you worried excessively about everyday matters (e.g., work, school, family, and finances) most of the day more days than not for at least 6 months?" Consider the other disorders in the decision tree (e.g., panic disorder, major depression) first. Consider an antidepressant such as venlafaxine or imipramine first; the nonbenzodiazepine anxiolytic buspirone second; use benzodiazepines sparingly, especially in patients with cognitive impairment or a psychoactive substance use disorder; and discontinue medications that fail to work. Although nonmedication treatments do not yet have established value, interventions are now being studied which target the hallmark feature of worry.

References

American Psychiatric Association. Diagnostic and statistical manual of mental disorders. 4th ed. Washington, DC: American Psychiatric Association, 1994.

Hyman SE, Arana GW. Handbook of psychiatric drug therapy. 3rd ed. Boston: Little, Brown, 1995.

Barlow DH. Anxiety and its disorders: the nature and treatment of anxiety and panic. New York: Guilford Press, 1988.

Reiman EM. Anxiety. In: Gelenberg AJ, Bassuk EL, eds. Practitioner's guide to psychoactive drugs. 4th ed. New York: Plenum, 1997.

Roth WT, Yalom D. Treating anxiety disorders. Boston: Jossey-Bass, 1996.

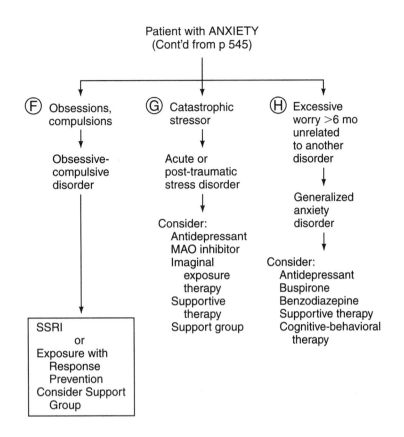

Patient with ANXIETY
(Cont'd from p 545)

Ⓕ Obsessions, compulsions

Obsessive-compulsive disorder

SSRI
or
Exposure with Response Prevention
Consider Support Group

Ⓖ Catastrophic stressor

Acute or post-traumatic stress disorder

Consider:
Antidepressant
MAO inhibitor
Imaginal exposure therapy
Supportive therapy
Support group

Ⓗ Excessive worry >6 mo unrelated to another disorder

Generalized anxiety disorder

Consider:
Antidepressant
Buspirone
Benzodiazepine
Supportive therapy
Cognitive-behavioral therapy

DEPRESSION

Iris R. Bell

Mood disorders, especially dysphoria, occur in 5% of the general population, with women and persons aged 25–44 years most at risk. The full syndrome of major depression carries significant morbidity and mortality in terms of suicide risk and poorer outcome of concomitant medical disorders. Many patients with depression present first to the primary care physician with somatic concerns and seek a medical diagnosis or treatment for anxiety or "nerves," while the proper diagnosis and treatment often are overlooked.

A. Depression is a clinical syndrome without a specific laboratory test to confirm the diagnosis; comprehensive clinical assessments provide the main data.

B. Criteria for diagnosis of major depression include at least five of nine symptoms present daily or almost daily during the same 2-week period and indicative of a change from previous functioning. Symptoms are (1) depressed mood, (2) markedly reduced interest or pleasure in activities, (3) significant weight loss or gain or decrease or increase in appetite, (4) insomnia or hypersomnia, (5) psychomotor agitation or retardation, (6) fatigue or low energy, (7) feelings of worthlessness or inordinate guilt, (8) difficulty concentrating or indecisiveness, and (9) recurrent thoughts of death or suicide or a suicide attempt. Broad differential diagnosis must include organic mood disorder, depressed, and a major depression.

C. A screening battery of laboratory tests helps rule out specific organic causes. In combination with the history and physical examination, findings may suggest more specific laboratory studies (see D). Specialized tests sensitive but not specific to major depression include the dexamethasone suppression test, the thyrotropin-releasing hormone stimulation test, and polysomnography.

D. Differential diagnosis for organic causes includes substance abuse and prescription drugs such as antihypertensives, hormones, analgesics, anticancer drugs, antiparkinsonian drugs, antianxiety and hypnotic drugs, GI drugs; endocrine and metabolic disorders (especially thyroid and adrenal); nutritional deficiencies (vitamins B_1, niacin, folate, B_{12}); and heavy metal toxicity (e.g., lead). Depression in alcoholics may resolve with abstinence. Depressive symptoms follow stroke in up to 60% of cases within 2 years. Treatment of underlying medical problems may lead to resolution of depression; if not, standard antidepressant treatment strategies often are effective.

E. Initial antidepressant regimens often involve selective serotonin reuptake inhibitors (SSRIs: fluoxetine, sertraline, paroxetine), especially in medically complex patients. Secondary amine tricyclics (nortriptyline, desipramine), whose side effects are better tolerated than those of amitriptyline or doxepin, are an important alternative, especially for comorbid chronic pain. If SSRIs and tricyclics fail or are contraindicated, other choices include bupropion, nefazodone, venlafaxine, or monoamine oxidase inhibitors (MAOIs: phenelzine, tranylcypromine). Low-dose trazodone is sometimes used for insomnia, in combination with activating agents such as fluoxetine. Choose medication to target symptoms (e.g., agitated vs. retarded) and address side effect profile. Watch for drug interactions with fluoxetine and MAOIs. MAOIs necessitate a tyramine free diet. Stimulants may mobilize apathetic, medically ill patients, but their long-term efficacy for major depression is uncertain.

F. Up to 50% of unipolar depressed patients with partial or no response to an antidepressant alone may respond more fully to the addition of lithium. More controversial augmentation strategies include buspirone supplementation (especially in agitated depression), thyroid supplementation, combination fluoxetine with tricyclic, and combination MAOI with tricyclic; the last two approaches involve a significant risk of drug interactions.

G. Growing evidence suggests that bright light therapy may suffice in some cases of winter depression; more standard somatic therapies also are effective.

H. Recent studies have shown the need for a combination of antidepressant and antipsychotic drugs rather than single-agent therapy to treat psychotic depression.

I. Bipolar patients may switch into manic episodes during treatment with antidepressant medications alone. This may necessitate concomitant coverage with lithium or another mood-stabilizing agent (e.g., divalproex, carbamazepine). Anecdotal evidence suggests possible usefulness of bupropion in treating bipolar depressions.

J. Electroconvulsive therapy is the most effective treatment for major depression, especially the subtype with psychotic features. It is the treatment of choice for acute suicidality, severe cachexia and dehydration secondary to poor intake, many medically complex major depressions, and antidepressant medication failures.

K. A chronic course of at least 2 years and a less severe depressive picture suggests a dysthymic disorder, which can co-occur with major depression. Dysphoria or fluctuating mood instability are characteristic of a range of chronic personality disorders that vary in their responsiveness to psychotherapeutic interventions.

L. An identifiable stressor, maladaptive symptoms lasting <6 months, and a generally less severe depressive picture suggest an adjustment disorder with depressed mood, which usually resolves with time and supportive psychotherapy.

(Continued on page 550)

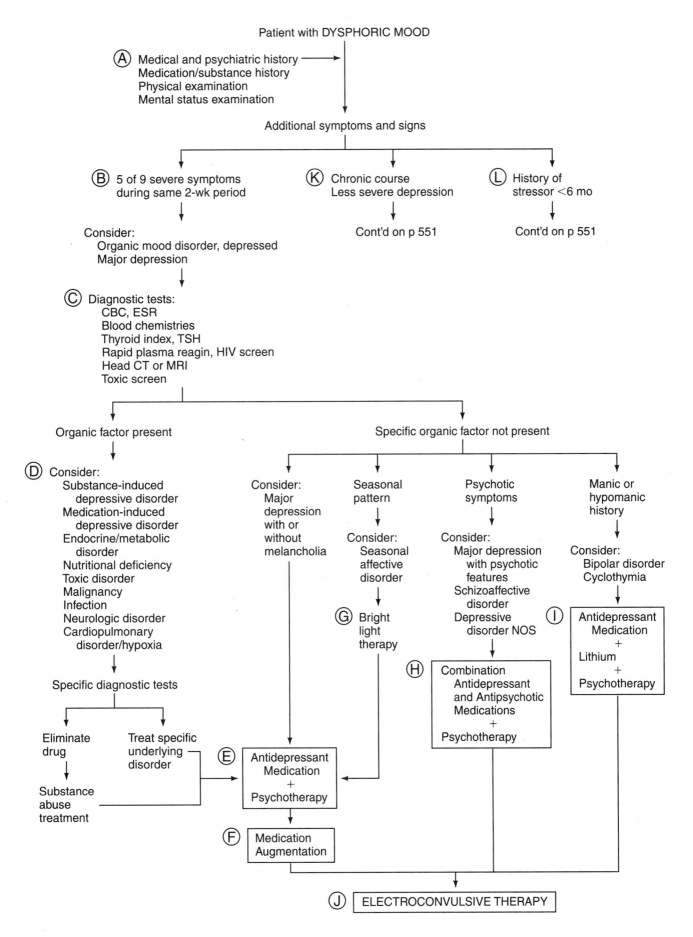

Patient with DYSPHORIC MOOD

Ⓐ Medical and psychiatric history
Medication/substance history
Physical examination
Mental status examination

Additional symptoms and signs

Ⓑ 5 of 9 severe symptoms
during same 2-wk period

Ⓚ Chronic course
Less severe depression

Cont'd on p 551

Ⓛ History of
stressor <6 mo

Cont'd on p 551

Consider:
Organic mood disorder, depressed
Major depression

Ⓒ Diagnostic tests:
CBC, ESR
Blood chemistries
Thyroid index, TSH
Rapid plasma reagin, HIV screen
Head CT or MRI
Toxic screen

Organic factor present

Specific organic factor not present

Ⓓ Consider:
Substance-induced
depressive disorder
Medication-induced
depressive disorder
Endocrine/metabolic
disorder
Nutritional deficiency
Toxic disorder
Malignancy
Infection
Neurologic disorder
Cardiopulmonary
disorder/hypoxia

Consider:
Major
depression
with or
without
melancholia

Seasonal
pattern

Consider:
Seasonal
affective
disorder

Psychotic
symptoms

Consider:
Major depression
with psychotic
features
Schizoaffective
disorder
Depressive
disorder NOS

Manic or
hypomanic
history

Consider:
Bipolar disorder
Cyclothymia

Specific diagnostic tests

Ⓖ Bright
light
therapy

Ⓘ Antidepressant
Medication
+
Lithium
+
Psychotherapy

Eliminate
drug

Treat specific
underlying
disorder

Ⓗ Combination
Antidepressant
and Antipsychotic
Medications
+
Psychotherapy

Substance
abuse
treatment

Ⓔ Antidepressant
Medication
+
Psychotherapy

Ⓕ Medication
Augmentation

Ⓙ ELECTROCONVULSIVE THERAPY

References

Brown SA, Inaba RK, Gillin JC, et al. Alcoholism and affective disorder: clinical course of depressive symptoms. Am J Psychiatry 1995; 152:45.

Charney DS, Miller HL, Licinio J, Salomon R. Treatment of depression. In: Schatzberg AF, Nemeroff CB, eds. Textbook of psychopharmacology. Washington, DC: American Psychiatric Press, 1995:575.

Cole S, Raju M. Making the diagnosis of depression in the primary care setting. Am J Med 1996; 101:10S.

Fava GA, Grandi S, Zielezny M, et al. Four-year outcome for cognitive behavioral treatment of residual symptoms in major depression. Am J Psychiatry 1996; 153:945.

Klerman GL, Weissman MM. The course, morbidity, and costs of depression. Arch Gen Psychiatry 1992; 49:831.

McCoy DM. Treatment considerations for depression in patients with significant medical comorbidity. J Fam Practice 1996; 43(6 suppl):S35.

Nierenberg AA. Treatment choice after one antidepressant fails: a survey of Northeastern psychiatrists. J Clin Psychiatry 1991; 52:383.

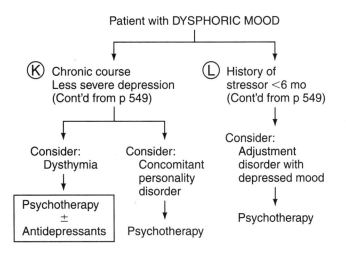

Patient with DYSPHORIC MOOD

Ⓚ Chronic course
Less severe depression
(Cont'd from p 549)

Consider:
Dysthymia

Psychotherapy
±
Antidepressants

Consider:
Concomitant
personality
disorder

Psychotherapy

Ⓛ History of
stressor <6 mo
(Cont'd from p 549)

Consider:
Adjustment
disorder with
depressed mood

Psychotherapy

EMOTIONAL DISORDERS WITH SOMATIC EXPRESSION

John Misiaszek

Patients with emotionally based somatic complaints are largely unaware of their emotional conflicts. Often labeled as "crocks," they receive poor and fragmented treatment, although their tendency to express their emotional conflicts through somatizing behavior does not immunize them against bona fide physical illness. Furthermore, many physical disorders such as thyroid disease, multiple sclerosis, and temporal lobe epilepsy may initially or primarily present as an emotional disorder, causing delays in diagnosis and treatment. The physical, emotional, and iatrogenic morbidity of patients who somaticize their psychic distress can be largely reduced by having a physician provide consistency, support, and reassurance while minimizing invasive procedures and redundant evaluations. These patients are emotionally impaired; rejection serves only to heighten their impairment.

A. The medical history should include a review for similar, previously undiagnosed disorders in the patient and family members. Often the somaticizing coping behavior has been modeled or reinforced earlier in life. Early traumatic emotional development may result in more severe somatoform expression such as a factitious disorder. Personal or family history also may suggest a proclivity for one of the major psychiatric disorders.

B. Patients with acute or chronic psychoses may have bizarre somatic complaints (e.g., an alien force has turned their intestines inside out). Their overall thought disturbance is readily manifest in their report. It is sometimes difficult to differentiate between the complaint as a delusion or a symbolic and personalized interpretation of a genuine physical discomfort. Patients with psychotic depression or monodelusional disorders (e.g., delusions of parasitosis) may have more focused or fixed somatic concerns that may or may not diminish when treated with high-potency antipsychotics such as haloperidol or pimozide.

C. Although delirious or demented patients may misperceive or fabricate somatic symptoms, their primary psychiatric problem is differentiated from "functional psychosis" by the presence of periodic or persistent confusion and disorientation. Antipsychotic medication may decrease the somatic delusions and behavioral difficulties, but treatment of the underlying disorder may be curative.

D. Depression may be masked by a complaint of headache or generalized fatigue. Vegetative signs of depression may be variably present, along with diminished self-esteem and a depressive affect; these often precede or coincide with somatic sensations. A primary depression must be distinguished from a secondary (or reactive) depression that is a result, not the cause, of a somatic problem.

E. Patients with a generalized anxiety disorder have a variety of somatic symptoms: tachycardia, motor tension, autonomic hyperactivity. Patients with panic attacks may fear cardiac or pulmonary disorders. A primary anxiety disorder needs to be differentiated from a secondary apprehension about a physical symptom.

F. A hypochondriacal reaction is distinguished from classical hypochondriasis in that it follows a recent stressful event, is short-lived, and responds to reassurance. Examples include an individual who is concerned about minor chest discomfort after a cardiac-related death of a close friend, a medical student who has a phobia about the "disease of the day," and a luncheon crowd's hysteria in response to the erroneous report of a food-poisoning victim in their midst.

G. Conversion disorder is likely if there is loss or alteration in physical function after a stressful event. The resultant psychic conflict is not readily apparent to the individual or evaluator. The diagnosis also requires that the physical problem cannot be explained by a known physical disorder. "La belle indifference" has been widely overstated as a characteristic symptom and is of little diagnostic value. Use caution when assigning this diagnosis. Studies show that 13–30% of patients so diagnosed later develop physical problems that could have explained their original physical complaint.

H. Conscious deceit is subdivided into malingering when secondary gain is apparent, and factitious disorder when reasons for the deceit are not understood by the patient or the physician. A military draft inductee who feigns a disorder to avoid conscription is malingering, whereas patients with factitious disorders (e.g., Munchausen's syndrome) have complex, convoluted reasons for faking somatic disorders, are angry and emotionally traumatized, have unsettled lives, and displace hostility onto others. They are difficult patients to treat either medically or psychiatrically; confrontation in the absence of a comprehensive medical psychiatric treatment plan rarely works and risks escalating maladaptive behavior.

I. Hypochondriasis is the misinterpretation of physical signs or sensations as serious disease. Patients typically are fearful, do not respond readily to support and reassurance, return for further evaluation and treatment, or seek other physicians. These patients have been described as hostile, masochistic, and demanding individuals who deny their needs for dependence, or (less commonly) individuals who are clinging, passive, and overtly dependent in their relationship with their doctor. Related terms are *somatization disorder,* in which patients develop multiple "review of systems" complaints as an early life-coping mechanism, and

Patient with ILL-DEFINED PHYSICAL COMPLAINTS
(Previous or Recent Evaluations Are Noncontributory)

Ⓐ Review medical and psychiatric history →
Physical examination

- Evidence of major psychiatric disorder
  - Bizzarre complaints or behavior
    - Sensorium clear
      - Ⓑ Consider:
        Acute psychosis
        Schizophrenia
        Delusional disorder
        Psychotic depression
        ↓
        Psychiatric referral
    - Sensorium confused
      - Ⓒ Consider:
        Delirium
        Dementia
        ↓
        Identify and treat underlying cause
  - Plausible complaints
    - Ⓓ Primary depression
      - Antidepressant Medication Trial
        ↓
        Psychiatric consultation if no response
    - Ⓔ Primary anxiety disorder
      - Stress management
        Relaxation exercises
        Judicious use of benzodiazepines or buspirone trial
- No evidence of major psychiatric disorder

- Recent stress
  - Ⓕ Reactive hypochondriasis
    - Removal from stress
      Emotional support and reassurance
  - Ⓖ Conversion disorder
    - Removal from stress
      Supportive emotional and physical interventions
      Positive suggestion
- No recent stress
  - Ⓗ Evidence of deceit
    - Evidence of secondary gain
      ↓
      Malingering
      ↓
      Confrontation
      Notification of involved health providers
    - No obvious secondary gain
      ↓
      Factitious disorder
      ↓
      Avoidance of unnecessary procedures
      Firm but supportive management
      Psychiatric consultation
  - No evidence of deceit
    - Ⓙ Undiagnosed physical disorder
    - Ⓘ Hypochondriasis or related disorder
      ↓
      Support and reassurance
      Avoidance of procedures or multiple physician contacts

References

somatoform pain disorder, when pain is the specific hypochondriacal concern.

J. The absence of a physical finding or inability to establish a physical diagnosis by itself is insufficient for a diagnosis of a major psychiatric or somatoform disorder. These diagnoses can be made only when the associated psychiatric characteristics are present and when the dysfunction and somatic problems are a consequence of such characteristics. Because life stress or misfortune is found in most medical patients and nonpatients alike, take care not to magnify such occurrences when there is no obvious connection to the physical impairment.

Barsky AJ. Hypochondriasis: medical management and psychiatric treatment. Psychosomatics 1996; 37:48.

Barsky AJ, Stern TA, Greenberg DB, Cassem NH. Functional somatic symptoms and somatoform disorders. In: Cassem NH, ed. Massachusetts General Hospital handbook of general hospital psychiatry. 4th ed. St Louis: Mosby, 1997:305.

Ekkehard D. Somatization disorder. Psychiatr Ann 1988; 18:330.

Ford CV. The somatizing disorders: illness as a way of life. New York: Elsevier, 1983.

Gerdes TT, Noyes R Jr, Kathal RG, et al. Physician recognition of hypochondriacal patients. Gen Hosp Psychiatry 1996; 18:106.

GRIEF

Gail L. Schwartz

A. Normal grief responses vary. The process of grieving may be seen as occurring in three stages: initial shock or numbing, acute mourning, and a period of resolution or recovery. A lack of perceived social support is one predictor of difficulty in recovery. Those seen as grieving most intensely early in the bereavement may have a poorer outcome after 1 year than those with a relative absence of mourning. There is little evidence to support the efficacy of treatment for people experiencing uncomplicated bereavement.

B. Neurovegetative symptoms of depression are common in bereavement. Sleep disturbance may last for up to 1 year. Appetite usually returns within 4 months after the loss. However, motor retardation, ruminative guilt, and a feeling of worthlessness are not typical symptoms of bereavement and suggest the need for psychiatric evaluation and treatment.

C. Persistent symptoms of anxiety and depression warrant a more detailed psychiatric evaluation. Clinically depressed patients are most often treated with a combination of antidepressant medication and psychotherapy.

D. More than 40% of bereaved spouses have at least one type of anxiety disorder during the first year of bereavement. A history of anxiety disorder is a strong predictor of its presenting during bereavement. Anxiety symptoms include somatic distress, obsessions and compulsions, phobias, and panic attacks.

E. Antidepressants are useful in the treatment of most anxiety disorders and may be preferred to benzodiazepines because of the lack of dependence potential.

F. A history of an addictive disorder is a strong predictor of substance abuse during grieving. Because there is a significant risk of morbidity and mortality with substance abuse, it is imperative that a careful history be taken and that bothersome symptoms of anxiety and sleeplessness be treated nonpharmacologically or with medications that have minimal addiction potential.

G. In normal grief the intensity of the emotional pain gradually decreases; significant resolution occurs by 1 year. Theories of attachment behavior have been used to explain the difficulties that complicate the grieving process for some people (Table 1).

H. It is suggested that expressive psychotherapy is most appropriate for conflicted grief syndromes, cognitive treatment may be particularly useful for dependent grief syndrome, and treatments developed specifically for persons with post-traumatic stress disorder may be most useful for those who have had a sudden, unexpected loss.

References

Clayton PJ. Bereavement and depression. J Clin Psychiatry 1990; 51(suppl):34.

Crow HE. How to help patients understand and conquer grief: avoiding depression in the midst of sadness. Postgrad Med 1991; 89:117.

Kim K, Jacobs S. Pathologic grief and its relationship to other psychiatric disorders. J Affect Disord 1991; 21:257.

Middleton W. Bereavement. Psychiatr Clin North Am 1987; 10:329.

Rosenzweig A, Prigerson H, Miller MD, Reynold CF 3rd. Bereavement and late-life depression: grief and its complications in the elderly. Annu Rev Med 1997; 48:421.

Rynearson EK. Psychotherapy of pathologic grief. Psychiatr Clin North Am 1987; 10:487.

Zisook S. Anxiety and bereavement. Psychiatr Med 1990; 8:83.

Zisook S, Schuchter SR, Sledge PA, et al. The spectrum of depressive phenomena after spousal bereavement. J Clin Psychiatry 1994; 55(suppl):29.

TABLE 1 Pathologic Grief Syndromes

Dependent	A stable sense of self depends on presence of the lost person
Unexpected loss	A post-traumatic stress syndrome with hyper-reactivity, intrusive memories, and nightmares alternating with affect constriction and numbing
Conflicted	Ambivalence toward the lost person is unacceptable, and the grieving person turns the negative feelings on himself or herself

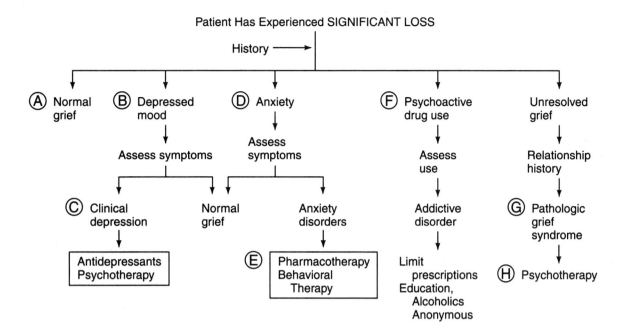

PSYCHOSIS

Alan J. Gelenberg

A psychotic episode is typified by deranged thinking, speech, and behavior, often manifesting as hallucinations (false sensory impressions: visual, auditory, olfactory, gustatory, tactile), delusions (false fixed beliefs), difficulty distinguishing reality from fantasy, disorganized thinking, and strange and inappropriate behavior.

A. Confronted with an acutely psychotic patient, the first task is to ensure the safety of the patient and others against injury or possible death. A calm, low-stimulus environment with nonthreatening behavior by staff is essential. Force should not be threatened unless overwhelming force is available. The patient should not be left alone and an examining physician should be accompanied by at least one other person. Some patients may need to be restrained. Patients should be questioned about any thoughts of suicide or injuring others, which must be taken extremely seriously.

B. A medical history is essential in the evaluation of a psychotic patient. Given the patient's mental status, the most valuable information will probably come from others who know him or her. Inquire about the time course of the emerging bizarre behavior and possible relation to any medical conditions, recent-onset physical symptoms, exposure to infectious or toxic agents, medication use, drug abuse, or recent surgery or trauma.

C. Possible medical causes of acute psychotic behavior should be considered and ruled out immediately. Despite the difficulties, perform as complete a physical examination as possible, including pupils and, to the extent possible, fundi. Examine carefully the patient's entire body for evidence of trauma, substance abuse, or disease. Staring or stereotypic motor behavior may suggest a seizure-related state and the advisability of obtaining an EEG.

D. Address such readily treatable (and potentially hazardous) conditions as hypoglycemia by such means as immediate drawing of blood followed by IV injection of a concentrated dextrose solution.

E. If the history (usually from others), a careful physical examination, and indicated laboratory tests fail to reveal any organic causes of psychosis, consider a psychiatric differential diagnosis.

F. Schizophrenia is a lifelong chronic condition marked by acute psychotic episodes interspersed with periods of less disturbed but still abnormal behavior. Between episodes, schizophrenics often show poor motivation and social awkwardness. Acute schizophrenic episodes are typically treated with antipsychotic agents, which usually are maintained at lower dosages to mitigate the likelihood and severity of future episodes. Now, more patients with schizophrenia are taking newer-generation antipsychotic drugs such as clozapine (Clozaril), risperidone (Risperdal), olanzapine (Zyprexa), and quetiapine (Seroquel). It is unclear whether these drugs are as able as traditional antipsychotics to suppress acutely emergent psychotic behavior. Moreover, to date, newer agents do not come in parenteral form. Use benzodiazepine sedation as needed as an adjunct to antipsychotic drugs during acute episodes.

G. Mania often presents as an acute psychosis. A history typically reveals past episodes of mania or major depression. A mental status examination shows the patient to be highly excited, emotionally labile, overtalkative, pressured in speech, hypersexual, and with grandiose ideas. Acute treatment consists of antipsychotic drugs as needed, often with adjunctive lithium. Divalproex (Depakote) increasingly is being used to suppress acute symptoms of mania. Lithium is the mainstay therapy for most bipolar (manic-depressive) patients. Carbamazepine (Tegretol and others) and newer anticonvulsants (notably gabapentin [Neurontin] and lamotrigine [Lamictal]) are coming into use also. Electroconvulsive therapy (ECT) usually is effective for patients who fail to benefit or cannot tolerate these medications. Use benzodiazepines adjunctively to control an acute episode.

H. Psychotic depression may become manifest either as a recurrent mood disorder itself or as an episode in the course of a bipolar illness. Delusions and hallucinations commonly manifest such depressive themes as guilt and punishment. Effective treatments include ECT and combined antipsychotic and antidepressant drugs. Clozapine and possibly other new antipsychotics may be especially helpful in treating psychotic depression. Guard against suicide, an omnipresent hazard in these patients.

I. Delusional (paranoid) disorder is a chronic condition characterized by a fixed and focused delusional system in the midst of otherwise intact thinking. It often is refractory to biologic and psychologic treatments.

J. Demented patients often manifest psychotic behaviors that can complicate long-term management. Rule out acute medical conditions, and if possible, handle disruptive behaviors through behavioral and environmental means. If this is not possible, low dosages of antipsychotic drugs may assist management.

References

American Psychiatric Association. Treatment of psychiatric disorders: a task force of the American Psychiatric Association. Washington, DC: American Psychiatric Association, 1989:1485, 1655, 1725.

Gelenberg AJ, Keith SJ: Psychosis. In: Gelenberg AJ, Bassak EL, eds. The practitioner's guide to psychoactive drugs. 4th ed. New York: Plenum, 1997.

Kaplan HI, Sadock BJ, eds. Comprehensive textbook of psychiatry. 6th ed. Baltimore: Williams & Wilkins, 1994.

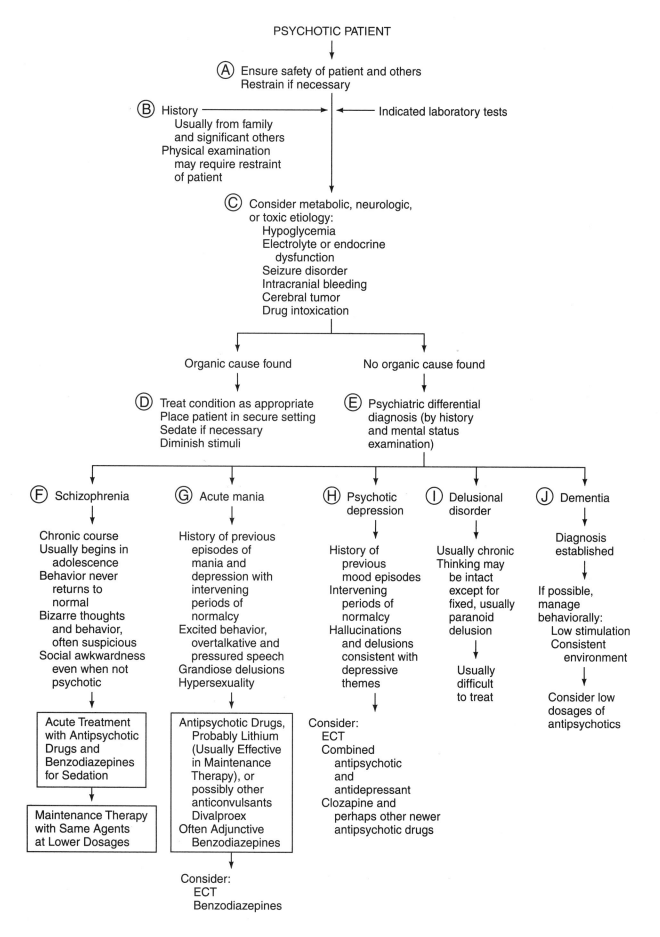

PSYCHOTIC PATIENT

Ⓐ Ensure safety of patient and others
Restrain if necessary

Ⓑ History ⟶ ← Indicated laboratory tests
Usually from family
and significant others
Physical examination
may require restraint
of patient

Ⓒ Consider metabolic, neurologic,
or toxic etiology:
Hypoglycemia
Electrolyte or endocrine
dysfunction
Seizure disorder
Intracranial bleeding
Cerebral tumor
Drug intoxication

Organic cause found   No organic cause found

Ⓓ Treat condition as appropriate   Ⓔ Psychiatric differential
Place patient in secure setting   diagnosis (by history
Sedate if necessary   and mental status
Diminish stimuli   examination)

Ⓕ Schizophrenia   Ⓖ Acute mania   Ⓗ Psychotic   Ⓘ Delusional   Ⓙ Dementia
                                      depression   disorder

Chronic course   History of previous   History of   Usually chronic   Diagnosis
Usually begins in   episodes of   previous   Thinking may   established
  adolescence   mania and   mood episodes   be intact
Behavior never   depression with   Intervening   except for   If possible,
  returns to   intervening   periods of   fixed, usually   manage
  normal   periods of   normalcy   paranoid   behaviorally:
Bizarre thoughts   normalcy   Hallucinations   delusion   Low stimulation
  and behavior,   Excited behavior,   and delusions   Consistent
  often suspicious   overtalkative and   consistent with Usually   environment
Social awkwardness   pressured speech   depressive   difficult
  even when not   Grandiose delusions   themes   to treat   Consider low
  psychotic   Hypersexuality   dosages of
                                                                                antipsychotics

Acute Treatment   Antipsychotic Drugs,   Consider:
with Antipsychotic Probably Lithium   ECT
Drugs and   (Usually Effective   Combined
Benzodiazepines   in Maintenance   antipsychotic
for Sedation   Therapy), or   and
                     possibly other   antidepressant
Maintenance Therapy anticonvulsants   Clozapine and
with Same Agents   Divalproex   perhaps other newer
at Lower Dosages   Often Adjunctive   antipsychotic drugs
                     Benzodiazepines

                    Consider:
                     ECT
                     Benzodiazepines

557

SMOKING CESSATION

Harry L. Greene II
Lawrence A. Garcia

The Surgeon General has determined that the leading preventable cause of death and disability in the United States is cigarette smoking. Annually, 3 million deaths worldwide are attributed to smoking. This toll is expected to reach 10 million by 2025. Although 75% of all adults visit a physician at least once a year, smokers visit more often because of increased illness. The first step in smoking cessation is to identify the smoker by simply asking: "Do you smoke?" Although a few may be evasive about their smoking, most admit it, and surveys show that 80% say they would like to quit.

A. Congratulate patients who are nonsmokers. Counsel preteenagers and teenagers about peer pressure, targeted advertising, and the fallacy of smoking as a way to be more grown-up. Encourage those who have quit to maintain their cessation.

B. Inform smokers of the adverse health consequences of smoking and the benefits of stopping, emphasize the damage or disease already present, motivate them to consider quitting, and give firm and unequivocal advice to quit. Judith Ockene of the University of Massachusetts recommends using guided questions such as "Are you aware of the effects of smoking on your health?" Make the patient aware of any physical findings that are present and related to smoking, in an effort to personalize the effects of smoking. Mention the benefits of quitting now, including lower risk of cancer, sudden death, or myocardial infarction (MI) and longer active life (at any age). Many smokers are fatalistic and unaware of the reversibility of smoking-related disease and risk. Make a statement such as: "As your physician, I must advise you that smoking is bad for your health."

C. One can sense whether a patient is contemplating quitting by asking questions such as: "How do you feel about being a smoker? What reasons do you have to quit? Were you able to stop smoking in the past? How did you do it that time? What caused you to start again? If you had that chance again what would you do differently?" The purpose of these questions is to allow insight, build confidence, problem solve, and begin a plan for a new successful cessation attempt. A critical series of questions are next posed: "Have you thought about stopping? Do you think you can stop now? How will you do it?"

D. At this point, some patients do not show adequate motivation or are unwilling to discuss or plan a cessation attempt. These people often lack the confidence that they can be successful and are unwilling to risk their self-esteem if they fail. Some investigators believe that these patients should sign a waiver stating they have been informed of the risks and for the moment are choosing to smoke against the physician's advice. They can be given a brochure to read and the subject can be broached again on subsequent visits. Watch for a possible critical incident (e.g., acute illness; MI in patient, friend, or relative; cancer; pregnancy; death of a valued person) as a time when contemplation can be changed to action.

E. Ambivalent patients often are unwilling to choose a quit date or sign a contract to quit but may be willing to do other things. A smoking diary can help document when, where, what they were doing, with whom, and the value of the cigarette from 1 (crucial) to 5 (not very important). The diary helps build awareness. It can be accompanied by tapering (i.e., eliminating the not very important cigarettes). Other techniques include switching to cigarettes with lower tar and nicotine content and smoking fewer each day. These measures are mainly directed at building confidence for a successful cessation attempt. Until patients are ready to change it is better not to court failure.

F. For patients ready to quit, a quit date should be set and a contract signed. These can be preprinted or simply written in the chart. The contract can serve as an additional reminder if it is on duplicate paper with a chart copy and another copy placed in a prominent location selected by the patient (e.g., refrigerator, mirror). Some patients may keep a smoking diary for a few days to increase awareness of when, where, and why they smoke. Once the quit date is chosen, develop an action plan in conjunction with the patient to determine who will be the support people at home and at work and how weight gain will be handled (increased exercise, low-calorie diet). As the lungs return to normal, patients often begin to cough; it is worth emphasizing this in a positive light (i.e., cleansing of the lungs). Tell patients to use a cough suppressant only as a last resort to help them sleep.

G. The decision to use nicotine replacement therapy is based on whether the patient is heavily addicted to nicotine. This can be ascertained by the response to two questions: "Do you smoke within 30 minutes after arising in the morning?" and "Do you smoke more than 25 cigarettes a day?" These patients may do better with nicotine replacement therapy. The choice of whether to use nicotine policricex gum or transdermal patches is a matter of choice by the physician and patient. Some patients cannot chew gum because of dental work or temporomandibular joint problems or because they have tried the gum before and lack confidence in it. For these patients transdermal patches may be indicated. Others may be smoking a small number of cigarettes each day or may prefer not to use nicotine replacement; for these patients a trial of cessation without replacement therapy may be appropriate.

(Continued on page 560)

Patient for SMOKING PREVENTION OR CESSATION

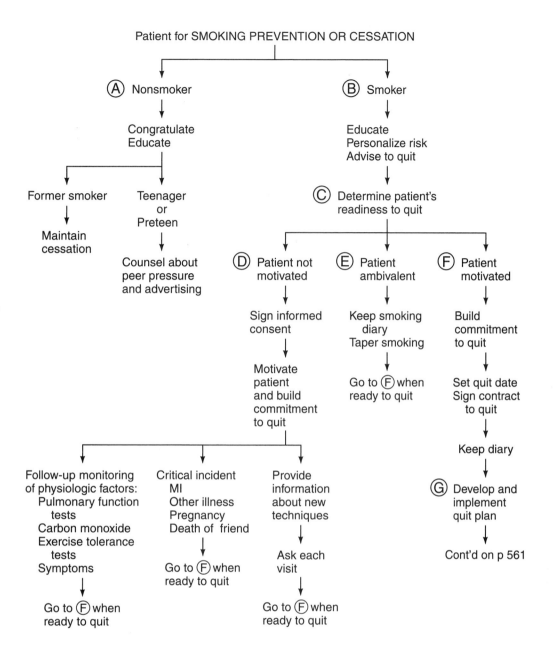

(A) Nonsmoker

Congratulate
Educate

Former smoker

Maintain
cessation

Teenager
or
Preteen

Counsel about
peer pressure
and advertising

(B) Smoker

Educate
Personalize risk
Advise to quit

(C) Determine patient's
readiness to quit

(D) Patient not
motivated

Sign informed
consent

Motivate
patient
and build
commitment
to quit

Follow-up monitoring
of physiologic factors:
   Pulmonary function
      tests
   Carbon monoxide
   Exercise tolerance
      tests
   Symptoms

Go to (F) when
ready to quit

Critical incident
   MI
   Other illness
   Pregnancy
   Death of friend

Go to (F) when
ready to quit

Provide
information
about new
techniques

Ask each
visit

Go to (F) when
ready to quit

(E) Patient
ambivalent

Keep smoking
diary
Taper smoking

Go to (F) when
ready to quit

(F) Patient
motivated

Build
commitment
to quit

Set quit date
Sign contract
to quit

Keep diary

(G) Develop and
implement
quit plan

Cont'd on p 561

H. For heavily addicted patients, offer nicotine (Nicorette) gum. This can be done on a timed schedule and gradually tapered after the psychologic aspects of addiction have abated. Many people who are unsuccessful in stopping do not use enough Nicorette gum or may use it incorrectly. For all patients beginning cessation, maintain close follow-up or contact over the first several days or weeks. This can be accomplished by a call from a staff member or by having patients call in with a report of how they are doing. The purpose of this is to identify slips (brief relapses) early and plan how to manage them and start the cessation attempt again. One slip is not a failure, and most patients who are successful have had to deal with three or four relapses.

I. For successful patients, praise and support should be part of the maintenance plan.

J. For those who relapse, starting again at F makes sense, or they can be referred to a more specialized program. Two forms of Nicorette are available, 2 or 4 mg. Depending on patients' overall pack-year history and smoking pattern, an initial 2-mg dose helps taper craving for the nicotine in the cigarettes. David Sachs of Stanford suggests that a rule of four's be followed with an eventual taper (i.e., 1 pack per day [ppd], 12 pieces Nicorette/day; 1.5 ppd, 16 pieces/day; 2 ppd, 20 pieces/day). He also suggests a chew, stop, and park regimen for the user (i.e., chew slowly until a tingle is felt, stop chewing and park the medication between cheek and gum, restart chewing when the tingle is gone, and stop when the tingle returns).

K. All future physician visits should include follow-up questions on cessation with reinforcement and praise for continued success.

L. For individuals who are addicted and for whom the transdermal nicotine patches are appropriate, the first dose is determined by amount of smoking and patient size.

M. Those weighing <105 lbs or smoking <20 cigarettes per day or who have frequent angina attacks should be considered for a 14-mg starting dose. Those who do not tolerate the 21-mg patch because of excess nicotine symptoms may do better on the lower dosage. The 14-mg dose is continued for at least 1 month.

N. Most smokers who are heavily addicted (with the exceptions noted in M) should begin with the 21-mg transdermal patch. This is continued for 1 month. Patients often comment on vivid, altered, or increased dreaming while using the 21-mg patch. Erythema develops beneath the patch in most patients. Patches should be moved to a new location each day. The manufacturer's instructions should be carefully followed. The patient must not smoke and use patches because this can lead to nicotine toxicity, increased angina, or MI. A small percentage of patients develop severe skin reactions (1–3%) at the patch site. These patients should be managed using gum.

O. After 1 month these patients should be given a 14-mg patch and this continued for 4–6 weeks, depending on how well the habit and psychologic components of smoking are doing.

P. Finally a 7-mg patch should be used for 2–4 weeks and then discontinued. Continue close follow-up and support as outlined under I and K. The patient who relapses while using patches should stop using them, pick a new quitting date, and start again at F. Nicotine via nasal spray or inhaler is being tested and may become available soon.

Q. Bupropion (Wellbutrin, Zyban) has recently been shown to produce 20–23% 1-year cessation rates when used at a dosage of 150 mg twice a day. The recommended duration is 7 weeks. Adverse effects included headache, insomnia, dry mouth, and anxiety. The drug should not be used in those with history of seizures. It seems to be able to ameliorate some of the dysphoric symptoms of smoking cessation. Bupropion can be used with nicotine replacement therapy.

References

Bartecchi CE, MacKenzie TD, Schrier RW. The human costs of tobacco use. N Engl J Med 1994; 330:907.

Benowitz NL. Treating tobacco addiction: nicotine or no nicotine? N Engl J Med 1997; 337:1230.

Bronson DL, Flynn BS, Solomon LJ, et al. Smoking cessation counseling during periodic health examinations. Arch Intern Med 1989; 149:1653.

Coates TJ, Cummings SR. Behavior modification. In: Kassirer JP, Greene HL II, eds. Current therapy in adult medicine. 4th ed. St Louis: Mosby, 1997:26.

DeNelsky GY. Smoking cessation: strategies that work. Cleve Clin J Med 1990; 57:416.

Greene HL II. Smoking cessation. In: Kassirer JP, Greene HL II, eds. Current therapy in adult medicine. 4th ed. St Louis: Mosby, 1997:35.

Guise BJ, Goldstein MG, Clark MM, Thebarge RW. Behavior change: the example of smoking. In: Noble J, Greene HL, Levenson W, eds. Primary care medicine. St Louis: Mosby, 1996:1650.

Hurt RD, et al. Comparison of sustained-release bupropion and placebo for smoking cessation. N Engl J Med 1997; 337:1195.

Joseph AM, Norman SM, Ferry LH. The safety of transdermal nicotine as an aid to smoking cessation in patients with cardiac disease. N Engl J Med 1996; 335:1792.

Ockene JK, Kristeller J, Goldberg R, et al. Increasing the efficacy of physician-delivered smoking interventions: a randomized clinical trial. J Gen Intern Med 1991; 6:1.

Patient for SMOKING PREVENTION OR CESSATION
(Cont'd from p 559)

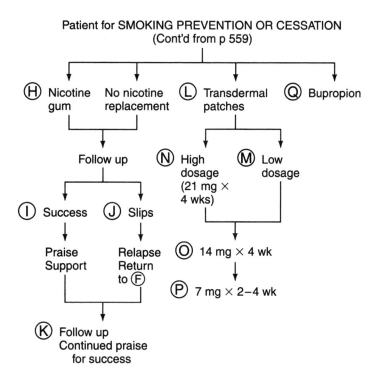

SUICIDAL PATIENT

Rebecca L. Potter

Most suicidal persons communicate their self-destructive intentions to those around them, including their physicians. As many as two thirds of those who commit suicide have seen a doctor in the weeks to months before their death. Medical students and primary care physicians should therefore know how to evaluate the suicidal patient. Does a patient look or feel depressed and talk of "not being able to go on," giving up, and losing interest in activities? If so, a more detailed assessment of suicidal risk is in order.

A. Psychiatric disorders associated with an increased risk of suicidal ideation and attempt include depression, bipolar disorder, alcohol or drug abuse, panic attacks, and panic disorders.

B. The following psychosocial factors place people at an increased risk of committing suicide: single, divorced, widowed, or separated marital status; unemployment; decreased social supports; humiliating life events (e.g., the recent loss of a job or an important relationship); a chronic medical illness; or a family history of suicide. A previous suicide attempt is a predictor of future completed suicide.

C. Do not ignore or minimize references to suicide: taking risks, talk of guilt over past events, talk of "ending it all," making a will, giving away prized possessions. Ask patients directly whether they are suicidal, and if so what plan they have; assess their understanding of the lethality of the plan. Do they have the means to carry out the plan? Have there been earlier attempts? Determine patients' mood, changes in appetite and sleep, the presence of hallucinations or delusions, and quality of speech. Patients with "command" hallucinations to commit suicide are at particularly high risk. A physical examination and laboratory studies to consider contributory or concomitant physical illness are necessary.

D. If the patient has serious immediate suicidal intent, consider psychiatric consultation and voluntary or involuntary hospitalization. If the risk is not as imminent, establish and make available a therapeutic relationship. The forming of a no-suicide contract, frequent appointments, and provision of reassurance and hope are important. Allow the patient to ventilate feelings and help him or her problem solve, communicating empathy and caring. Treat any underlying psychiatric or medical disorder.

References

Blumenthal SJ. Suicide: a guide to risk factors, assessment, and treatment of suicidal patients. Med Clin North Am 1988; 72:937.

Hirschfeld JM, Russell JM. Assessment and treatment of suicidal patients. N Engl J Med 1997; 337:910.

Malone KM, Szanto K, Corbitt EM, Mann JJ. Clinical assessment versus research methods in the assessment of suicidal behavior. Am J Psychiatry 1995; 152:1601.

Roy A. Suicide. In: Kaplan HI, Sadock BJ, eds. Comprehensive textbook of psychiatry. 6th ed. Baltimore: Williams & Wilkins, 1995.

Weissman MM, Kierman GL, Markowitz JS, Ouellette R. Suicidal ideation and suicide attempts in panic disorder and attacks. N Engl J Med 1989; 321:1209.

SUICIDAL PATIENT

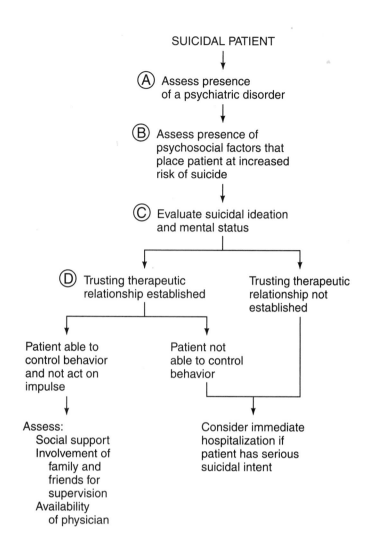

(A) Assess presence
of a psychiatric disorder

(B) Assess presence of
psychosocial factors that
place patient at increased
risk of suicide

(C) Evaluate suicidal ideation
and mental status

(D) Trusting therapeutic
relationship established

Trusting therapeutic
relationship not
established

Patient able to
control behavior
and not act on
impulse

Patient not
able to control
behavior

Assess:
    Social support
    Involvement of
        family and
        friends for
        supervision
    Availability
        of physician

Consider immediate
hospitalization if
patient has serious
suicidal intent

PHARMACOLOGY

ACUTE ANTICOAGULATION

Michael D. Katz

Thromboembolic disorders and medical procedures that may require anticoagulation therapy include proximal deep venous thrombosis (DVT), pulmonary embolism (PE), atrial fibrillation with embolism, acute myocardial infarction, and placement of mechanical heart valves. In situations of apparent thromboembolic disorders (as opposed to prophylaxis) that are potentially life-threatening (e.g., PE with shock), initiate heparin therapy before performing diagnostic tests.

A. Diagnostic tests vary in sensitivity and specificity. In patients with PE, a high degree of clinical suspicion may necessitate therapy even when the ventilation-perfusion scan is negative.

B. Contraindications to heparin are relative: The risks must be weighed against the potential benefits. In most cases, patients with previous hypersensitivity or heparin-induced thrombocytopenia, active bleeding, intracranial hemorrhage, GI bleeding, hemophilia, thrombocytopenia, severe hypertension, or recent surgery of the brain, spinal cord, or eye should not receive heparin therapy. In PE patients in whom there are contraindications to heparin therapy, consider placement of an inferior vena cava (IVC) filter.

C. In patients with massive PE or those with hemodynamic compromise, consider thrombolytic therapy with streptokinase, urokinase, or tissue plasminogen activator (TPA). However, clinical trials have shown no clear advantage of thrombolytic therapy over heparin in most patients with venous thromboembolism.

D. Several studies show that a weight-based approach to administering heparin achieves more rapid anticoagulation without increased risk of bleeding. Many institutions have developed heparin dosing protocols to facilitate the appropriate use of heparin. However, use of such protocols does not obviate the need for close clinical and laboratory monitoring by the physician. Check partial thromboplastin time (PTT) no sooner than 6 hours after any bolus; PTT checked sooner may be falsely elevated.

(Continued on page 568)

SIGNIFICANT THROMBOEMBOLIC DISORDER Suspected

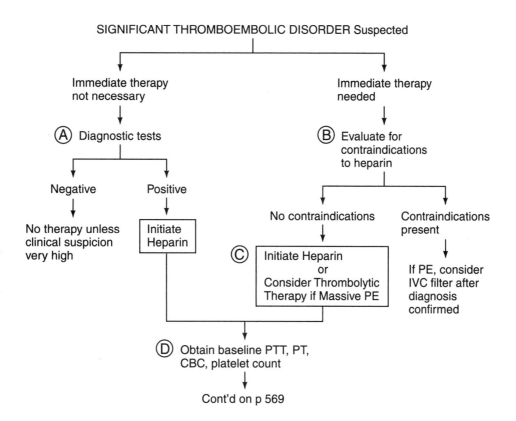

Cont'd on p 569

E. A variety of low-molecular-weight heparin (LMWH) products such as enoxaparin have been marketed. These agents appear to be at least as effective as unfractionated heparin (UH), do not require PTT monitoring, and can be administered by intermittent SC injection. However, these products are much more expensive than UH and offer no particular advantage in the hospitalized patient. Several studies show that LMWH can be administered safely to outpatients with DVT or PE. A patient who is medically stable and has the appropriate home environment and insurance coverage may be discharged on LMWH (e.g., enoxaparin 1 mg/kg SC q12h). Such therapy is continued until the level of long-term anticoagulation (warfarin) is therapeutic.

F. If long-term anticoagulation is indicated and there are no contraindications to warfarin, initiate warfarin as soon as the PTT is therapeutic. The initial warfarin dose should be the same as the expected maintenance dose. Continue heparin therapy for at least 4 days after the initiation of warfarin. Earlier rises in the PT/INR are due primarily to depletion of factor VII. Patients are not truly anticoagulated until significant depletion of factors II and X has occurred.

References

The Columbus Investigators. Low-molecular-weight heparin in the treatment of patients with venous thromboembolism. N Engl J Med 1997; 337:657.

Hirsh J, Rashke R, Warkentin TE, et al. Heparin: mechanism of action, pharmacokinetics, dosing considerations, monitoring, efficacy and safety. Chest 1995; 108(suppl):258S.

Hyers TM, Hull RD, Weg JG. Antithrombotic therapy for venous thromboembolic disease. Chest 1995; 108(suppl):335S.

Levine M, Gent M, Hirsh J, et al. A comparison of low-molecular-weight heparin administered primarily at home with unfractionated heparin administered in the hospital for proximal deep-vein thrombosis. N Engl J Med 1996; 334:677.

Raschke RA, Reilly BM, Guidry JR, et al. The weight-based heparin dosing nomogram compared with a "standard care" nomogram. A randomized controlled trial. Ann Intern Med 1993; 119:874.

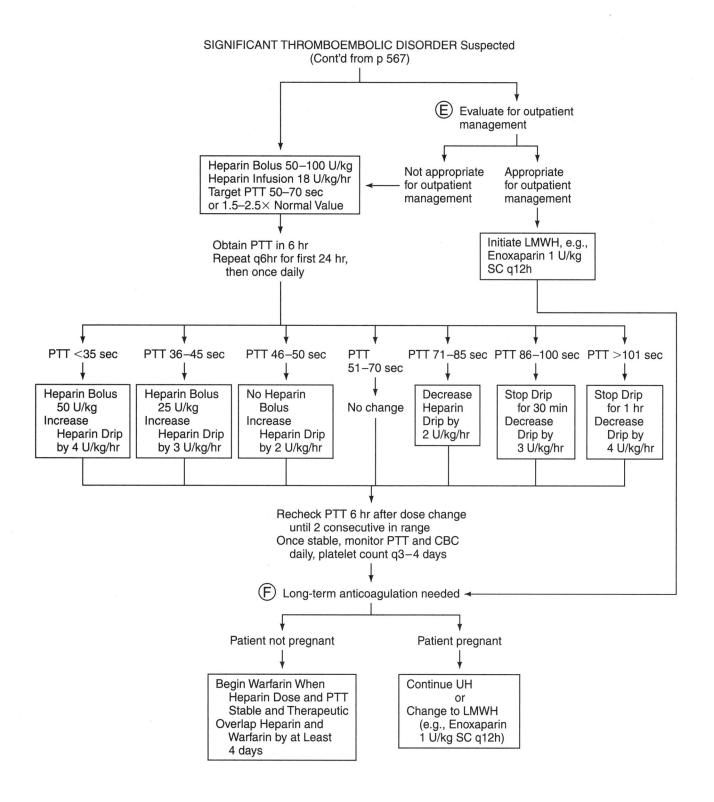

SIGNIFICANT THROMBOEMBOLIC DISORDER Suspected
(Cont'd from p 567)

E Evaluate for outpatient management

Heparin Bolus 50–100 U/kg
Heparin Infusion 18 U/kg/hr
Target PTT 50–70 sec
or 1.5–2.5× Normal Value

Not appropriate for outpatient management

Appropriate for outpatient management

Obtain PTT in 6 hr
Repeat q6hr for first 24 hr, then once daily

Initiate LMWH, e.g., Enoxaparin 1 U/kg SC q12h

PTT <35 sec

PTT 36–45 sec

PTT 46–50 sec

PTT 51–70 sec

PTT 71–85 sec

PTT 86–100 sec

PTT >101 sec

Heparin Bolus 50 U/kg Increase Heparin Drip by 4 U/kg/hr

Heparin Bolus 25 U/kg Increase Heparin Drip by 3 U/kg/hr

No Heparin Bolus Increase Heparin Drip by 2 U/kg/hr

No change

Decrease Heparin Drip by 2 U/kg/hr

Stop Drip for 30 min Decrease Drip by 3 U/kg/hr

Stop Drip for 1 hr Decrease Drip by 4 U/kg/hr

Recheck PTT 6 hr after dose change
until 2 consecutive in range
Once stable, monitor PTT and CBC
daily, platelet count q3–4 days

F Long-term anticoagulation needed

Patient not pregnant

Patient pregnant

Begin Warfarin When Heparin Dose and PTT Stable and Therapeutic Overlap Heparin and Warfarin by at Least 4 days

Continue UH
or
Change to LMWH
(e.g., Enoxaparin 1 U/kg SC q12h)

LONG-TERM ANTICOAGULATION

Michael D. Katz

A. Contraindications to long-term anticoagulant therapy include those listed under acute anticoagulation (p 566), as well as patients who are severely debilitated and malnourished, those who fall or undergo significant trauma, alcoholics, and those who are unlikely to understand or comply with therapy. As always, the risk-benefit ratio must be considered. Pregnancy is an absolute contraindication to warfarin. Women of childbearing age who receive warfarin must be given an effective contraceptive method.

B. Patients with recurrent thromboembolism on warfarin therapy should first be evaluated for compliance and adequacy of anticoagulation. If low-intensity anticoagulation was used, consider high-intensity therapy. Alternatively, consider subcutaneous low-molecular-weight heparin (LMWH) therapy. In patients with frequent recurrences of thromboembolism, consider the presence of malignancy or other hypercoagulable state.

C. The level of anticoagulation during warfarin therapy is determined by the International Normalized Ratio (INR). This calculated value corrects for the widely varying thromboplastin reagents used to determine the prothrombin time (PT). Warfarin therapy cannot be safely or effectively managed without use of the INR. For most clinical indications, the target INR is 2.0–3.0. For patients with mechanical prosthetic heart valves or those who failed lower-intensity anticoagulation, a target INR of 2.5–3.5 is desired. These INR ranges serve as clinical guidelines, not absolute values. The target INR for a specific patient is based on the risk of bleeding, age, and concomitant drug therapy.

D. Warfarin therapy must be closely monitored. Frequent monitoring is needed as therapy is titrated; less frequent visits are needed as the patient becomes stable. Initially, patients should be evaluated at weeks 1, 2, and 4. If the INR remains in the target range, the patient may be monitored every 4–8 weeks. Studies have shown that patient outcomes are consistently improved if patients are monitored by an anticoagulation clinic. All patients who are given warfarin must receive education and counseling regarding the underlying thromboembolic disorder, how to take the warfarin, possible side effects, and significant drug interactions. This information must be reviewed at each patient encounter.

(Continued on page 572)

Patient for LONG-TERM ANTICOAGULATION

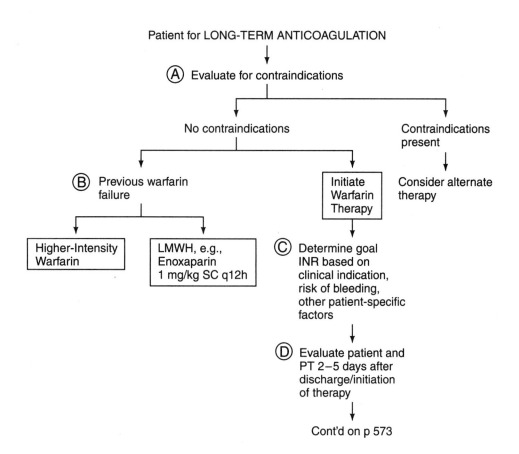

Ⓐ Evaluate for contraindications

No contraindications

Contraindications present

Ⓑ Previous warfarin failure

Initiate Warfarin Therapy

Consider alternate therapy

Higher-Intensity Warfarin

LMWH, e.g., Enoxaparin 1 mg/kg SC q12h

Ⓒ Determine goal INR based on clinical indication, risk of bleeding, other patient-specific factors

Ⓓ Evaluate patient and PT 2–5 days after discharge/initiation of therapy

Cont'd on p 573

E. If the INR is not in the target range, evaluate the patient for noncompliance, drug interactions, or change in cardiac or hepatic function. Many drugs, including over-the-counter products, vitamins, and alternative agents, have significant interactions with warfarin. Any new drug should be initiated with great caution. If a correctable factor is identified, the patient may continue on the previous warfarin dose. In a previously stable patient with a minor fluctuation in INR and no change in clinical status, the warfarin dose may be continued and the INR rechecked in 1 week. Patients with a very high INR, e.g., >6–10, should be assessed for bleeding complications. In the absence of bleeding, holding the warfarin dose may be the best approach. The INR can be reduced quickly by administering vitamin K 2.5 mg PO or 0.5–1 mg SC without causing warfarin resistance.

F. The duration of anticoagulant therapy is determined by the underlying disease and risk of recurrent thromboembolism. For patients with a first deep venous thrombosis (DVT) or pulmonary embolism (PE), 3–6 months of therapy is adequate. However, in patients with recurrent DVT or PE, atrial fibrillation with embolism or mechanical valves will require long-term therapy.

G. Bleeding complications may occur with a therapeutic or elevated INR. The risk of future anticoagulation must be weighed against the risk of future bleeding episodes. The management of warfarin-associated bleeding generally consists of holding the drug and administering vitamin K and/or fresh frozen plasma. Full reversal of anticoagulation may not be desired in patients with mechanical heart valves. Administration of large doses of vitamin K (>5 mg SC/IV) will cause resistance to future warfarin therapy for several weeks. In patients who develop GI bleeding or hematuria with a therapeutic INR, a GI or urinary tract lesion may be present.

References

Ansell JE, Hughes R. Evolving models of warfarin management: anticoagulation clinics, patient self-monitoring and patient self-management. Am Heart J 1996; 132:1095.

Ansell JE, Oertel LB, Wittkowsky AK. Managing Oral Anticoagulation Therapy. Gaithersburg, MD: Aspen 1997.

Hirsh J. Substandard monitoring of warfarin in North America: time for a change. Arch Intern Med 1992; 152:257.

Hirsh J, Dalen JE, Deykin D, et al. Oral anticoagulants: mechanism of action, clinical effectiveness, and optimal therapeutic range. Chest 1995; 108(Suppl):231S.

Levine MN, Raskob G, Landefeld S, Hirsh J. Hemorrhagic complications of anticoagulant treatment. Chest 1995; 108(Suppl):276S.

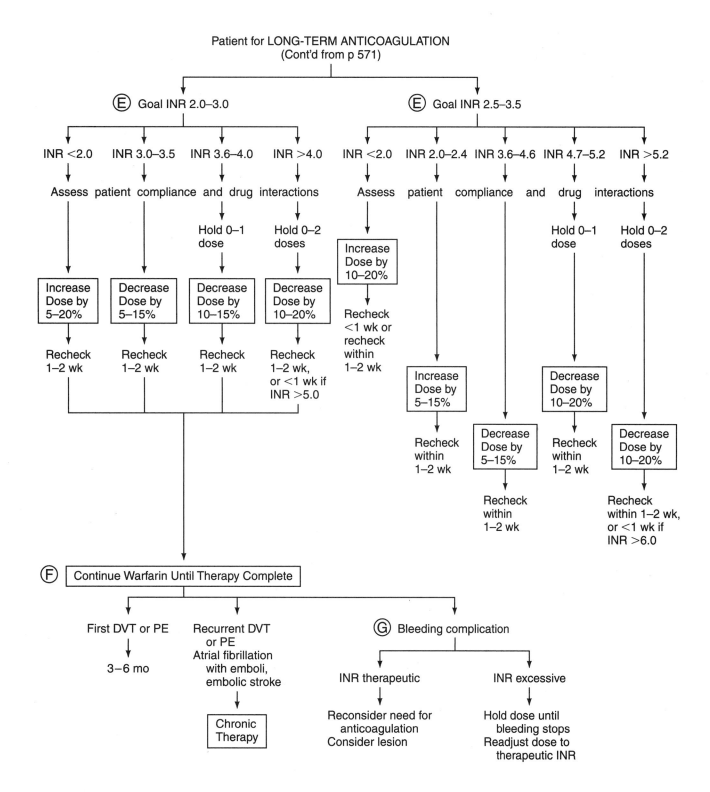

Patient for LONG-TERM ANTICOAGULATION
(Cont'd from p 571)

Ⓔ Goal INR 2.0–3.0

INR <2.0 | INR 3.0–3.5 | INR 3.6–4.0 | INR >4.0

Assess patient compliance and drug interactions

Hold 0–1 dose

Hold 0–2 doses

Increase Dose by 5–20%

Decrease Dose by 5–15%

Decrease Dose by 10–15%

Decrease Dose by 10–20%

Recheck 1–2 wk

Recheck 1–2 wk

Recheck 1–2 wk

Recheck 1–2 wk, or <1 wk if INR >5.0

Ⓔ Goal INR 2.5–3.5

INR <2.0 | INR 2.0–2.4 | INR 3.6–4.6 | INR 4.7–5.2 | INR >5.2

Assess patient compliance and drug interactions

Increase Dose by 10–20%

Recheck <1 wk or recheck within 1–2 wk

Hold 0–1 dose

Hold 0–2 doses

Increase Dose by 5–15%

Recheck within 1–2 wk

Decrease Dose by 5–15%

Recheck within 1–2 wk

Decrease Dose by 10–20%

Recheck within 1–2 wk

Decrease Dose by 10–20%

Recheck within 1–2 wk, or <1 wk if INR >6.0

Ⓕ Continue Warfarin Until Therapy Complete

First DVT or PE
↓
3–6 mo

Recurrent DVT or PE
Atrial fibrillation with emboli, embolic stroke
↓
Chronic Therapy

Ⓖ Bleeding complication

INR therapeutic
↓
Reconsider need for anticoagulation
Consider lesion

INR excessive
↓
Hold dose until bleeding stops
Readjust dose to therapeutic INR

ANAPHYLAXIS

Michael D. Katz

The common signs and symptoms of anaphylaxis include an aura, rhinitis, cough, pruritus, urticaria, laryngeal edema, generalized edema, decreased sensorium, shock, bronchospasm, GI cramps, and vomiting. Rarely, patients may develop heart failure, pulmonary edema, and disseminated intravascular coagulation. Other conditions such as vasovagal reactions, hyperventilation, globus hystericus, and hereditary angioedema may mimic aspects of anaphylaxis and should be ruled out before initiating aggressive therapy.

A. Anaphylaxis is associated with a variety of factors, including foods, drugs, insect bites and stings, latex, and exercise. More than one third of cases have no identifiable cause. Drugs associated with anaphylaxis include β-lactam antibiotics, sulfonamides, anesthetics, chymopapain, protamine, dextran, and radiocontrast media. In any patient with anaphylaxis, obtain a complete exposure history, including any previous reactions.

B. Local reactions usually consist of redness, swelling, and pain at the site of injection. Systemic signs and symptoms may develop rapidly. Measures to slow absorption of the antigen from the injection site, such as application of ice or use of a venous- (not arterial) occluding tourniquet, may be useful in the field until the patient reaches medical attention.

C. Base the initial management of anaphylaxis on support of vital signs. Place all patients in the Trendelenburg position and give supplemental oxygen. In patients with cardiac or respiratory arrest or serious arrhythmias, initiate basic and advanced cardiac life support measures.

D. Epinephrine is the mainstay of therapy for anaphylaxis; no other drug has proved as effective. Epinephrine reverses the effects of the mediators of anaphylaxis and may reduce the further release of these mediators. In most adults, give 0.3 ml of 1:1000 solution by subcutaneous (SC) injection (in children, the dose is 0.01 ml/kg). However, if the patient is in shock, give epinephrine through a central vein or instill into the endotracheal tube. If the desired response is not achieved and no adverse effects occur, repeat epinephrine in 10 minutes. Monitor elderly patients, especially those with underlying cardiac disease, very closely.

(Continued on page 576)

Patient with SIGNS AND SYMPTOMS OF ANAPHYLAXIS

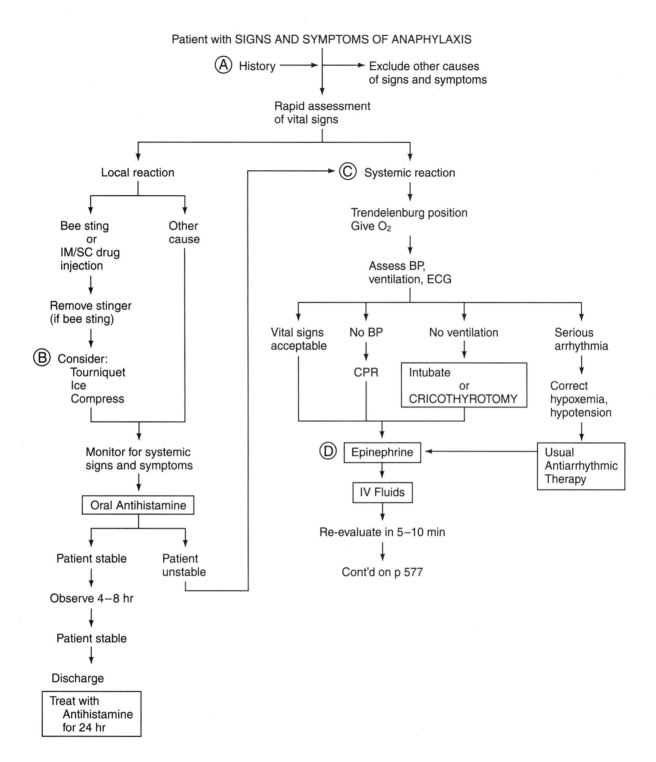

Cont'd on p 577

E. In patients with severe bronchospasm, epinephrine and inhaled β_2 agonists (e.g., albuterol) are the most effective treatment. There is no evidence that IV theophylline is effective in the treatment of acute, severe bronchospasm, and it may increase the risk of cardiac arrhythmias. However, in a patient with refractory bronchospasm, a loading dose of theophylline (5 mg/kg) may be administered.

F. Antihistamines serve as second-line therapy when a prolonged course is expected. Agents such as diphenhydramine or hydroxyzine may be especially useful in treating pruritus. Corticosteroids are not helpful in the immediate management but may be useful in treating late-phase immune reactions. Methylprednisolone in IV doses of 50–125 mg every 6 hours has been used. In less severe cases, oral prednisone may be appropriate. In patients with a prolonged or refractory course, the addition of the H_2 blocker cimetidine may be helpful.

G. Instruct all patients with anaphylaxis in ways to avoid future exposure to the inciting agent. The cause of the episode, if known, should be clearly documented in the patient's medical record, especially in drug-induced anaphylaxis.

H. In some instances specific preventive therapy may be indicated. Consider patients with bee sting allergy who cannot easily avoid future exposures for desensitization. In patients with frequently recurrent idiopathic anaphylaxis, prophylactic therapy with corticosteroids and antihistamines has proved effective. Autoinjectors containing epinephrine also may be used by the patient at risk for another serious reaction.

References

Bochner B, Lichtenstein I. Anaphylaxis. N Engl J Med 1991; 324:1785.

Corren J, Schocket AL. Anaphylaxis: a preventable emergency. Postgrad Med 1990; 87:167.

deShazo RD, Kemp SF. Allergic reactions to drugs and biologic agents. JAMA 1997; 278:1895.

Wong S, Yarnold PR, Yango C, et al. Outcome of prophylactic therapy for idiopathic anaphylaxis. Ann Intern Med 1991; 114:133.

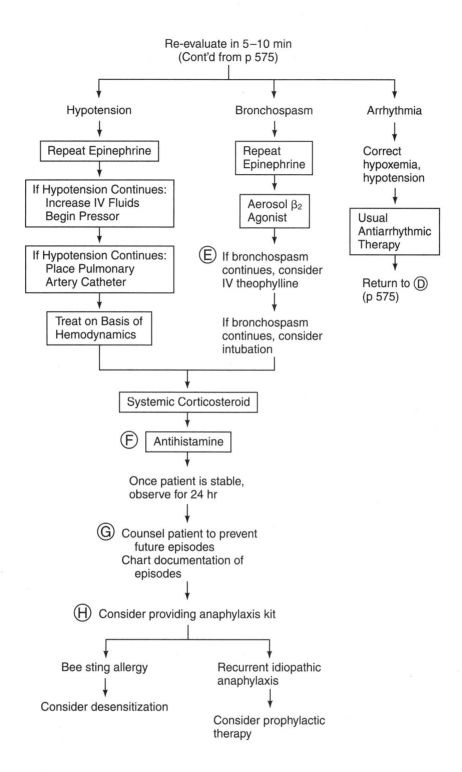

Re-evaluate in 5–10 min
(Cont'd from p 575)

Hypotension

Repeat Epinephrine

If Hypotension Continues:
Increase IV Fluids
Begin Pressor

If Hypotension Continues:
Place Pulmonary
Artery Catheter

Treat on Basis of
Hemodynamics

Bronchospasm

Repeat
Epinephrine

Aerosol β₂
Agonist

Ⓔ If bronchospasm
continues, consider
IV theophylline

If bronchospasm
continues, consider
intubation

Arrhythmia

Correct
hypoxemia,
hypotension

Usual
Antiarrhythmic
Therapy

Return to Ⓓ
(p 575)

Systemic Corticosteroid

Ⓕ Antihistamine

Once patient is stable,
observe for 24 hr

Ⓖ Counsel patient to prevent
future episodes
Chart documentation of
episodes

Ⓗ Consider providing anaphylaxis kit

Bee sting allergy

Consider desensitization

Recurrent idiopathic
anaphylaxis

Consider prophylactic
therapy

EVALUATION OF ADVERSE DRUG REACTIONS

Robert J. Lipsy
Michael D. Katz

A. An adverse drug reaction (ADR) is any unexpected, unintended, undesired, or excessive response to a drug or medication that (1) requires discontinuing the medication; (2) requires changing the medication; (3) requires modifying the dosage; (4) necessitates hospital admission; (5) prolongs stay in a health care facility; (6) necessitates supportive treatment; (7) significantly complicates diagnosis; (8) negatively affects prognosis; or (9) results in temporary or permanent harm, disability, or death. The concept of medication misadventures includes medication errors as well as ADRs.

ADRs are far more common than many clinicians believe. A recent meta-analysis of 39 prospective studies concluded that serious ADRs occur in 6.7% of hospitalized patients, with a fatality rate of 0.32%. Annually, 2.2 million hospitalized patients experience serious ADRs, with 106,000 deaths per year, making ADRs the fifth leading cause of death. The elderly are especially prone to ADRs.

B. Evaluate any patient receiving a pharmacologically active substance (including diagnostic agents and alternative products) who has any adverse event for a possible ADR. Medication errors, including improper prescribing, dispensing, or administration of a drug, are one possible cause of ADRs.

C. Establishing a temporal association is often the most difficult part of the evaluation. Most ADRs manifest within the first day or two of treatment, and nearly all by the second week of therapy. The temporal relationship is drug, patient, and reaction specific. To establish a clear-cut temporal relationship, compare the time of onset of the reaction with that expected based on previous reported reaction or the known or proposed pathophysiologic mechanism. If the reaction has not been seen with the suspected drug, compare similar agents or drugs within the same class. Take into account patient specificity: for example, type I hypersensitivity reactions may be immediate in nature in a previously exposed patient, or delayed 5–10 days in a naive patient.

D. Discontinue all potential offending agents, if possible. However, the decision to discontinue agents depends on the severity of the reaction, the effectiveness of the agent, the need for continued therapy, and the availability of therapeutic alternatives. If an alternative agent is used, choose one that is unlikely to cause the same ADR.

E. Like the onset of a reaction, resolution varies according to the specific nature of the reaction and the patient. Be aware that some adverse reactions, such as ototoxicity from aminoglycosides or nephrotoxicity from amphotericin B, may resolve only after long periods or may have permanent sequelae.

F. Rechallenge should not be undertaken unless the benefits outweigh the risks and should not be used merely to confirm the association between the ADR and the suspected drug. Be aware that there may be a different manifestation of the adverse reaction upon rechallenge, particularly in cases of allergic reactions. These changes may be in the temporal relationship or in the severity of the reaction.

G. The FDA MedWatch program is a voluntary system to report adverse events and products problems. The FDA is especially interested in serious or unusual reactions, reactions to new drugs, and reactions to herbal and other alternative medicine products. For more information, call 800-FDA-1088.

References

Kessler DA. Introducing MedWatch: a new approach to reporting medication and device adverse effects and product problems. JAMA 1993; 269:2765.

Lazarou J, Pomeranz BH, Corey PN. Incidence of adverse drug reactions in hospitalized patients: a meta-analysis of prospective studies. JAMA 1998; 279:1200.

Naranjo CA, Busto U, Sellers EM, et al. A method for estimating the probability of adverse drug reactions. Clin Pharmacol Ther 1981; 30:239.

Proceedings of the Interdisciplinary Conference on Understanding and Preventing Drug Misadventures. Am J Health-Syst Pharm 1995; 52:369.

Awareness of Possible ADVERSE DRUG REACTIONS (ADRs)

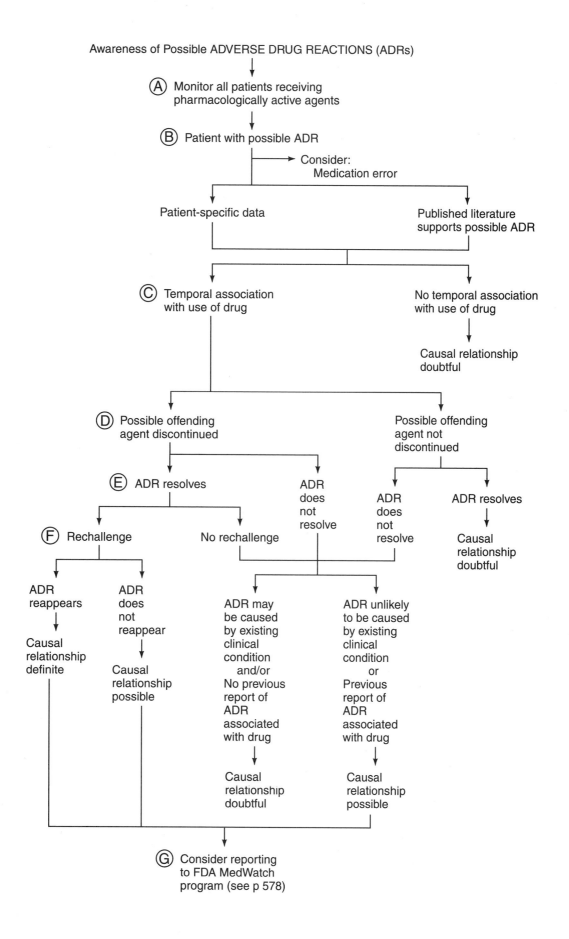

NONSURGICAL ANTIMICROBIAL PROPHYLAXIS

Collin Freeman

A. Patients undergoing surgery who require bacterial endocarditis prophylaxis include those with prosthetic valves, previous bacterial endocarditis, congenital cardiac malformations, acquired valvular dysfunction, hypertrophic cardiomyopathy, and mitral valve prolapse with valvular regurgitation.

B. Dental procedures in which prophylaxis is indicated are those known to cause gingival or mucosal bleeding, including cleaning. Surgical procedures in which prophylaxis may be required include tonsillectomy and adenoidectomy, bronchoscopy performed with a rigid bronchoscope, sclerotherapy performed for esophageal varices, surgical procedures involving mucosa of the respiratory or intestinal tracts, gallbladder surgery, cystoscopy, urethral dilatation, urethral catheterization or urinary tract surgery, vaginal hysterectomy, vaginal delivery with an infection of the birth canal, and incision and drainage of infected tissue.

C. Fluoroquinolones (FQ) include some that are active for systemic infections (e.g., ciprofloxacin, ofloxacin, sparfloxacin) and some that are indicated only for urinary and digestive tract infections (e.g., lomefloxacin, norfloxacin). Dosing is normally b.i.d. or once daily. Check prescribing information to determine the appropriate dose and frequency when using these antibiotics.

D. Prophylaxis against *Pneumocystis carinii* pneumonia (PCP) is given to HIV-positive patients who have a history of PCP, a CD4 cell count $<200/mm^3$, unexplained fever for ≥ 2 weeks, or a history of oropharyngeal candidiasis. Consult the most recent CDC guidelines.

E. Traveler's diarrhea is likely in persons traveling to countries where hygiene is poor. Most diarrheal illnesses of this type are self-limiting. It is best to avoid foods that are not fully cooked and unboiled water (even ice) in underdeveloped countries. If medications are used, they should be continued for the duration of the trip and for 2 days to 2 weeks after leaving the underdeveloped country.

F. Influenza prophylaxis is given in the fall and winter months to (1) persons ≥ 65 years old; (2) residents of nursing homes and other chronic-care facilities that house persons of any age with chronic medical conditions; (3) adults and children with chronic disorders of the pulmonary or cardiovascular systems, including children with asthma; (4) adults and children who have required regular medical follow-up or hospitalization during the preceding year because of chronic metabolic diseases (including diabetes mellitus), kidney dysfunction, various blood abnormalities, or immunosuppression (including immunosuppression caused by medications, e.g., organ and bone marrow transplant patients); and (4) health-care workers in close contact with other high-risk patients. People not meeting these criteria may also receive flu shots. People with egg-allergy should not receive influenza vaccine.

(Continued on page 582)

NONSURGICAL ANTIMICROBIAL PROPHYLAXIS

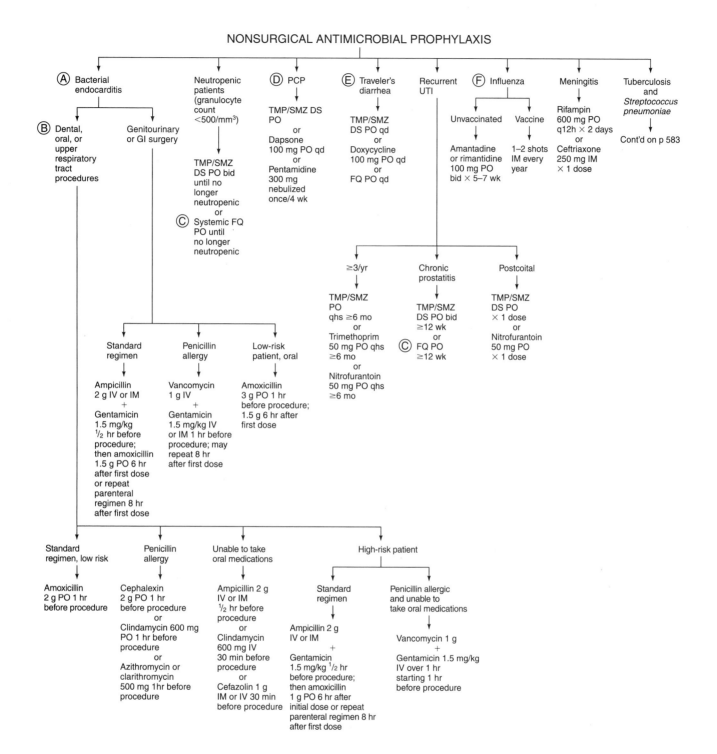

(A) Bacterial endocarditis

(B) Dental, oral, or upper respiratory tract procedures

Genitourinary or GI surgery

Neutropenic patients (granulocyte count <500/mm³)

TMP/SMZ DS PO bid until no longer neutropenic

or

(C) Systemic FQ PO until no longer neutropenic

(D) PCP

TMP/SMZ DS PO

or

Dapsone 100 mg PO qd

or

Pentamidine 300 mg nebulized once/4 wk

(E) Traveler's diarrhea

TMP/SMZ DS PO qd

or

Doxycycline 100 mg PO qd

or

FQ PO qd

Recurrent UTI

(F) Influenza

Unvaccinated

Amantadine or rimantidine 100 mg PO bid × 5–7 wk

Vaccine

1–2 shots IM every year

Meningitis

Rifampin 600 mg PO q12h × 2 days

or

Ceftriaxone 250 mg IM × 1 dose

Tuberculosis and *Streptococcus pneumoniae*

Cont'd on p 583

≥3/yr

TMP/SMZ PO qhs ≥6 mo

or

Trimethoprim 50 mg PO qhs ≥6 mo

or

Nitrofurantoin 50 mg PO qhs ≥6 mo

Chronic prostatitis

TMP/SMZ DS PO bid ≥12 wk

or

(C) FQ PO ≥12 wk

Postcoital

TMP/SMZ DS PO × 1 dose

or

Nitrofurantoin 50 mg PO × 1 dose

Standard regimen

Ampicillin 2 g IV or IM
+
Gentamicin 1.5 mg/kg ½ hr before procedure; then amoxicillin 1.5 g PO 6 hr after first dose or repeat parenteral regimen 8 hr after first dose

Penicillin allergy

Vancomycin 1 g IV
+
Gentamicin 1.5 mg/kg IV or IM 1 hr before procedure; may repeat 8 hr after first dose

Low-risk patient, oral

Amoxicillin 3 g PO 1 hr before procedure; 1.5 g 6 hr after first dose

Standard regimen, low risk

Amoxicillin 2 g PO 1 hr before procedure

Penicillin allergy

Cephalexin 2 g PO 1 hr before procedure

or

Clindamycin 600 mg PO 1 hr before procedure

or

Azithromycin or clarithromycin 500 mg 1hr before procedure

Unable to take oral medications

Ampicillin 2 g IV or IM ½ hr before procedure

or

Clindamycin 600 mg IV 30 min before procedure

or

Cefazolin 1 g IM or IV 30 min before procedure

High-risk patient

Standard regimen

Ampicillin 2 g IV or IM
+
Gentamicin 1.5 mg/kg ½ hr before procedure; then amoxicillin 1 g PO 6 hr after initial dose or repeat parenteral regimen 8 hr after first dose

Penicillin allergic and unable to take oral medications

Vancomycin 1 g
+
Gentamicin 1.5 mg/kg IV over 1 hr starting 1 hr before procedure

G. Indications for tuberculosis (TB) prophylaxis include (1) close contact with a person with known active TB for <2 months; (2) a recent skin test (<2 years) that has now converted to positive (≥10 mm); and (3) a skin test that has been positive for an unknown length of time in a patient who also is immunocompromised or shows lesions on chest films. People exposed to patients with known isoniazid (INH)- and rifampin-resistant strains, or who reside in a known multidrug-resistant TB area, should receive ethambutol (ETB) and pyrazinamide (PZA) or PZA and ciprofloxacin.

H. Pneumococcal vaccine prophylaxis is given to patients at high-risk for *Streptococcus pneumoniae* infection. These include (1) every person ≥65 years old; (2) anyone ≥2 years old who has a chronic illness that would predispose to a pneumococcal infection (e.g., diabetes mellitus, alcoholism, liver cirrhosis, or various unspecified heart and lung diseases, (such as emphysema or severe congestive heart failure); (3) people who have immunocompromised disorders, including those who have had spleen removal, chronic kidney failure, or cancers (lymphoma, multiple myeloma), have undergone transplantation of an organ or bone marrow, or have HIV infection; and (4) any person who lives in a special environment or social setting (e.g., Native Americans).

References

Centers for Disease Control and Prevention. Guidelines for preventing the transmission of *Mycobacterium tuberculosis* in health-care facilities, 1994. MMWR 1994; 43 (RR-13):1.

Centers for Disease Control and Prevention. USPHS/IDSA guidelines for the prevention of opportunistic infections in persons infected with human immunodeficiency virus: a summary. MMWR 1995; 44 (RR-8):1.

Dajani AS, Taubert KA, Wilson W, et al. Prevention of bacterial endocarditis: recommendations by the American Heart Association. JAMA 1997; 277:1794.

Dickinson GM, Bisno AL. Antimicrobial prophylaxis of infection. Infect Dis Clin North Am 1995; 9:783.

Ericsson CD, DuPont HL. Traveler's diarrhea: approaches to prevention and treatment. Clin Infect Dis 1993; 16:616.

Falagas ME, Gorbach SL. Practice guidelines: urinary tract infections. Infect Dis Clin Pract 1995; 4:241.

Fiebach N, Beckett W. Prevention of respiratory infections in adults. Influenza and pneumococcal vaccines. Arch Intern Med 1994; 154:2545.

Giarmarellou H. Empiric therapy for infections in the febrile, neutropenic, compromised host. Med Clin North Am 1995; 79:559.

NONSURGICAL ANTIMICROBIAL PROPHYLAXIS
(Cont'd from p 581)

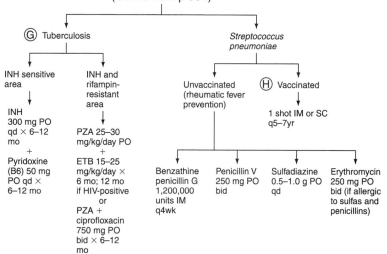

Ⓖ Tuberculosis

INH sensitive area

INH
300 mg PO
qd × 6–12
mo
+
Pyridoxine
(B6) 50 mg
PO qd ×
6–12 mo

INH and rifampin-resistant area

PZA 25–30
mg/kg/day PO
+
ETB 15–25
mg/kg/day ×
6 mo; 12 mo
if HIV-positive
or
PZA +
ciprofloxacin
750 mg PO
bid × 6–12
mo

Streptococcus pneumoniae

Unvaccinated (rheumatic fever prevention)

Benzathine
penicillin G
1,200,000
units IM
q4wk

Penicillin V
250 mg PO
bid

Sulfadiazine
0.5–1.0 g PO
qd

Erythromycin
250 mg PO
bid (if allergic
to sulfas and
penicillins)

Ⓗ **Vaccinated**

1 shot IM or SC
q5–7yr

ANTIMICROBIAL PROPHYLAXIS IN SURGICAL PATIENTS

Brian L. Erstad

A. A classification system for expected postoperative wound infection rates related to surgical procedures was developed by the National Academy of Sciences–National Research Council in the 1960s. This system categorized surgery as clean (Cl), clean-contaminated (CC), unknown contamination (UC), contaminated (CO), or dirty (D), depending on associated infection rates; rates of infection are generally <2% for clean and about 40% for dirty procedures. However, infection rates for the same operation may vary at different institutions; physician- and institution-specific rates should be recorded and used in the consideration of prophylaxis. Other factors predictive of postoperative infection, including risks within particular categories, are described elsewhere (see reference by Page, et al.). In addition to the antimicrobials listed in the decision tree, mechanical bowel cleansing (e.g., oral polyethylene glycol solution, sodium phosphate with or without bisacodyl) is routinely used the day before elective colorectal surgery. For abdominal trauma, prophylaxis is indicated until the exact site and extent of injury can be determined during surgery. Treatment, not prophylaxis, is needed for contaminated or dirty surgical procedures, as well as complicated trauma (e.g., colon injury with delayed surgery). Local antimicrobial prophylaxis with irrigations, impregnated beads or cement, and bonded grafts may provide protection equivalent to IV prophylaxis in some types of surgery, but well-designed trials are needed before recommendations can be made with confidence.

B. Do not base the decision to use antimicrobial prophylaxis solely on postoperative wound infection rates. Total hip replacement is classified as a clean operative procedure according to criteria developed by the National Academy of Sciences–National Research Council, but a postoperative infection of the prosthesis may be catastrophic. Hence, a clinically significant decrease in the incidence of an unacceptable complication may be sufficient justification for prophylaxis. Such justification often is used for the prophylaxis of bacterial endocarditis.

C. Cefazolin is the standard with which other antimicrobials should be compared for most surgical procedures. Cefazolin is inexpensive, has a moderately long half-life, has a spectrum against most predominant pathogens, and has demonstrated activity in clinical trials. Vancomycin may be used for surgery involving prosthetic materials or devices (including total hip replacement) *if* a high rate of methicillin-resistant *Staphylococcus aureus* or *epidermidis* infection has been documented, but its use is not indicated for routine prophylaxis, given the increasing incidence of vancomycin-resistant enterococcal infection.

TABLE 1 Drug Dosages for Surgical Antimicrobial Prophylaxis

Cefazolin	1–2 g IV
Cefoxitin	1–2 g IV
Vancomycin	1 g IV
Clindamycin	600–900 mg IV
Gentamicin	1.7 mg/kg IV
Penicillin	1 million units IV
Erythromycin	1 g PO × 3 doses*
Neomycin	1 g PO × 3 doses*

*Give at 1 PM, 2 PM, and 11 PM the day before surgery.

D. Antimicrobials with aerobic and anaerobic activity (e.g., second-generation cephalosporins, ampicillin/sulbactam, ticarcillin/clavulanate, trovafloxacin) are indicated for prophylaxis when mixed pathogens are common, as in surgery for diabetic foot infections and abdominal trauma. In colorectal surgery it is unclear whether IV antimicrobials provide benefits beyond mechanical cleansing and oral antimicrobial prophylaxis, but a single dose of an agent with combined aerobic/anaerobic activity is often used. Give IV antimicrobials within 30 minutes of the first incision to ensure adequate concentrations. Additional doses of the antimicrobial may be needed during extended procedures, depending on its pharmacokinetic properties: for example, a second dose of cefazolin should be given 4 hours and cefoxitin 2 hours from the start of an operation. With the possible exceptions of coronary bypass and arthroplastic procedures, there is little benefit from antimicrobial administration beyond a single preoperative dose (unless treatment, not prophylaxis, is indicated). Recommended dosages are listed in Table 1.

References

Antimicrobial prophylaxis in surgery. Med Lett Drugs Ther 1993; 35:91.

Cruse PJE, Foord R. A five-year prospective study of 23,649 surgical wounds. Arch Surg 1973; 107:206.

Culver DH, Horan TC, Gaynes RP, et al. National Nosocomial Infections Surveillance System. Surgical wound rates by wound class, operative procedure, and patient risk index in US hospitals, 1986–1990. Am J Med 1991; 3B(suppl):152.

Davis JM, Huycke MM, Wells CL, et al. Surgical Infection Society position on vancomycin-resistant enterococcus. Arch Surg 1996; 131:1061.

Martin C, Viviand X, Potie F. Local antibiotic prophylaxis in surgery. Infect Control Hosp Epidemiol 1996; 17:539.

Nichols RL, Smith JW, Garcia RY, et al. Current practices of preoperative bowel preparation among North American colorectal surgeons. Clin Infect Dis 1997; 24:609.

Page CP, Bohnen JMA, Fletcher JR, et al. Antimicrobial prophylaxis for surgical wounds: guidelines for clinical care. Arch Surg 1993; 128:79.

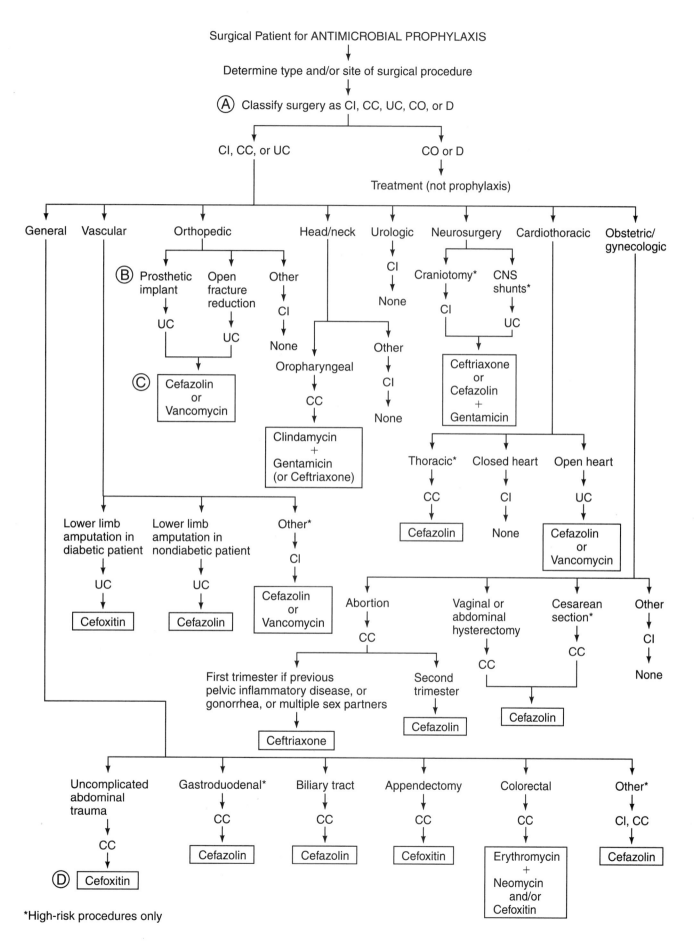

Surgical Patient for ANTIMICROBIAL PROPHYLAXIS

Determine type and/or site of surgical procedure

Ⓐ Classify surgery as CI, CC, UC, CO, or D

CI, CC, or UC

CO or D

Treatment (not prophylaxis)

General   Vascular   Orthopedic   Head/neck   Urologic   Neurosurgery   Cardiothoracic   Obstetric/gynecologic

Ⓑ Prosthetic implant   Open fracture reduction   Other

UC   UC

Ⓒ Cefazolin or Vancomycin

CI

None

Oropharyngeal

CC

Clindamycin + Gentamicin (or Ceftriaxone)

CI

None

Other

CI

None

Craniotomy*   CNS shunts*

CI   UC

Ceftriaxone or Cefazolin + Gentamicin

Thoracic*   Closed heart   Open heart

CC   CI   UC

Cefazolin   None   Cefazolin or Vancomycin

Lower limb amputation in diabetic patient   Lower limb amputation in nondiabetic patient   Other*

UC   UC   CI

Cefoxitin   Cefazolin   Cefazolin or Vancomycin

Abortion

CC

Vaginal or abdominal hysterectomy   Cesarean section*   Other

CC   CC   CI

None

First trimester if previous pelvic inflammatory disease, or gonorrhea, or multiple sex partners   Second trimester

Ceftriaxone   Cefazolin   Cefazolin

Uncomplicated abdominal trauma   Gastroduodenal*   Biliary tract   Appendectomy   Colorectal   Other*

CC   CC   CC   CC   CC   CI, CC

Ⓓ Cefoxitin   Cefazolin   Cefazolin   Cefoxitin   Erythromycin + Neomycin and/or Cefoxitin   Cefazolin

*High-risk procedures only

585

CHOOSING APPROPRIATE ANTIMICROBIAL THERAPY

Michael D. Katz

The choice of appropriate antimicrobial therapy should be based on several factors, including pathogens being treated, the antimicrobial spectrum, and a variety of patient-specific factors. Antibiotic choices should be based on a sound rationale.

A. Empiric therapy is based on a presumptive diagnosis of infection or clinical syndrome. Especially in the hospital setting, empiric therapy is broad in spectrum, designed to cover the most likely pathogens in the specific patient. Before initiating empiric therapy, obtain appropriate specimens for culture and sensitivity. Empiric therapy is indicated when the infection is potentially rapidly life threatening (sepsis, pneumonia) or causes significant morbidity (urinary tract infection, otitis media).

B. The most likely pathogens at a site of infection may be based on normal flora at that site, tropism of certain pathogens for various tissues or organs, and patient-specific factors such as previous antimicrobial therapy, nosocomial versus community-acquired infection, and patient immune status. Not every possible pathogen requires coverage; just those that are most likely. Recent emergence of drug resistance in common bacterial pathogens such as *Streptococcus pneumoniae, Staphylococcus aureus,* and *Enterococcus* has made antibiotic decision making more complex. The clinician must know current local resistance patterns of common pathogens as well as factors driving increased resistance. The use of certain drugs such as vancomycin should be based on strict guidelines to reduce the development and spread of resistance.

C. Patient-specific factors include history of previous adverse reactions to antimicrobials, patient age, pregnancy or lactation, concomitant drugs, excretory organ function, immune status, and site of infection. For very ill patients, IV administration is preferable to ensure adequate drug concentrations at the site of infection.

D. Combination therapy is indicated when broad-spectrum coverage is desired (sepsis), in polymicrobial infections (intraperitoneal abscesses), to prevent the emergence of resistance (tuberculosis), or to provide antimicrobial synergy (streptococcal endocarditis, β-lactam/aminoglycoside for *Pseudomonas aeruginosa* infections, amphotericin/5- flucytosine for cryptococcal meningitis).

E. The cost of drug therapy is based not only on the drug cost but on the cost of administration, supplies, and monitoring. If all else is equal, choose the least expensive regimen. However, therapeutic efficacy is of primary importance.

F. Definitive therapy occurs when a microbiologic as well as a clinical diagnosis is confirmed. Definitive therapy is narrow in spectrum and generally requires only one drug. If the patient was previously receiving empiric therapy, determine the need for continued treatment.

G. Sensitivity data are useful in determining definitive data, but there are pitfalls. If the reported sensitivities do not fit usual patterns for that organism, the reliability of the information is suspect. If minimal inhibitory concentrations (MICs) are present, in general, any drug in the sensitive MIC range will be effective.

H. Even with positive cultures, broad-spectrum therapy may be indicated. Base the choice of antimicrobial regimen on clinical judgment as well as laboratory data.

I. A variety of drug-specific factors must be considered. Certain agents do not penetrate well into certain tissues (aminoglycosides in CNS infections). If a relatively new antimicrobial is considered, there should be clinical trials documenting efficacy compared with the conventional regimen for that infection. Consider drug toxicity; reserve more toxic drugs (aminoglycosides, amphotericin B) for higher-risk patients.

J. If the patient is not very ill and has adequate GI tract function, give oral antimicrobials as soon as possible. However, in some cases, long-term or home IV antimicrobial therapy is indicated if oral agents are not available for the specific infection.

References

Kim JG, Gallis HA. Observations on spiraling empiricism: its causes, allure, and perils with particular reference to antibiotic therapy. Am J Med 1989; 87:201.

Moellering RC. Principles of anti-infective therapy. In: Mandell GL, Bennett JE, Dolin R, eds. Principles and practice of infectious diseases. 4th ed. New York: Churchill Livingstone, 1995:199.

Shales DM, Gerding DN, John JF, et al. Society for Healthcare Epidemiology of America and Infectious Disease Society of American Joint Committee on the Prevention of Antimicrobial Resistance: guidelines for the prevention of antimicrobial resistance in hospitals. Clin Infect Dis 1997; 25:584.

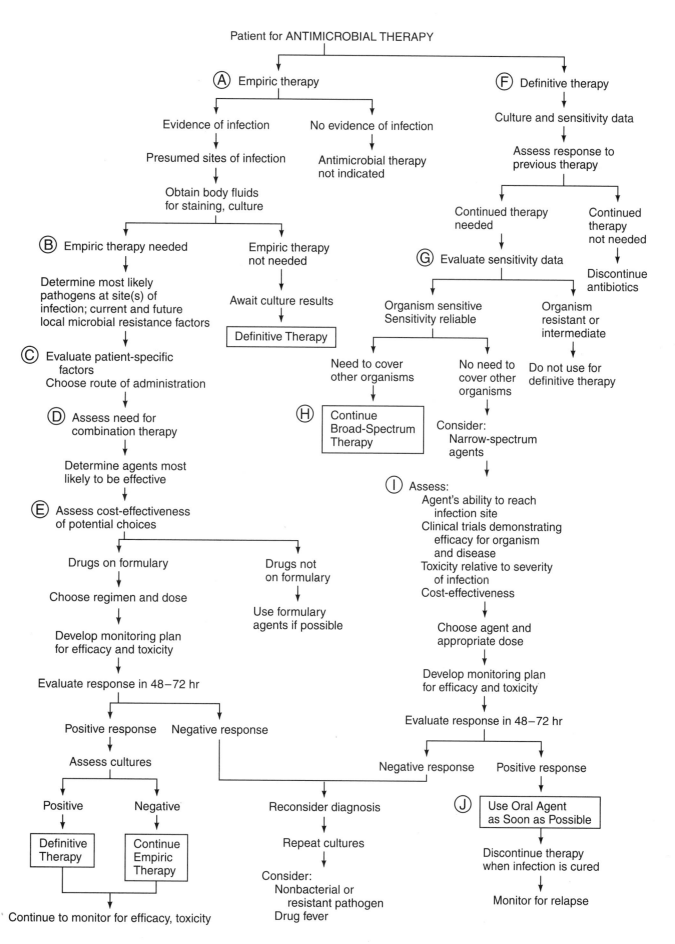

Patient for ANTIMICROBIAL THERAPY

(A) Empiric therapy

Evidence of infection

No evidence of infection

Presumed sites of infection

Antimicrobial therapy not indicated

Obtain body fluids for staining, culture

(B) Empiric therapy needed

Empiric therapy not needed

Determine most likely pathogens at site(s) of infection; current and future local microbial resistance factors

Await culture results

Definitive Therapy

(C) Evaluate patient-specific factors
Choose route of administration

(D) Assess need for combination therapy

Determine agents most likely to be effective

(E) Assess cost-effectiveness of potential choices

Drugs on formulary

Drugs not on formulary

Choose regimen and dose

Use formulary agents if possible

Develop monitoring plan for efficacy and toxicity

Evaluate response in 48–72 hr

Positive response   Negative response

Assess cultures

Positive   Negative

Definitive Therapy

Continue Empiric Therapy

Reconsider diagnosis

Repeat cultures

Consider:
Nonbacterial or resistant pathogen
Drug fever

Continue to monitor for efficacy, toxicity

(F) Definitive therapy

Culture and sensitivity data

Assess response to previous therapy

Continued therapy needed

Continued therapy not needed

(G) Evaluate sensitivity data

Discontinue antibiotics

Organism sensitive
Sensitivity reliable

Organism resistant or intermediate

Need to cover other organisms

No need to cover other organisms

Do not use for definitive therapy

(H) Continue Broad-Spectrum Therapy

Consider:
Narrow-spectrum agents

(I) Assess:
Agent's ability to reach infection site
Clinical trials demonstrating efficacy for organism and disease
Toxicity relative to severity of infection
Cost-effectiveness

Choose agent and appropriate dose

Develop monitoring plan for efficacy and toxicity

Evaluate response in 48–72 hr

Negative response   Positive response

(J) Use Oral Agent as Soon as Possible

Discontinue therapy when infection is cured

Monitor for relapse

USE AND MONITORING OF AMINOGLYCOSIDE ANTIBIOTICS

Brian L. Erstad

Gentamicin (G), tobramycin (T), netilmicin (N), and amikacin (A) are members of a class of anti-infectives known as the aminoglycosides. They are injectable antimicrobials primarily used for their excellent activity against gram-negative aerobic bacteria, with a few important exceptions (e.g., *Stenotrophomonas maltophilia*). These agents tend to have similar spectra, although tobramycin may be particularly useful for *Pseudomonas aeruginosa* in institutions with gentamicin-resistant strains. The aminoglycosides are particularly useful for their additive or synergistic actions with other antimicrobials in serious infections. They are commonly used in combination with penicillins for synergism when treating enterococcal infections. Many infectious disease experts also recommend the addition of an aminoglycoside to β-lactam therapy for serious infections caused by organisms such as *P. aeruginosa.*

A. Although the loading dose of an aminoglycoside can be readily calculated on the basis of body weight, the subsequent maintenance doses need to be calculated with consideration of the patient's renal function. Equations and computer programs have been developed for dosing the aminoglycosides, but less complicated nomograms can be used until blood levels are obtained. The nomograms of Sarubbi and Hull (for traditional multiple-dose daily regimens) and Nicolau et al. (for single-dose daily regimens) are widely used. Once-daily regimens involve less complicated dosing calculations and are probably less labor intensive than traditional dosing methods yet have similar efficacy in most populations. However, some groups have not been well studied (e.g., transplant, pregnant, burn, and pediatric patients), and others (e.g., geriatric patients) may be more prone to toxicity with once-daily dosing.

B. One interaction between aminoglycosides and penicillins deserves special mention. Aminoglycoside concentrations may be lowered in vivo and in vitro by concomitant administration of penicillins. The schedules of these antimicrobials should be spread as far apart as possible to avoid this interaction.

C. Remember to monitor the patient and not just the serum aminoglycoside levels. Potential nephro- and ototoxicity concerns have led to use of aminoglycoside assays at many hospitals. When used appropriately, these assays can be valuable monitoring tools. However, they are not a substitute for clinical evaluation. Aminoglycoside levels may be in the therapeutic range, but the patient may not be clinically improving, which may require a change or re-evaluation of therapy. Aminoglycoside levels may not be needed for expected therapy <5 days in patients with stable renal function and fluid balance. When aminoglycoside levels are needed, diligent attention to their collection and analysis is crucial. Aminogly-coside doses may be skipped or given at unexpected times. Blood may be drawn from a line containing the aminoglycoside or not drawn at all. The draw may not be at the proper time. If the level is ordered and drawn correctly, the specimen may not be properly stored before analysis.

D. The definitions of the pharmacokinetic terms *peak* and *trough* have not been standardized in the medical literature. In this chapter peak level refers to the blood concentration of an aminoglycoside drawn 30 minutes after a 30-minute infusion. The trough level is the concentration 30 minutes before a dose of the aminoglycoside. For once-daily dosing a single level is drawn 6–14 hours after the dose is administered, with subsequent adjustment by nomogram (see Nicolau reference).

E. The introduction of antimicrobials with enhanced gram-negative activity has allowed the clinician more choices for treating such infections. Fears of aminoglycoside toxicity have limited the use of these compounds in many institutions. However, with proper selection and monitoring of patients, the incidence of major toxicity is acceptable. It is thought that the nephrotoxicity associated with aminoglycosides primarily is related to multiple daily doses given for prolonged periods. Other factors associated with aminoglycoside toxicity include liver disease, shock, and congestive heart failure, as well as the age and sex of the patient (higher in the elderly and females). Fortunately, when nephrotoxicity does occur, it usually presents as a reversible, nonoliguric renal failure. Ototoxicity usually occurs in patients with renal failure who receive aminoglycosides for prolonged periods.

F. The optimal duration of aminoglycoside therapy has not been well studied. In general, extended courses (weeks) are necessary for more severe infections such as osteomyelitis caused by gram-negative bacteria. Uncomplicated wound or urinary tract infections often resolve after 3–5 days of taking the aminoglycosides. Consider the site, severity, and clinical response in deciding when to discontinue therapy.

References

Hatala R, Dinh T, Cook DC. Once-daily aminoglycoside dosing in immunocompetent adults: a meta-analysis. Ann Intern Med 1996; 124:717.

Henderson JL, Polk RE, Kline BJ. In vitro interaction of gentamicin, tobramycin, and netilmicin by carbenicillin, azlocillin, or mezlocillin. Am J Hosp Pharm 1981; 38:1167.

Marra F, Partovi N, Jewesson P. Aminoglycoside administered as a single daily dose. Drugs 1996; 52:344.

USE OF AMINOGLYCOSIDE ANTIBIOTIC INDICATED

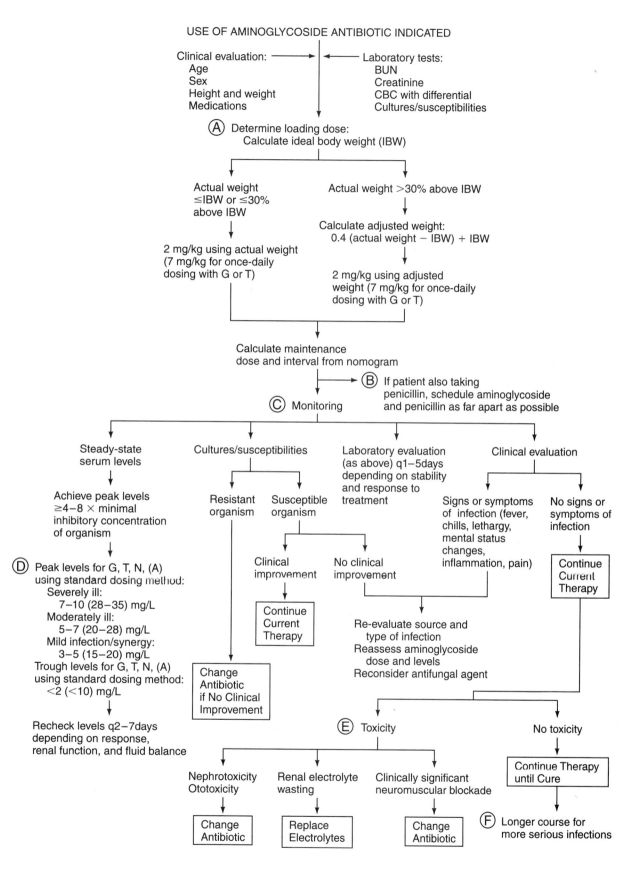

Nicolau DP, Freeman CD, Belliveau PP, et al. Experience with a once-daily aminoglycoside program administered to 2,184 adult patients. Antimicrob Agents Chemother 1995; 39:650.

Sarubbi FA, Hull JH. Amikacin serum concentrations: prediction of levels and dosage guidelines. Ann Intern Med 1978; 89:612.

USE AND EVALUATION OF SERUM DRUG LEVELS

Collin Freeman
Brian L. Erstad

A. Certain medications have a pharmacokinetic characteristic known as a narrow therapeutic index (NTI). This means there is a narrow range, or window, between a serum level at which a drug will have a minimal therapeutic effect and a minimal toxic effect. Some examples of these medications include but are not limited to theophylline, phenytoin, carbamazepine, digoxin, procainamide, quinidine, and aminoglycoside antibiotics (see p 588 for specific evaluation and dosing of aminoglycoside antibiotics). These drugs generally have a relationship between the effect of the drug and the patient's serum drug level (SDL). Not all drugs with an assay for obtaining an SDL have this relationship (e.g., benzodiazepines). Other drugs may be monitored by SDLs only under certain circumstances (e.g., aspirin in Kawasaki's syndrome).

B. Therapeutic drug monitoring (TDM) involves patients receiving drugs with an NTI and requires obtaining SDLs at appropriate times to maximize efficacy and minimize toxicity of that particular drug therapy. The use of pharmacokinetics often is helpful to develop a personal drug-dosing regimen based on SDLs. Obtain a patient's specific parameters (weight, height, age, sex, renal and hepatic laboratory values) because these factors can all affect an SDL and the response to drug therapy.

C. Most therapeutic ranges of NTI drugs are based on a trough level, which usually is defined as an SDL obtained 30 minutes or less before the next scheduled dose of the drug. Reference ranges for SDLs in the literature usually are based on trough levels. It is therefore difficult to judge what an SDL means clinically when it is drawn too early. Drawing an SDL too early may also cause an erroneously high level to be reported (e.g., digoxin). This can occur if the blood is drawn during the distribution phase of the drug (the period in which the drug in the plasma is equilibrating with the tissues and other fluids into which it will distribute). An SDL is more useful when the patient's blood is drawn after it has achieved steady state (SS). Steady state is that condition in which the rate of the drug administered is equal to the rate of its elimination. Drawing blood and determining an SDL before the drug has reached SS usually results in a lower level being reported than will occur at SS. Four to five half-lives is the time frame considered necessary before a drug achieves SS. Therefore, to calculate when a drug will reach SS, the clinician must first obtain the appropriate half-life of the drug for the particular patient.

D. It is important that the patient's response to the medication be considered rather than the reported SDL.

E. Changing a drug dosage regimen on the basis of an SDL should be carefully considered. All benefits and risks of a dosage change need to be taken into account (e.g., when a theophylline level has been reported correctly as 19.0 [therapeutic 10-20] µg/ml but the patient has not experienced clinical benefit). It is probably more prudent to try an additional therapy or discontinue the theophylline and try another kind of bronchodilating therapy rather than attempt to obtain an SDL of 20 µg/ml.

References

Postelnick M. Therapeutic drug monitoring: where have we been and where are we going? J Pharm Pract 1995; 8:1.

Schumacher GE. TDM: therapeutic drug monitoring. Norwalk, CT: Appleton & Lange, 1995.

Taylor WJ, Diers-Caviness MH, eds. A textbook for the clinical application of therapeutic drug monitoring. Irving, TX: Abbot Laboratories, Diagnostic Division, 1986.

EVALUATION OF SERUM DRUG LEVEL Requested

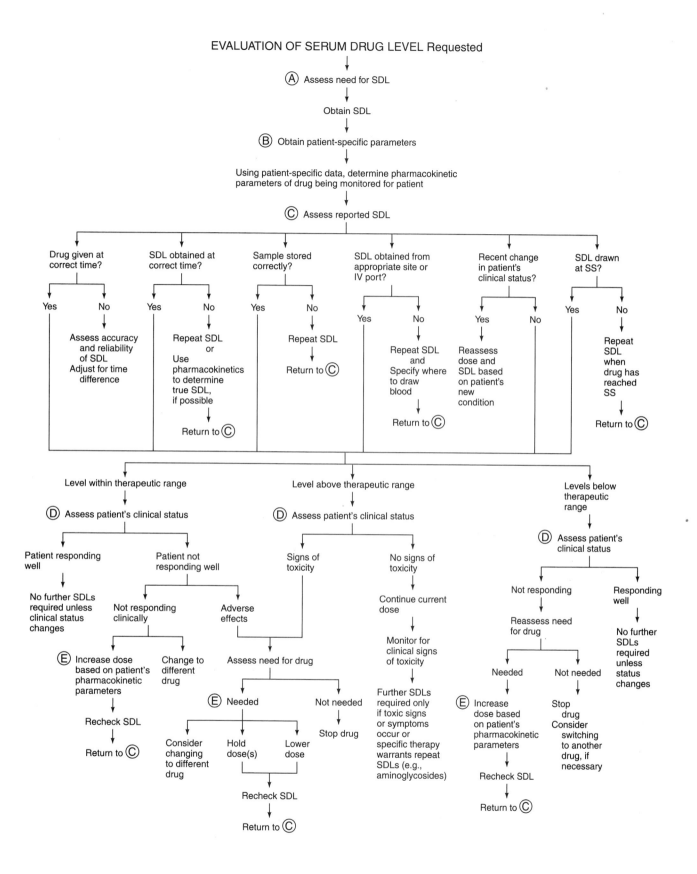

EVALUATION OF A DRUG FOR CLINICAL USE OR INCLUSION IN A FORMULARY

Terra A. Robles

The systematic evaluation of the impact of drug therapy is the basis for guiding clinicians in selecting safe, effective agents for disease treatment. As new drugs become available, more effective agents should replace those found less effective in well-designed clinical trials. FDA approval covers a drug's safety and efficacy for its labeled indications. However, the FDA does not address whether a drug is safer or more effective than other agents for a given indication. Systems for maximizing rational drug use are necessary in organized health care settings because of the multiplicity of drugs, the complexities of their use, and the necessity of cost-effective practices. Pharmacy and Therapeutics (P&T) Committees were developed to assist as advisory and educational bodies to medical staffs on issues concerning the therapeutic use of drugs. The Joint Commission on Accreditation of Healthcare Organizations (JCAHO) requires hospitals to have a functioning P&T Committee, as does the National Committee for Quality Assurance (NCQA) for managed-care organizations. The formulary is a list of pharmaceuticals that in the judgment of the P&T Committee and the medical staff, permits high-quality yet cost-effective therapy. The P&T Committee continuously evaluates agents for comparative efficacy and safety and develops and enforces policies that prevent the use of agents likely to lead to suboptimal, hazardous, or unnecessarily costly health outcomes. As fragmented health care moves toward treatment based on illnesses, P&T Committees must likewise move toward evaluating drug use within the scope of disease management, including total quality and economic impact. This process involves the evaluation of drug studies.

A. A drug or drug class is selected for evaluation because (1) a new drug entity has been introduced; (2) a drug has a newly approved or changed use; (3) a drug has a new approved dosage form, a new method of administration, or a new combination of active ingredients; (4) there has been a significant change in the drug's profile: pharmacology, pharmacokinetics, or cost; (5) prescribing has been inappropriate, drug cost is high, or drug monitoring requires the development of specific guidelines or criteria of use; (6) local practice standards warrant evaluation of a drug for an unlabeled use; (7) a drug has decreased usefulness; (8) the use or cost of the drug is greater than expected; or (9) the prescriber has requested consideration of the drug's addition to the formulary.

B. Appropriate medical literature documenting the safety and efficacy of the drug to be evaluated must be available. Pharmaceutical manufacturer-provided information must not be the sole source for such data. Non-biased, blinded, randomized, controlled studies offer credibility. Pharmacoeconomic and cost-effectiveness studies also should be included.

C. Decide whether an entire disease state review or only portions of a review are required. It is important to include all areas that will provide the evaluator with the information necessary for a comprehensive review.

D. When a summary of information is presented to the P&T Committee, it should be organized in a format that can easily be critiqued and assimilated, including all the areas decided on in C.

E. The FDA classifies drugs as "P," priority review drug (a drug that appears to represent an advantage over available therapy); "S," standard review drug (a drug that appears to have therapeutic qualities similar to those of an already marketed drug); "AA," AIDS drug (a drug indicated for treating AIDS or other HIV-related disease); "E," subpart E drug (a drug developed or evaluated under special procedure for drugs to treat life-threatening or severely debilitating illnesses); and "V," designated orphan drug.

F. Determine whether the differences between the new agent and other similar agents are clinically significant. Consider any information that may affect outcomes (e.g., drug interactions, increased hospitalizations). Address additional costs or quality-of-care issues associated with incorrect use or ineffectiveness; assess any increased costs versus increased safety, efficacy, and outcome.

G. Summarize well-designed clinical trials that evaluate therapeutic outcomes. Are only in vitro data available, or is there meaningful clinical information? Identify studies that address total impact on the treatment of the disease. This will assist in distinguishing all costs and benefits, which may not be realized if only the drug agent is evaluated.

H. An older drug may have much documentation on its adverse drug reactions (ADRs), whereas a new agent in the same class may not. Keep in mind the potential that a new agent may have an unreported ADR. Evaluating a drug's pharmacology and pharmacokinetics will assist in identifying potential ADRs.

I. Consider a drug's potential to reduce overall cost (e.g., decreased length of stay). This should be determined for all therapeutically similar agents as compared with the new drug being reviewed. Consider whether the additional cost of an agent associated with marginal benefit justifies its use. Pharmacoeconomic evaluations can assist in identifying impact beyond acquisition costs (e.g., polypharmacy of less effective agents, cost of ADRs, monitoring, dosage escalation).

REQUEST TO P&T COMMITTEE FOR FORMULARY ADDITION OR DRUG REVIEW

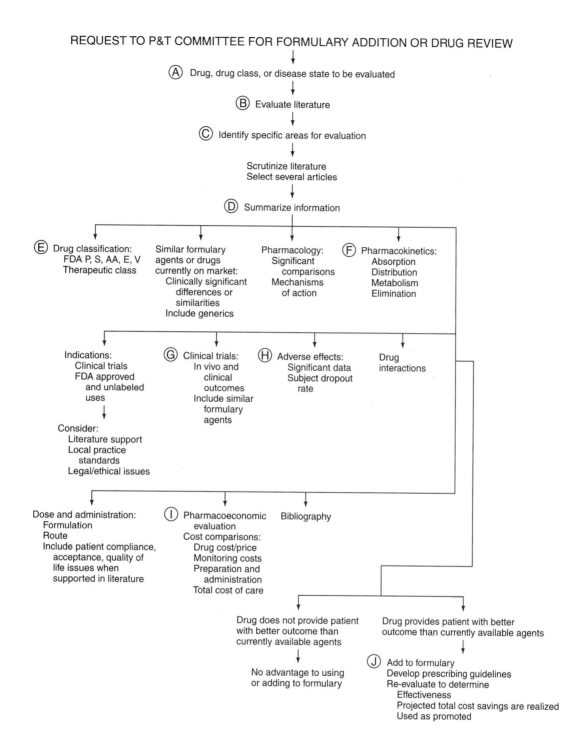

J. Follow-up is necessary, especially for drugs that require monitoring or surveillance programs. Delete from the formulary, if possible, drugs that the new agent is replacing.

References

American Society of Health Systems Pharmacists. ASHP statement on medication-use evaluation. Am J Health Syst Pharm 1996; 53:1953.

Liang FZ, Greenberg RB, Hogan GF. Legal issues associated with formulary product selection when there are two or more recognized drug therapies. Am J Hosp Pharm 1988; 45:2372.

Pilkington MA, Dolinsky D. Selecting alternate drug therapies. Med Care 1991; 29:152.

Schumacher GE. Multiattribute evaluation in formulary decision making as applied to calcium-channel blockers. Am J Hosp Pharm 1991; 48:301.

Sesin GP. Therapeutic decision-making: a model for formulary evaluation. Drug Intell Clin Pharm 1986; 20:581.

INDEX

A

Abdominal pain
    acute, 154-155
    chronic, 156-157
    and gas, 196
    in women, 470-471
ABO compatibility
    in granulocyte transfusion, 228
    in platelet transfusion, 224
Abortion, spontaneous, 466
Abscess
    brain, 262
    intra-abdominal, 296
    prostatic, 512
Acanthosis nigricans, 122
Achalasia, 162, 166
ACHES mnemonic, 494
Acid ingestion, 528
Acidosis
    metabolic, 310-311
    respiratory, 312
Acoustic neuroma, 38
Acoustic stapedius reflex testing, 42
Acromegaly, 148
Acromioclavicular separations, 422
Acute abdomen, 154-155, 470-471
Acute interstitial nephritis, 300
Acute myocardial infarction, 78, 98-101
Acute promyelocytic leukemia, 216
Acute renal failure, 50, 300-301
Acute tubular necrosis, 300
Acyclovir, 460
Adenocarcinoma, 244
Adenomas
    adrenocortical, 76
    parathyroid, 128
    pituitary, 146, 148
Adenopathy, mediastinal, 232, 400-401
Adenosine, 64
Adrenal glands
    and gynecomastia, 152
    mass in, 144-145
    postoperative suppression of, 52-53
Adrenal insufficiency, fatigue in, 4
α-Adrenergic agents
    for prostatodynia, 512
    for urinary incontinence, 514
β₂-Adrenergic agonists, 576
β-Adrenergic antagonists; *see* β Blockers
Adrenocorticotropic hormone excess, 146
Adriamycin, bleomycin, vinblastine, and dacarbazine
        (ABVD), 232
Adverse drug reactions, 578-579, 592
Ageusia, 382
Agoraphobia, 544
AIDS dementia complex, 380
Airway obstruction, foreign body, 526
Akathisia, 370
Albumin
    ascites and, 174
    in edema, 18

Alcohol
    acute behavioral change from, 376
    confusional states from, 380
    gynecomastia from, 152
    hypoglycemia from, 120
    myopathy from, 358
    and transaminase levels, 200
Alcoholism, 542-543
    anorexia and weight loss from, 160
    hypomagnesemia in, 322
    and liver disease, 202
    memory loss from, 344
Aldosteronism, 76
Alkali burns, 528
Alkaline phosphatase, 454-455
    and osteopenia, 440
Alkalosis
    metabolic, 312-313
    respiratory, 310
Allergy
    conjunctivitis from, 30
    rhinitis from, 34
    transfusions and, 230
Allograft rejection, renal transplant, 330
Alloimmunization, and platelet transfusions, 224
Allopurinol
    for chronic myelogenous leukemia, 234
    for gout, 442
    for kidney stones, 306
Alport's syndrome, 40
Alzheimer's disease, 346, 378
Amantadine, 364
Amaurosis fugax, 338
Amenorrhea, 462-463
Amikacin, 588
Aminoglycosides
    in neutropenic patient, 246
    use and monitoring of, 588-589
Amiodarone, hyperpigmentation from, 104
Amnesia, 344-347
Amoxicillin/clavulanate, 476
Amphotericin B, 247
Ampicillin, 528
Amylase, elevated serum, 204-205
Amylase/creatinine clearance ratio, 204
Amyl nitrate, 72
Amyloidosis, 238
Amyotrophic lateral sclerosis, 356
Analgesic rebound headache, 334
Anaphylaxis, 574-577
Anegrelide, 211
Anemia, 206-209
    and neutropenia, 214
    transfusion and, 226
Aneurysm, aortic, 178
Angina
    stable, 66-67
    unstable, 68-70
    in women, 472-475
Angioedema, 108

Angioplasty, percutaneous coronary
  for acute myocardial infarction, 98
  unstable angina and, 66
Angiotensin-converting enzyme inhibitors, 98
Animal bites, 530-531
Anion gap acidosis, 310
Ankylosing spondylitis, 414, 416
Anorectal disorders
  constipation from, 188
  and fecal incontinence, 198
Anorectal pain, 192-193
Anorexia, 160-161
Anorexia nervosa, 8, 160
Anorgasmia, 16
Anosmia, 382
Anovulation, 462
Antibiotics
  for genital herpes, 460
  for meningitis, 262, 264, 266, 268
  in neutropenic patient, 246-247
  for prostatitis, 512
  for red eye, 30
  for rhinitis, 32
  for salpingitis, 460
  for *S. aureus* bacteremia, 292
  for sepsis, 288
  for urinary tract infections, 476
  use and monitoring of, 588-589
Antibodies
  anticoagulant, 220
  antinuclear, 452-453
  in CREST syndrome, 434
  thyroid, 130
  transfusions and, 230
Anticentromere antibody, 452
Anticholinergics, 372
Anticoagulants, endogenous, 220
Anticoagulation therapy
  acute, 566-569
  long-term, 570-573
  for stroke, 340, 342
  for transient ischemic attacks, 336-337
Antidepressants
  for anxiety disorders, 554
  for depression, 548
  for eating disorders, 8
Antiepileptic drugs, 350
Antihistamines, 576
Antihistone antibodies, 452
Antimicrobials
  for acute meningitis, 262, 264
  for bite wounds, 530
  choice of, 586-587
  in neutropenic patients, 246-247
  prophylactic, 580-585
Antinuclear antibody test, 452-453
α_2-Antiplasmin deficiency, 216
Antiplatelet therapy, 336
Antipsychotic drugs, 556
Antiretroviral therapy, 276, 278
Antispasmodics
  for flatulence, 196
  for prostatodynia, 512
  for urinary incontinence, 514
Antithrombin III
  and deep venous thrombosis, 218
  disseminated intravascular coagulation and, 217

Antithyroglobulin antibodies, 130
Antithyroidal medications, 134, 136
Antivenin, 532
Anxiety, 544-547
  in bereavement, 554
  somatic symptoms of, 552
Aorta
  aneurysm in, 178
  coarctation of, 76
Aortic regurgitation, 72
Aortic stenosis, 70
Aortoenteric fistula, 178
Apnea
  in brain death, 386
  in near-drowning, 536, 538
Arrhythmias, 60-65
  cardiac arrest from, 94
  hypotension from, 78
  palpitations from, 80
Arteriography
  bronchial, 388
  for gastrointestinal bleeding, 180-181
  for pulseless extremity, 522
Arteriovenous malformations
  and guaiac-positive stools, 194
  and pulmonary nodules, 404
Arteritis
  giant cell, 444-445
  temporal, 332, 338
Arthritis
  foot, 432
  in hand and wrist, 428
  knee, 430
  monoarticular, 412-413
  polyarticular, 414-415
  seronegative, 416-417
  in temporomandibular joint, 450
Arthrography, knee, 430
Asbestos exposure, 410-411
Ascites, 174-175
Aspergillus, 247
Aspiration; *see also* Joint aspiration; Needle aspiration
  fluid, 536
  foreign body, 524
Aspirin, 336
Asterixis, 362
Asthma, 392
Ataxia, 348, 360
Atheromatous stenosis, 76
Athetosis, 370
Atopic dermatitis, 110
Atrial fibrillation, 134
Atrial premature contractions, 80
Atrial tachycardia, 62
Atrioventricular block, 60
Atrioventricular re-entrant tachycardia, 62
Atropine, 60
Atypical squamous cells of undetermined significance, 486
Austin Flint murmur, 72
Autoantibodies, factor VIII, 220
Autoimmune disorders
  fever from, 296-297
  hearing loss from, 40
  leukopenia in, 214
Autologous bone marrow transplantation, 252
Autologous transfusions, 226

Axillary lymph nodes
    breast cancer and, 480, 482
    carcinoma in, 244
    enlarged, 240
Azithromycin
    for *Chlamydia* infections, 461, 506
    in HIV-infected patient, 278
Azoospermia, 518
AZT; *see* Zidovudine

B

Babinski sign, 360
Back pain, lower, 424-425
Bacteremia, *Staphylococcus aureus,* 292-293
Bacteria
    drug resistance of, 586
    rhinitis from, 32
Bacteriuria, 512
Baker's cyst, 430
Balanitis circumscripta, 416
Ballismus, 370
Barium enema
    for belching causes, 168
    for constipation, 188
Barium esophagography, 162
Barotrauma, hearing loss from, 42
Barrett's esophagus, 164
Barrier contraceptive methods, 492
Battery ingestion, 524, 528
Battle's sign, 384
Becker's muscular dystrophy, 358
Becker's nevus, 104
Behavioral therapy
    for anxiety attacks, 544
    for obesity, 12
Behavior change
    acute, 376-377
    chronic, 378-381
Belching, 168-169
Bell's palsy, loss of taste in, 382
Benign paroxysmal positional vertigo, 348
Benign prostatic hyperplasia, 506, 510
Benzodiazepines, 38
Bereavement, 554-555
Bernstein test, 166
Bile acid malabsorption, 190
Biliary cirrhosis, pruritus in, 110
Biliary colic, 176-177
Biopsy
    bone, 250
    bone marrow, 214
    of brain and meninges, 266
    breast, 478
    cervical, 460
    endometrial, 464
    liver, 200
    lymph node, 240, 244
    muscle, 456
    nerve, 366
    prostate, 510-511
Birth control methods, 490-493
Birthmarks, 104
Bites, human and animal, 530-531
Bladder
    calculi of, 506
    cancer of, 254, 506

Bladder outlet obstruction
    prostate enlargement and, 510
    and urinary incontinence, 516
Bleeding
    abnormal vaginal, 464-465
    disorders of, 220
    disseminated intravascular coagulation and, 216
    gastrointestinal, 178-181
    in pregnancy, 466-469
    rectal, 182-183
    warfarin-associated, 572
Blepharitis, 30
β Blockers
    for acute myocardial infarction, 98
    and thyroid, 54, 140
Blood cultures, 288
Blood gases, in near-drowning victim, 538
Blood pressure
    gastrointestinal bleeding and, 178, 180
    measurement of, 2, 74
    oral contraceptives and, 496
Blood transfusion; *see* Transfusion therapy
Blood urea nitrogen, gastrointestinal bleeding and, 180
Bone disease
    alkaline phosphatase and, 454
    metastatic, 248, 250
Bone marrow
    biopsy of, 214
    chronic myelogenous leukemia and, 234
    transplantation of, 252-253
Bone scanning, 248, 430
Boric acid, 459
Botulinum toxin injection, 372
Bowel disease, 178
Bradycardia, 60-61, 80
Brain abscess, 262
Brain death, 386-387
Brain trauma, confusional states from, 380
Breakthrough bleeding, oral contraceptives and, 494, 495, 496
Breast
    biopsy of, 478
    discharge from, 484-485
    examination of, 2
    oral contraceptives and, 496
Breast cancer, 244
    adjuvant therapy choices in, 480-483
    breast masses and, 478-479
    vs. gynecomastia, 152
    metastatic, chemotherapy for, 248
Breast conservation surgery, 480
Breast milk, oral contraceptives and, 494
Bretylium, 64
Bronchial arteriography, 388
Bronchial artery embolization, 388
Bronchitis, 394
Bronchoscopy
    for pulmonary nodules, 402, 404
    for stridor, 390
Bronchospasm, in anaphylaxis, 576
Brown-Séquard hemisection, 356
Bulimia, 8, 160
Bumetanide, 88
Bupropion, 560
Burns, acid and alkali, 528
Burping, 168-169
Bursitis, 418

Bursitis—cont'd
  knee, 430
  trochanteric, 426
Busulfan, 234

C

Café-au-lait spots, 104
Calcinosis, 434
Calcium
  hypercalcemia from, 128
  for hypocalcemia, 126
Calcium gluconate, for hydrofluoric acid burns, 528
Calcium pyrophosphate deposition, 412, 414
Calf vein thrombosis, 218
Campylobacter diarrhea, 260
Cancer
  adrenal, 144
  cervical, 466, 486
  colorectal, 182, 188, 194-195
  and Cushing's syndrome, 146
  gastric, 168
  hypercalcemia in, 128
  neutropenia in, 246-247
  and neutrophilia, 212
  obesity and, 12
  polyneuropathy from, 368
  prostate, 510, 512
  pulmonary nodules, 402-403, 404-405
  screening for, 2
  skeletal metastases of, 248
  squamous cell carcinoma, 244
  and superior vena caval syndrome, 256
  therapy-induced secondary malignancy in, 254-255
  thyroid, 138, 140
  of unknown primary site, 242-245
  uterine, 464
Candida
  in neutropenic patient, 247
  vulvovaginitis from, 458
Candidiasis, 272
Captopril stimulation test, 76
Carbapenems, 246
Carcinoma; *see* Cancer
Cardiac arrest, 94-95
Cardiac dyspnea, 96-97
Cardiac risk index, 44
Cardiac tamponade, 78
Cardiomegaly, 18, 84-85
Cardiomyopathies, 88
Cardiopulmonary resuscitation, 94, 536
Cardiovascular disease, oral contraceptives and, 494
Carnitine palmityl transferase deficiency, 374
Carotid artery disease, visual loss from, 338
Carotid stenosis, 336
Carpal tunnel syndrome, 428
Catecholamines
  hypoglycemia and, 120
  pheochromacytoma and, 76
Catheter
  Foley, 526
  Swan-Ganz, 78
Cauda equina lesions, 356-357
Caustic ingestion and exposure, 528-529
CD4 lymphocyte number, 276, 278
Cefazolin, 584
Cefepime, 246

Cefixime, 506
Cefoxitin, 584
Ceftazidime, 246
Ceftriaxone, 460, 506
Central nervous system
  infection in, 286-287
  tumors, 160
Cephalosporins, 246
Cephaloxin, 476
Cerclage, cervical, 466
Cerebellopontine angle tumors, 38
Cerebrospinal fluid analysis, 262, 264, 266, 268
Cerebyx; *see* Phosphenytoin
Cervical biopsy, 460
Cervical cancer
  Pap smear and, 486
  in pregnancy, 466
Cervical cap, 492
Cervical cytologic screening, 2
Cervical polyps, in pregnancy, 466
Cervical radiculopathy, 422
Cervical spine
  near-drowning and, 536, 538
  and neck pain, 420
Cervicitis, 460-461, 486
  chlamydial, 270
  in pregnancy, 466
Chalazion, 30
Chancres, syphilitic, 270
Charcot-Marie-Tooth disease, 368
Chemicals
  injury from, 30, 528-529
  sweating from, 24
Chemotherapy, 244
  for breast cancer, 480, 482
  for Hodgkin's disease, 232
  for metastatic bone disease, 248
  for multiple myeloma, 236
  neutropenia from, 246-247
  and secondary malignancies, 254
Chest pain
  esophageal, 162
  noncardiac, 166-167
  in women, 472-475
Chest radiography
  for cardiac dyspnea, 96
  of cor pulmonale, 90
  for cough, 394
  for dyspnea, 396
  of right ventricular failure, 92
Childs' index of liver disease, 56
Chlamydia
  cervicitis from, 460-461
  nongonococcal urethritis from, 506
  in STDs, 270, 272
Chloroquine, 260
Cholangiography, 172
Cholecystectomy, 176
Cholelithiasis, 176
Cholera vaccine, 260
Cholesterol levels
  and coronary artery disease, 116, 118
  screening of, 2
Chorea, 370
Christmas disease, 222
Chronic fatigue syndrome, 4, 6, 7

Chronic inflammatory demyelinating polyradiculo-
  neuropathy, 366, 368
Chronic myelogenous leukemia, 212, 234-235
Chronic obstructive pulmonary disease, postoperative, 46-47
Chronic renal failure, 298-299
  pruritus in, 110
Churg-Strauss syndrome, 112
Cimetidine, 576
Ciprofloxacin
  for gonorrhea, 506
  for urinary tract infections, 476
Cisplatin, and hypomagnesemia, 322
Clarithromycin, 278
Clenched fist injury, 530
Clindamycin
  prophylactic, 584
  for vaginal infections, 458
Clomiphene citrate, 500
Clonazepam, 352
Clonic-tonic seizures, 350
Clopidogrel, 336
Clotrimazole, 458
Clotting factors
  deficiencies, 220, 222
  disseminated intravascular coagulation and, 216-217
Clue cells, 272
Cluster headaches, 334
Coagulation abnormalities, 220-223
Coarctation of aorta, 76
Cocaine, rhinitis from, 32
Coccidioidomycosis, 4
Coccygodynia, 192
Cognitive-behavioral therapy, 544
Colchicine, 442
Colic, biliary, 176-177
Colitis
  Emtamoeba histolytica, 260
  and gastrointestinal bleeding, 178
Collagen vascular disease
  and deep venous thrombosis, 218
  peripheral neuropathy of, 366
  Raynaud's phenomenon and, 438
Colon
  cancer of, 182, 188, 194-195
  transit times of, 188
Colonoscopy
  for colon cancer, 194
  for constipation, 188
  for diarrhea causes, 186
  for gastrointestinal bleeding, 181
  for rectal bleeding, 182
Colorectal surgery, antimicrobial prophylaxis for, 584
Coma, 384-385
Common bile duct stones, 176-177
Completed stroke, 340-341
Compulsions, 546
Computed tomography
  for acute headache, 332
  for lymphadenopathy, 240
  of mediastinal adenopathy, 400
Condoms, 492
Conductive hearing loss, 40, 42
Confusional state, 376-377, 380
Congenital adrenal hyperplasia, 150
Congestive heart failure, 86-87
  from transfusions, 230
Conjunctivitis, 30

Conn's syndrome, 76
Constipation, 188-189, 190
Contraceptive methods, 490-493
Contractures, 374
Conversion disorder, 552
Coombs test, 206
Cornea
  abrasions of, 30
  alkali burns of, 528
  ulceration of, 28
Coronary artery bypass grafting, 66
Coronary artery disease
  congestive heart failure from, 86
  dyslipidemia and, 116, 118
  in women, 472-474
Coronary heart disease, prevention of, 102
Cor pulmonale, 90-91, 92
Corticosteroids
  for anaphylaxis, 576
  for gout, 442
  obesity from, 12
  for thyroiditis, 140
Cortisol levels, in Cushing's syndrome, 146
Cosyntropin stimulation test, 120
Cotton wool spots, 280
Cough, 394-395
Counseling
  for HIV-infected patient, 276
  after myocardial infarction, 102-103
  recommendations for, 2
CPR; see Cardiopulmonary resuscitation
CPR drug dependence mnemonic, 542
Cramps, muscle, 374-375
Cranial nerve palsy, and red eye, 26
Craniopharyngiomas, 462
Creatine kinase level, 456-457
CREST syndrome, 434
Crixivan; see Indinavir
Crohn's disease, 196
Cryptococcal meningitis, 262, 264
CT scan; see Computed tomography
Cushing's disease, 144, 146-147
  hypertension with, 76
Cu-T 380A, 492, 493
Cutis laxa, 448
Cystitis, 476
Cysts
  Baker's, 430
  ovarian, 470
  renal, 308-309
Cytarabine arabinoside, 234
Cytology, in pleural effusion, 398
Cytomegalovirus
  in HIV-infected patient, 280
  in renal transplant recipients, 330
Cytoxan, 254

D

Darkfield examination for syphilis, 270
ddC; see Zalcitabine
ddI; see Didanosine
Decongestants, 32
Deep venous thrombosis, 218-219
  anticoagulation therapy for, 566-569, 572
  postoperative, 48
Defecography, 188-189, 198

Defibrillation, 94
Degenerative joint disease
    in hand and wrist, 428
    in temporomandibular joint, 450
Dehydroepiandrosterone sulfate, 150
Déjérine-Sottas disease, 368
Delaviradine, 278
Delusional disorder, 556
Dementia, 378-381
    anorexia and weight loss from, 160
    memory loss in, 346
    psychotic behaviors in, 556
Demyelinating neuropathies, 368
Dental procedures, antimicrobial prophylaxis
        for, 580
Depacon; see Sodium valproate
Depo-Provera, 492
Depression, 548-549, 551
    anorexia and weight loss from, 160
    in bereavement, 554
    memory loss in, 346
    from oral contraceptives, 496
    psychotic, 556
    somatic symptoms of, 552
de Quervain's tenosynovitis, 428
Dermatitis, 110
Dermatofibromas, 104
Dermatologic manifestations
    arthritis and, 416
    in HIV-infected patient, 280
    of toxic shock syndrome, 290
Dermatomyositis, 358
Dermographism, 108
Desbuquois' syndrome, 446
Desipramine, 8
Desogestrel, 494
Dexamethasone, 258
Dexamethasone suppression test, 76
    for Cushing's syndrome, 146
d4T; see Stavudine
Diabetes mellitus, 122-125
    arthritis from, 412
    and obesity, 12
    and oral contraceptives, 494
    in perioperative evaluation, 52, 53
    peripheral neuropathy of, 366
    and proteinuria, 302
    pruritus in, 110
    and taste disturbances, 382
Diabetic ketoacidosis, 122, 124
Dialysis, 326-327
    perioperative, 50
    pruritus from, 110
Diaphragm, contraceptive, 492
Diarrhea
    acute, 184-185
    chronic, 186-187
    in HIV-infected patient, 280
    in irritable bowel syndrome, 190
    traveler's, 260, 580
Diastolic murmur, 72-73
Diazepam
    for prostatodynia, 512
    for status epilepticus, 352
Dicyclomine, 196
Didanosine, 278

Diet
    for dyslipidemia, 118
    goiter from, 136
    and intestinal gas, 196
    in irritable bowel syndrome, 190
    for obesity, 12
Diethylstilbestrol, 493
Diffuse esophageal spasm
    chest pain in, 166
    dysphagia with, 162
Dihydrotachysterol, 126
1,25-Dihydroxyvitamin D, 128
Disc herniation, 424
Dislocations
    in joint hypermobility, 446
    shoulder, 422
Disseminated intravascular coagulation, 216-217
Diuretics
    hypokalemia from, 318
    for pulmonary edema, 88
Diverticulosis, 156
Dizziness, 348-349
DNA antibodies, 452
Dobutamine, 88
Domestic violence, 502-505
Dopamine
    for pulmonary edema, 88
    and TSH suppression, 142
Doxycycline
    for Chlamydia infections, 461, 506
    for gonorrhea, 506
    for malaria, 260
Drowning, 536-539
Drugs; see also Medications
    abuse of, 542
    adverse reactions to, 330, 578-579
    coma from, 384
    gynecomastia from, 152
    nausea and vomiting from, 158
Duchenne's muscular dystrophy, 358
Dupuytren's contractures, 428
DVT; see Deep venous thrombosis
Dysbetalipoproteinemia, 116
Dysgeusia, 382
Dyslipidemia, 116-119
Dysosmia, 382
Dyspareunia, 16
Dyspepsia, 170-171
Dysphagia, 162-163, 280
Dysphoria, 548
Dyspnea
    cardiac, 96-97
    pulmonary, 396-397
Dysproteinemias, 368
Dysthymic disorder, 548
Dystonia, 370, 372
Dystrophies, 358, 359
Dysuria, 476, 506-507

E

Eating Attitudes Test, 8
Eating disorders, 8-9, 160
ECG; see Electrocardiography
Echocardiography
    for cardiac dyspnea, 96
    for chest pain in women, 472, 474

Echocardiography—cont'd
    of cor pulmonale, 90
    of right ventricular failure, 92
    for syncope, 82
Ectopic pregnancy, 466
Edema, 18-21
    acute pulmonary, 88-89
    in stroke, 342
EEG; see Electroencephalography
Ehlers-Danlos syndrome, 446, 448
Eldepryl; see Selegiline
Elderly
    anorexia and weight loss in, 160
    transfusion reactions in, 230
Electrocardiography
    for chest pain in women, 472
    of cor pulmonale, 90
    of right ventricular failure, 92
    for syncope, 82
Electroconvulsive therapy
    for depression, 548
    for psychosis, 556
Electroencephalography of seizures, 350
Electromechanical dissociation, 94
Electromyography
    and creatine kinase, 456
    for neck pain, 420
    for peripheral neuropathies, 366, 368
Electrophoresis, abnormal serum protein, 236-239
Electrophysiologic study
    after acute myocardial infarction, 98
    for syncope, 82
Embolism
    in foot, 432
    pulmonary; see Pulmonary embolism
    pulseless extremity from, 522
    stroke from, 342
Embolization, bronchial artery, 388
EMG; see Electromyography
Emotional disorders, 552-553
Encephalitis, herpes simplex, 344
Endocarditis
    antimicrobial prophylaxis for, 580
    arthritis in, 414
    fever from, 296
Endocrine disorders
    and chronic diarrhea, 186
    myopathies of, 358
    postoperative, 52-53
    and sweating, 24
Endometrial biopsy, 464
Endometrial carcinoma, 464
Endoscopic retrograde cholangiopancreatography, 172, 176
Endoscopy
    for belching causes, 168
    and gastrointestinal bleeding, 178, 180
    for heartburn, 164
    for noncardiac chest pain, 166
Endotracheal intubation, for asthma, 392
End-stage renal disease
    dialysis for, 326-327
    and renal transplantation, 328-329
Enoxaparin, 48
Entamoeba histolytica, 260
Enzymatic defects, anemia from, 206
Enzyme-linked immunosorbent assay, 276
Eosinophilic fasciitis, 434

Eosinophilic myalgia syndrome, 434
Ependymoma, 192
Epididymitis, 508
Epilepsy, 350; see also Seizures
Epinephrine
    for anaphylaxis, 574, 576
    for cardiac arrest, 94
    for stridor, 390
Epipodophyllotoxins, 254
Episcleritis, 30
Epivir; see Lamivudine
Erdheim's disease, 446
Erectile dysfunction, 14
Ergocalciferol, 126
Ergotamine, withdrawal headache from, 334
Eructation, 168-169
Erythroderma, toxic shock syndrome and, 290
Erythromycin, 507
Erythropoietin, polycythemia and, 210
Escherichia coli
    diarrhea from, 260
    in neutropenic patient, 246
Esophageal manometry, 162
Esophagitis, 164
Esophagogastroduodenoscopy, 162, 194
Esophagus
    acid and alkali burns of, 528
    disorders of, 162, 166, 434
    foreign body in, 526
Estrogen
    and amenorrhea, 462
    and gynecomastia, 152
    in oral contraceptives, 490, 494-495, 496
Estrogen-progestin challenge test, 462
Estrogen receptor status, in breast cancer, 480, 482
Ethinyl estradiol, 494
Ethynodiol diacetate, 494
Eustachian tube, patulous, 36
Exercise
    and cramps, 374
    urticaria after, 108
Exercise testing
    for chest pain in women, 472, 473, 474
    after myocardial infarction, 98, 102
    for stable angina, 66
    for syncope, 82
Exposure
    asbestos, 410-411
    caustic substance, 528-529
    to hepatitis, 294-295
Extragonadal germ cell syndrome, 244
Extremity, pulseless, 522-523
Exudates, in pleural effusion, 398

F

Factitious disorder, 552
Factor V deficiency, 222
Factor VII deficiency, 222
Factor VIII
    deficiency of, 222
    disseminated intravascular coagulation and, 216-217
Factor IX deficiency, 222
Familial benign hypercalcemia, 128
Familial combined hyperlipidemia, 116

Familial hypercholesterolemia, 116
Fasciitis, eosinophilic, 434
Fatigue, 4-7
FDA MedWatch program, 578
Fecal impaction, 186
Fecal incontinence, 198-199
Fecal occult blood testing, 194
Femur fractures, 426
Ferritin, hemochromatosis and, 202
Fertility awareness methods, 492
Fever
    in HIV-infected patient, 280
    in neutropenic cancer patient, 246-247
    in renal transplant recipient, 330-331
    and sweating, 24
    during transfusion, 230
    of unknown origin, 296-297
Fibrin, 217
Fibrinogen, 217
    clotting factor deficiencies and, 222
    and deep venous thrombosis, 218
Fibrin split products, 216
Fibromuscular dysplasia, renal, 76
Fibromyalgia
    fatigue in, 4
    soft tissue pain of, 418
Fibrositis, 418
Finkelstein's test, 428
Fistula
    aortoenteric, 178
    gastrocolic, 168
    vesicovaginal, 514
Flatulence, 196-197
Fluconazole
    in neutropenic patient, 247
    for yeast infections, 458
Fluid aspiration, 536
Fluoroquinolones, 580
Fluoxitene, 8
Folate deficiency, 208
Foley catheter, 526
Follicle-stimulating hormone
    and amenorrhea, 462
    and fertility, 498, 518
Foot pain, 432-433
Foreign body
    aspiration of, 390
    in eye, 30
    ingestion of, 524-526
Foreign travel, infection and immunization considerations
        for, 260-261
Formulary, drug, 592-593
Fractures
    cervical, 420
    femur, 426
    pathologic, 248-251
    pelvic, 426
    shoulder, 422
    temporal bone, 40
Freckles, 104
Free thyroxine (FT$_4$), 130
    hyperthyroidism and, 134
    hypothyroidism and, 131
    in nonthyroidal illness, 142
Free thyroxine index, 130, 142
Frostbite, 534

FSH; see Follicle-stimulating hormone
FT$_4$; see Free thyroxine
Furosemide, 88

G

Gait disturbances, 360-361
Galactography, 484
Galactorrhea, 484-485
Gallbladder disease, 168
Gallstones
    belching and, 168
    colic from, 176-177
Gammopathy, monoclonal, 236-239
Ganglions, 428
Ganser's syndrome, 380
Gardnerella vaginalis, 458
Gas, intestinal, 196-197
Gastric outlet obstruction, 168
Gastric surgery, for obesity, 12
Gastrocolic fistula, 168
Gastroesophageal reflux disease, 164-165, 166
Gastrointestinal disorders
    anorexia and weight loss from, 160
    chest pain in, 166
    in CREST syndrome, 434
    dyspepsia in, 170
    dysphagia with, 162
Gastrointestinal system
    bleeding in, 178-181
    endoscopy of, 168
    foreign bodies in, 524, 526
Genital herpes, 460
Genital ulcers, 270
Genital warts, 460
Gentamicin
    in surgical prophylaxis, 584
    use and monitoring of, 588
Gestational diabetes, 122
Giant cell arteritis, 444-445
Giddiness, 348
Glasgow Coma Scale, 384
Glaucoma, 28
Glenohumeral dislocation, 422
Glomerulonephritis
    hematuria in, 304
    and proteinuria, 302
    rapidly progressive, 300
Glucagon, for food bolus removal, 526
Glucocorticoids
    and Cushing's syndrome, 146
    and hyperglycemia, 122
    and TSH suppression, 142
Glucose control, perioperative, 52, 53
Glucose tolerance test, 122
Goiter, 136-137, 140
Gonococcal infection, 270
    endocervicitis, 460
    septic arthritis from, 412
    urethritis, 506
Gout, 442-443
    vs. rheumatoid arthritis, 414
Graham Steel murmur, 72
Granulocyte transfusion, 228-229
Granuloma inguinale, 270
Granulomatosis, 112

Graves' disease
  hyperthyroidism from, 134
  orbitopathy in, 26
  thyroid pain in, 140
Grief, 554-555
Growth hormone, and galactorrhea, 484
Guaiac-positive stools, 194-195
Guillain-Barré syndrome, 368
Gynecomastia, 152-153

H

H₂-receptor antagonists, 164, 170
Haemophilus ducreyi, 270
Haemophilus influenzae, meningitis from, 262
Hamman's sign, 528
Hand pain, 428-429
Hashimoto's thyroiditis, 131, 140
β-hCG; *see* β-Human chorionic gonadotropin
Headache
  acute, 332-333
  chronic, 334-335
  from oral contraceptives, 496
Head trauma
  amnesia from, 344
  anosmia after, 382
  bacterial meningitis in, 262
Head-up tilt test, 82
Hearing loss, 38, 40-43
Hearing tests, 38, 40
Heartburn, 164-165
Heart failure
  congestive, 86-87, 230
  right ventricular, 92-93
Heart murmurs
  diastolic, 72-73
  systolic, 70-71
Heart valves, prosthetic, 570
Heimlich maneuver, in near-drowning victim, 536
Helicobacter pylori, 170
Hemarthrosis, 412
Hematemesis, 178, 180
Hematochezia, 178, 182-183
Hematocrit, transfusion and, 226
Hematologic disorders
  and neutrophilia, 212
  postoperative, 48-49
Hematuria, 304-305
  prostate enlargement and, 510
Hemoccult test, 194
Hemochromatosis
  serum iron in, 202
  and transaminase levels, 200
Hemodialysis, 326, 327
Hemoglobin
  defects of, 206
  polycythemia and, 210
Hemolysis
  in anemia, 206
  in transfusion reaction, 230
Hemophilia A, 222
Hemophilia B, 222
Hemoptysis, 388-389
Hemorrhage
  disseminated intravascular coagulation and, 216
  spinal subarachnoid, 192
  stigmata of recent, 180

Hemorrhage—cont'd
  in stroke, 342
  subarachnoid, 332
  subconjunctival, 30
Henoch-Schönlein purpura, 112
Heparin, 566-569
  for acute myocardial infarction, 98
  for deep venous thrombosis, 218, 219
  for pulseless extremity, 522
  in surgical prophylaxis, 48
  for transient ischemic attacks, 336
Hepatic iron index, 202
Hepatitis
  exposure to, 294-295
  in perioperative evaluation, 56-57
  and transaminase levels, 200
  vaccine for, 260
Hereditary disorders
  of hearing loss, 40
  motor and sensory neuropathy, 368
Herpes simplex encephalitis, amnesia from, 344
Herpes simplex keratitis, 28
Herpes simplex virus
  and cervicitis, 460
  urethritis from, 507
  vulvovaginitis from, 458
Hip pain, 426-427
Hip replacement, antimicrobial prophylaxis for, 584
Hirschsprung's disease, 188
Hirsutism, 150-151
HIV; *see* Human immunodeficiency virus
HIV-1 RNA levels, 276, 278
Hives, 108-109
Hivid; *see* Zalcitabine
HLA immunization, 224
Hodgkin's disease, 232-233
  cancer therapy-induced, 254
  pruritus in, 110
Homan sign, 218
Homocystinuria, 446
Hordeolum, 30
Hormone replacement therapy, 2
Human bites, 530-531
β-Human chorionic gonadotropin
  and ectopic pregnancy, 466, 470
  and gynecomastia, 152-153
Human diploid vaccine, 260
Human immunodeficiency virus
  acutely ill patient with, 280-281
  approach to, 276-279
  CNS infection in, 286-287
  foreign travel and, 260
  P. carinii pneumonia prophylaxis in, 580
  pulmonary infiltrates in, 282-285
Human papillomavirus, 270, 460
  and abnormal Pap smear, 486
  vulvovaginitis from, 458
Hydrocele, 508
Hydrocephalus, in stroke, 342
Hydrofluoric acid exposure, 528
Hydroxychloroquine, hyperpigmentation from, 104
Hydroxyurea
  for chronic myelogenous leukemia, 234
  and polycythemia, 210-211
Hyperamylasemia, 204-205
Hypercalcemia, 128-129
Hyperglycemia, 122-125

Hyperhidrosis, 24-25
Hyperkalemia, 50, 320-321
Hyperkinesias, 370-373
Hypermobility of joints, 446-449
Hypernatremia, 316-317
Hypernephroma, 248
Hyperparathyroidism, 128
Hyperpigmentation, 104-105
Hyperprolactinemia, 148, 462
Hypersplenism, 206
Hypertension, 74-77
    adrenal masses and, 144
    congestive heart failure from, 86
    portal, 174
    pulmonary, 84
Hyperthyroidism, 134-135
    with goiter, 136
    and gynecomastia, 152
    myopathy of, 358
    pruritus in, 110
    thyroid pain in, 140
Hypertrichosis, 150
Hypertriglyceridemia, 116
Hypertrophic cardiomyopathy, 70
Hyperuricemia, 442-443
Hyphema, 28
Hypoalbuminemia, 126
Hypocalcemia, 126-127
Hypochondriasis, 552
Hypocomplementemia, 112
Hypogeusia, 160
Hypoglycemia, 120-121
Hypogonadism, 518
Hypokalemia, 318-319
Hypomagnesemia, 126, 322-323
Hyponatremia, 314-315
Hypoparathyroidism, 126
Hypophosphatemia, 324-325
Hypopyon, 28
Hypotension, 78-79
Hypothermia, 534-535, 536, 538
Hypothyroidism, 131, 133
    galactorrhea from, 484
    with goiter, 136
    in perioperative evaluation, 54-55
    thyroid pain in, 140
Hypoxia
    in near-drowning victim, 536, 538
    polycythemia and, 210

I

^{125}I, 218
^{131}I
    for Graves' disease, 134
    thyroid pain from, 140
Imipramine, 514
Immunization
    of HIV-infected patient, 276
    HLA, 224
    for travel, 260-261
Immunoassays
    enzyme, 276
    β-hCG, 152-153
    thyroid, 130
Immunoglobulin M levels, monoclonal gammopathy
        and, 238

Immunosuppression, in renal transplant recipient, 330
Impedance plethysmography
    for deep venous thrombosis, 218
    for edema, 20
Incontinence
    fecal, 198-199
    urinary, 514-517
Indinavir, 278
Infections
    arthritis from, 412
    and aseptic meningitis, 268
    cervicitis from, 460-461
    chemotherapy-induced neutropenia and, 246-247
    conjunctivitis from, 30
    diarrhea from, 184, 186
    and fever of unknown origin, 296
    foot pain from, 432
    foreign travel and, 260-261
    granulocyte transfusion for, 228
    headache from, 332
    hearing loss from, 42
    in HIV-infected patient, 280
    leg ulcers from, 106
    leukopenia from, 214
    lymphadenopathy from, 240
    and multiple pulmonary nodules, 404
    and neutrophilia, 212
    postoperative, 584
    in pregnancy, 466
    prophylaxis against, 278
    in renal transplant recipient, 330
    rhinitis from, 34
    sexually transmitted, 270-275
    of thyroid, 140
    from transfusions, 230
    urinary tract, 330, 476-477, 506, 510
    urticaria from, 108
Infertility
    female, 498-501
    male, 518-519
Inflammation
    and neutrophilia, 212
    in polyarthritis, 414
    shoulder, 422
Inflammatory bowel disease, 184, 186
Influenza prophylaxis, 580
Ingrown toenail, 432
Inguinal nodes
    enlarged, 240
    metastasis in, 244
Insulin, perioperative concerns of, 52, 53
Insulin-dependent diabetes mellitus, 122, 124
Insulinomas, 120
α-Interferon, 234
International Normalized Ratio, 570, 572
Intestinal gas, 196-197
Intrauterine devices, 492, 493
Intubation, in near-drowning victim, 536, 538
Invirase; see Saquinavir
Iodine
    for deep venous thrombosis, 218
    and goiter, 136
    for Graves' disease, 134
    painful thyroid from, 140
Iritis, 28
Iron, elevated serum, 202-203
Iron deficiency anemia, 208

Irritable bowel syndrome, 190-191
    abdominal pain with, 156
    diarrhea in, 186
Ischemia
    of bowel, 178
    lower extremity, 522-523
    mesenteric, 156
    stroke from, 340-341
Isoniazid
    in HIV-infected patient, 278
    for tuberculosis, 408
Isoproterenol
    in head-up tilt test, 82
    for tachycardia, 64

J

Jaundice, 172-173
Joint aspiration
    for hip pain, 426
    for monarthritis, 412
Joint hypermobility, 446-449
Jugular venous pressure, edema and, 18, 20

K

Kallmann's syndrome, 382
Kaposi's sarcoma, 280
Keratoconjunctivitis sicca, 436-437
Keratoderma blennorrhagica, 416
Keratoses, seborrheic, 104
Ketoconazole, 458, 459
Kidney disease, polycystic, 308
Kidney stones, 306-307
Kidney transplantation
    and fever, 330-331
    patient selection for, 328-329
Klebsiella, 246
Kleihauer-Betke test, 468
Klinefelter's syndrome, 152
Klonopin; see Clonazepam
Knee pain, 430-431
Knuckle sandwich, 530
Korsakoff's syndrome, 344

L

Labyrinthitis, 348
Lactate dehydrogenase, 398
Lactation, as birth control method, 492
Lactic acidosis, 310
Lactose intolerance
    dyspepsia in, 170
    and intestinal gas, 196
Lamivudine, 278
Laparotomy, for Hodgkin's disease, 232
Laryngoscopy
    for foreign body ingestion, 524
    for stridor, 390
Laxatives, diarrhea from, 186
Lead toxicity, 368
Leg cramps, 374
Leg ulcers, 106-107, 114
Lentigo, 104
Leptospirosis, 290

Leukemia
    acute promyelocytic leukemia, 216
    cancer therapy-induced, 254
    chronic myelogenous, 212, 234-235
    pruritus in, 110
Leukocyte alkaline phosphate score, 234
Leukocytes
    in cerebrospinal fluid, 264
    filters, 224, 226
Leukocytosis, 212-213, 234
Leukopenia, 214-215
Levodopa
    for dystonias, 372
    hyperkinesia from, 370
    for Parkinson's disease, 364
Levonorgestrel, 494
Lidocaine
    for acute myocardial infarction, 98
    for status epilepticus, 354
    for tachycardia, 64
    for tinnitus, 38
Light therapy, 548
Lipoprotein lipase deficiency, 116
Listeria monocytogenes, 262
Lithium
    for depression, 548
    goiter from, 136
    for psychosis, 556
Livedo reticularis, 114-115
Liver disease
    alcoholic, 202
    clotting times and, 216, 217
    and gynecomastia, 152
    in perioperative evaluation, 56-57
    and transaminase levels, 200
Liver function tests, 18
Liver spots, 104
Lo-Ovral, 492-493
Lorazepam, 352
Low back pain, 424-425
Lower extremity ischemia, 522-523
Lower motor neuron signs of weakness, 356
Low-molecular-weight heparin, 568
Lumbar spine disorders, hip pain from, 426
Lung disorders
    asbestos exposure and, 410-411
    diffuse interstitial disease, 406-407
    pulmonary nodules, 404-405
Lupus anticoagulant, 220
Luteinizing hormone, 462
Lyme disease, fatigue in, 4
Lymphadenopathy, 240-241, 254
Lymph nodes, axillary
    breast cancer and, 480, 482
    carcinoma in, 244
    enlarged, 240
lymphogranuloma venereum, 270
Lymphomas
    cancer therapy-induced, 254
    monoclonal gammopathy and, 238
Lymphopenia, 214

M

Macroamylasemia, 204
Macrocytic anemias, 208

Magnesium
  for hydrofluoric acid ingestion, 528
  and hypomagnesemia, 322
  for tachycardia, 64
Magnetic resonance imaging
  for knee pain, 430
  for neck pain, 420
  of pituitary, 148
  for spinal cord lesions, 258
Malabsorption syndromes, 160
Malaria, 260
Malignancy
  gastrointestinal, 160
  hearing loss from, 42
  hypercalcemia in, 128
  and neutrophilia, 212
  and pulmonary nodules, 404-405
  and sweating, 24
  therapy-induced secondary, 254-255
  thyroid, 138
Malingering, 552
Mallory-Weiss mucosal tear, 178
Mammography, 2, 478, 484
Mania, 556
Mannerisms, 370
Manometry
  anorectal, 198
  esophageal, 162, 166
  gastrointestinal, 170
Mantoux test, 408
Marfan's syndrome, 446
Mastocytosis, 108
Maturity-onset diabetes of the young, 122
McMurray's test, 430
Measles, 290
Mediastinal adenopathy, 400-401
Mediastinal masses, 232
Mediastinoscopy, 402, 404
Medications; see also specific agents
  acute behavioral change from, 376
  adverse reactions to, 330, 578-579, 592
  anaphylaxis from, 574
  anosmia from, 382
  for anxiety disorder, 544, 546
  asthma from, 392
  chronic abdominal pain from, 156
  coma from, 384
  confusional states from, 380
  for depression, 548
  diarrhea from, 186
  formulary of, 592-593
  hearing loss from, 40, 42
  hirsutism from, 150
  hypercalcemia from, 128
  hyperkinesias from, 370
  hypoglycemia from, 120
  hypothyroidism from, 131
  interstitial nephritis from, 300
  leukopenia from, 214
  lupus from, 452
  and migraine, 334
  nausea and vomiting from, 158
  in near-drowning victim, 538
  neutrophilia from, 212
  and obesity, 12
  pancreatitis from, 204
  polyneuropathy from, 368

Medications—cont'd
  and prolactin level, 462
  and Raynaud's phenomenon, 438
  and rhinitis, 32, 34
  serum levels of, 590-591
  sweating from, 24
  taste changes from, 382
  for tinnitus, 38
  and transaminase levels, 200
  urticaria from, 108
  warfarin interactions with, 572
Medroxyprogesterone acetate, 462
Mefloquine, 260
Melanoma, 104
Melanosis coli, 188
Melasma, 104
Melena, 178, 180
Melphalan, 238
Memory loss, 344-347
Meniere's disease
  dizziness in, 348
  tinnitus in, 38
Meningiomas, 462
Meningismus, 384-385
Meningitis
  aseptic, 268-269
  bacterial, 262-265
  chronic, 266-267
Menkes' syndrome, 448
Mesenteric ischemia, 156
Mestranol, 494
Metabolic disorders
  with abdominal pain, 156
  acidosis, 310-311
  alkalosis, 312-313, 318
  amnesia from, 344
  anemia from, 208
  neuropathies of, 368
  tinnitus in, 36
Metastases
  bone, 248, 250
  inguinal node, 244
Methimazole, goiter from, 136
Methylprednisolone, 576
Methylprednisone, 528
Metronidazole, 458
Metyrapone stimulation test, 148
Miconazole, 458
Microangiopathic hemolytic anemia, 206, 216
Microcytic anemias, 208
Migraine headache, 332, 334, 335
Milk-alkali syndrome, 128
Minocycline, hyperpigmentation from, 104
Mitral regurgitation, 70
Mitral stenosis, 72
Mitral valve prolapse, 70
Mobitz I atrioventricular block, 60
Molar pregnancy, 466
Moles, 104
Monarthritis, 412-413
Mongolian spots, 104
Monitoring
  of palpitations, 80
  for syncope, 82
Monoamine oxidase inhibitors, 548
Monoclonal gammopathy, 236-239
Mononeuritis multiplex, 366

Mononeuropathies, 366
Morphea, 434
Morphine, 88
Morton's neuroma, 432
Motility disorders
    chest pain in, 166
    dyspepsia in, 170
    dysphagia with, 162
MRI; *see* Magnetic resonance imaging
Mucor, 247
Multidisciplinary pain center, 22
Multifocal atrial tachycardia, 62
Multifocal mononeuropathy, 366
Multinodular goiter, 136
Multiple endocrine neoplasia, pheochromocytoma in, 144
Multiple myeloma, 236, 237
Multiple sclerosis, vertigo in, 348
Murphy's sign, 176
Muscle
    biopsy of, 456
    cramps and aches, 374-375
Muscular dystrophy, 358, 359
Myasthenia gravis, 358
Mycobacterium avium complex, prophylaxis against, 278
Mycobacterium tuberculosis, 408
    meningitis from, 262
    prophylaxis against, 278
Myelography
    for neck pain, 420
    for spinal cord lesions, 258
Myelopathies, 356
Myocardial infarction
    acute, 78, 98-101
    counseling after, 102-103
Myoglobinuria, 374
Myopathies, 358-359, 456
Myotonic dystrophy, 358

N

Naloxone, 534
Narcotic bowel syndrome, 156
Narrow QRS complex tachycardia, 62-63
Narrow therapeutic index, 590
Nasogastric tube, 180
Nausea, 158-159
    from oral contraceptives, 496
Near-drowning, 536-539
Neck pain, 420-421
Neck trauma, and coma, 384
Necrosis, avascular
    arthritis from, 412
    in knee, 430
Needle aspiration
    of breast masses, 478
    of pulmonary nodules, 402, 404
Neisseria gonorrhoeae, 270
    cervicitis from, 460, 461
Neisseria meningitidis, 262
Nelfinavir, 278
Neonatal hyperparathyroidism, 128
Neonatal lupus syndrome, 452
Neoplasia
    knee pain from, 430
    multiple endocrine, 144

Neoplasm
    fever from, 296
    hearing loss from, 40, 42
    testicular, 508
Nephritis, 300, 304
Nephrotic syndrome, 302
Nephrotoxicity, aminoglycoside, 588
Nerve biopsy, 366
Nerve conduction studies, 366, 368
Nerve roots, cervical, 420
Netilmicin, 588
Neuroglycopenia, 120
Neuronitis, vestibular, 348
Neuropathies
    and creatine kinase, 456
    peripheral, 356-357, 366-369
Neutropenia, 214
    and fever in cancer patient, 246-247
    granulocyte transfusion for, 228
Neutrophilia, 212
Nevi, 104
Nevirapine, 278
Nevus of Ota, 104
Niacin, for dyslipidemia, 118
Nicotine replacement therapy, 558, 560
Nipple discharge, 484-485
Nitrofurantoin, 476
Nitroglycerin
    for acute myocardial infarction, 98
    for pulmonary edema, 88
Nitroprusside, 88
Nocturnal penile tumescence test, 14
Nongonococcal urethritis, 270, 506, 507
Non–insulin-dependent diabetes mellitus, 122, 124
Non-nucleoside reverse transcriptase inhibitors, 278
Nonoxynol-9, 492
Nonsteroidal anti-inflammatory drugs, 442
Norethindrone acetate, 494
Norethynodrel, 494
Norfloxacin, 476
Norgestrel, 494
Norplant, 492
Nortriptyline, 38
Norvir; *see* Ritonavir
Nucleoside reverse transcriptase inhibitors, 278
Nutcracker esophagus
    chest pain in, 166
    dysphagia with, 162

O

Obesity, 12-13
    Cushingoid, 146
    and transaminase levels, 200
Obsessions, 546
Occipital horn syndrome, 448
Odynophagia, 280
Ofloxacin, 506
Oligoasthenospermia, 518
Opportunistic infection prophylaxis, 278
Oral cholecystography, 176
Oral contraceptives, 490, 494-497
    and abnormal vaginal bleeding, 464
    postcoital, 492-493
    for premenstrual syndrome, 488
Oral disorders, and taste disturbances, 382
Oral glucose tolerance test, 122

Orbital cellulitis, 26
Ortho-Novum 777, 494
Osgood-Schlatter disease, 430
Osteitis fibrosa cystica, 440
Osteoarthritis, 412, 414
Osteomalacia, 250, 440
Osteopenia, 440-441
Osteoporosis, 250, 440
Otosclerosis, 42
Ototoxicity, aminoglycoside, 588
Ovary
    cysts of, 470
    failure of, 462
    polycystic disease of, 150
    tumor of, 150
Overweight, definition of, 12
Ovral, 492-493
Ovulation, 498
Oxybutynin, 514
Oxygen, for pulmonary edema, 88
Oxygen-hemoglobin dissociation curve, in near-drowning
        victim, 538
Oxygen saturation
    polycythemia and, 210
    pulmonary infiltrates and, 282

P

Pacemaker, 60
Pain
    abdominal; *see* Abdominal pain
    anorectal, 192-193
    chest; *see* Chest pain
    chronic, 22-23, 156-157
    with deep venous thrombosis, 218
    diffuse muscle, 444-445
    emotional, 554
    foot, 432-433
    in hand and wrist, 428-429
    hip, 426-427
    knee, 430-431
    low back, 424-425
    lower extremity ischemic, 522
    neck, 420-421
    noncardiac chest, 166-167
    shoulder, 422-423
    soft tissue, 418-419
    temporomandibular, 450-451
    thyroid, 140-141
Palatal myoclonus, tinnitus in, 36
Palpitations, 80-81
Palsies, 366, 382
Pancreas, and ascites, 174
Pancreatitis
    hypocalcemia in, 126
    serum amylase in, 204
Panic disorder, 544
Papain, 526
Papillary carcinoma, 138
Papillomavirus; *see* Human papillomavirus
Pap smear, 464, 486-487
Paraldehyde, 354
Paralysis, 522
Paranoid disorder, 556
Paraproteinemias, 368
Parathyroid adenoma, 128
Parathyroid hormone deficiency, 126

Paresthesia, 522
Parkinson's disease, 364-365
Parosmia, 382
Paroxysmal supraventricular tachycardia, 62
Partial seizures, 350
Partial stroke, 342
Partial thromboplastin time, 220
    disseminated intravascular coagulation and, 216
    monitoring, in heparin therapy, 566, 568
Pasteurella multocida, 530
Pelvic inflammatory disease, 272
    acute abdominal pain in, 470
    vs. cervicitis, 460
Pelvis
    examination of, 192
    fractures of, 426
    pain in, 156
Pemberton's sign, 136
Penicillin
    aminoglycoside interaction with, 588
    for bite wounds, 530
    in neutropenic patient, 246
    in surgical prophylaxis, 584
Pentobarbital, 354
Peptic ulcer
    dyspepsia with, 170
    and serum amylase elevation, 204
Percutaneous coronary angioplasty
    for acute myocardial infarction, 98
    unstable angina and, 66
Percutaneous transhepatic cholangiography, 172
Perioperative evaluation, 44-57
    of cardiac patient, 44-45
    endocrine complications in, 52-53
    hematologic complications in, 48-49
    liver complications in, 56-57
    morbidity and mortality risk in, 44
    pulmonary complications in, 46-47
    renal complications in, 50-51
    thyroid disease in, 54-55
Peripheral neuropathy, 356-357, 366-369
Peritoneal dialysis, 326, 327
Peritonitis, 174
pH, fecal, 186
Phalen's sign, 428
Pharmacoeconomics, 586, 592
Pharmacokinetics, 588, 590
Pharmacotherapy; *see* Medications; *specific agents*
Pharmacy and Therapeutics Committees, 592
Phenobarbital, 352
Phenothiazines, hyperpigmentation from, 104
Pheochromocytoma, 76, 144
Philadelphia chromosome, 234
Phlebotomy, 210
Phobias, 544
Phosphate level, hypocalcemia and, 126
Phosphenytoin, 352
Pick's disease, 378
Pigmented lesions, 104-105
Pingueculae, 30
Pituitary adenomas, 146
Pituitary tumor, 148-149
Placental abruption, 468
Placenta previa, 468
Plasma, for coagulation abnormalities, 222
Plasmacytoma, 236
Plasmodium falciparum, 260
Plasmodium vivax, 260

Platelets
   in disseminated intravascular coagulation, 216
   transfusion of, 224-225
Pleural effusion, 398-399, 410
Pleural lesions, 410
Plexopathies, 357
Plummer's disease, 136
Pneumococcal vaccine, 582
Pneumocystis infections
   prophylaxis against, 278, 580
   in renal transplant recipients, 330
Pneumonia
   and pleural effusion, 398
   Pneumocystis carinii, 280, 282, 580
Pneumothorax, 78
Podagra, 442
Poisoning, snake venom, 532-533
Polyarteritis nodosa, 112
Polycystic kidney disease, 308
Polycystic ovarian disease, 150
Polycythemia, 210-211
Polycythemia vera, 110
Polymyalgia rheumatica, 444-445
Polymyositis, 358
Popliteal cyst, 430
Positive end-expiratory pressure, in near-drowning
   victim, 538
Postpartum thyroiditis, 131
Post-traumatic stress disorder, 546
Potassium balance
   and hyperkalemia, 320-321
   and hypokalemia, 318-319
Pravastatin, 116, 118
Prednisone
   for amyloidosis, 238
   for anaphylaxis, 576
   for chronic myelogenous leukemia, 235
   for giant cell arteritis, 444
   for gout, 442
Pregnancy
   acute abdominal pain in, 470
   anticoagulant antibodies in, 220
   vaginal bleeding in, 466-469
Premature ejaculation, 14
Premature infants, transfusion in, 226
Premature rupture of membranes, 468
Premenstrual dysphoric disorder, 488
Premenstrual syndrome, 488-489
Preterm labor, 468
Preventive health services, 2-3
Probenecid, 442
Procainamide, 64
Proctalgia fugax, 192
Proctitis, and fecal incontinence, 198
Proctoscopy, 198
Progestasert, 492
Progesterone, 490
Progestin, 494, 495, 496
Progestin challenge test, 462
Progestin-only contraceptives, 492, 494
Progressing stroke, 342-343
Prolactin
   and amenorrhea, 462
   and galactorrhea, 484
Prolactinomas, 148
Propylthiouracil, goiter from, 136

Prostate
   biopsy of, 510-511
   cancer, 248
   enlargement of, 506, 510-511
   examination of, 510, 512
Prostate-specific antigen, 510
Prostatitis, 512-513
Prostatodynia, 512
Prosthetic heart valves, anticoagulation for, 570
Prosthetic replacements, for pathologic
   fractures, 248
Protease inhibitors, 278
Protein C deficiency, 218
Protein electrophoresis, abnormal serum,
   236-239
Protein S deficiency, 218
Proteinuria, 18, 302-303
Prothrombin time
   clotting factor deficiencies and, 222
   disseminated intravascular coagulation
     and, 216
Provera; *see* Medroxyprogesterone acetate
Pruritus, 110-111, 458
PSA; *see* Prostate-specific antigen
Pseudohypoparathyroidism, 126
Pseudomonas aeruginosa
   aminoglycosides for, 588
   in neutropenic patient, 246, 247
Pseudoxanthoma elasticum, 448
Psoriatic arthritis, 414, 416
Psychiatric disorders
   alcoholism with, 542
   chronic fatigue in, 7
   confusion and inattention in, 376
   vs. premenstrual syndrome, 488
   psychoses, 552, 556-557
   and suicide risk, 562
Psychotherapy, for grief syndromes, 554
Pterygium, 30
Pulmonary complications, postoperative, 46-47
Pulmonary disease, in HIV-infected patient,
   282-285
Pulmonary dyspnea, 396-397
Pulmonary edema, 88-89
Pulmonary embolism
   anticoagulation therapy for, 566-569
   in deep venous thrombosis, 218
   postoperative, 48
   warfarin therapy for, 572
Pulmonary hypertension
   in cardiomegaly, 84
   and cor pulmonale, 90
Pulmonary nodules
   multiple, 404-405
   solitary, 402-403
Pulmonic regurgitation, 72
Pulmonic stenosis, 70
Pulseless extremity, 522-523
Puncture wounds, 530
Purpura, 112-113
P waves, 62
Pyelonephritis
   in renal transplant recipients, 330
   in urinary tract infections, 476
Pyoderma gangrenosum, 416
Pyuria, 304, 506-507

Q

QRS complex tachycardias, 62-65
Quinolone
   in neutropenic patient, 246-247
   for traveler's diarrhea, 260

R

Rabies, 530
Rabies vaccine, 260
Raccoon eyes, 384
Radial nerve dysfunction, 428
Radiation therapy, 244
   for breast cancer, 480
   for Hodgkin's disease, 232
   for metastatic bone disease, 248
   for monoclonal gammopathy, 236
   and secondary malignancies, 254
   for superior vena caval syndrome, 256
Radiculopathies, 357
Radioactive iodine uptake test, 130, 134, 140
Radiography
   for belching causes, 168
   for foreign body ingestion, 524
   hip and pelvis, 426
   of osteopenia, 440
   temporomandibular, 450
Radionuclide scan, 180
Radiopaque marker study, 188
Random-donor unit, 224
Rash
   in HIV-infected patient, 280
   of toxic shock syndrome, 290
Raynaud's phenomenon, 434, 438-439
Rectal bleeding, 182-183
Rectal disorders; see Anorectal disorders
Rectal examination of prostate, 510, 512
Red blood cells
   in anemia, 206, 208
   in diarrhea, 184
   transfusion with, 226-227
Red eye, 26-31
Reflexes
   acoustic stapedius, testing of, 42
   and gait disturbances, 360
Refsum's disease, 368
Regurgitation, 158
Rehabilitation, cardiac, 102
Reiter's syndrome, 414, 416
Renal disorders
   carcinoma, 308
   cysts and masses, 308-309
   and gynecomastia, 152
   postoperative, 50-51
Renal failure
   acute, 300-301
   chronic, 298-299
Renal insufficiency
   bladder outlet obstruction and, 510
   serum amylase elevation in, 204
Renal transplantation
   fever and, 330-331
   patient selection for, 328-329
Renovascular hypertension, 76
Rescriptor; see Delaviradine
Respiratory acidosis, 312
Respiratory alkalosis, 310

Resuscitation of near-drowning victim, 536, 538
Retinitis, in HIV-infected patient, 280
Retrograde ejaculation, 518
Retrovir; see Zidovudine
Rhabdomyolysis, 300
Rheumatism, nonarticular, 418-419
Rheumatoid arthritis, 414
   in hand and wrist, 428
Rheumatoid factor, in Sjögren's syndrome, 436
Rhinitis, 32-35
Rhogam therapy, 468
Rhythm, contraceptive, 492
Ribonucleoprotein antibodies, 452
Ribot's law, 344
Right ventricular failure, 92-93
Right ventricular hypertrophy, 90
Rinne's test, 40
Risk
   in domestic violence cases, 504
   preventive health care and, 2
Ritonavir, 278
Rocky Mountain spotted fever, 290
Rome criteria for irritable bowel syndrome, 190
Rotator cuff tears, 422
RR intervals, 62, 64
RU486, 493

S

Sacral nerves, 192
Sacroiliac joint, arthritis in, 416
Salicylates, 140
Salmonella, 260
Saquinavir, 278
Scabies, 110, 280
Schirmer test, 436
Schizophrenia, 556
Schmorl's nodules, 440
Schober's test, 416
Sciatica, 424
Scleritis, 26
Sclerodactyly, 434
Scleroderma, 434-435
Scrotal mass, 508-509
Seborrheic keratoses, 104
Seizures, 350-355
   acute behavioral change from, 376
   coma from, 385
   dysosmia in, 382
Selective serotonin reuptake inhibitors
   for depression, 548
   for premenstrual syndrome, 488
Selegiline, 364
Selenium-75 homocholic acid taurine test, 190
Semen analysis, 518
Senile dementia of Alzheimer's type, 346, 378
Sensitive Thyroid-Stimulating Hormone test, 130, 142
Sensorineural hearing loss, 40-43
Sepsis, 112, 288-289
Septic arthritis, 412
Serum drug levels, 590-591
Serum protein electrophoresis, 236-239
Sexual dysfunction, 14-17
Sexual intercourse, and urinary tract infections, 476
Sexually transmitted diseases, 270-275
   and abnormal Pap smear, 486
   cervicitis from, 460-461

Sexually transmitted diseases—cont'd
  dysuria from, 506
  foreign travel and, 260
  and vaginal discharge, 458-459
Sharp objects, ingestion of, 524, 526
Shigella, 260
Shoulder pain, 422-423
Shunting vascularity, 84
Siderosis, alcoholic, 202
Sigmoidoscopy
  for colon cancer, 194
  for constipation, 188
  for diarrhea causes, 186
  for gastrointestinal bleeding, 181
  for rectal bleeding, 182
Simvastatin, 118
Single-donor apheresis unit, 224
Sinusitis, 32, 34, 332
Sinus node disease, 60
Sinus node re-entry tachycardia, 62
Sjögren's syndrome, 436-437
Skeletal metastases, 248
Skin test
  for antivenin reaction, 532
  tuberculin, 408-409
Smell dysfunction, 382-383
Smith antibodies, 452
Smoking
  anosmia from, 382
  and neutrophilia, 212
Smoking cessation, 558-561
Snake venom
  and fibrinogen, 217
  poisoning by, 532-533
Social phobia, 544
Sodium bicarbonate therapy, 310
Sodium urate crystals, 442
Sodium valproate, 352
Soft tissue pain, 418-419
Solitary pulmonary nodule, 402-403
Somatic disorders, 552-553
Spermatocele, 508
Spermicides, 492
Spinal cord disorders
  compression, 258-259
  sweating from, 24
  and weakness, 356
Spinal subarachnoid hemorrhage, 192
Spine
  arthritis in, 416
  cervical, 420, 536, 538
  hip pain from, 426
  stenosis of, 424
Spirometry, 394
Splenomegaly, 234
Spondyloarthropathies, 414, 416, 424
Spondyloepimetaphyseal dysplasia with joint
    laxity, 446
Sputum specimen, 282
Squamous cell carcinoma, 244
Squamous intraepithelial lesions, 486
Stapedial muscle spasm-induced tinnitus, 36
Staphylococcus aureus
  arthritis from, 412
  bacteremia, 292-293
  meningitis from, 262

Staphylococcus aureus—cont'd
  in neutropenic patient, 246
  toxic shock syndrome from, 290
Status epilepticus, 352-355, 385
Stavudine, 278
STDs; *see* Sexually transmitted diseases
Steady state, in pharmacokinetics, 590
Stem cell transplantation, 234, 235, 252-253
Stenoprophomonas maltophilia, 247
Steroids
  and adrenal suppression, 52
  for burn injuries, 528
  for hearing loss, 42
  myopathy from, 358
  in neutropenic patient, 246
Stickler's syndrome, 446, 448
Stigmata of recent hemorrhage, 180
Stool
  blood in, 178, 180
  guaiac-positive, 194-195
Stool culture, 184
Streptococcus pneumoniae
  meningitis from, 262
  prophylaxis against, 278, 582
Streptococcus pyogenes, 290
Streptokinase, 98
Stress disorder, 546
Stress echocardiography, 472, 474
Stress fractures, 426
Stress incontinence, 514
Stress testing
  after acute myocardial infarction, 98
  for stable angina, 66
Strictures, from burns, 528
Stridor, 390-391
Stroke
  completed, 340-341
  from oral contraceptives, 496
  progressing, 342-343
Stye, 30
Subarachnoid hemorrhage, 192, 332
Subconjunctival hemorrhage, 30
Substance abuse
  during bereavement, 554
  diagnostic criteria for, 542
  memory loss from, 344
Suicidal patient, 562-563
Superior vena caval syndrome, 256-257
Supraclavicular nodes, 240
Supraventricular arrhythmias, 80
Supraventricular tachycardia, 62-65, 80
Surgery
  antimicrobial prophylaxis for, 580, 584-585
  autologous transfusions in, 226
  perioperative evaluation in; *see* Perioperative evaluation
  and risk of deep venous thrombosis, 218
Swan-Ganz catheterization, 78
Sweating, 24-25
Sweet's syndrome, 234
Sympathetic nervous system lesions, sweating from, 24
Syncope, 82-83
Syphilis, 270, 280
Systemic lupus erythematosus
  antinuclear antibody test for, 452
  arthritis in, 414
Systolic murmur, 70-71

T

T₄; *see* Thyroxine
Tachycardia, 62-63, 64-65
Tamoxifen, 248, 480, 482
Tampons, toxic shock syndrome and, 290
Tardive dyskinesia, drug-induced, 370
Tarsal tunnel compression, 432
Taste dysfunction, 382-383
Telangiectasia, 434
Temporal arteritis
    headache from, 332
    visual loss from, 338
Temporal bone fractures, 40
Temporomandibular pain, 450-451
Tendinitis, 418
    rotator cuff, 422
Tendon rupture, hand and wrist, 428
Tenosynovitis, de Quervain's, 428
Tension headache, 334
Terconazole, 458
Testis
    and gynecomastia, 152
    measurement of, 152
    neoplasms in, 508
    ruptured, 508
Tetanus, 530
Tetany, 126
Tetracycline, 506-507
Thalassemias, 208
Theophylline, 576
Thiamine, in hypothermia resuscitation, 534
Thiazide, 306
Thoracentesis, 398
Thoracoscopy, 402, 404
Thoracotomy, 402, 404
3TC; *see* Lamivudine
Thrombectomy, 523
Thrombocytopenia, 214, 216
Thromboembolism
    anticoagulation therapy for, 566-569, 570-573
    surgical prophylaxis for, 48
Thrombolytic therapy, 566
    for acute myocardial infarction, 98
    for completed stroke patients, 340
    for pulseless extremity, 522
Thrombosis
    deep venous; *see* Deep venous thrombosis
    pulseless extremity from, 522
    stroke from, 342
Thrush, 280
Thyroid
    nodule, 138-139
    painful, 140-141
Thyroid antimicrosomal antibodies, 130
Thyroid disease, in perioperative evaluation, 54-55
Thyroid function tests, 130
    for hyperthyroidism, 134
    hypothyroidism and, 131
    in nonthyroidal illness, 142-143
Thyroid imaging-radionuclide scan, 130
Thyroiditis
    hyperthyroidism in, 134
    pain of, 140-141
Thyroid replacement therapy, in perioperative evaluation, 54
Thyroid-stimulating hormone
    and galactorrhea, 484
    and goiter, 136

Thyroid-stimulating hormone—cont'd
    hyperthyroidism and, 134
    hypothyroidism and, 131
Thyroid storm, 54
Thyrotoxicosis factitia, 134
Thyroxine
    free, 130, 131, 134
    in nonthyroidal illness, 142
Thyroxine therapy
    for goiter, 136
    for hypothyroidism, 131
    for thyroid nodules, 138
Ticlopidine, 336
Tics, 370
Tinea pedis, 432
Tinel's sign, 428
Tinnitus, 36-39
Tissue plasminogen activator
    for acute myocardial infarction, 98
    for completed stroke patient, 340
Tobramycin, 588
Toenail infections, 432
Tonic seizures, 350, 352
Torulopsis glabrata, 458
Toxic shock syndrome, 290-291, 492
Toxins
    acute behavioral change from, 376
    coma from, 384
    confusional states from, 380
    polyneuropathy from, 368
    and Raynaud's phenomenon, 438
Toxoplasma gondii, 278, 280
Transaminase levels, 200-201
Transferrin, hemochromatosis and, 202
Transfusion therapy
    with granulocytes, 228-229
    with platelets, 224-225
    reactions and complications in, 230-231
    with red blood cells, 226-227
Transient global amnesia, 345
Transient ischemic attacks, 336-337
Transient monocular visual loss, 338-339
Transplantation
    bone marrow, 252-253
    renal, 328-329, 330-331
    stem cell, 234, 235, 252-253
Transthoracic needle aspiration, 402, 404
Trauma
    brain, 380
    to foot or toes, 432
    head, 262, 344, 382
    neck, 384
Travel, infection and immunization considerations for, 260-261
Traveler's diarrhea, 260, 580
Tremor, 362-363
Trichomonads, 270
Trichomonas vaginalis, 458, 507
Tricuspid stenosis, 72
Tricyclen, 494
Triglyceride levels, 116
Triiodothyronine by RIA (T₃ RIA) test, 130, 142
Tri-Levelen, 494
Trimethoprim-sulfamethoxazole
    in HIV-infected patient, 278
    in neutropenic patient, 246-247
    for rhinitis, 32

Trimethoprim-sulfamethoxazole—cont'd
    for traveler's diarrhea, 260
    for urinary tract infections, 476
Tri-Norinyl, 494
Triphasil, 494
Trochanteric bursitis, 426
Trousseau's syndrome, 216
TSH; *see* Thyroid-stimulating hormone
Tubal ligation, 490
Tuberculosis
    fever from, 296
    prophylaxis for, 582
    pulmonary nodules in, 404
    skin test of, 408-409
Tuberculous cervicitis, 460
Tuberculous meningitis, 264
Tumors
    aldosterone-secreting, 144
    anosmia from, 382
    bone, 248, 250
    breast, 480, 482
    central nervous system, 24
    pituitary, 148-149
    plasma cell, 236
    small bowel, 194
    and spinal cord compression, 258
Typhoid vaccine, 260

U

Ulcers
    cervical, 460
    corneal, 28
    genital, 270
    leg, 106-107
    peptic, 170, 204
Ulnar nerve dysfunction, 428
Ultrasonography
    abdominal, 168, 470
    for biliary colic, 176
    for deep venous thrombosis, 218
Unfractionated heparin, 568
Uniform Determination of Death Act, 386
Unknown primary carcinoma, 242-245
Unstable angina, 68-70
Upper motor neuron signs of weakness, 356
Ureaplasma urealyticum, 506, 507
Uremia, 208
Urethral smear, 506
Urethritis, 270, 506, 507
Urge incontinence, 514, 516
Uric acid production, 442
Urinalysis
    for edema, 18
    microscopic examination, 506
    for prostatitis, 512
Urinary incontinence, 514-517
Urinary tract infection
    in men, 506, 510
    in renal transplant recipients, 330
    in women, 476-477
Urokinase, 522
Urticaria, 108-109, 112
Usher's syndrome, 40
Uveitis, 28

V

Vaccinations
    pneumococcal, 582
    recommendations for, 2
    for travel, 260-261
Vaginal bleeding
    abnormal, 464-465
    in pregnancy, 466-469
Vaginal discharge, 458-459
    in pregnancy, 466
Vaginal infections, sexually transmitted, 270-275
Vaginal prolapse, 514
Vaginismus, 16
Vaginitis, 458
    vs. cervicitis, 460
    in pregnancy, 466
Vaginosis, 272, 458
Valvular heart disease, 86
Vancomycin
    in neutropenic patient, 246
    in surgical prophylaxis, 584
Varicella virus, prophylaxis against, 278
Varicocele, 508, 518
Varicose veins, 432
Vascular disorders
    and acute behavioral change, 376
    in foot, 432
    in hand, 428
    hearing loss from, 40, 42
Vasculitis
    mesenteric, 156
    in neuropathies, 366
    purpura of, 112-113
Vasectomy, 490
Vasomotor rhinitis, 34
Vasopressin, 181
Venography
    for deep venous thrombosis, 218
    for edema, 20
Venom poisoning, 532-533
Venous insufficiency, 106
Ventricular arrhythmias, 98
Ventricular ectopy, 80
Ventricular failure, 92-93
Ventricular fibrillation, 94
Ventricular septal defect, 70
Ventricular tachycardia, 64
Verapamil, 64
Verruca plantaris, 432
Vertebrobasilar transient ischemic attacks, 336
Vertigo, 348
Very low calorie diets, 12
Vesicovaginal fistulae, 514
Vestibular disorders, 348-349
Vestibular neuronitis, 348
Videx; *see* Didanosine
Vincristine, 235
Viracept; *see* Nelfinavir
Viral meningitis, 264
Viramune; *see* Nevirapine
Virilization, 150
Visual loss, transient monocular, 338-339
Vitamin B_{12} deficiency, anemia from, 208
Vitamin D
    and hypercalcemia, 128
    and hypocalcemia, 126

Vitamin deficiencies
    anemia from, 208
    polyneuropathy from, 368
Vitamin K
    clotting times and, 216
    in warfarin therapy, 572
Vomiting, 158-159
von Willebrand disease, 222
Vulvovaginitis, 458

W

Waardenburg's syndrome, 40
Waldenström's macroglobulinemia, 238
Warfarin
    long-term anticoagulation with, 568, 570-573
    in surgical thromboembolism prophylaxis, 48
    for transient ischemic attacks, 336
Weakness, 356-359
Weber's test, 40
Wegener's granulomatosis, 112
Weight changes, oral contraceptives and, 496
Weight loss
    anorexia and, 160
    involuntary, 10-11
Wellbutrin; *see* Bupropion
Wernicke-Korsakoff syndrome, 344
Wheals, 108-109
Wheezing, 392-393
Whipple's triad, 120
White blood cells
    in chronic myelogenous leukemia, 234
    in diarrhea, 184
    in leukocytosis, 212

White blood cells—cont'd
    in leukopenia, 214
    in polycythemia, 210
Wide QRS complex tachycardia, 64-65
Wilson's disease, 200
Wing-beating tremor, 362
Withdrawal states, sweating from, 24
Wolff-Parkinson-White syndrome, 62
Women
    acute abdominal pain in, 470-471
    chest pain in, 472-475
    domestic violence against, 502-505
    incontinence in, 514
    urinary tract infections in, 476-477
Wrinkly skin syndrome, 448
Wrist pain, 428-429

X

Xanthomas, 116
Xerosis, 110
Xerostomia, 436

Y

Yeast infections, 458

Z

Zalcitabine, 278
ZDV; *see* Zidovudine
Zerit; *see* Stavudine
Zidovudine, 278
Zyban; *see* Bupropion